ATLAS OF
CANCER SURGERY

ATLAS OF CANCER SURGERY

Norman D. Bloom, M.D.
Chief, Surgical Oncology
Cabrini Medical Center
Clinical Professor of Surgery
New York Medical College
New York, New York

Edward J. Beattie, M.D. *(deceased)*
Medical Director, Comprehensive Cancer Center
Beth Israel Medical Center
Professor of Surgery
Albert Einstein College of Medicine
New York, New York

James C. Harvey, M.D.
Western Surgical Center
Asheville, North Carolina

Illustrations by:
Hugh A. Thomas

W.B. SAUNDERS COMPANY
A Harcourt Health Sciences Company
Philadelphia London New York St. Louis Sydney Toronto

W.B. SAUNDERS COMPANY
A Harcourt Health Sciences Company

The Curtis Center
Independence Square West
Philadelphia, Pennsylvania 19106

Library of Congress Cataloging-in-Publication Data

Bloom, Norman D.

　Atlas of cancer surgery / Norman D. Bloom, Edward J. Beattie, James C. Harvey; [illustrator] Hugh A. Thomas.

　　p.; cm.

　ISBN 0-7216-6199-8

　1. Cancer—Surgery—Atlases.　I. Beattie, Edward J.　II. Harvey, James C. III. Title. [DNLM: 1. Neoplasms—surgery—Atlases.　QZ 17 B655a 2000]

RD651.B575 2000

616.9994059—dc21　　　　　　　　　　　　　　　　　　　　　　　　　99-059399

Editor:　Richard H. Lampert
Editorial Assistant:　Beth LoGiudice
Project Manager:　Edna Dick
Production Manager:　Norman Stellander
Illustration Specialist:　Rita Martello
Book Designer:　Jonel Sofian

ATLAS OF CANCER SURGERY　　　　　　　　　　　　　　　　　　　　　　ISBN　0-7216-6199-8

Copyright © 2000 by W.B. Saunders Company

All rights reserved. No part of this publication may be reproduced or transmitted in any form or by any means, electronic or mechanical, including photocopy, recording, or any information storage and retrieval system, without permission in writing from the publisher.

Printed in the United States of America

Last digit is the print number:　9　8　7　6　5　4　3　2　1

In Memoriam

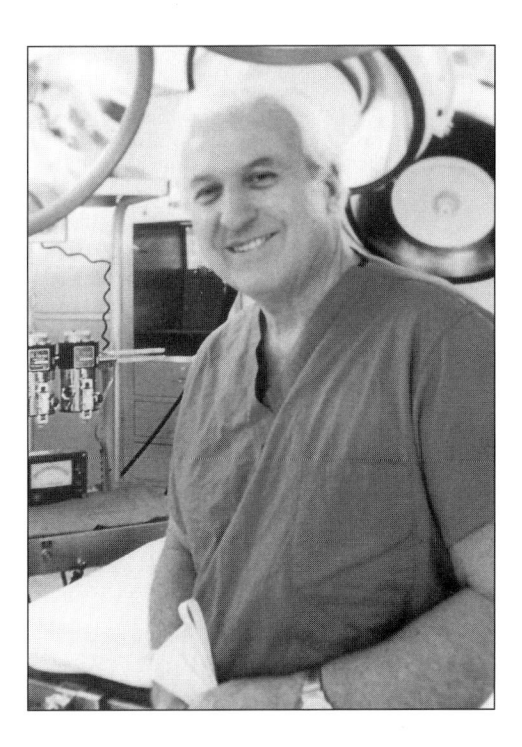

Edward J. Beattie died during the final stages of the preparation of this atlas. A 50-year career devoted to investigating "the cancer problem" was brought to an end by the enemy he fought long and hard against for the thousands of patients in his care.

Born in Philadelphia in 1918, Ted graduated with honors from Princeton and Harvard Medical School. After residency in surgery at Peter Bent Brigham and a fellowship in thoracic surgery at George Washington University, he became Chief of Thoracic Surgery at Gallinger Municipal Hospital and Director of Surgical Research at George Washington University Hospital.

Ted spent 11 years at the University of Illinois and became a full professor and Chairman of the Department of Surgery prior to moving to Memorial Sloan-Kettering Cancer Center in 1965. During the next 17 years he served as Chief of Thoracic Service, then Chairman of Surgery and finally Chief Medical Officer.

After sojourning in Miami, Ted returned to New York and became Chief of Thoracic Surgery at the David B. Kaiser Lung Cancer Center of Beth Israel Medical Center. He started the Beth Israel Medical Center Comprehensive Cancer Center, where he was Medical Director until his death.

Ted's legacy goes beyond the numerous articles and books that bear his name. Ted inspired hundreds of residents and fellows to recognize the importance of a multidisciplinary approach to cancer care and to continuously seek out scientific and technologic advances that would improve the end results in cancer management and be less disruptive to the patients' lives.

He taught us to always be positive and optimistic with our patients, to muster all resources available to us for their treatment, and to remember that each patient is an individual not a statistic. He approached every battle with a glint in his eye and spryness in his step.

Contributors

Michael Hausman, M.D.
Chief of Upper Extremity Surgery
Associate Clinical Professor of Orthopaedics
Mount Sinai School of Medicine
New York, New York

John Hoffman, M.D.
Professor of Surgery
Temple University School of Medicine
Chief Hepatobiliary and Pancreatic Surgery
Fox Chase Cancer Center
Philadelphia, Pennsylvania

Charles Miller, M.D.
Alfred and Florence Gross Professor of Surgery
Director, Recanati/Miller Transplant Patient Institute
Mount Sinai School of Medicine
New York, New York

Myron Schwartz, M.D.
Associate Professor Surgery
Mount Sinai School of Medicine
Deputy Director, Liver Transplantation and
   Chief of Hepatobiliary Surgery
Mount Sinai School of Medicine
New York, New York

Takashi Takahashi, M.D.
Chief Surgical Department
Cancer Institute Hospital
Japanese Foundation for Cancer Research
Tokyo, Japan

Harold Wanebo, M.D.
Professor of Surgery
Boston University School of Medicine
Chief of Surgery, Roger William's Medical Center
Providence, Rhode Island

Preface

In attempting to develop this Atlas of Cancer Therapy, considerable thought was given as to how to make this atlas different from its predecessors.

First and foremost, anatomic relationships are emphasized. To accomplish this, detailed anatomic drawings serve as an introduction to each section and provide the foundation on which each of the operative procedures is based. All the drawings are also placed in the orientation of the operating surgeon.

Secondly, all the illustrations have been created by a single illustrator to provide uniformity throughout the text.

Thirdly, to make each procedure as concise as possible and to avoid constant repetition of techniques, there are certain assumptions. One type of incision that can be utilized may be highlighted but can be varied according to individual surgical preferences. Similarly, the techniques used in creating a specific anastomosis may not be included because there can be many different approaches taken in a given situation. These and other individual surgical decisions are best left to the individual performing the procedure; these options are in the armanentarium of all well-trained surgeons.

Fourthly, a picture is worth a thousand words. A well-illustrated procedure allows for brevity in each accompanying legend.

Finally, one can always use help from friends and colleagues. The case illustrations show how the basic surgical oncologic principles can be integrated and expanded on in an attempt to adequately handle the situation that one can be confronted with.

NORMAN D. BLOOM

NOTICE

Medicine is an ever-changing field. Standard safety precautions must be followed, but as new research and clinical experience broaden our knowledge, changes in treatment and drug therapy become necessary or appropriate. Readers are advised to check the product information currently provided by the manufacturer of each drug to be administered to verify the recommended dose, the method and duration of administration, and the contraindications. It is the responsibility of the treating physician, relying on experience and knowledge of the patient, to determine dosages and the best treatment for the patient. Neither the Publisher nor the editor assumes any responsibility for any injury and/or damage to persons or property.

THE PUBLISHER

Contents

Part I HEAD AND NECK 1

1. Surgical Anatomy of the Thyroid 2
2. Thyroid Lobectomy 7
3. Surgical Anatomy of the Parotid Gland 21
4. Parotidectomy 23
5. Surgical Anatomy for Radical Neck Dissection 28
6. Radical Neck Dissection 31
7. Clinical Case: Desmoi Tumor Thoracic Inlet 43
   Michael Hausman

Part II CHEST 47

8. Surgical Anatomy of the Right Chest 48
9. Thoracic Incision 57
10. Right Upper Lobectomy 62
11. Right Lower Lobectomy 75
12. Surgical Anatomy of the Left Lung 81
13. Left Upper Lobectomy 87
14. Left Lower Lobectomy 93
15. Clinical Case: Thymoma 101
    Edward J. Beattie
16. Clinical Case: Chondrosarcoma Sternum 106
    James C. Harvey
17. Transhiatal Esophageal Resection and Gastric Pull-up 113
18. Thoracic Esophagectomy 126
19. Esophagogastrectomy 134

Part III UPPER ABDOMEN 145

20. Upper Abdomen Anatomy 146
21. Gastric Surgery 153
22. Clinical Case: Extended Gastrectomy With Radical Lymphadenectomy 168
    Takashi Takahashi
23. Right Hepatic Lobectomy 182
24. Left Hepatic Lobectomy 196
25. Trisegmentectomy 206
26. Clinical Case: Hepatic Lobectomy: Vascular Isolation Technique 218
    Charles Miller
    Myron Schwartz
27. Radical Cholecystectomy 232
28. Pancreatectomy (Whipple Procedure) 241
29. Distal Pancreatectomy 254
30. Clinical Case: Regional Pancreatectomy for a Retroperitoneal Sarcoma 258
    John Hoffman
31. Right Adrenalectomy 264
32. Left Adrenalectomy 268

Part IV LOWER ABDOMEN 273

33. Surgical Anatomy of the Abdomen 274
34. Right Hemicolectomy 279
35. Left Hemicolectomy 293
36. Transverse Colectomy 301
37. Sigmoid Colectomy 311
38. Low Anterior Resection 321
39. Surgical Anatomy of the Perineum 333
40. Abdominal Perineal Resection 335
41. Surgical Anatomy for Pelvic Exenteration (Female) 341
42. Pelvic Exenteration (Female) 347
43. Urinary Diversion 365
44. Surgical Anatomy for Pelvic Exenteration (Male) 369
45. Pelvic Exenteration (Male) 371
46. Clinical Case: Abdominosacral Resection 377
    Harold Wanebo

Part V RADICAL AMPUTATIONS 395

47. Surgical Anatomy for Radical Resection of the Upper Extremity 396
48. Forequarter Amputation 401
49. Tikoff-Lindberg Procedure 415
50. Surgical Anatomy of the Pelvis 429
51. Hemipelvectomy 432
52. Clinical Case: Chondrosarcoma of the Pubis 449
    Norman D. Bloom

53. Clinical Case: Chondrosarcoma of the Iliac Wing   455
    Norman D. Bloom

Part VI BREAST AND SOFT TISSUE TUMORS   461

54. Surgical Anatomy of the Breast   462
55. Modified Radical Mastectomy   465
56. Radical Mastectomy   476
57. Surgical Anatomy of the Groin   483
58. Groin Dissection   485
    Index   489

Part I

HEAD AND NECK

2 • Part I HEAD AND NECK

Chapter 1
Surgical Anatomy of the Thyroid

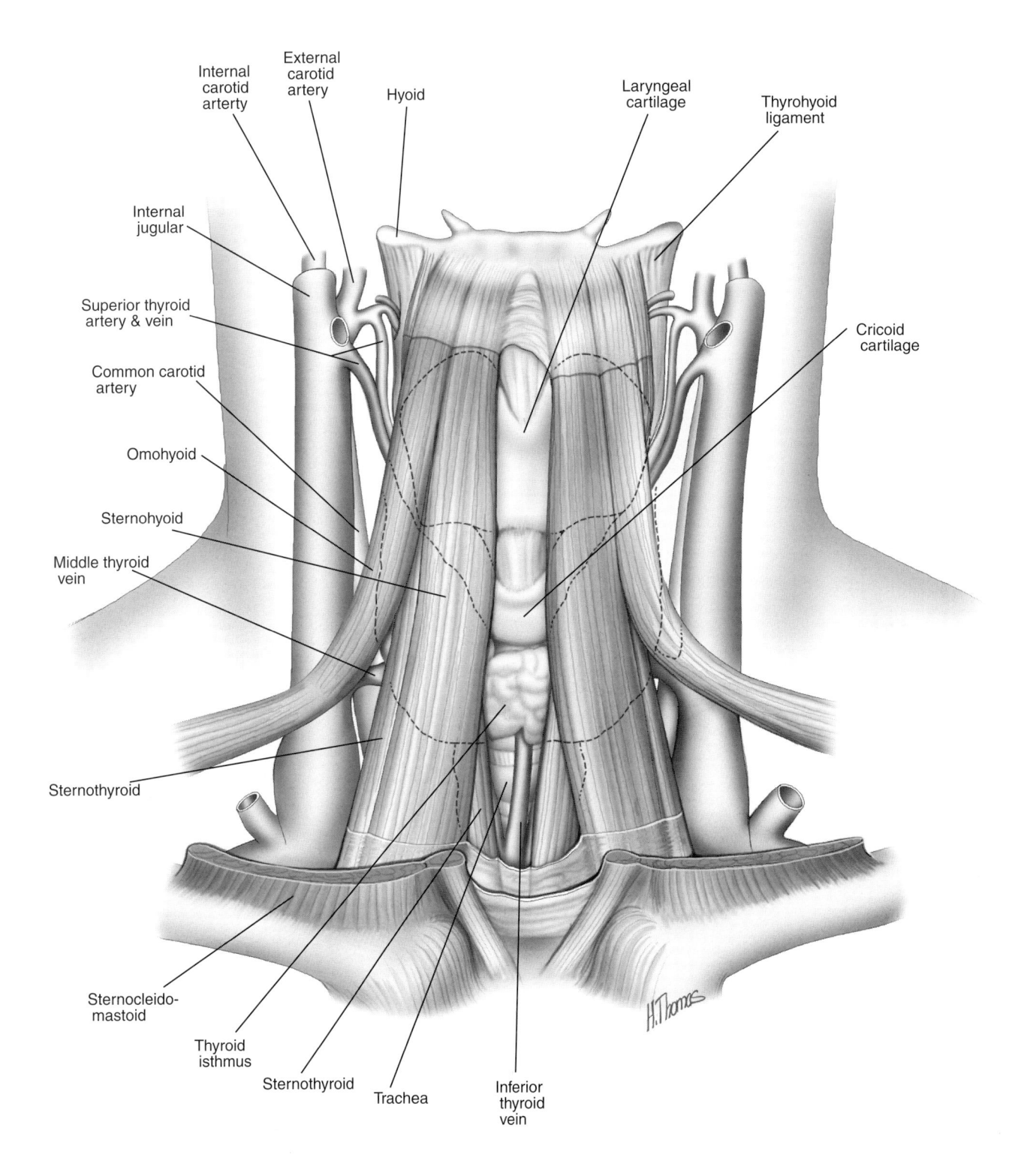

Figure 1–1 • The anatomic drawings in this chapter are meant to orient the surgeon to the anatomy of the central neck. An anteroposterior view of the neck reveals the sternohyoid, sternothyroid, omohyoid, and underlying thyroid gland.

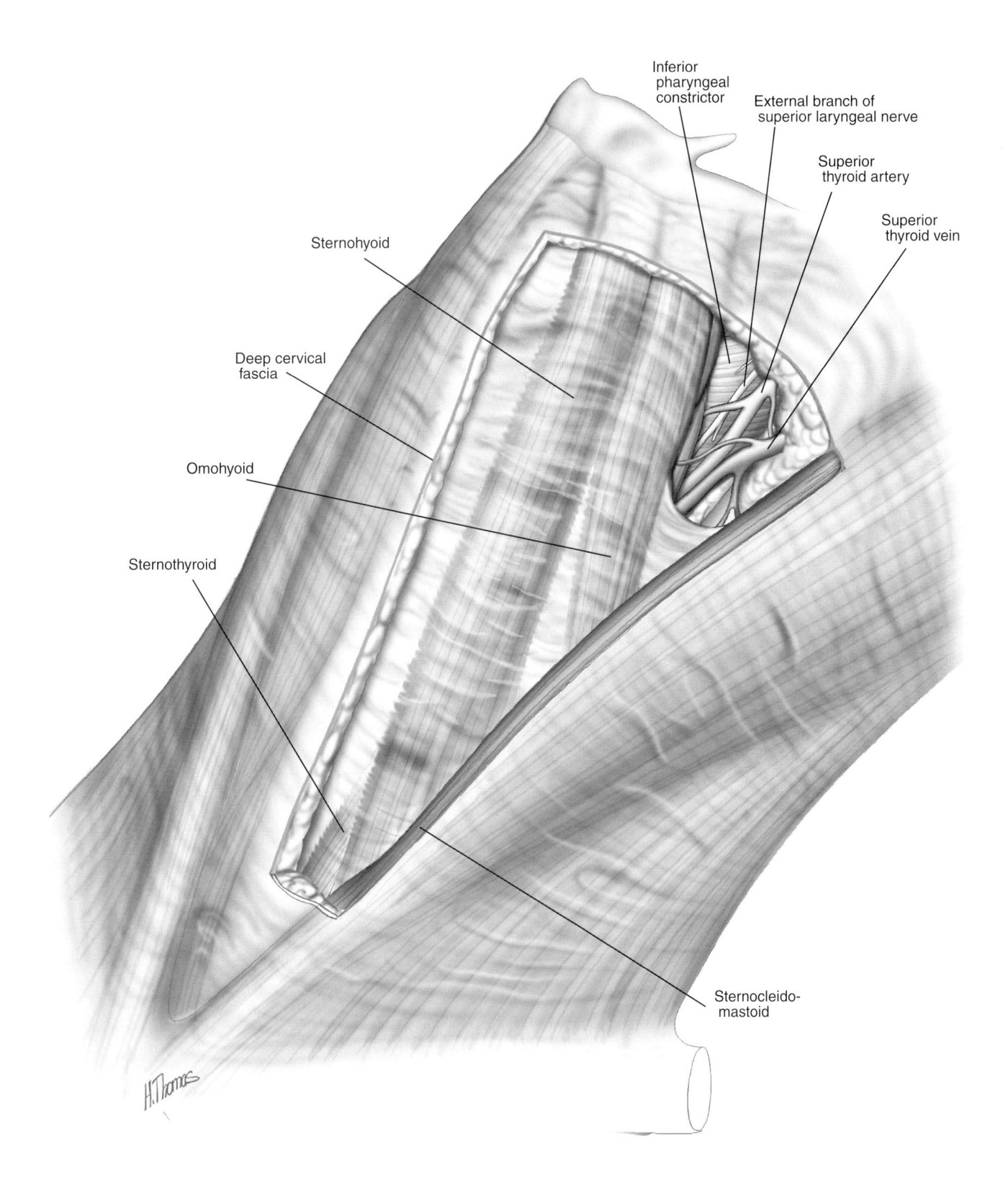

Figure 1–2 • An oblique view demonstrates also the origin of the superior thyroid artery off the external carotid and the vein off the internal jugular.

4 • Part I HEAD AND NECK

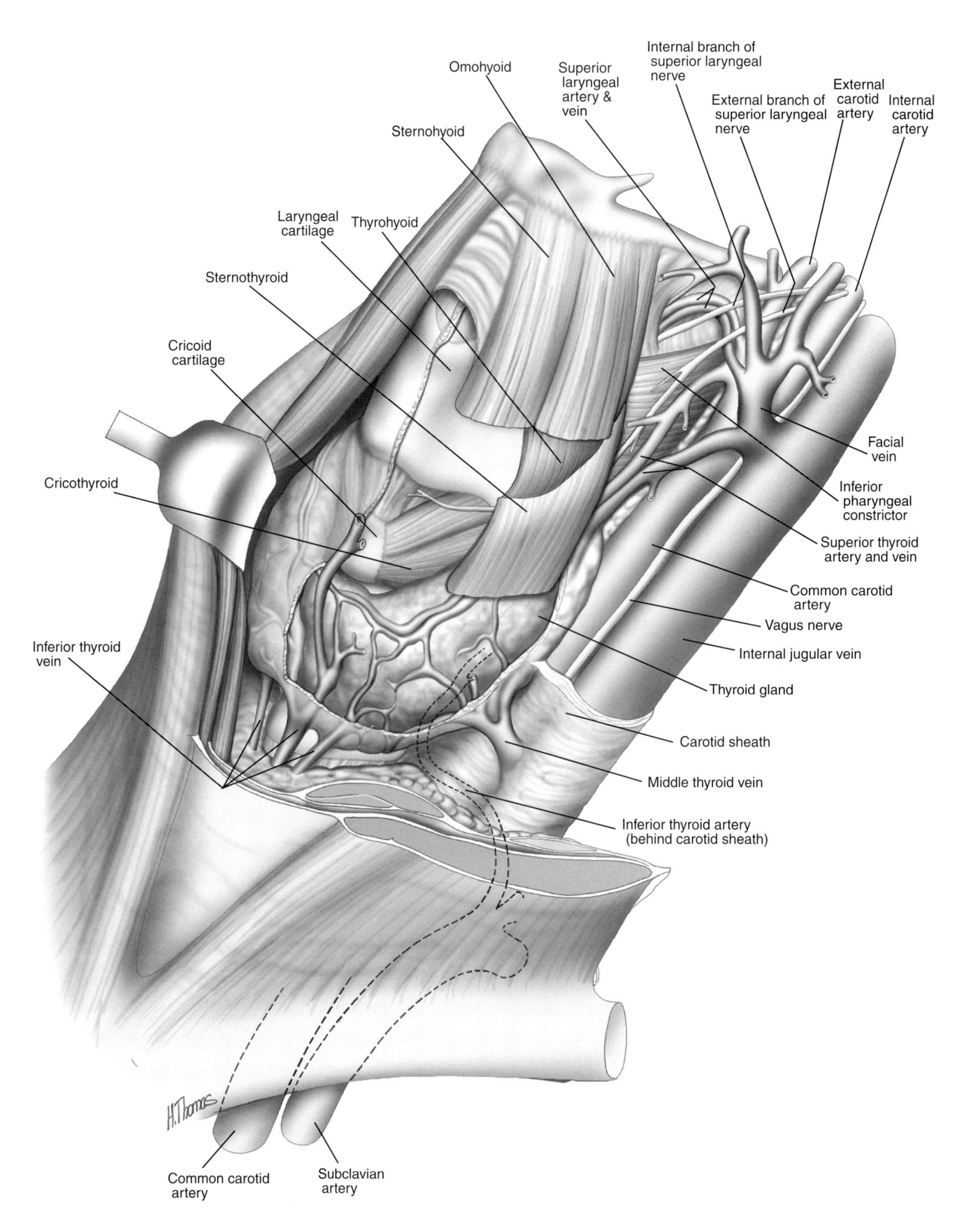

Figure 1–3 • With the strap muscles removed, the complete blood supply to the thyroid is illustrated.

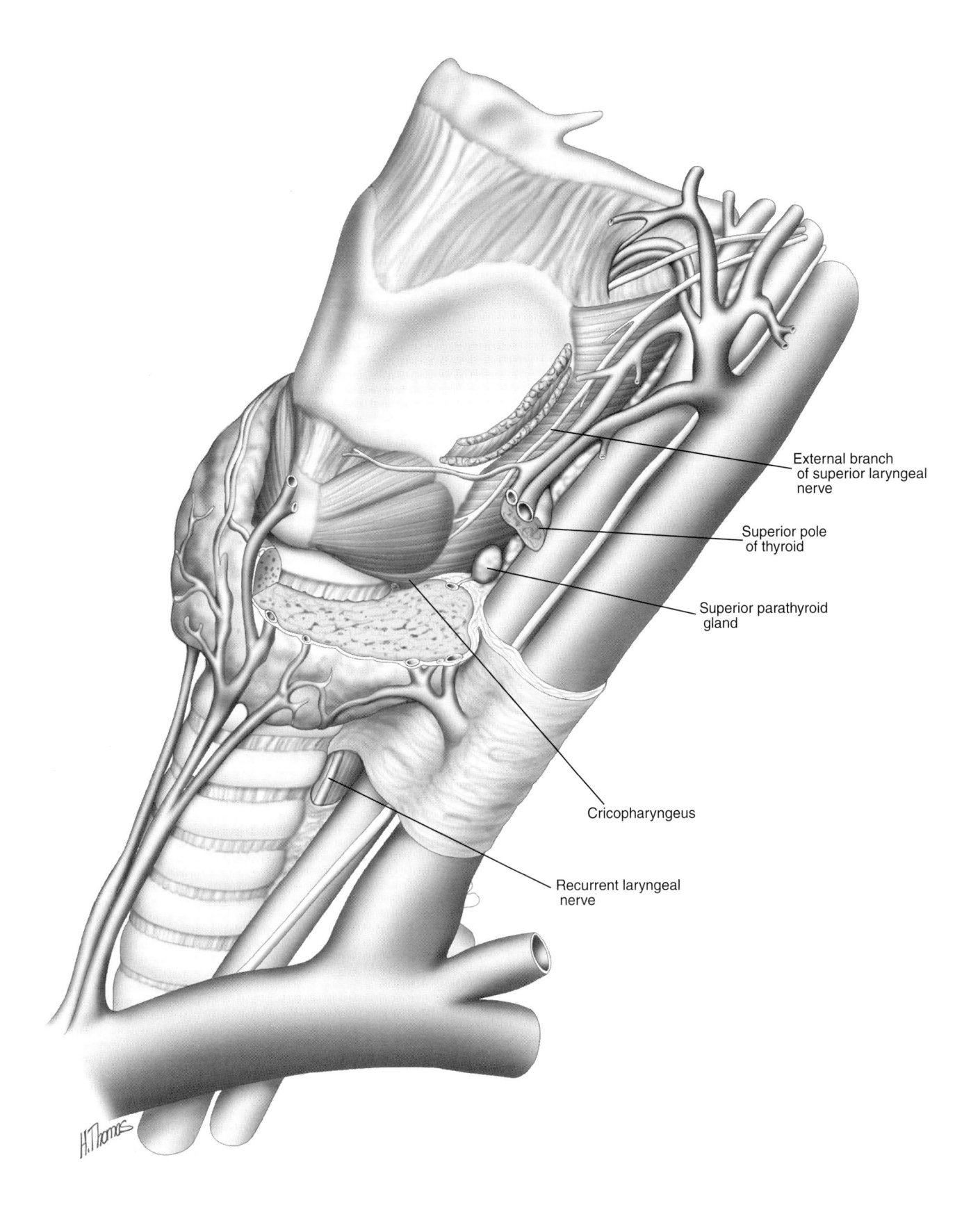

Figure 1–4 • The course of the superior laryngeal and recurrent laryngeal nerves is identified.

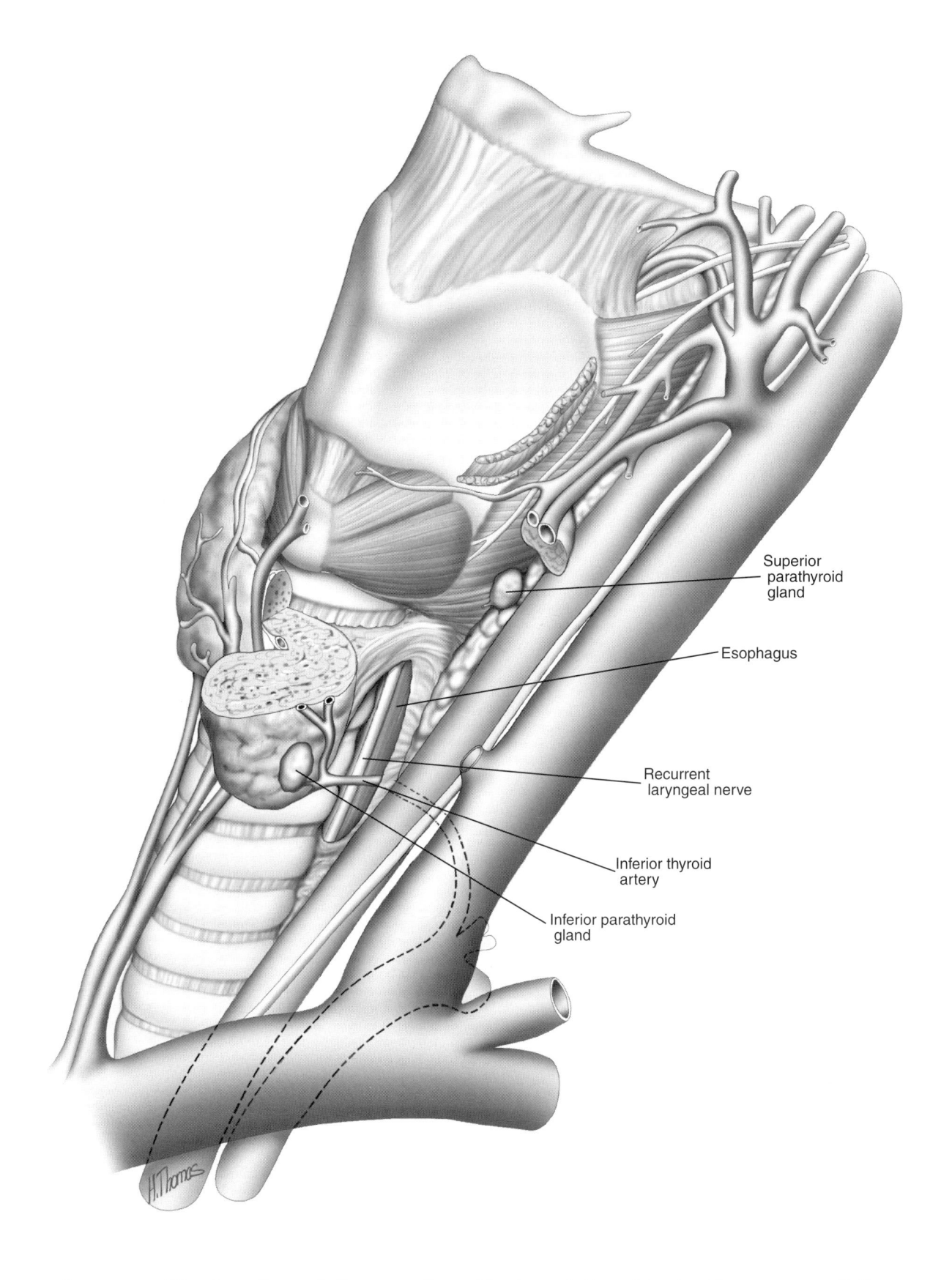

Figure 1–5 • The location of the parathyroids in relationship to the course of the recurrent laryngeal nerve is illustrated.

Chapter 2
Thyroid Lobectomy

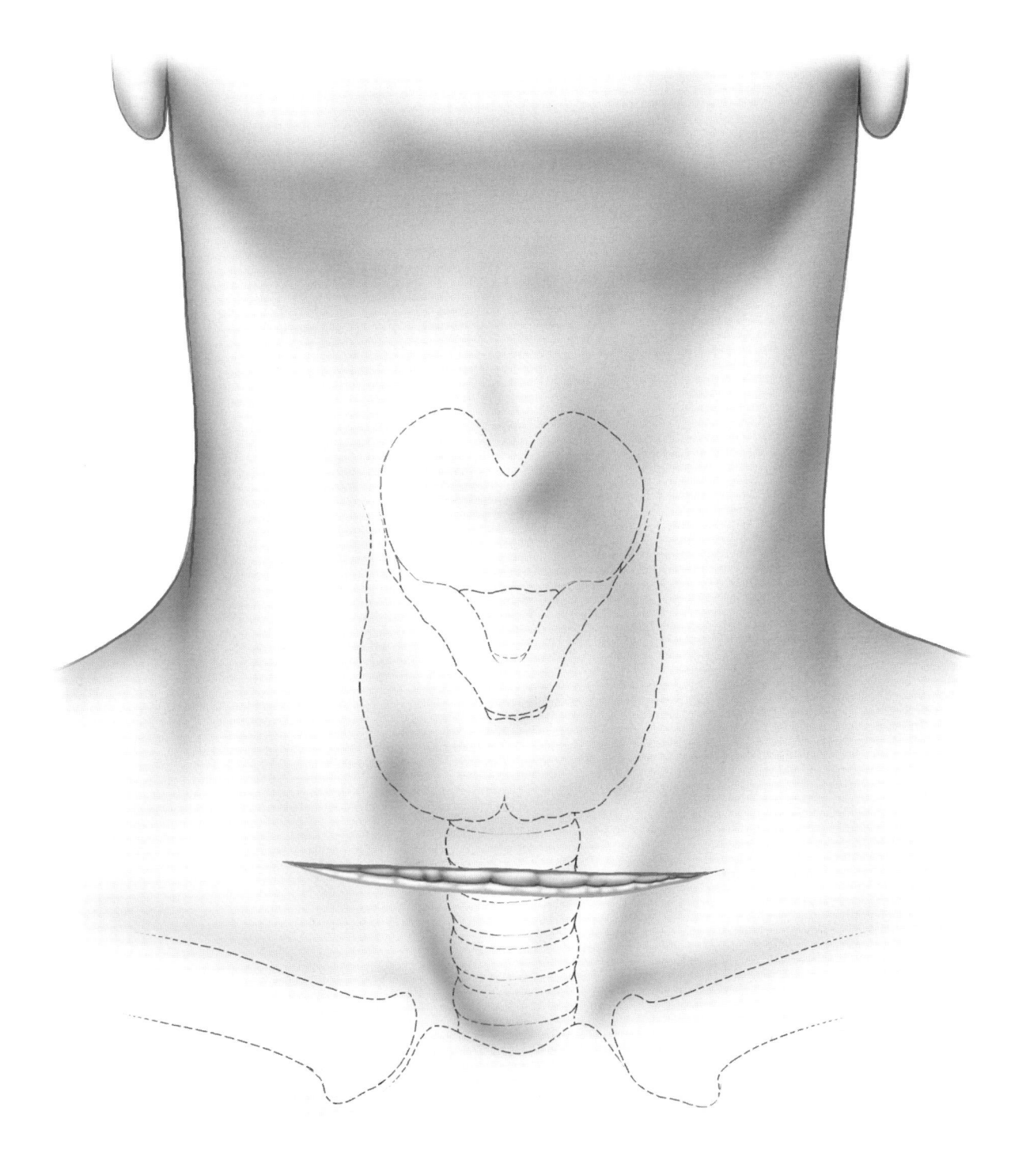

Figure 2–1 • A transverse cervical incision is placed in a skin crease two finger-breadths above the sternal notch between the edges of the sternocleidomastoid muscles.

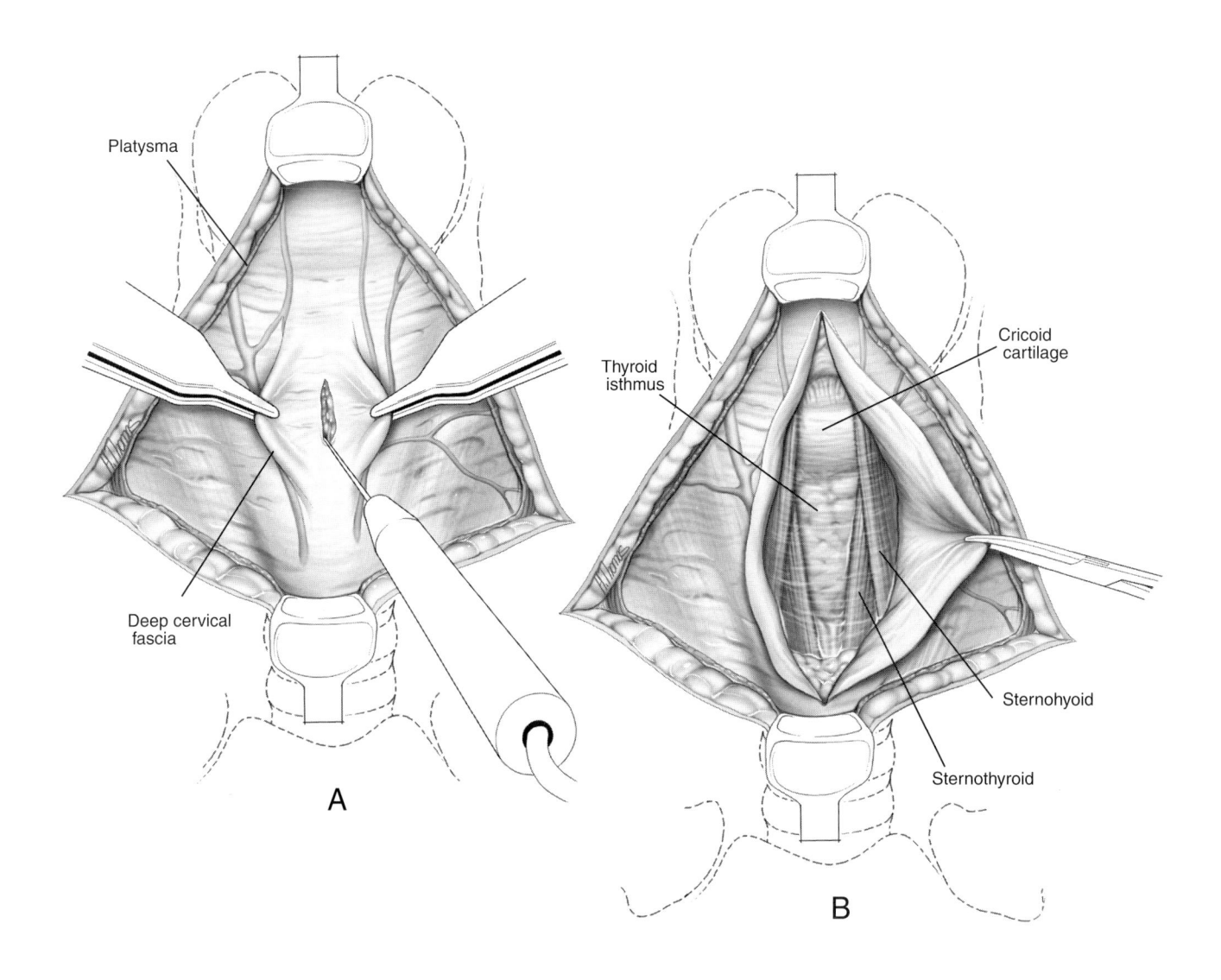

Figure 2–2 • **A,** The fascia between the strap muscles is divided after elevation of the skin flaps beneath the platysma.
  B, The thyroid gland is exposed in the midline.

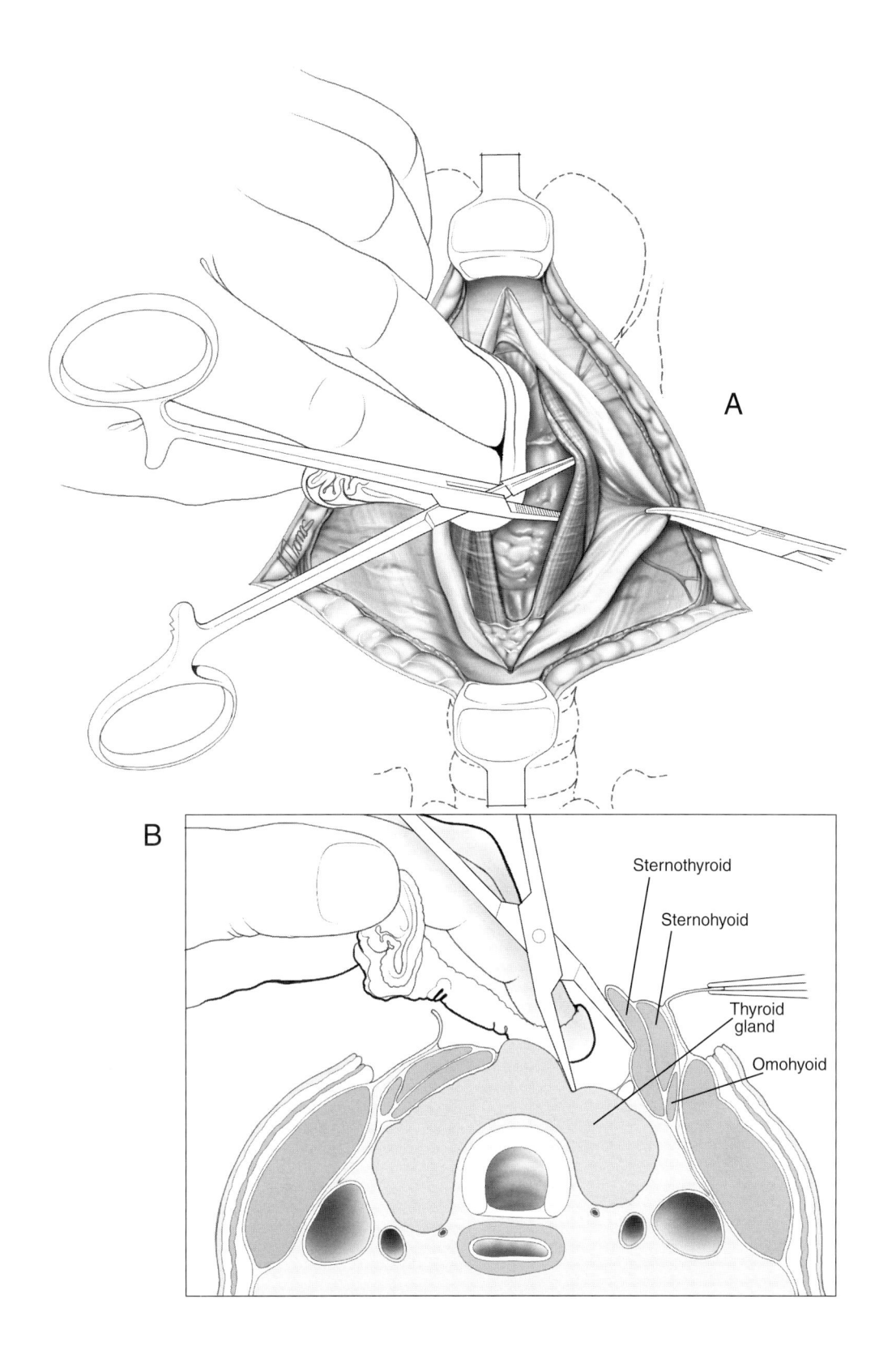

Figure 2-3 • **A,** The strap muscles are mobilized off the thyroid gland by blunt dissection.
B, A cross-sectional view depicting this technique.

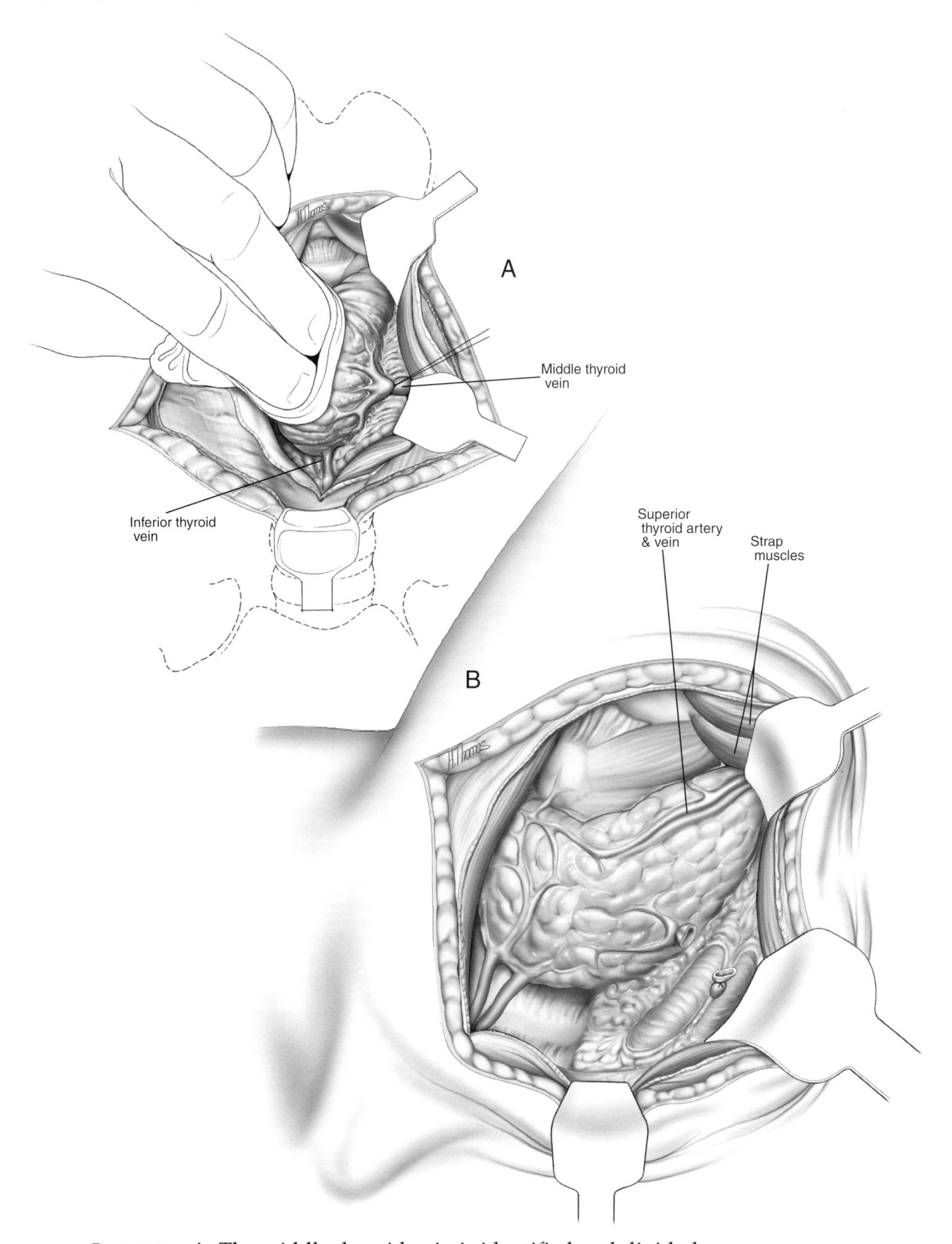

Figure 2–4 • **A,** The middle thyroid vein is identified and divided.
B, After division of the middle thyroid vein, the gland can be elevated and rotated medially.

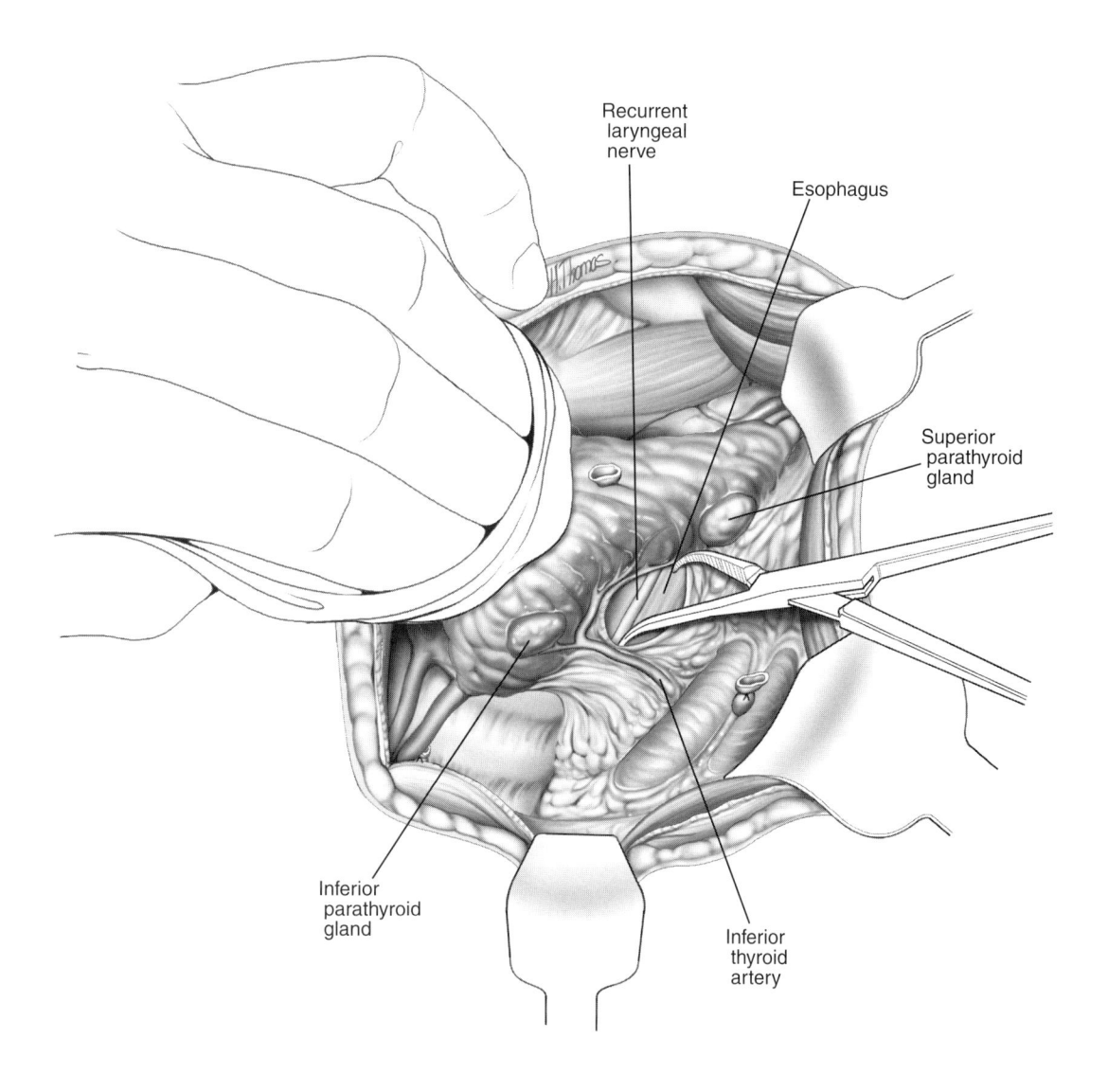

Figure 2–5 • The recurrent laryngeal nerve is identified by bluntly dissecting in the tracheoesophageal groove superior to the inferior thyroid artery.

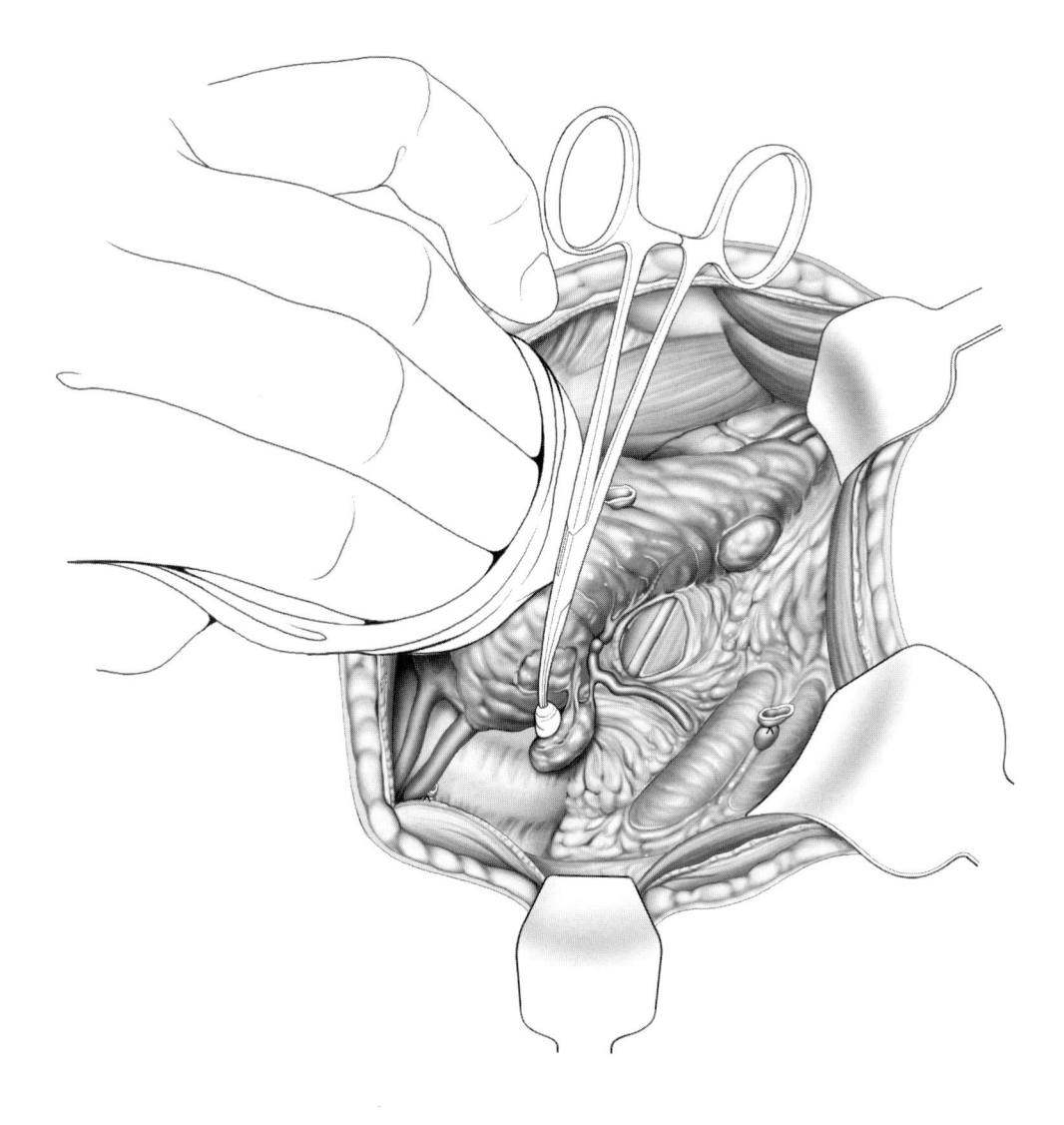

Figure 2-6 • The inferior parathyroid, which is anterior to the recurrent laryngeal nerve, is dissected off the gland and preserved. The blood supply to the gland off the inferior thyroid artery is preserved.

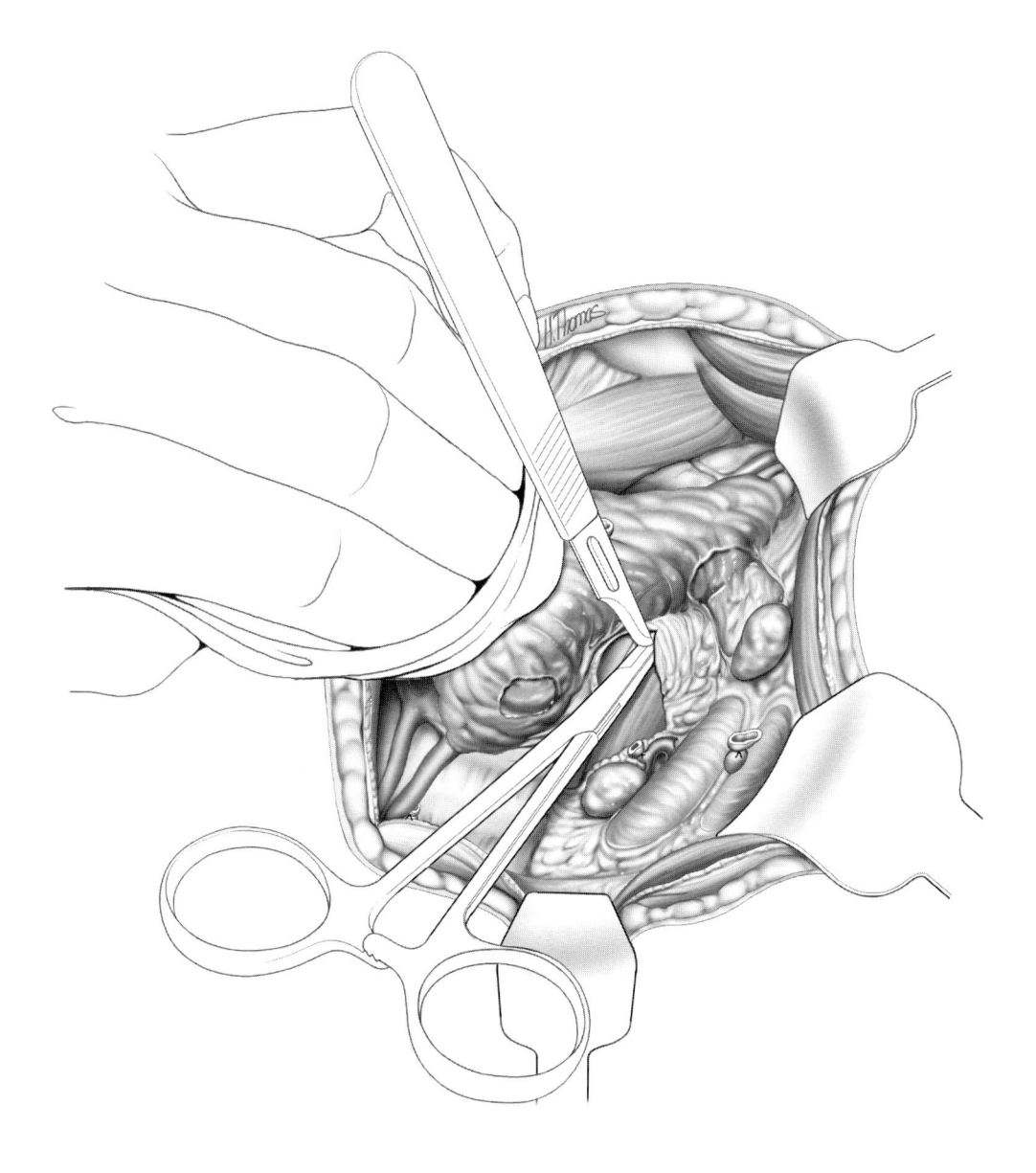

Figure 2–7 • The recurrent laryngeal nerve is dissected free along its entire course.

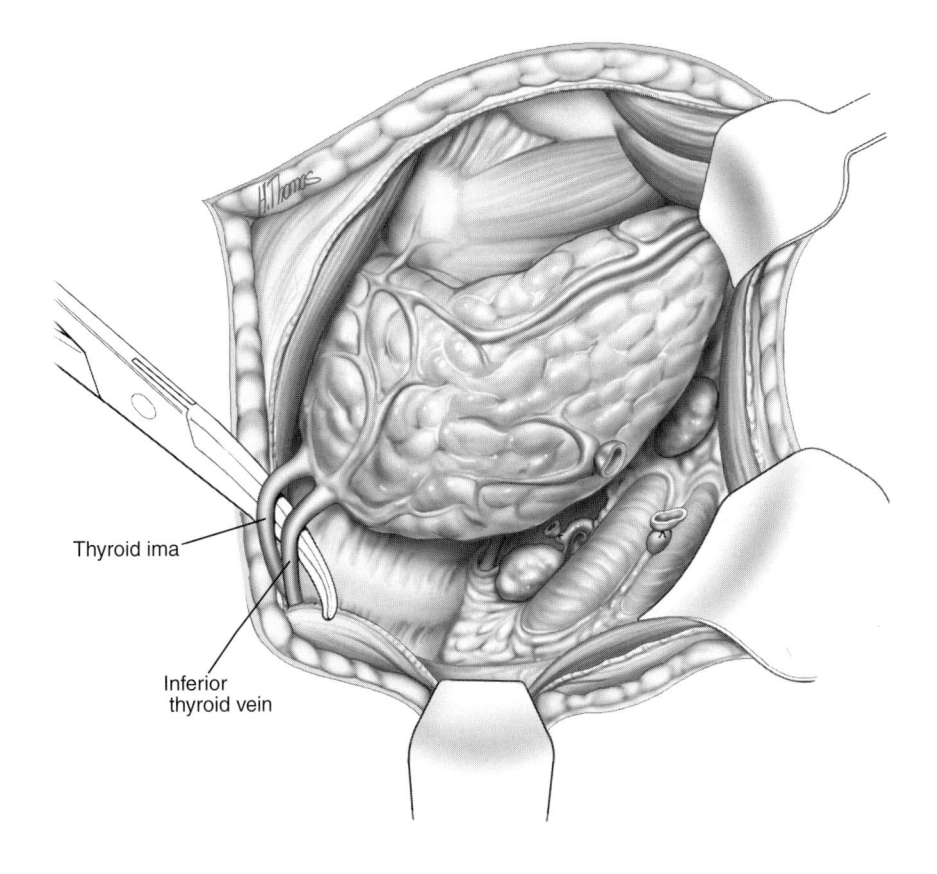

Figure 2-8 • The inferior thyroid vein and thyroid ima are divided to expose the trachea inferiorly.

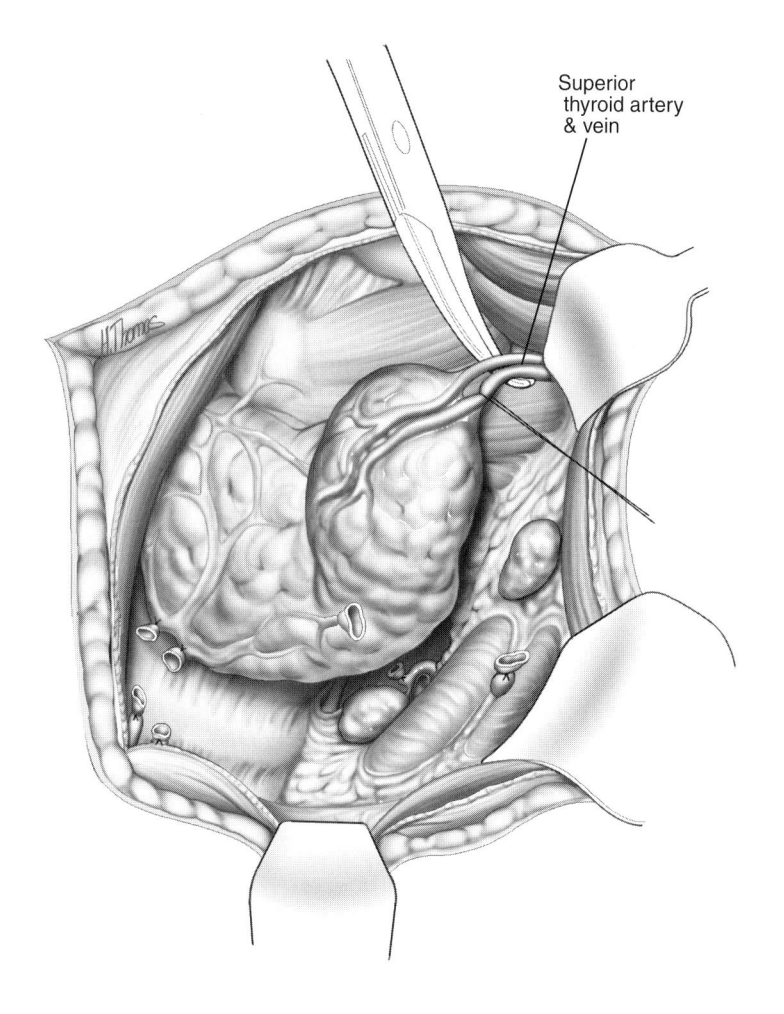

Figure 2–9 • The superior thyroid vessels are identified at the point where they enter the thyroid gland and are divided.

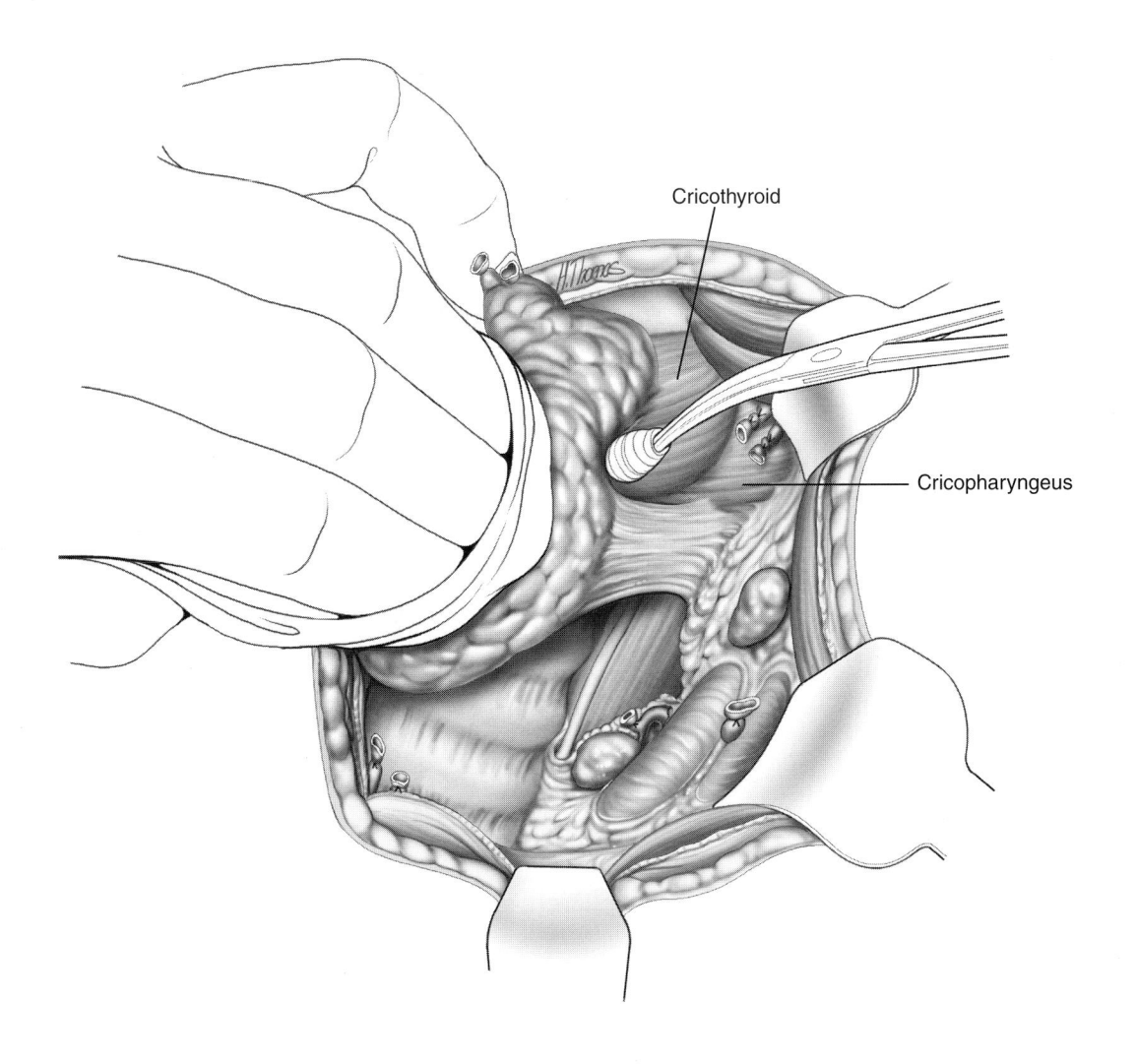

Figure 2-10 • The superior pole is now completely mobilized, avoiding any damage to the underlying musculature through which the superior laryngeal nerve runs.

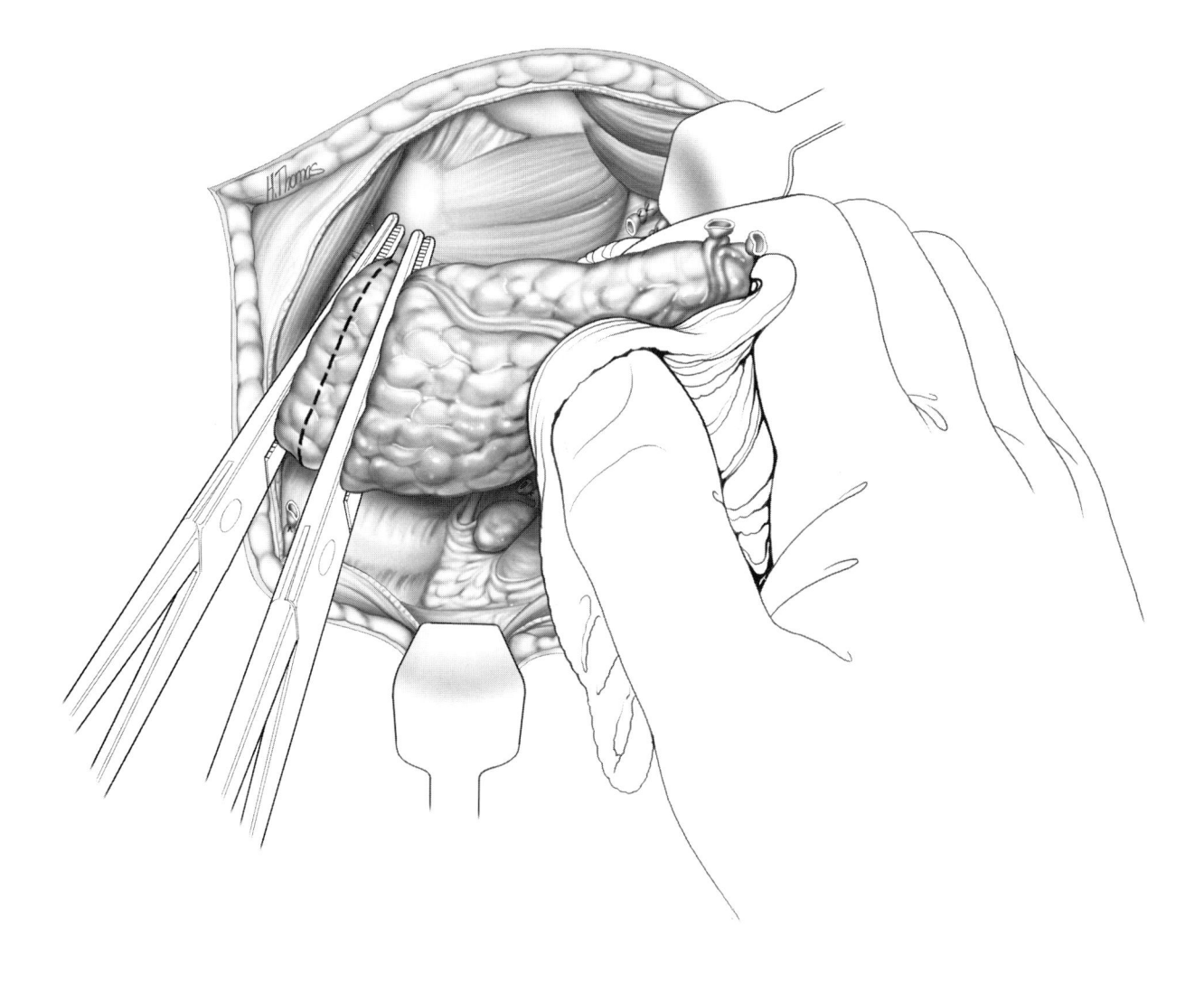

Figure 2–11 • If a lobectomy is to be performed, the isthmus is divided. If a total thyroidectomy is to be performed, the opposite half of the gland is dissected in a similar manner.

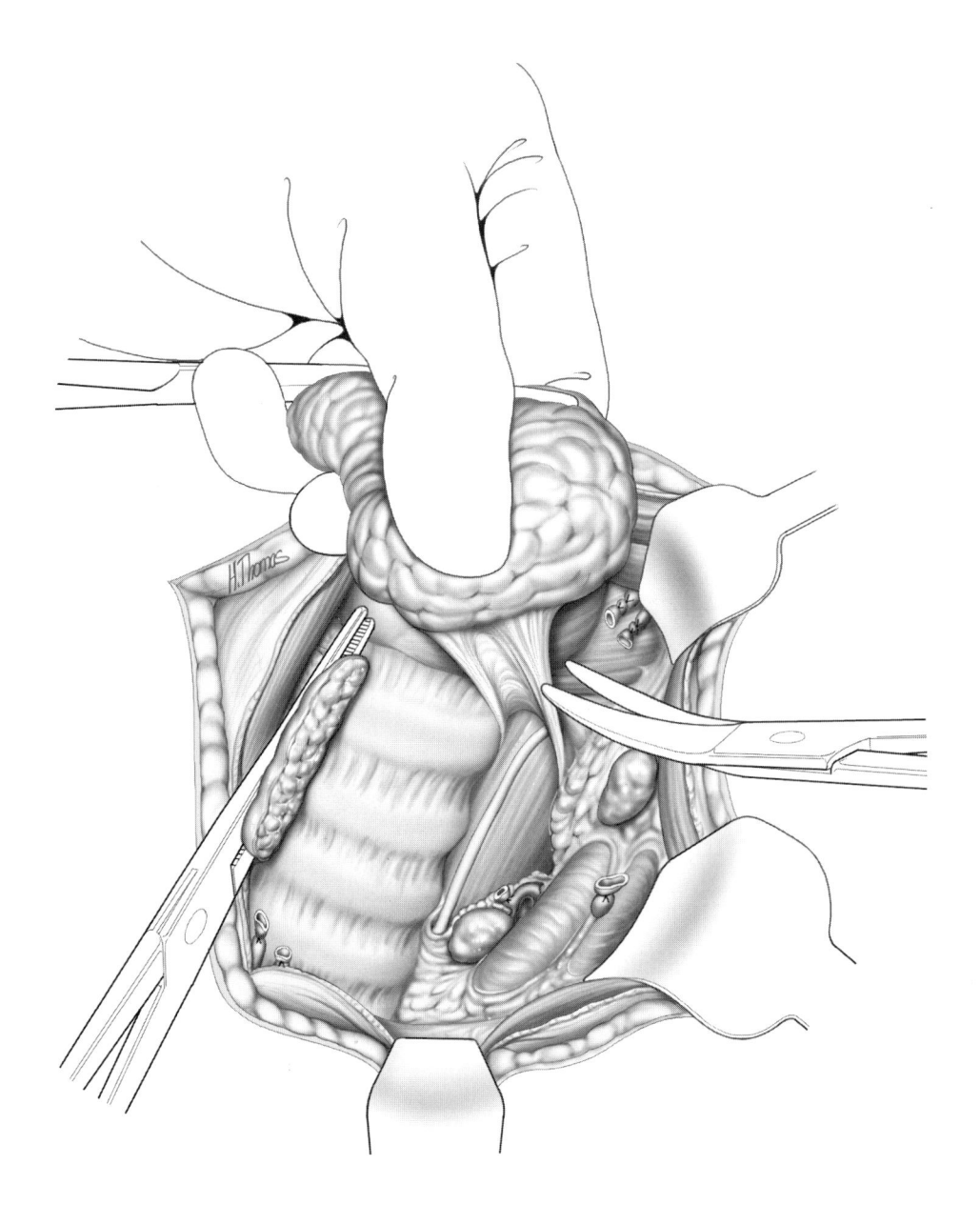

Figure 2–12 • The remaining attachments of the gland are then incised. This is the area where the greatest risk of injury to the recurrent laryngeal nerve exists.

Thyroid Lobectomy • 19

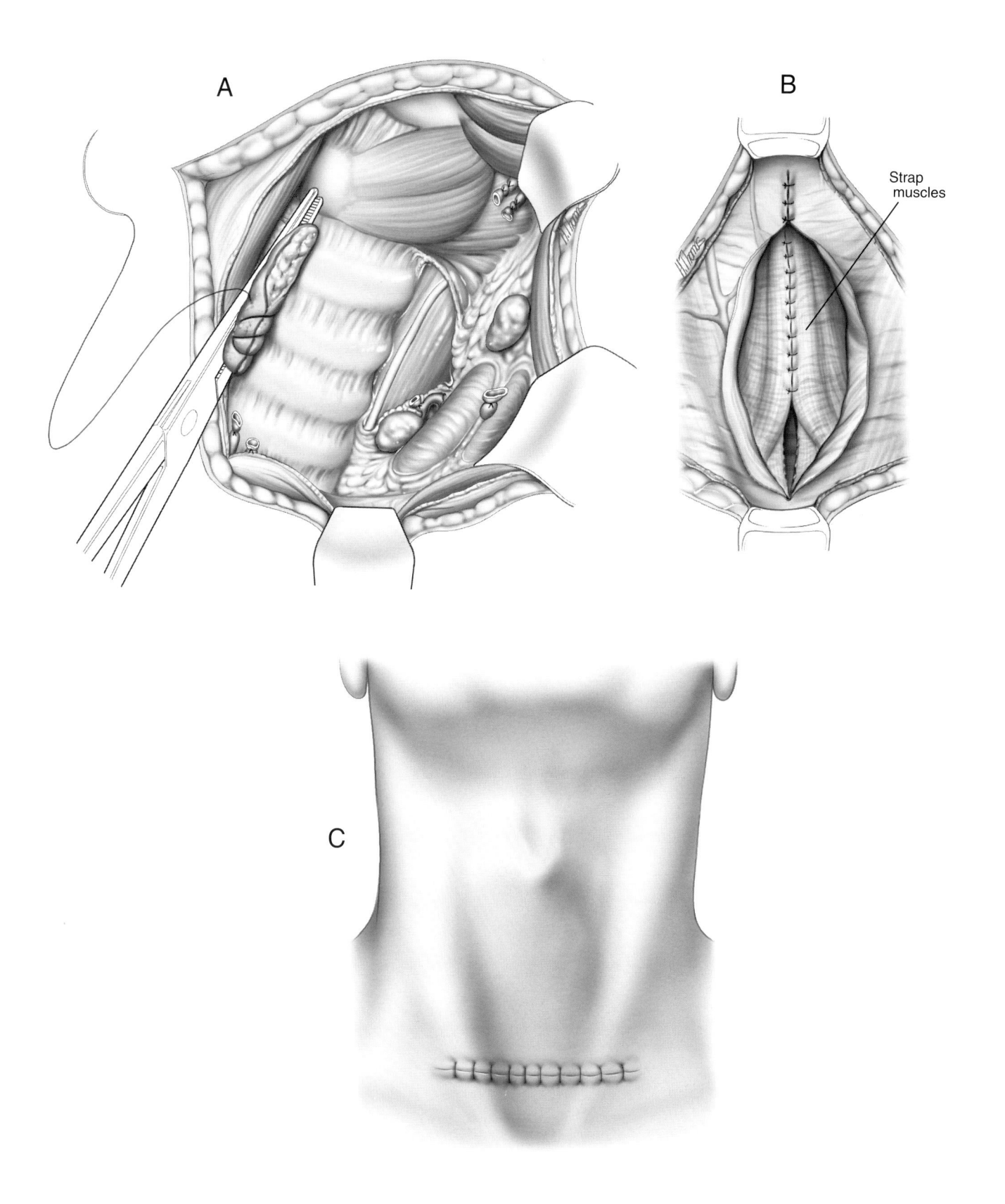

Figure 2–13 • **A,** The cut end of the isthmus is oversewn.
B, The wound is closed by reapproximating the strap muscles.
C, The platysma, and the skin are closed. A drain may be left or not.

Chapter 3
Surgical Anatomy of the Parotid Gland

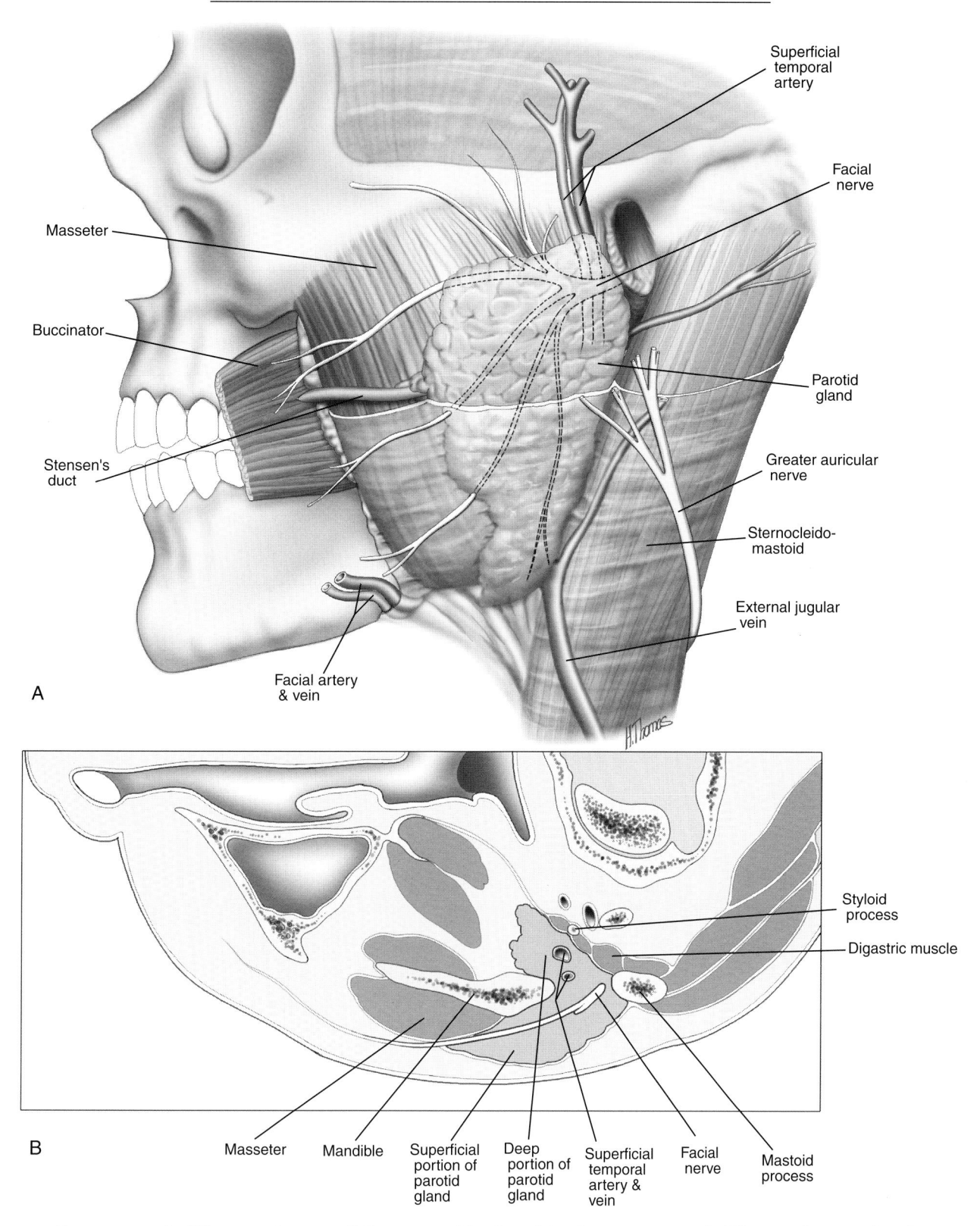

Figure 3–1 • **A,** The anatomy of the parotid gland is demonstrated. The main trunk of the facial nerve is within the substance of the gland.

B, Cross-sectional anatomy defining the deep parotid lobe and the plane of the facial nerve.

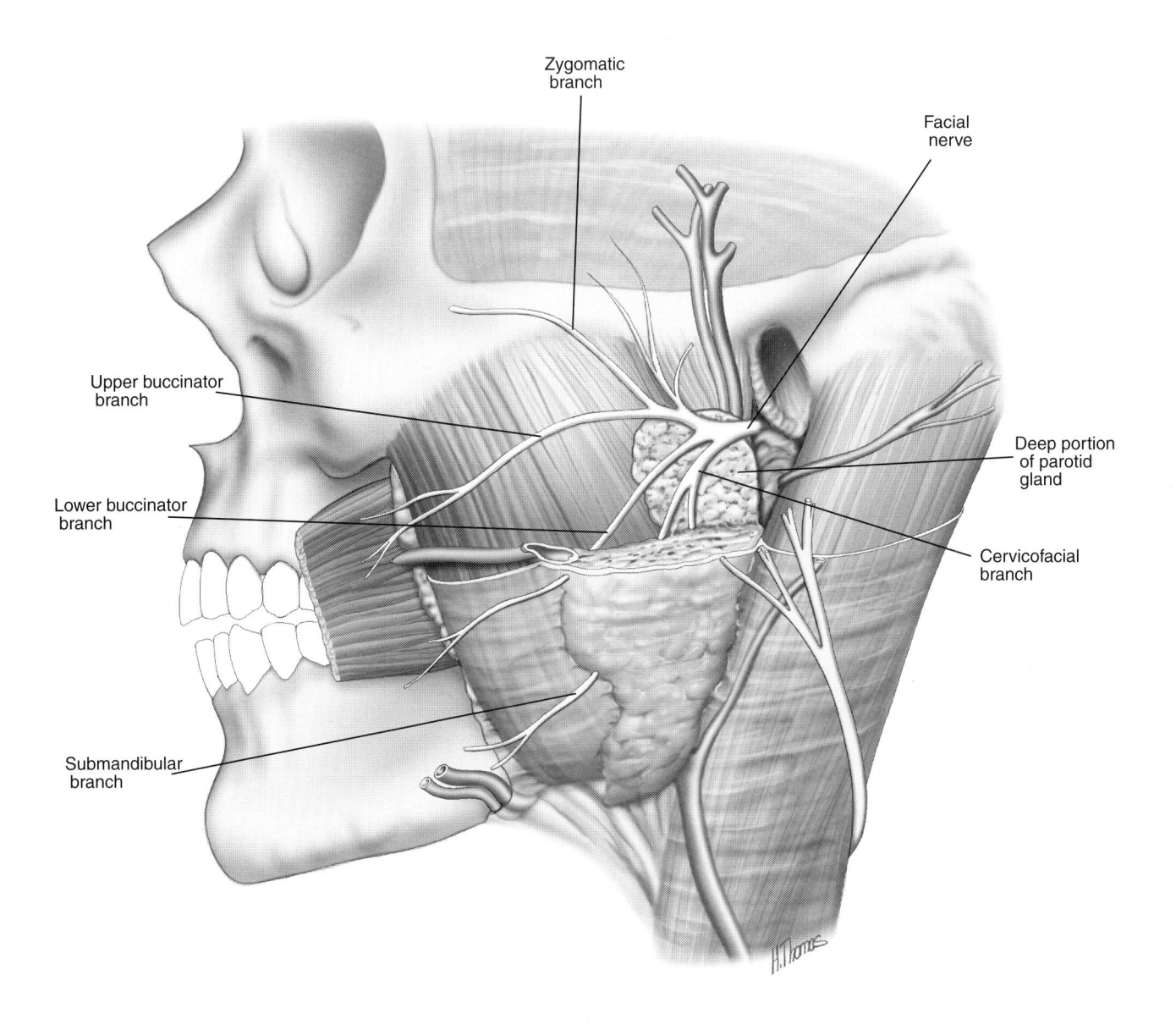

Figure 3–2 • The facial nerve is exposed in the depth of the parotid gland.

Chapter 4
Parotidectomy

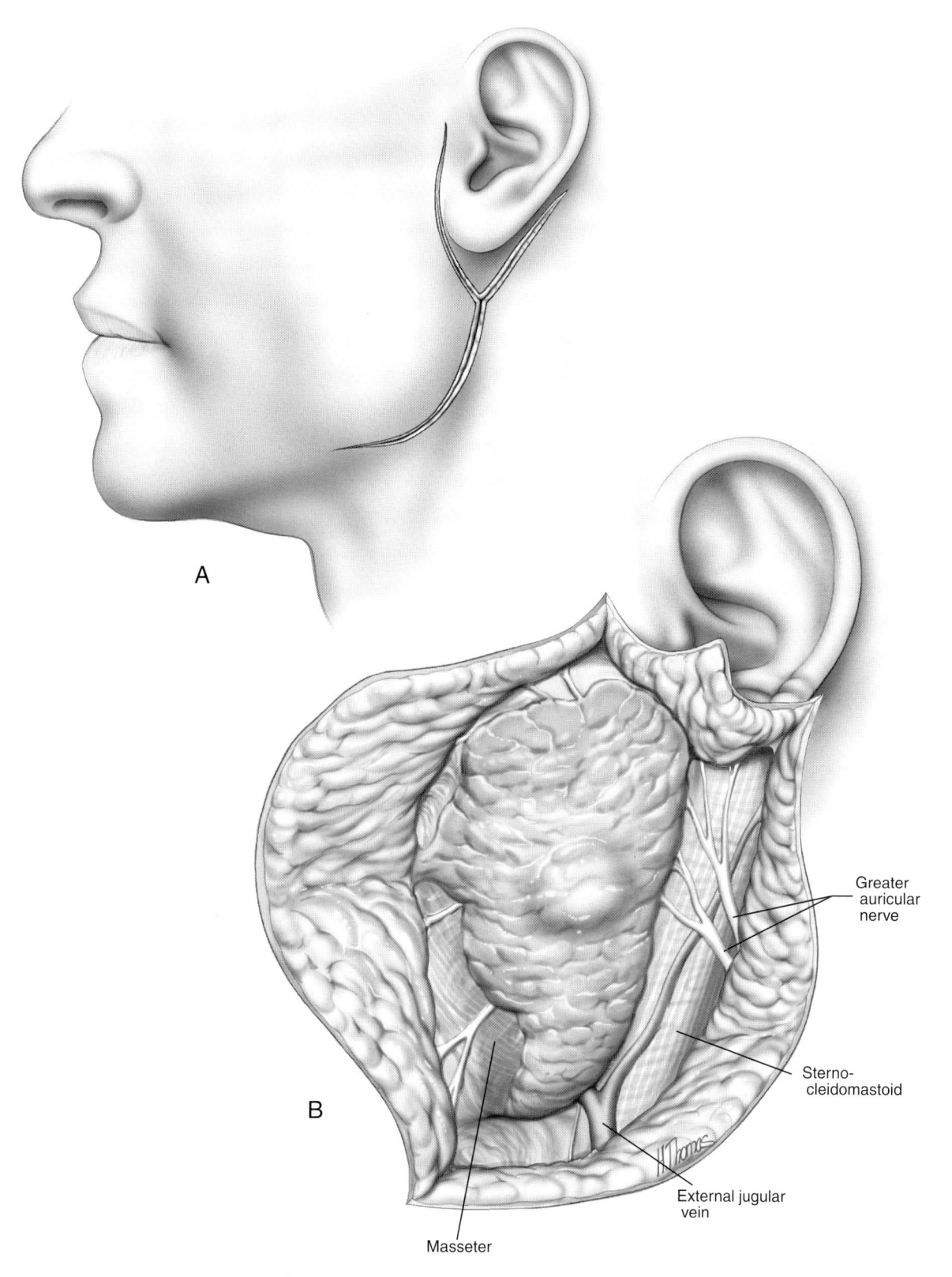

Figure 4–1 • **A,** The traditional skin incision.
B, The skin flaps are elevated, and the greater auricular nerve is exposed.

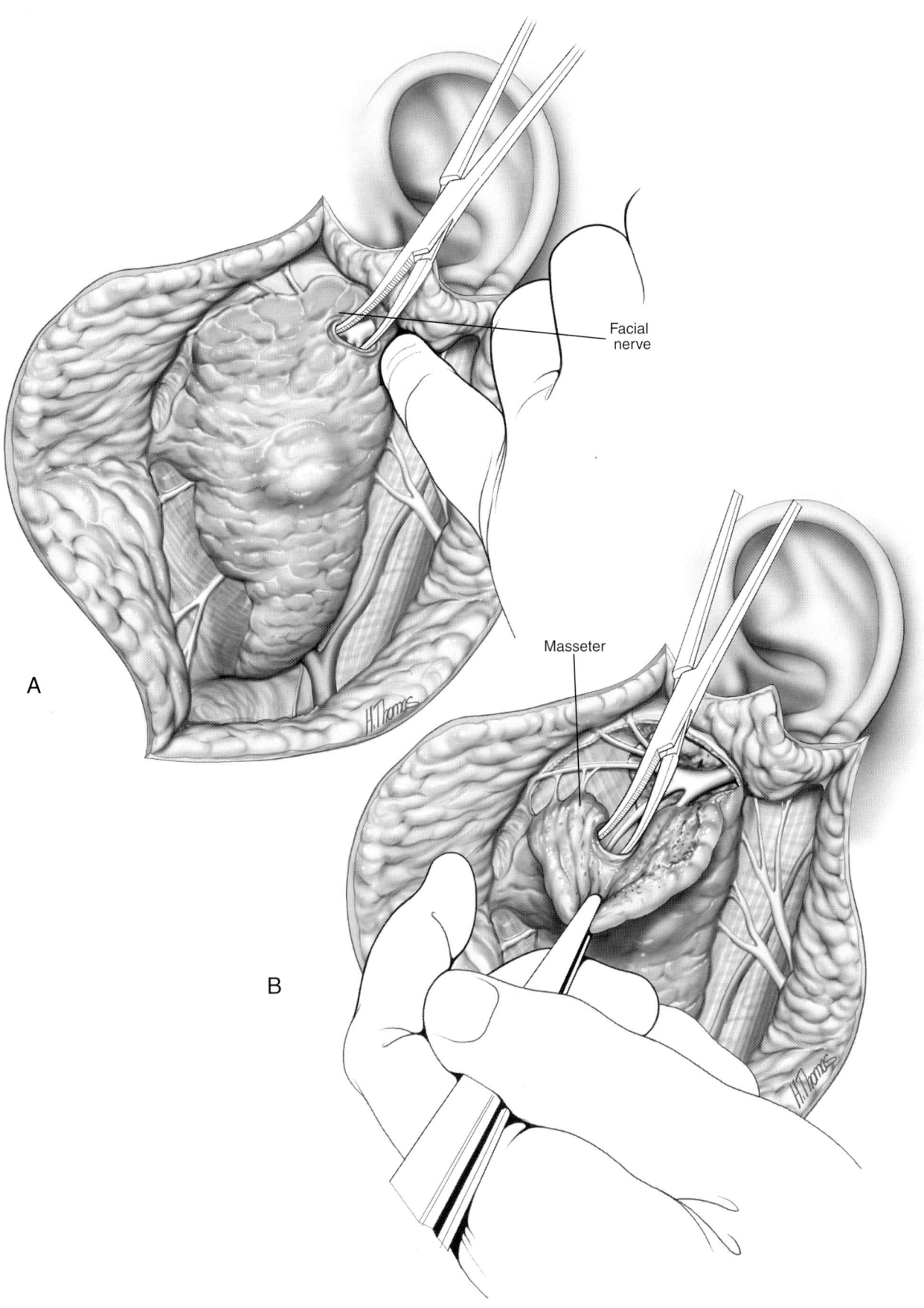

Figure 4–2 • **A,** The main trunk of the nerve is identified by placing the fifth digit on the mastoid and beginning to dissect bluntly the parotid tissue in front of the digit.
   B, After identifying the main trunk, the major branches are individually dissected by keeping the back of the mosquito clamp directly on the nerve trunk.

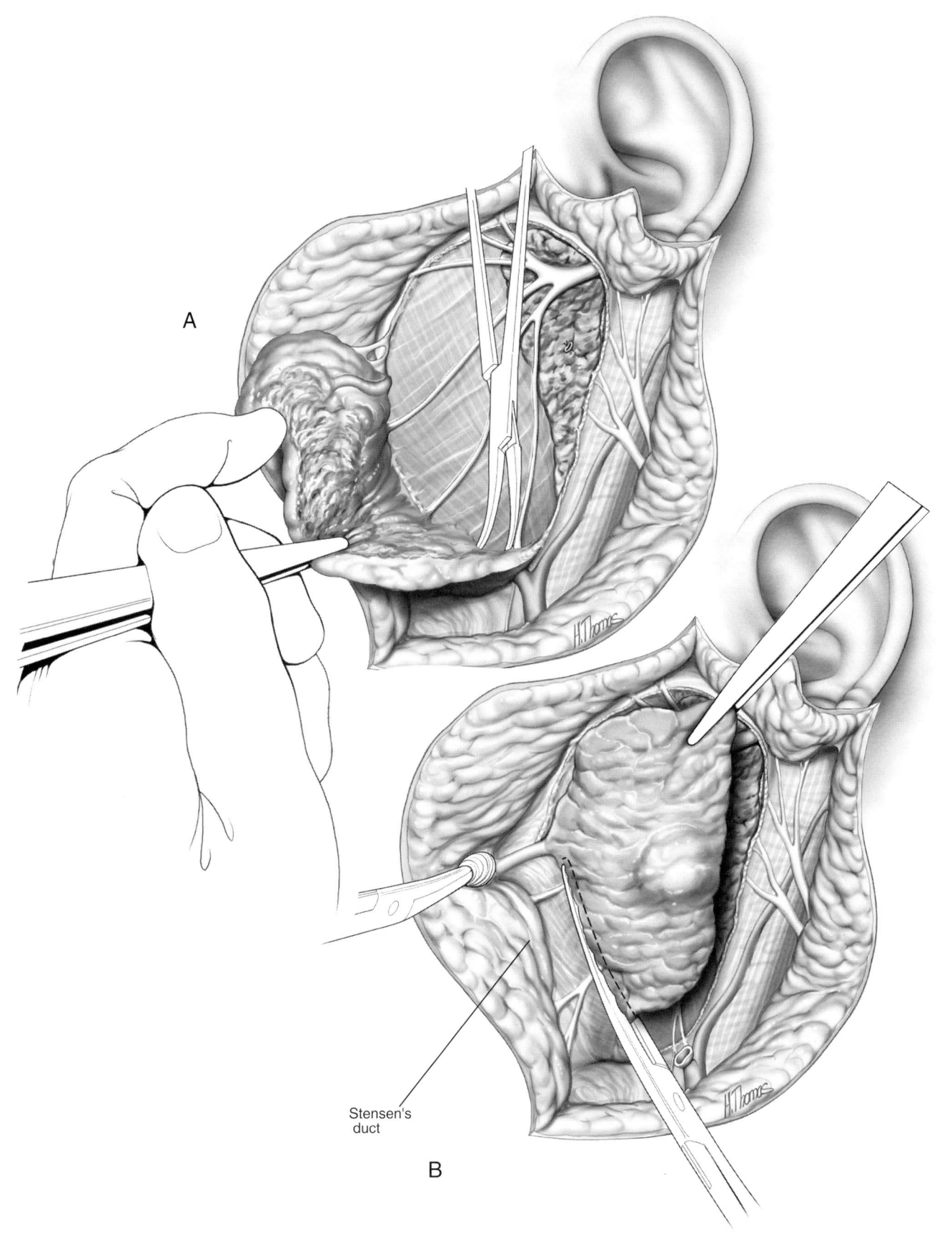

Figure 4–3 • **A,** The dissection between the superficial and deep lobes is completed by dissecting the mandibular branch.

B, The remaining glandular tissue is divided, and Stensen's duct is identified.

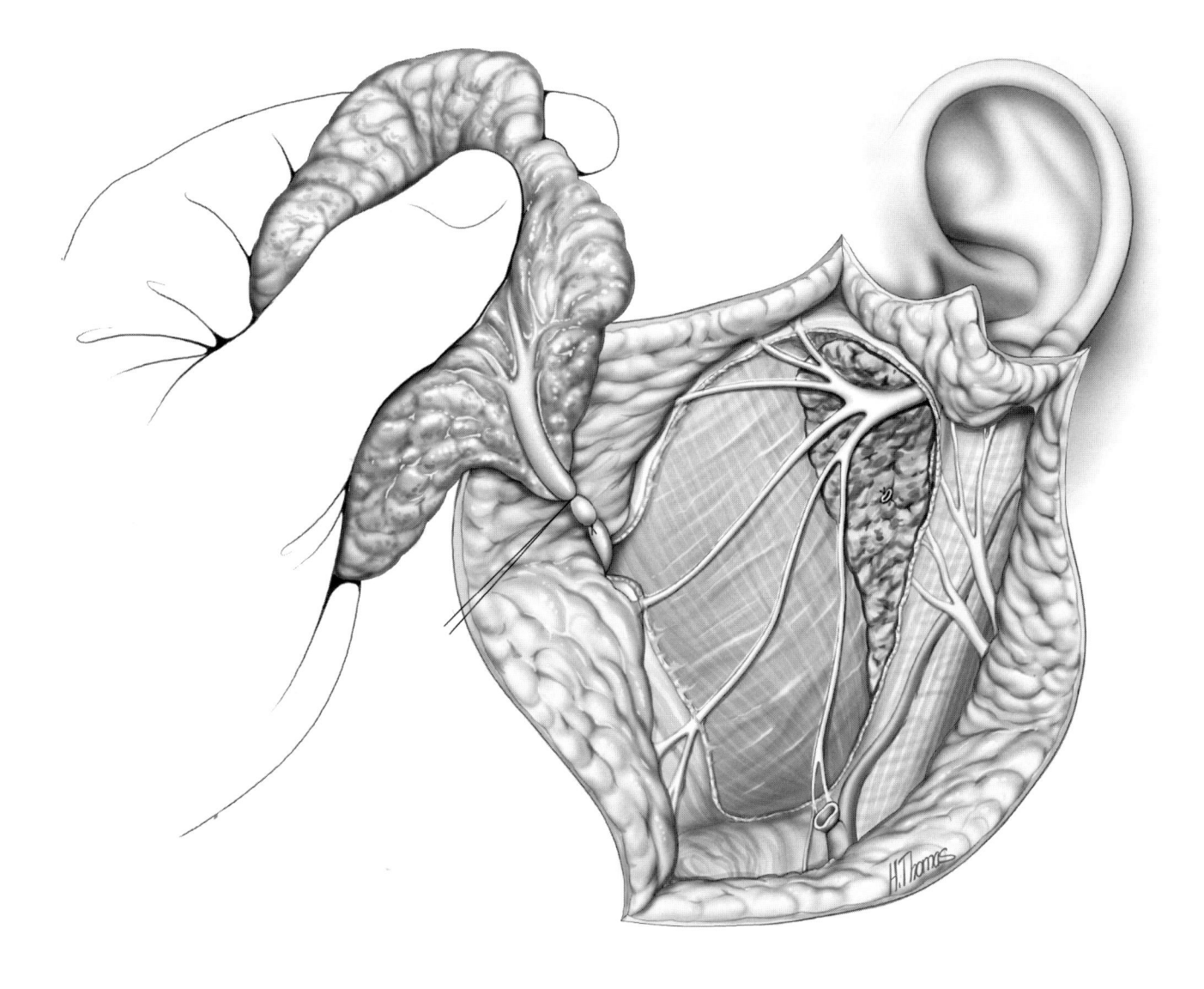

Figure 4–4 • Stensen's duct is ligated, and the superficial lobe is removed. All major trunks of the facial nerve are completely dissected and preserved.

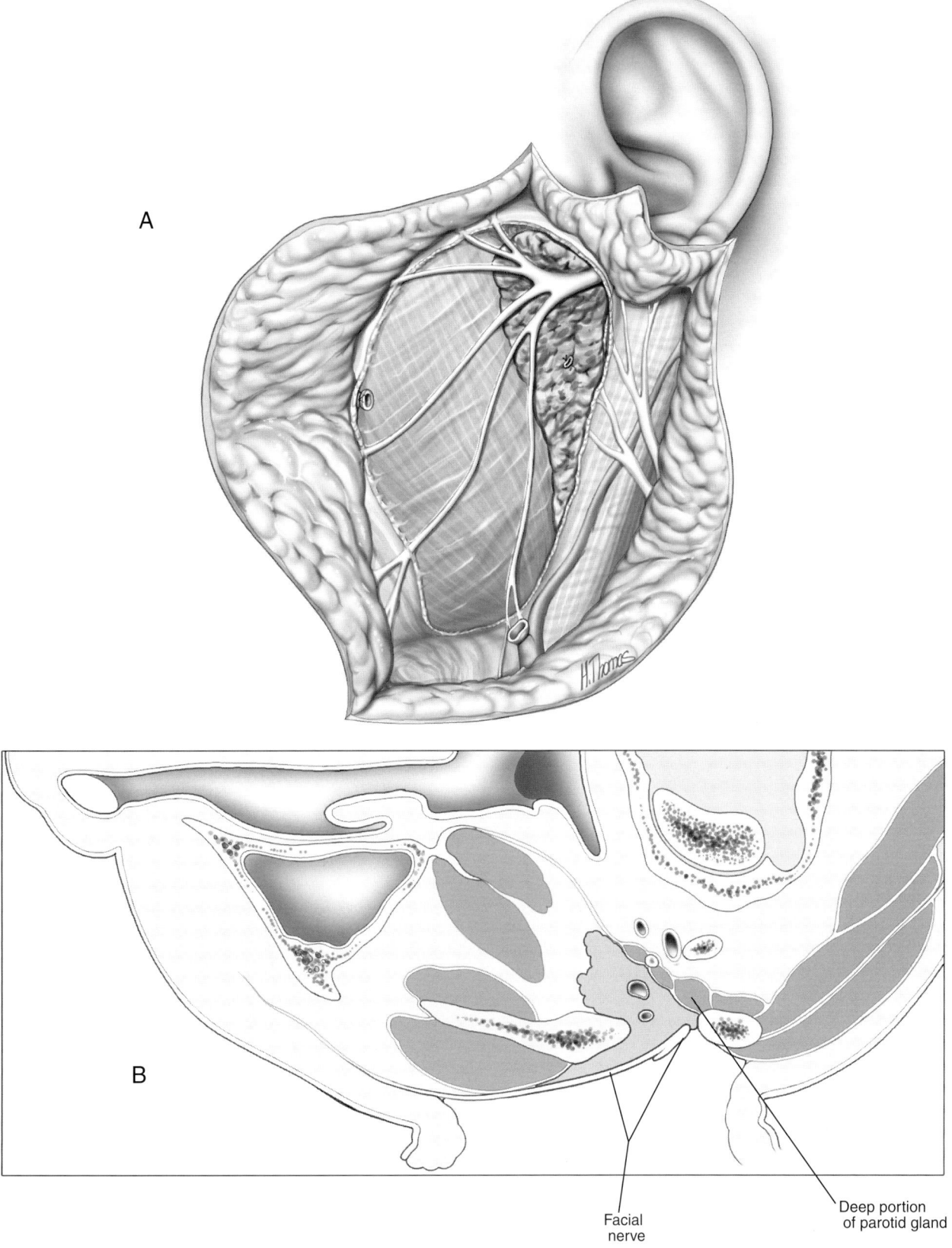

Figure 4–5 • **A,** The resected superficial lobe is absent, and the bed of the resection is depicted.
   B, A cross-sectional view showing the relationship of the facial nerve to the deep lobe of the parotid following a superficial parotidectomy.

Chapter 5
Surgical Anatomy for Radical Neck Dissection

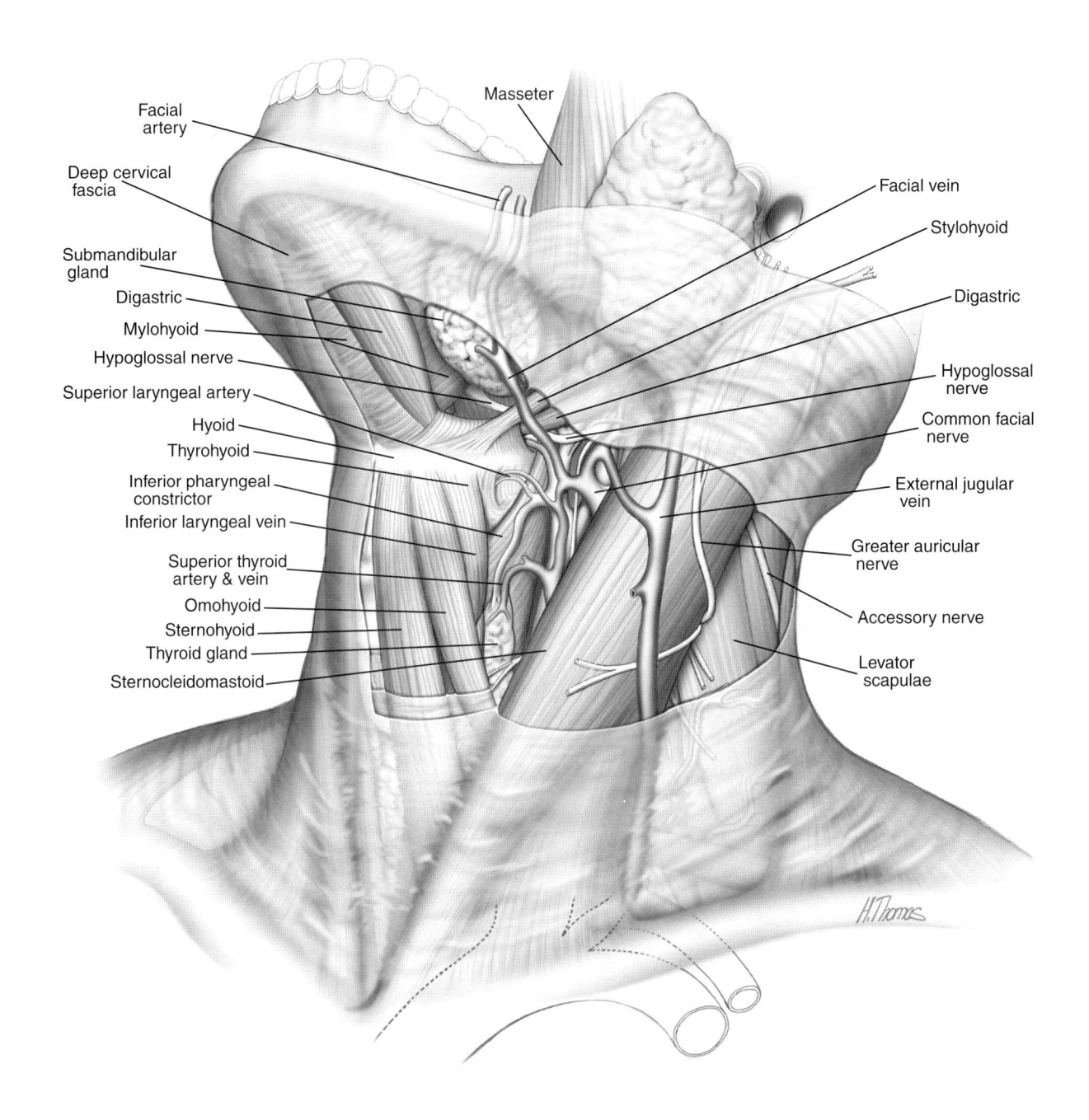

Figure 5–1 • The central anatomy of the neck is clearly displayed upon removal of the platysma and deep cervical fascia.

Surgical Anatomy for Radical Neck Dissection • 29

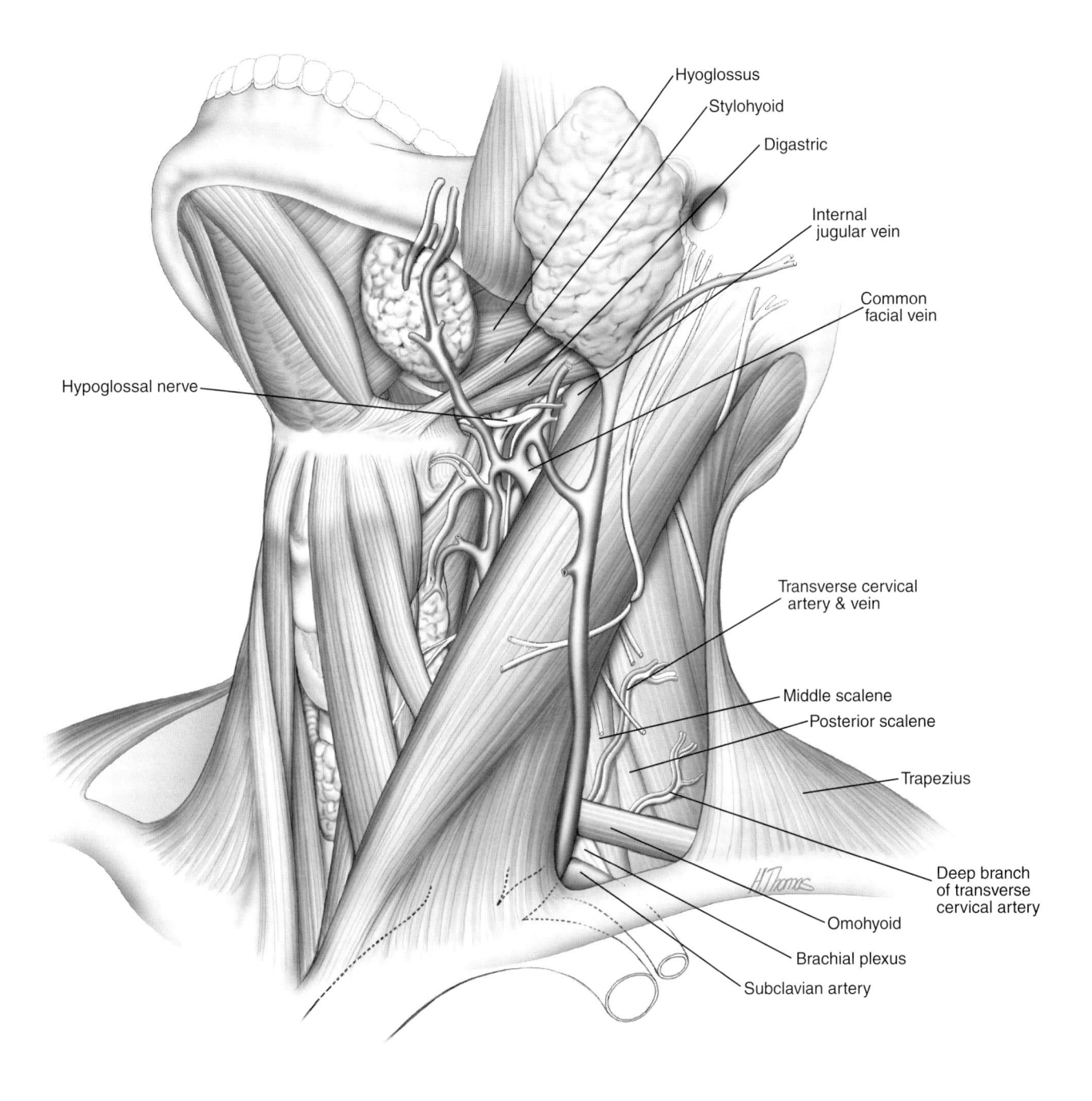

Figure 5–2 • The major anatomic structures comprising the submaxillary, anterior, and posterior triangles of the neck.

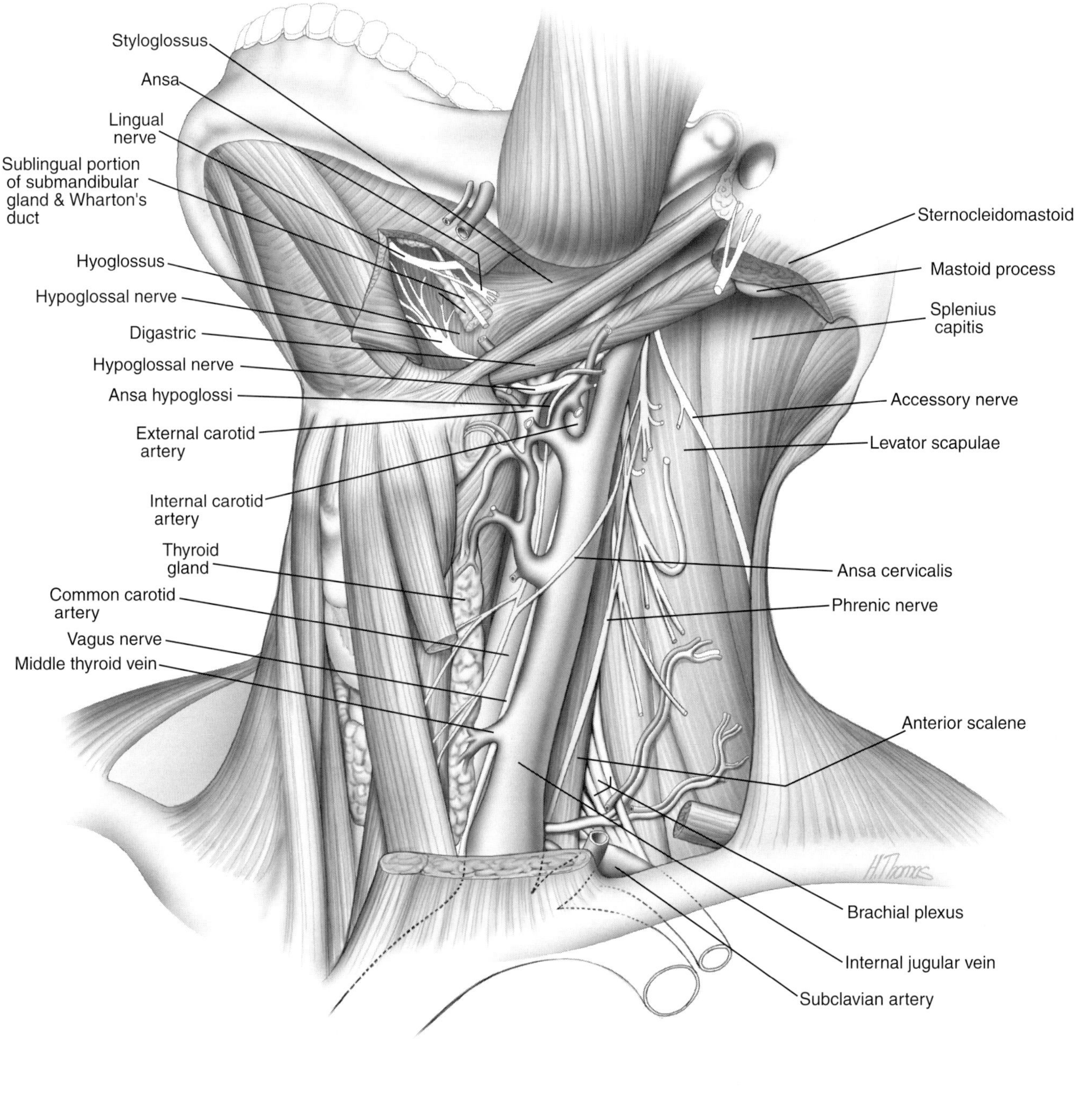

Figure 5–3 • The deep structures of the submaxillary triangle (gland removed) and central neck (sternocleidomastoid removed).

Chapter 6
Radical Neck Dissection

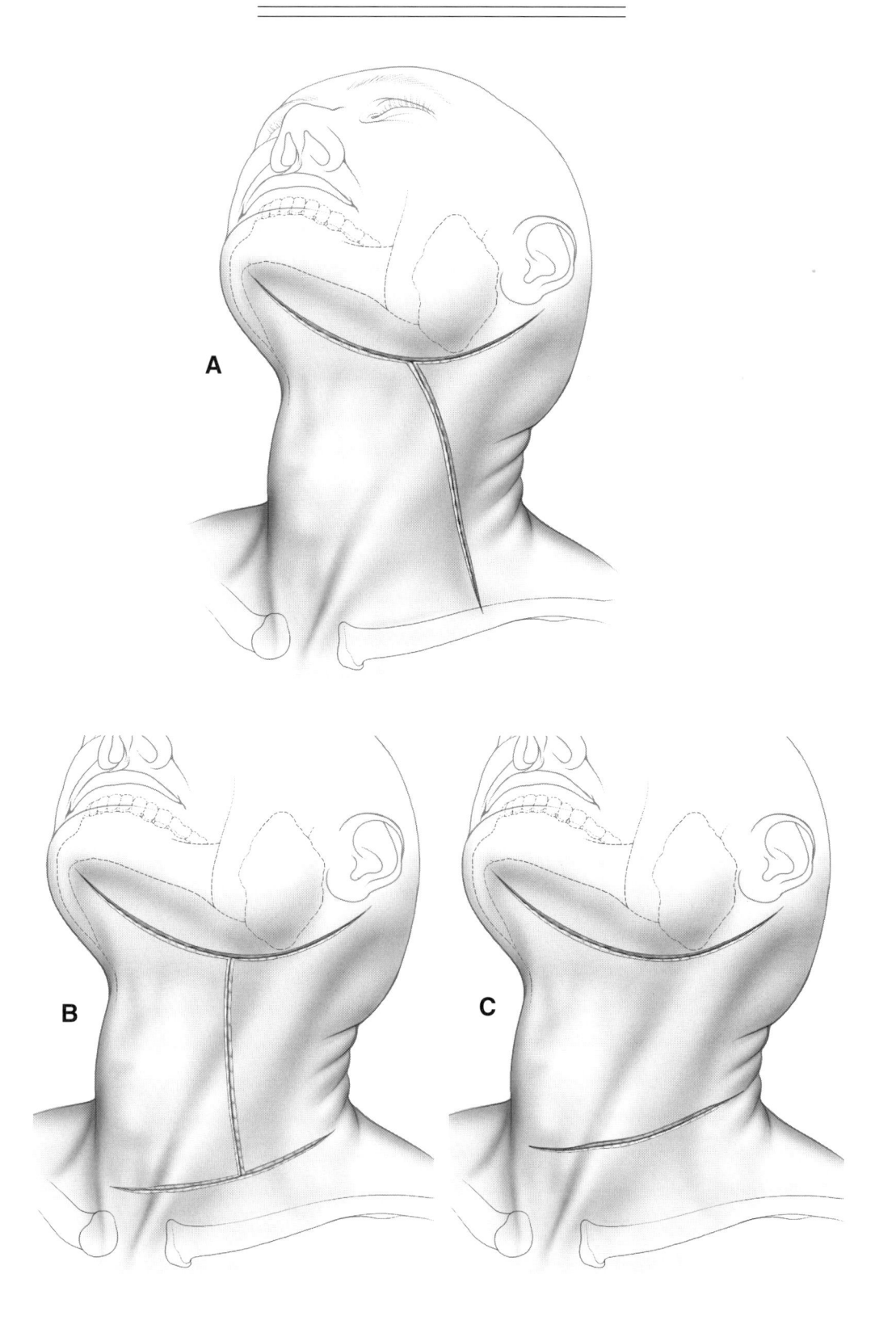

Figure 6–1 • **A–C,** One of several incisions can be employed in the performance of a radical neck dissection.

32 • Part I HEAD AND NECK

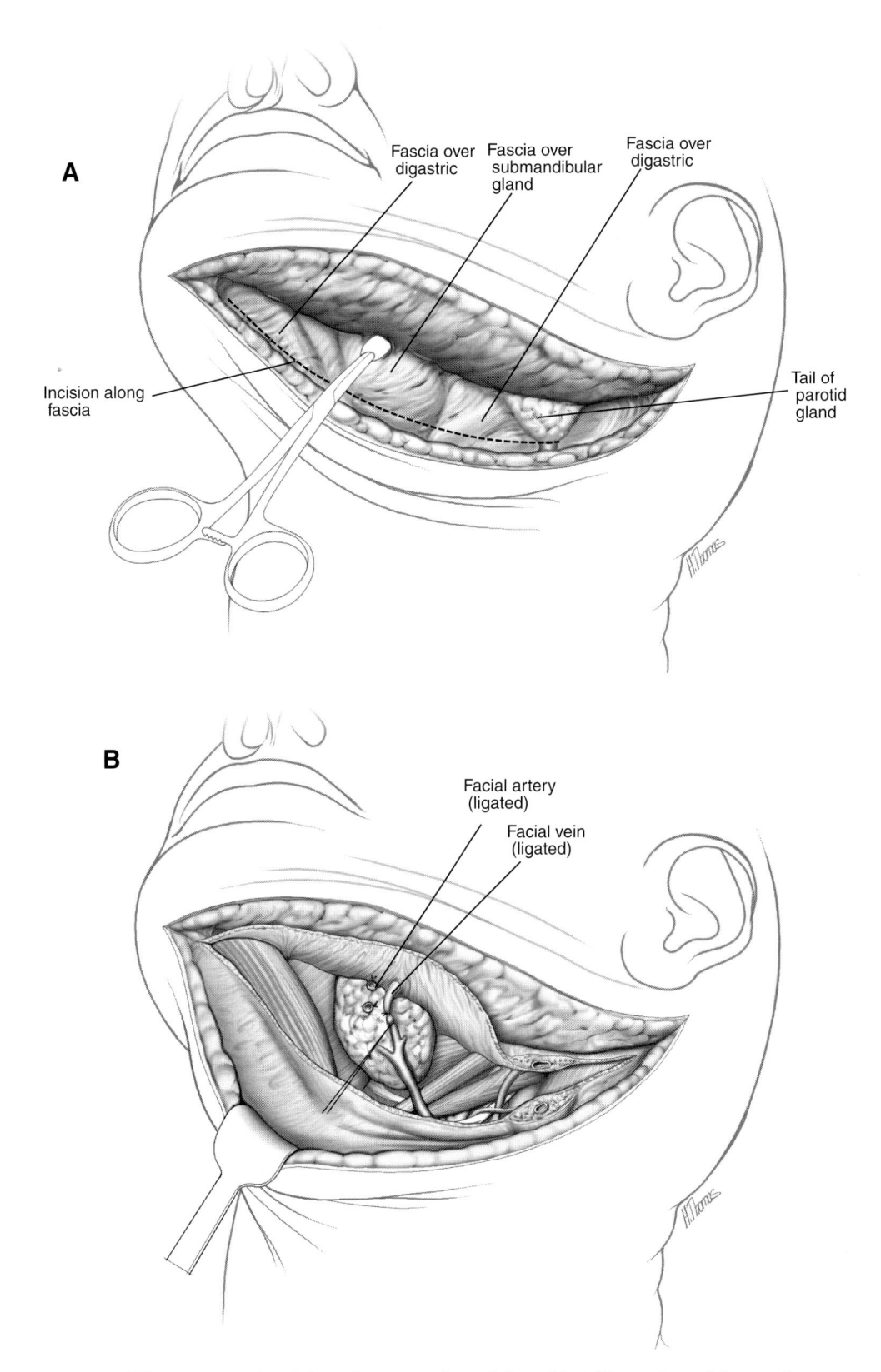

Figure 6–2 • **A,** The upper incision is completed by dividing the skin, subcutaneous tissue, platysma, and cervical fascia over the inferior edge of the submaxillary gland.
  B, The superior flap is elevated, exposing the facial artery and vein, which are ligated. The fat and nodal tissue in the submental area are mobilized off the digastric.

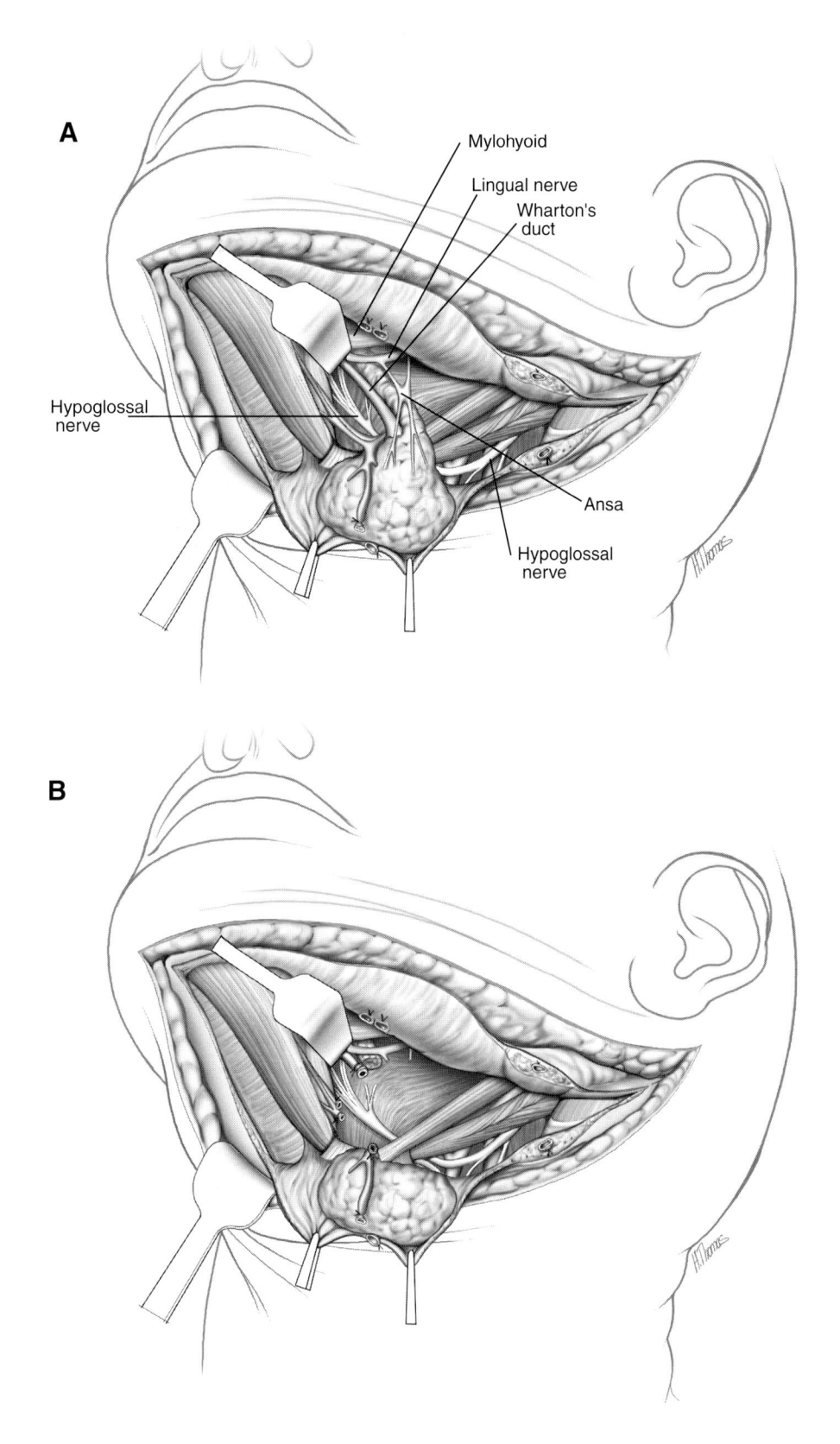

Figure 6–3 • **A,** The submaxillary triangle dissection is completed by identifying the lingual nerve and dividing the ansa cervicalis.
B, Wharton's duct is divided by elevating the mylohyoid and identifying the hypoglossal nerve as it passes under the digastric muscle.

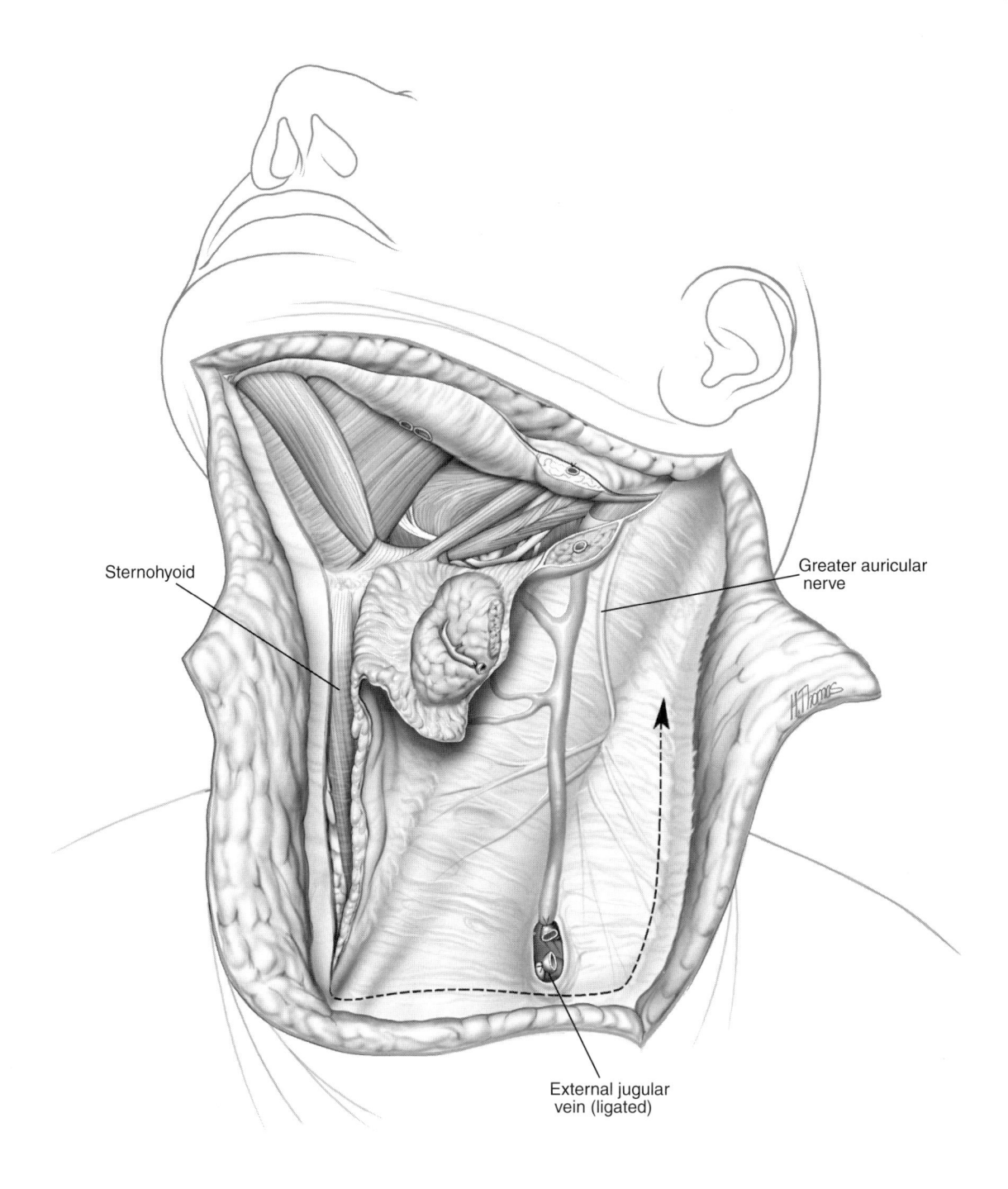

Figure 6–4 • The completed submaxillary gland dissection and resection of a portion of the tail of the parotid laterally is depicted. The remaining skin flaps are elevated under the cut platysma.

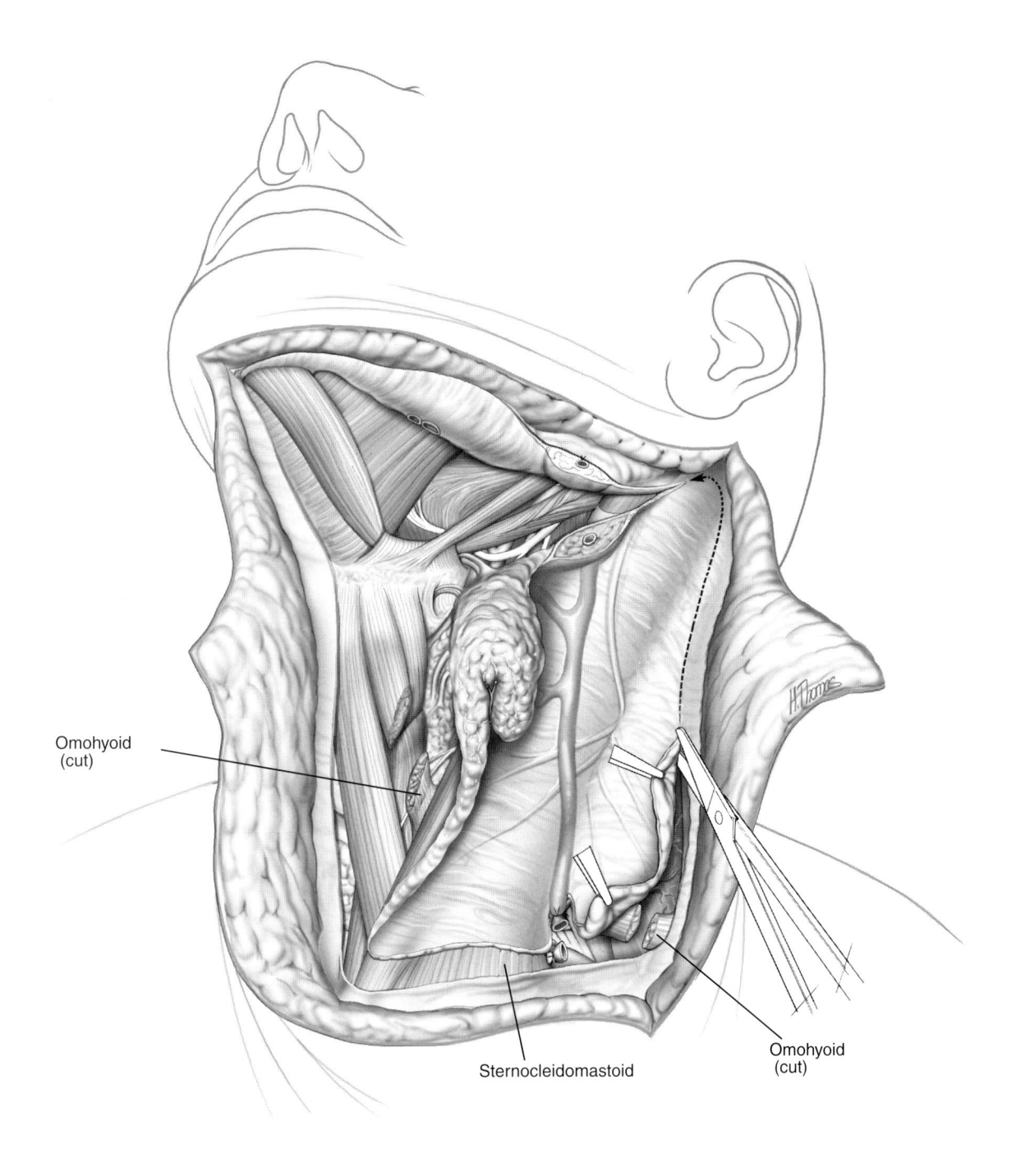

Figure 6–5 • The fascia overlying the strap muscles from the hyoid to the clavicle is cut and reflected laterally. Inferiorly, the fascia over the sternocleidomastoid is incised, the external jugular vein is divided, and the posterior triangle dissection is begun. The posterior belly of the omohyoid is divided.

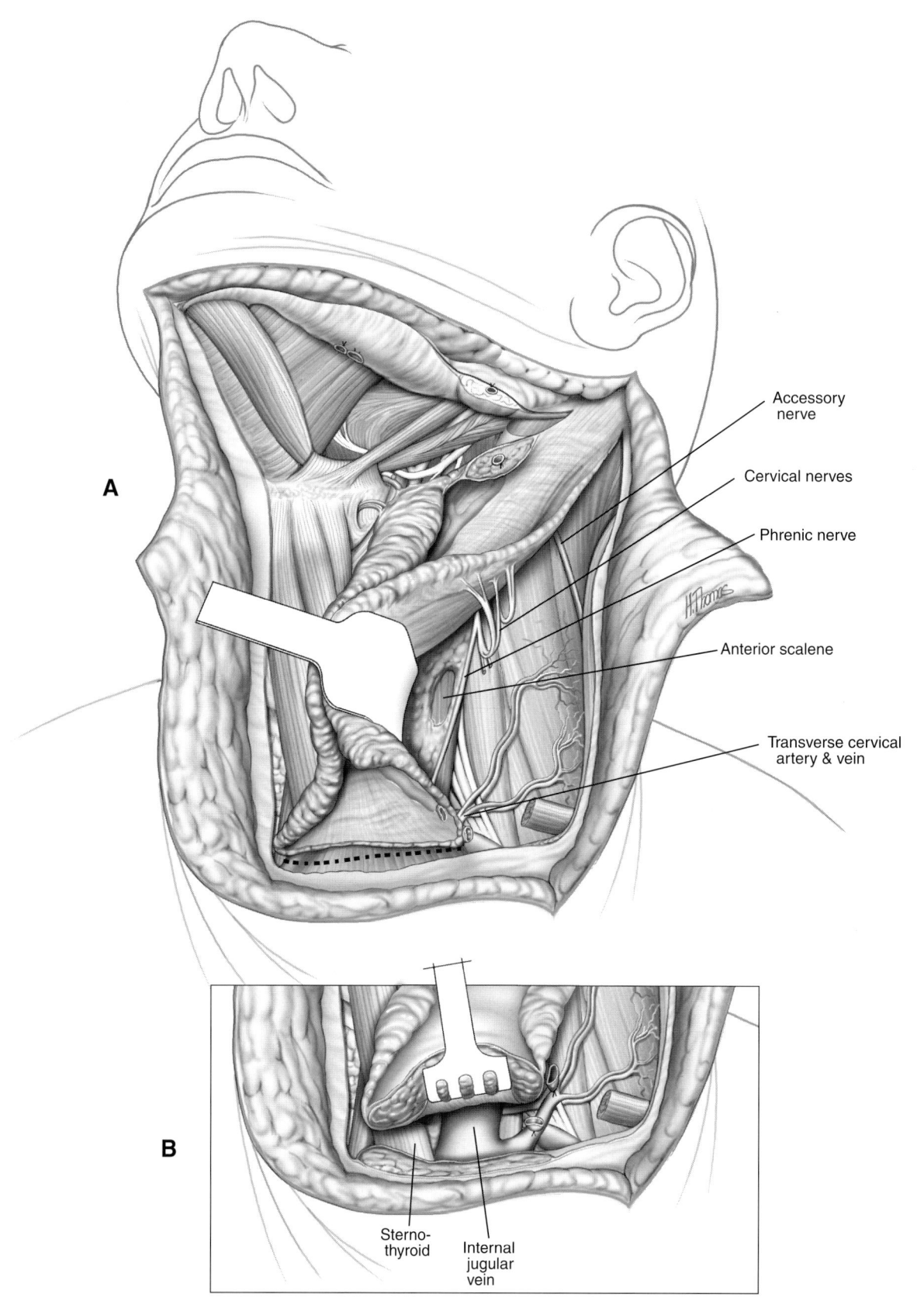

Figure 6–6 • **A,** The posterior triangle is dissected from lateral to medial, identifying and preserving the spinal accessory nerve, which is identified in the midneck and the phrenic nerve on the anterior scalene. The latter is usually elevated with the nodal tissue.

B, The sternocleidomastoid is divided.

Radical Neck Dissection • 37

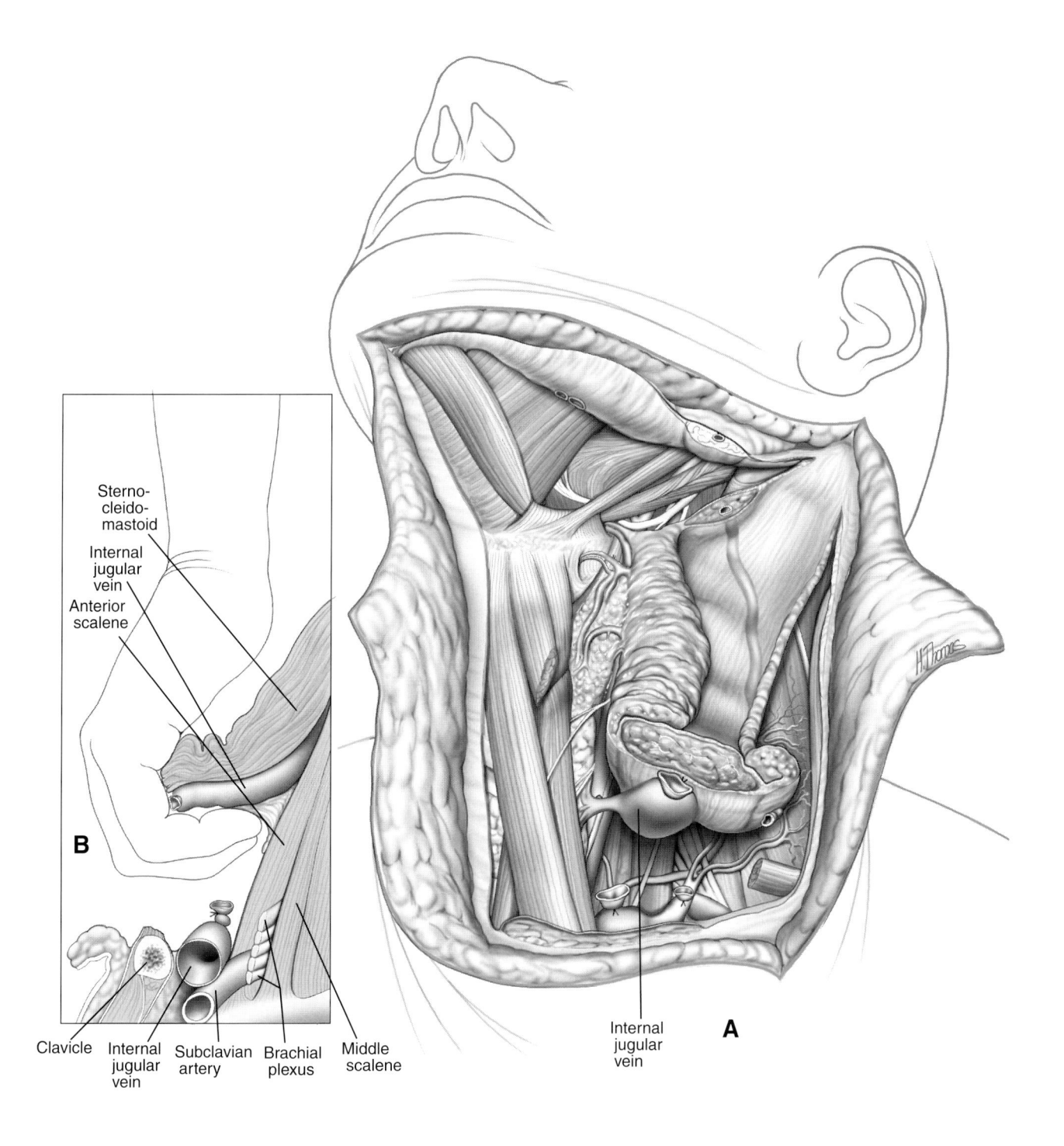

Figure 6–7 • **A,** The internal jugular vein is divided.
   B, By placing several fingers behind the divided vein, the vein is dissected bluntly off the underlying carotid sheath.

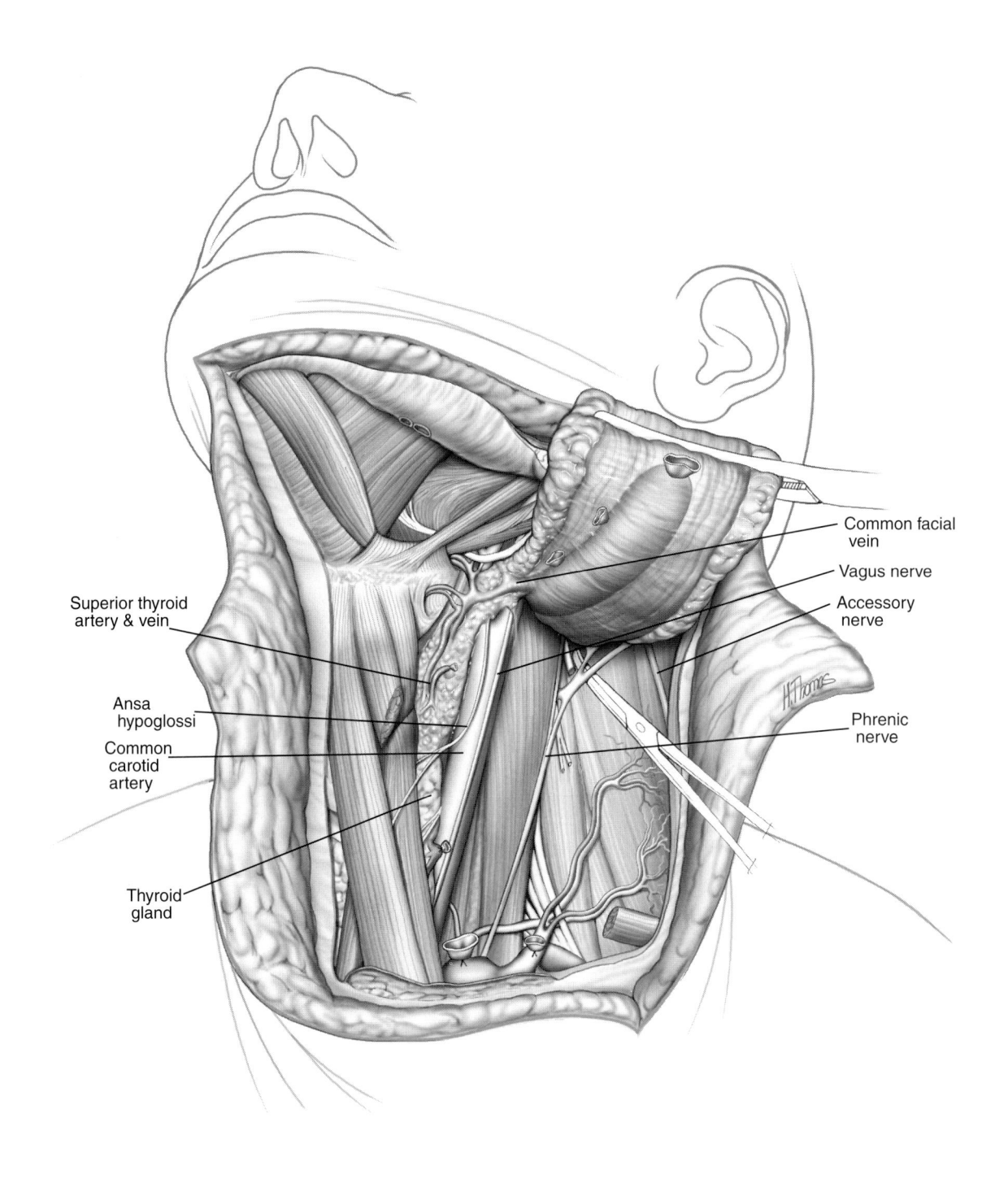

Figure 6–8 • All venous branches medially are divided, and the sensory cervical roots are divided, preserving the phrenic nerve.

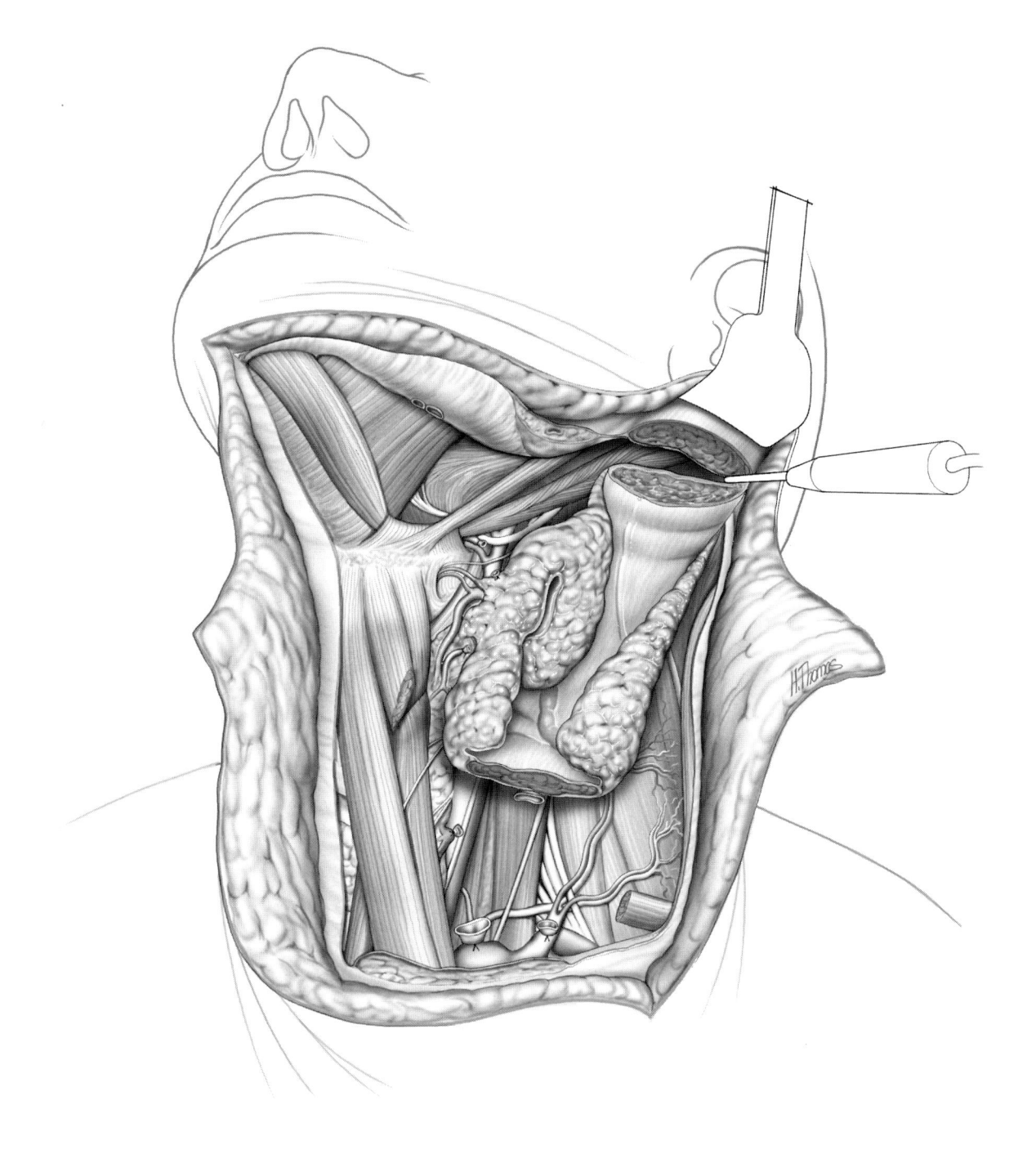

Figure 6–9 • The sternocleidomastoid is divided near its origin.

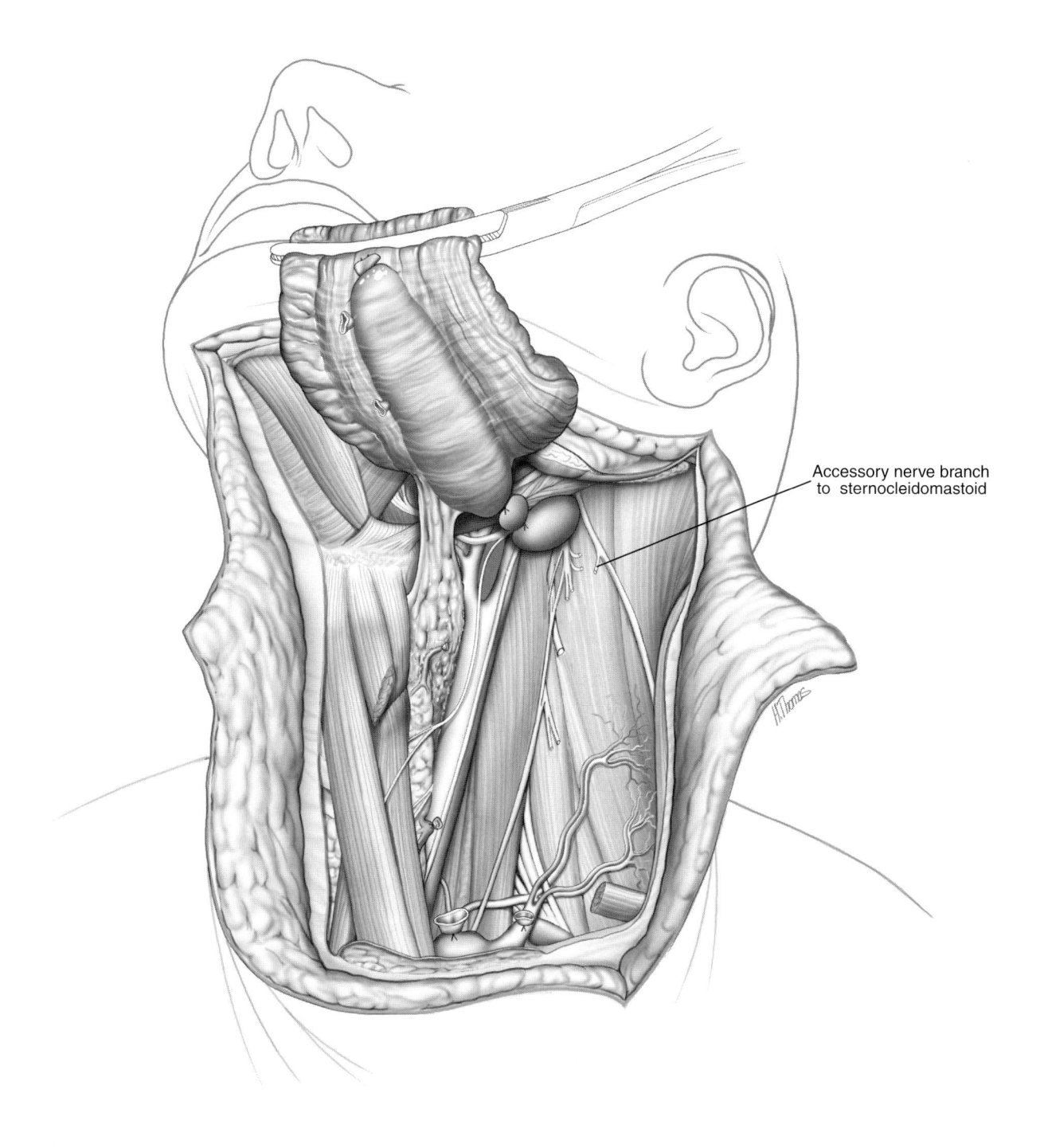

Figure 6–10 • The internal jugular vein is divided, and the spinal accessory nerve is preserved if feasible. Extensive nodal disease in the upper jugular region may preclude its preservation. A branch off the spinal accessory to the sternocleidomastoid is divided.

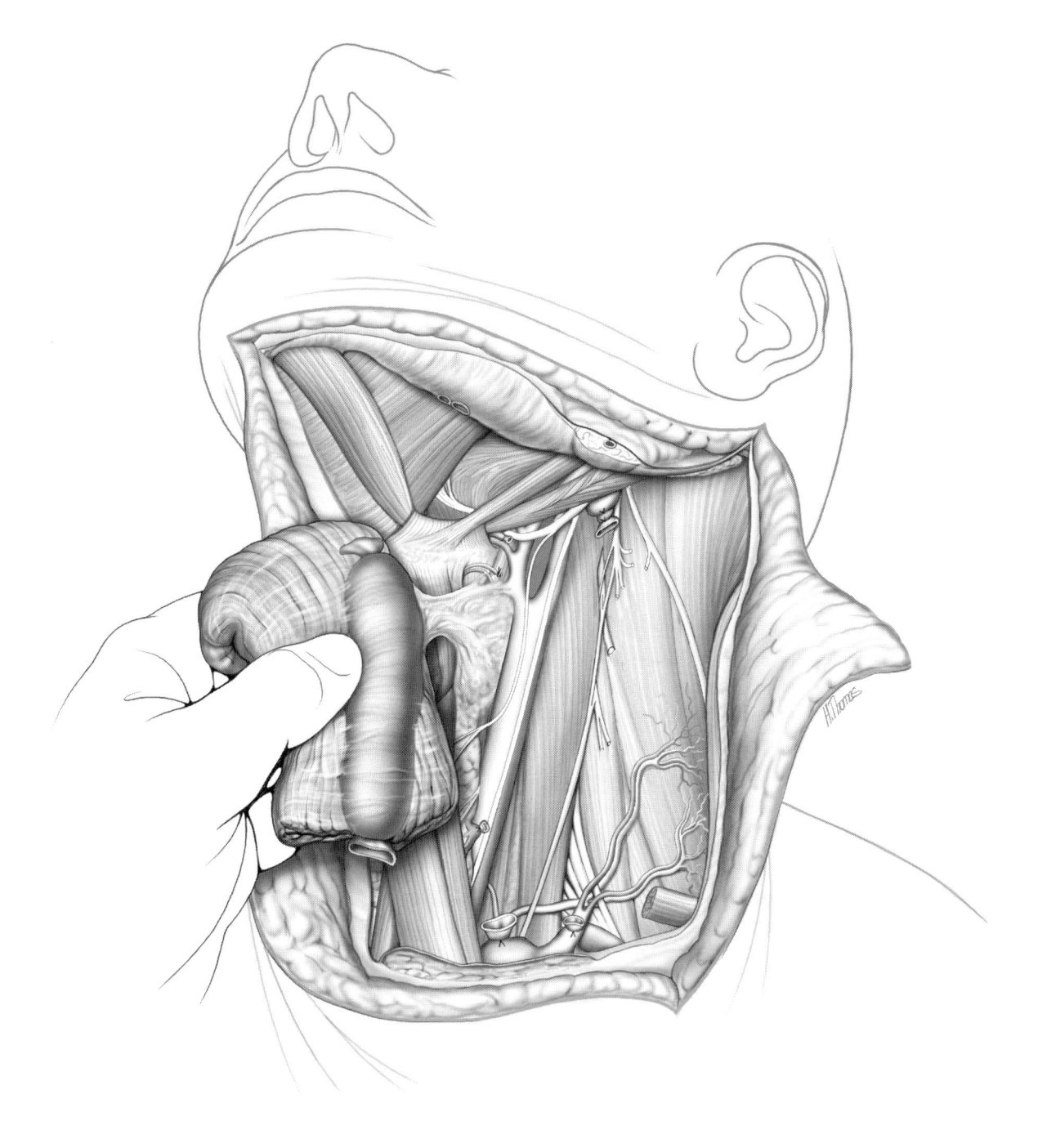

Figure 6–11 • To complete the neck dissection, the remainder of the medial attachments are divided.

42 • Part I HEAD AND NECK

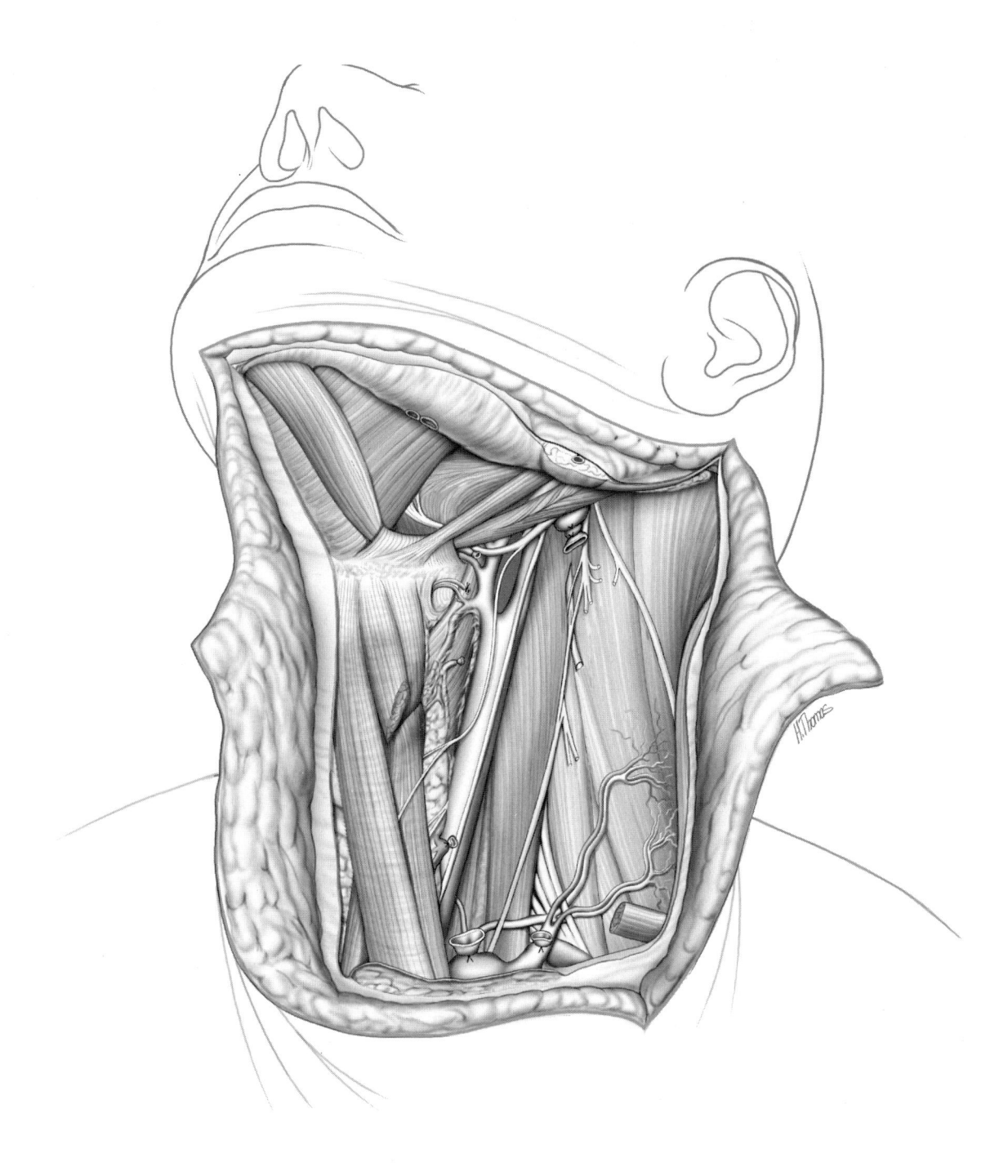

Figure 6–12 • After the neck dissection is completed, the skin flaps are closed and two drains are secured into position.

Chapter 7
Clinical Case: Desmoid Tumor Thoracic Inlet

Michael Hausman

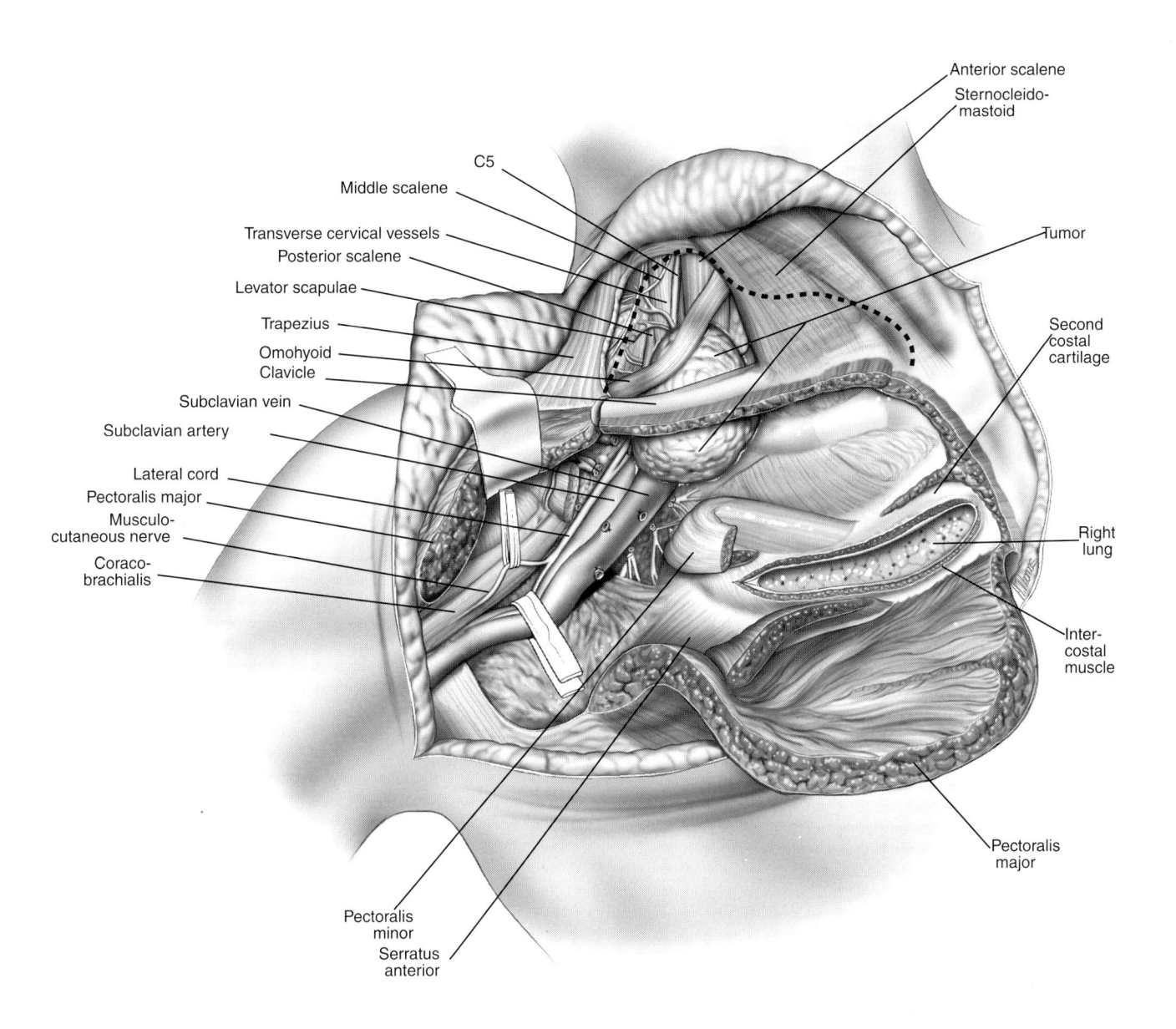

Figure 7–1 • A 26-year-old white woman presented with a desmoid tumor arising in the thoracic inlet in the root of the neck. The tumor was completely wrapped around the brachial plexus in the posterior triangle of the neck as well as around the subclavian artery and vein beneath the clavicle.

44 • Part I HEAD AND NECK

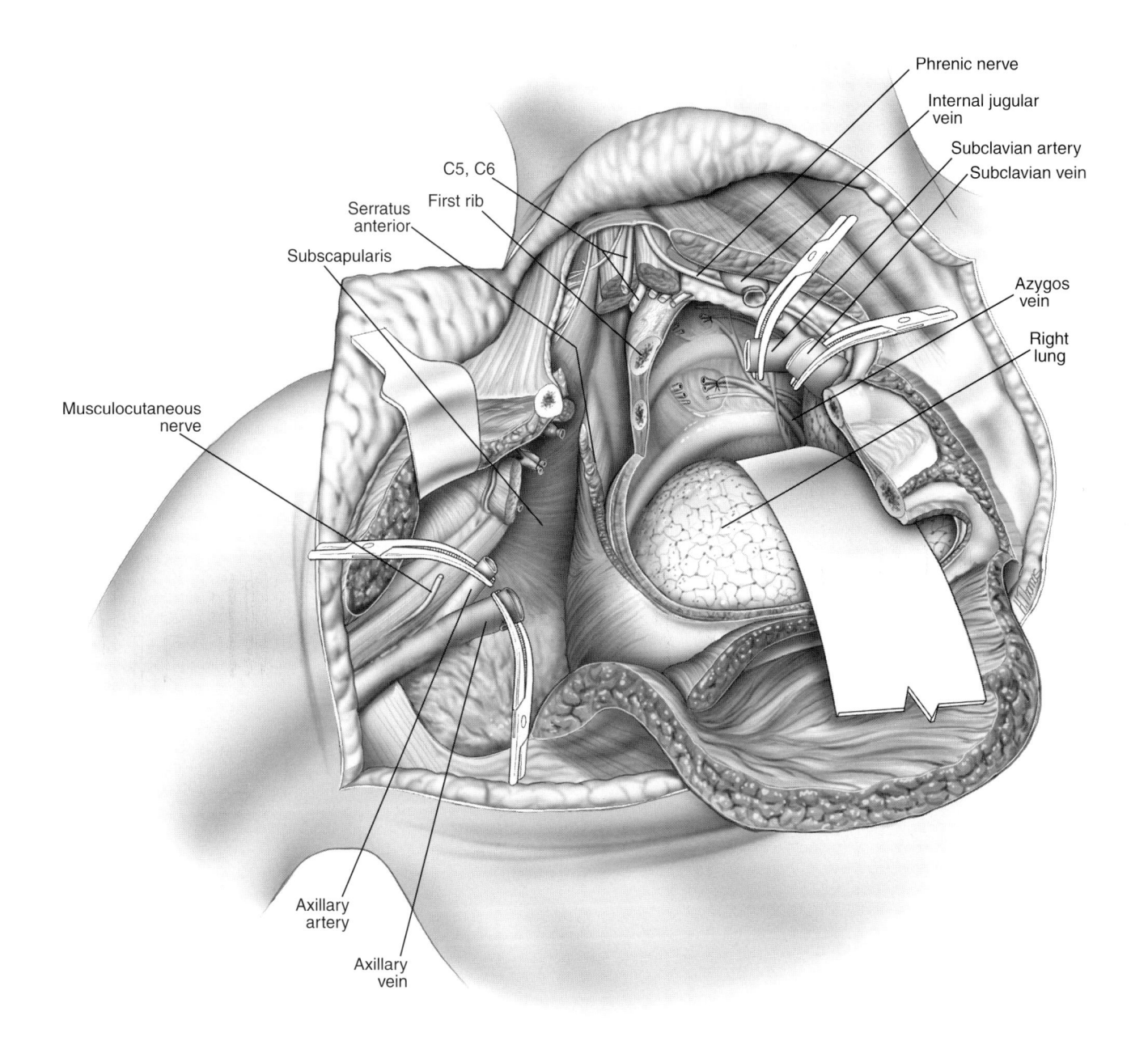

Figure 7–2 • The resection involved removing the brachial plexus, the clavicle and first and second ribs, and a segment of the subclavian artery and vein.

Clinical Case: Desmoid Tumor Thoracic Inlet • 45

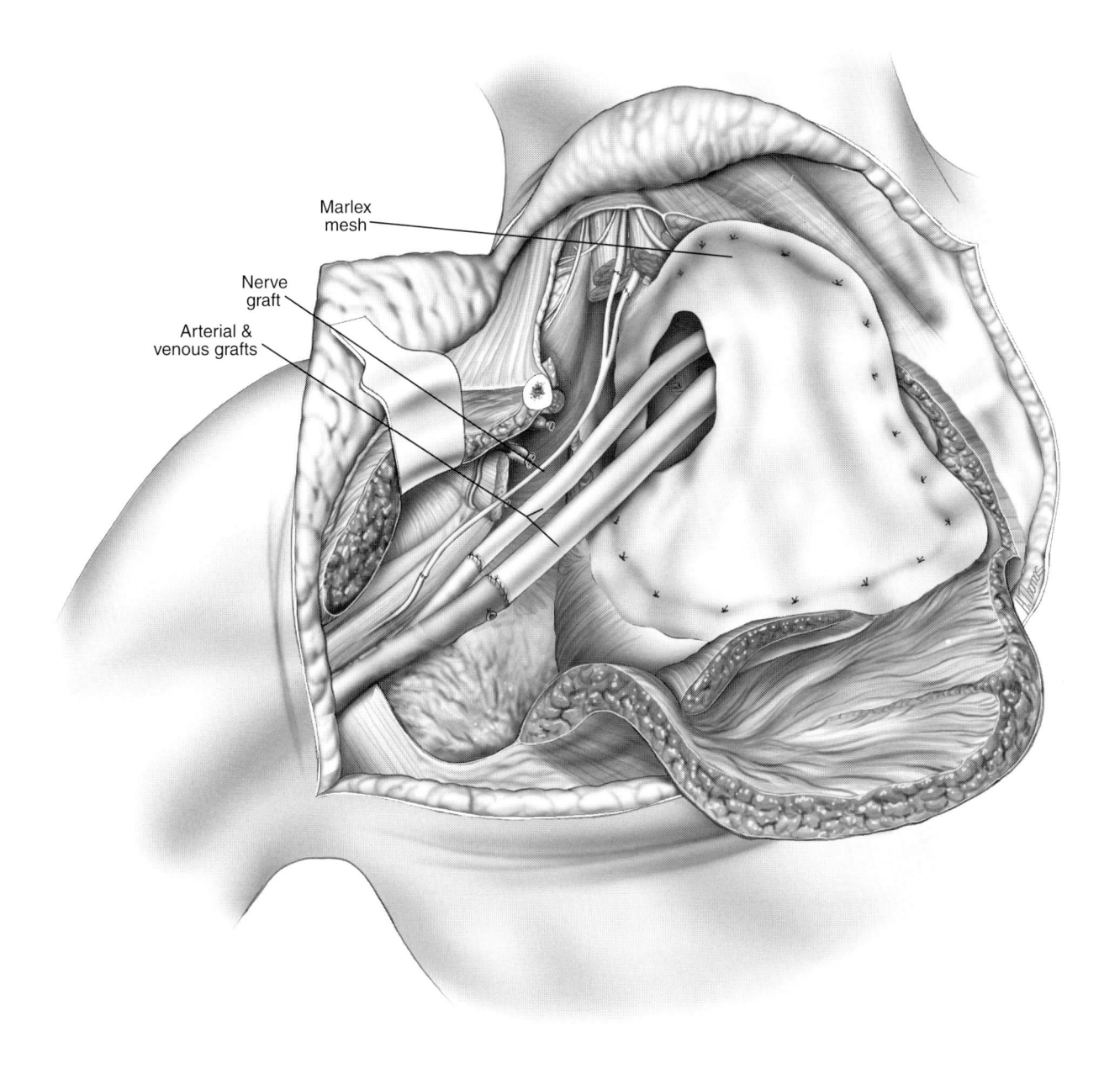

Figure 7–3 • Vascular grafts were created, as were nerve grafts to the musculocutaneous nerve. The chest wall defect was reconstructed utilizing Marlex mesh. The woman is 5 years postresection, with no evidence of recurrent disease. She has regained some elbow flexion.

Part II

CHEST

48 • Part II CHEST

Chapter 8
Surgical Anatomy of the Right Chest

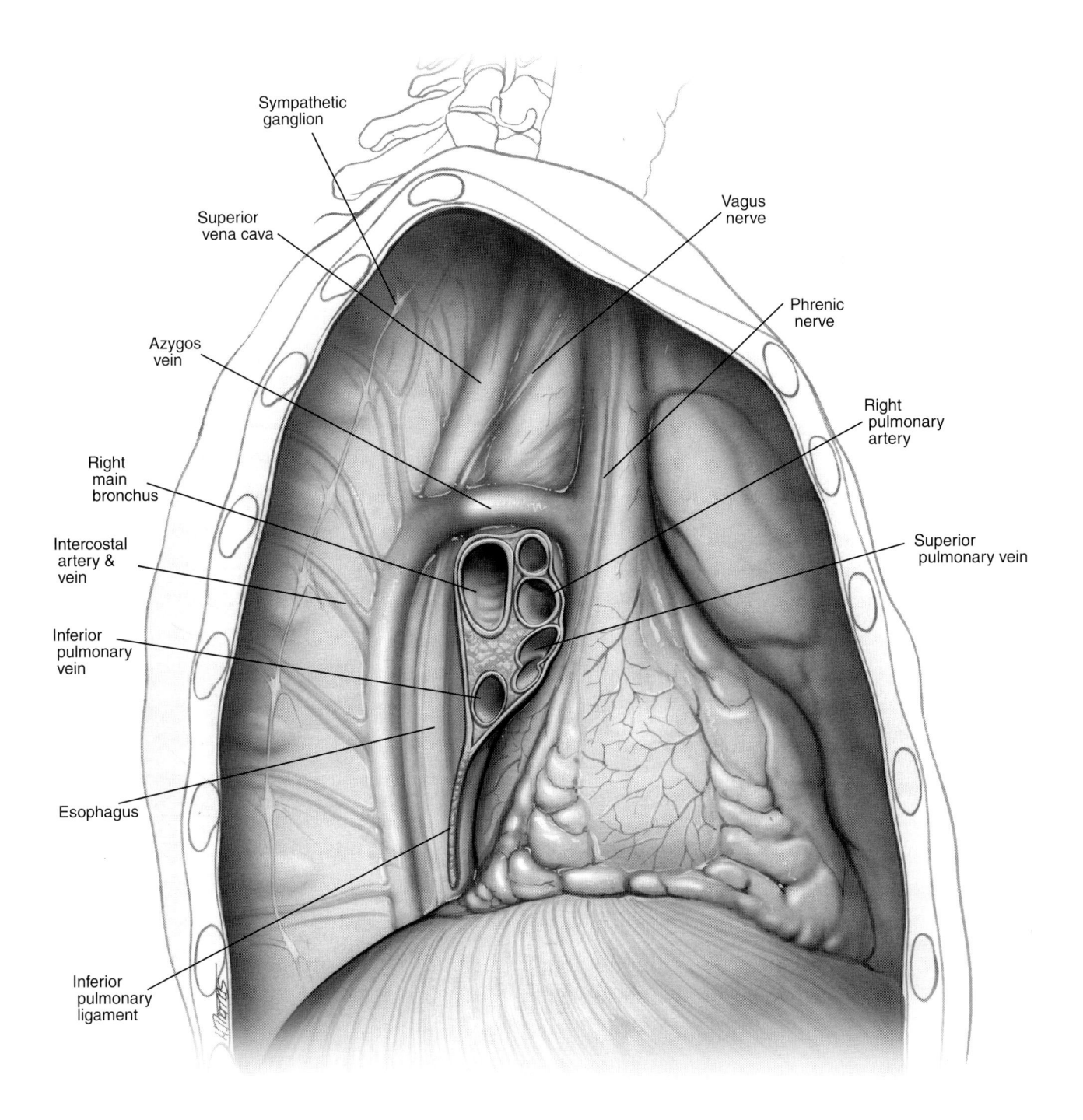

Figure 8–1 • *See legend on opposite page*

Figure 8–1 • The right lung has been removed to show the important anatomic landmarks. It can be seen that the intercostal veins overlying the vertebral bodies join the azygos vein. Just above the right hilum the azygos vein turns anteriorly and drains into the superior vena cava. The phrenic nerve runs along the side of the superior vena cava. More posteriorly, the vagus nerve can be seen entering the chest in the midmediastinum. The recurrent nerve branch is given off high in the chest, and it passes posteriorly and medially under the subclavian artery. The vagus nerve then continues downward, joins the esophagus, and runs along the lateral side of the esophagus to the abdomen.

The hilum of the lung is invested with mediastinal pleura, which with its two leaves extends down toward the diaphragm and forms the inferior pulmonary ligament. In the posterosuperior portion of this hilum is seen the right mainstem bronchus, and immediately caudad to that is the inferior pulmonary vein. In the anterior portion of the hilum and slightly cephalad to the mainstem bronchus can be seen two branches of the pulmonary artery, which in turn has come out of the mediastinum posterior to the superior vena cava. In approximately the same plane as the main pulmonary artery and immediately caudal to it is the superior pulmonary vein, shown here with two branches. This vein lies cephalad and anterior to the inferior pulmonary vein.

Surgical Anatomy of the Right Chest • 51

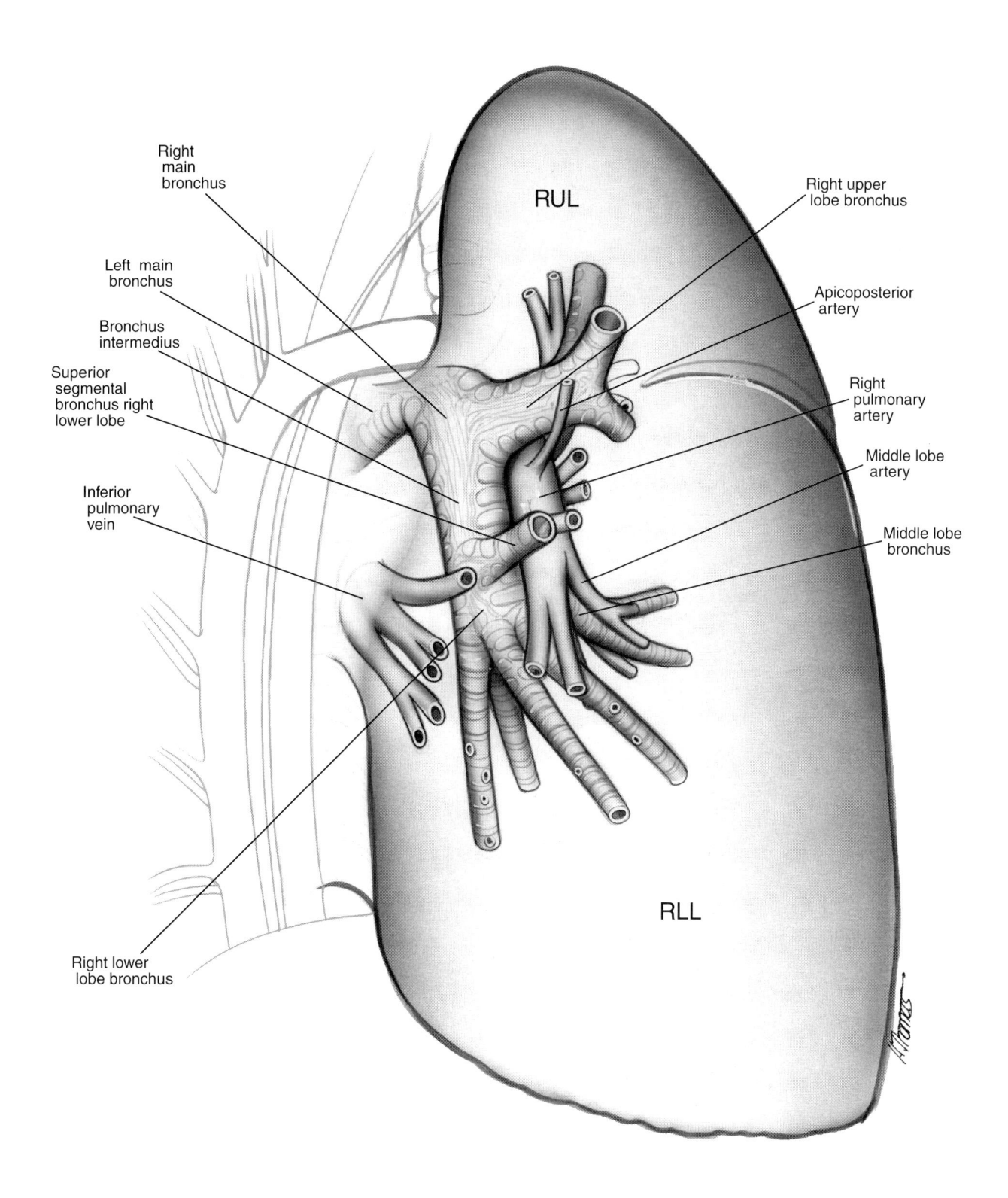

Figure 8–2 • This posterior view shows relatively clearly how one can approach the right upper lobe bronchus since the arterial and venous supplies to the right upper lobe are primarily anterior to the bronchus. It can also be seen that the main pulmonary artery runs lateral and anterior to the bronchus down the lung. The inferior pulmonary vein is primarily caudad to the bronchus intermedius. These veins drain from the intersegmental planes and tend to be caudal to the bronchi in this location.

52 • Part II CHEST

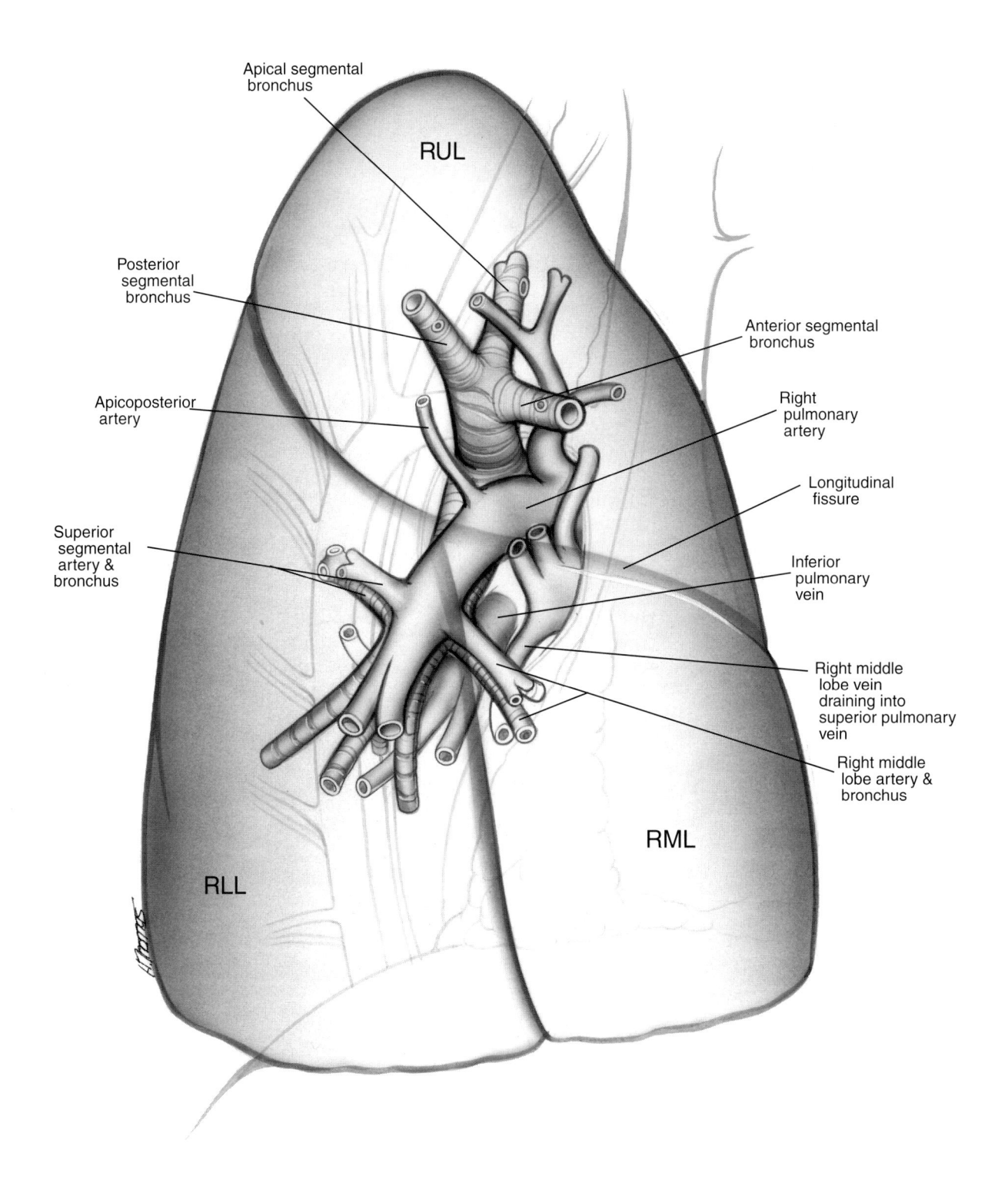

Figure 8–3 • *See legend on opposite page*

Figure 8–3 • It is important for the surgeon to develop a mind's-eye picture of the three-dimensional spatial relationship of the bronchi, arteries, and veins supplying the lung, the lung lobes, and the lung segments.

The bronchi and their branches are the key to the location of the various subdivisions of the lung. These subdivisions, or segments, have certain anatomic variations, but the standard location is as follows: after the right upper lobe bronchus has taken origin shortly below the tracheal carina, the right upper lobe bronchus trifurcates into an anterior branch, posterior branch, and apical branch. The bronchus intermedius then continues caudad and bifurcates into right middle lobe and right lower lobe bronchi. An important point is that the superior segmental bronchus of the right lower lobe comes off posteriorly almost even with or frequently only slightly more caudad than the right middle lobe bronchus. The right lower lobe bronchus continues downward and on the right side branches into four basal segments.

The pulmonary artery is anterior, for the most part, and slightly cephalad to these bronchi, so that if the various bronchial segments are identified, one or more arterial branches accompany the segment. The veins, however, form and collect in the intersegmental planes and pass from the intersegmental planes to the collecting veins, which lead to the superior and inferior pulmonary veins. The superior pulmonary vein drains primarily the right upper lobe but usually also has a branch draining the right middle lobe. Similarly, the inferior pulmonary vein drains primarily the lower lobe, but it often has a venous tributary from the middle lobe.

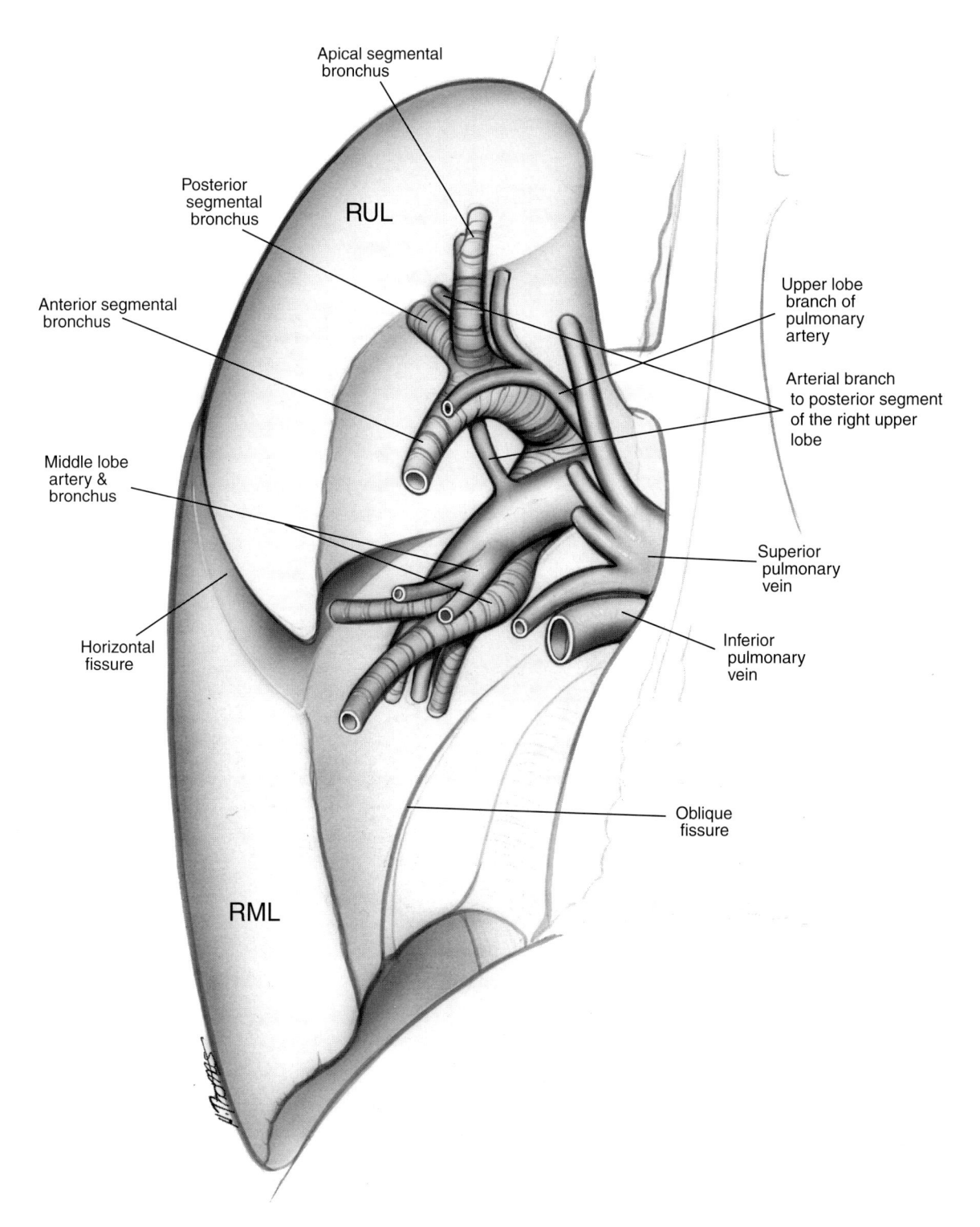

Figure 8–4 • From an anterior oblique view, we can see the bronchus to the right upper lobe with its trifurcation and its arterial blood supply. The posterior arterial branch to the posterior segment of the right upper lobe can be seen as it comes from the pulmonary artery caudad to the right upper lobe bronchus take-off near the longitudinal fissure. This branch moves posteriorly and cephalad to supply the posterior segment. This artery branch has to be looked for. It is sometimes hard to dissect and can be a source of trouble to the surgeon. The superior pulmonary vein is well seen anteriorly. The spatial configuration of the bronchi and arteries is shown, whereas the inferior pulmonary vein is seen as a main channel only.

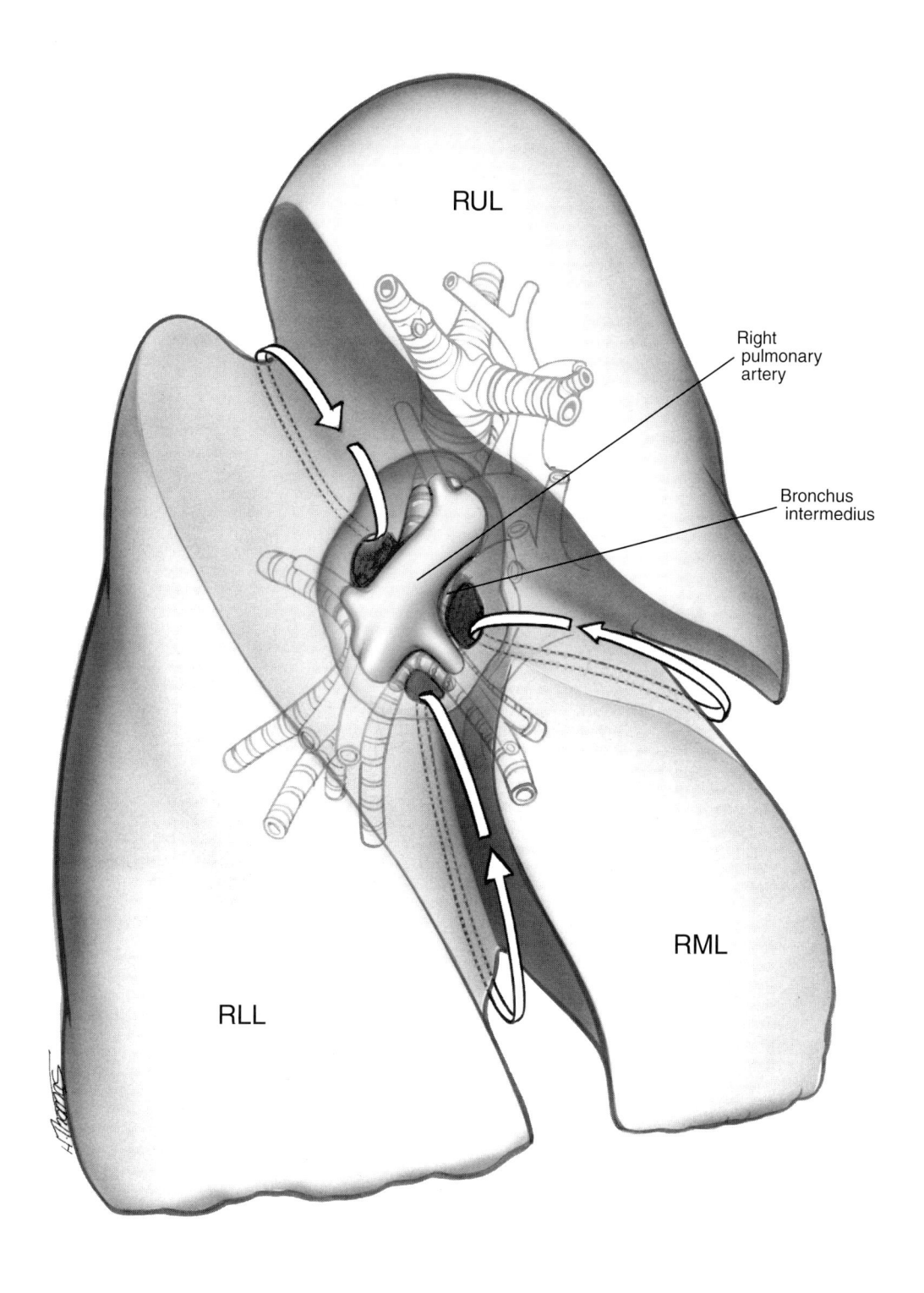

Figure 8–5 • This figure illustrates the incomplete fissures of the right lung, with the right pulmonary artery and bronchus intermedius exposed.

Chapter 9
Thoracic Incision

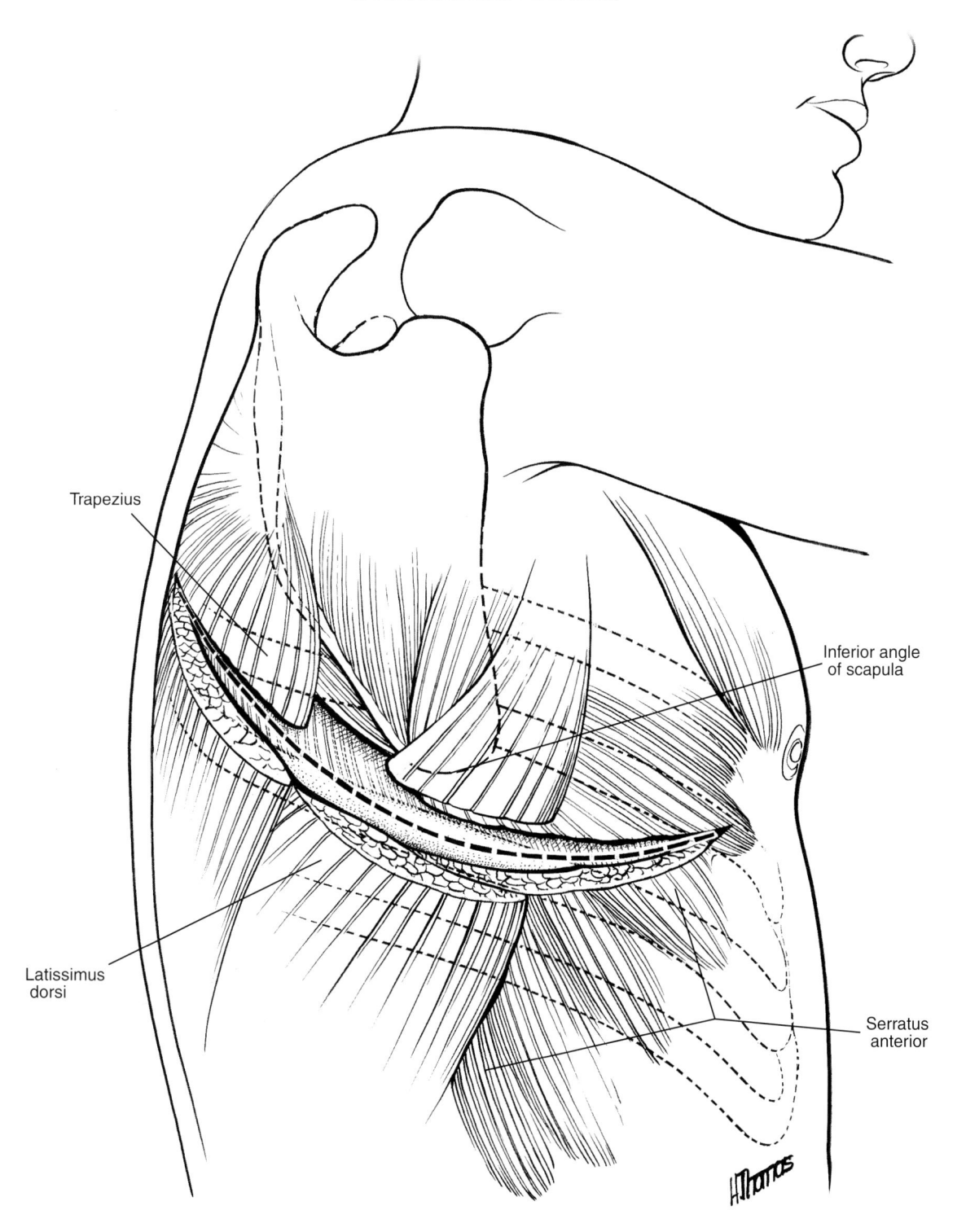

Figure 9–1 • The patient is in the left lateral position, with the right chest diagrammed. The incision is made just beneath the angle of the scapula. The anterior portion of the incision is curved toward the nipple in a man and toward the inframammary crease in a woman. The muscles to be cut are the latissimus dorsi and serratus anteriorly and the trapezius and rhomboids posteriorly.

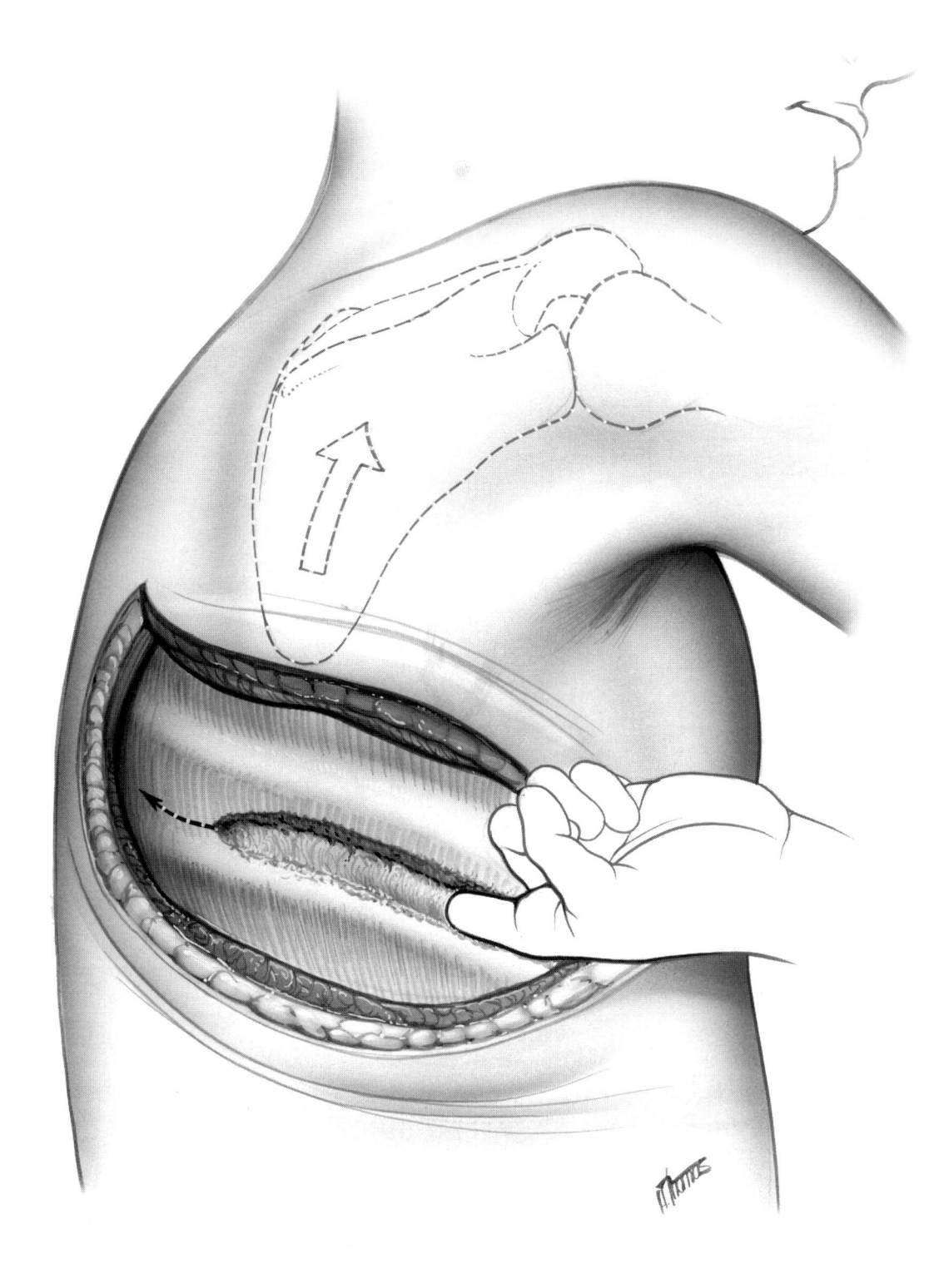

Figure 9–2 • The scapula is retracted cephalad, and the fifth or sixth interspace is determined as the point of entry. The intercostal muscles are divided, and the chest cavity is entered. The index finger is inserted to ascertain the presence or absence of adhesions.

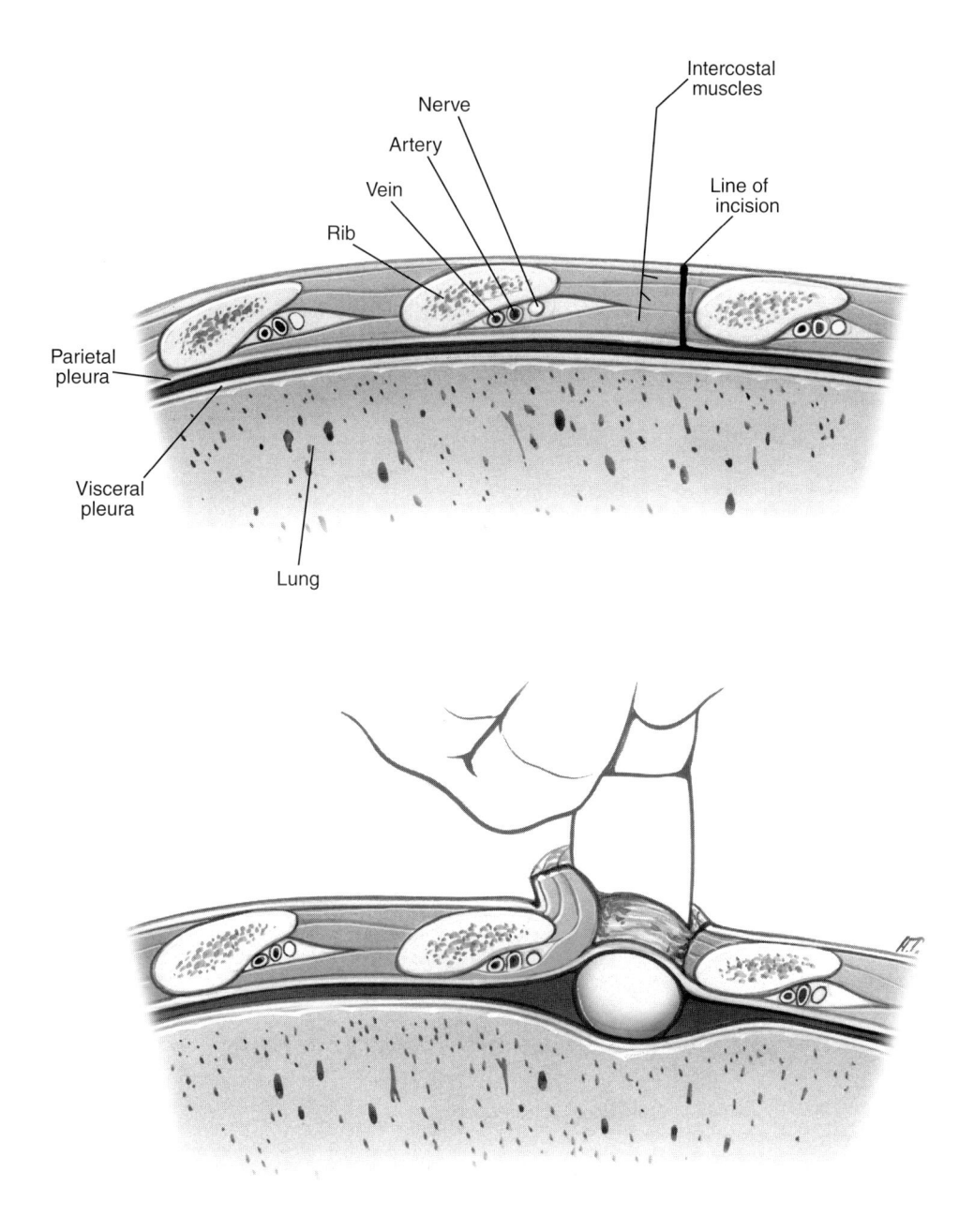

Figure 9–3 • This cross-sectional view demonstrates the relationship of the intercostal artery, vein, and nerve in relation to the rib and the line of division of the intercostal muscles.

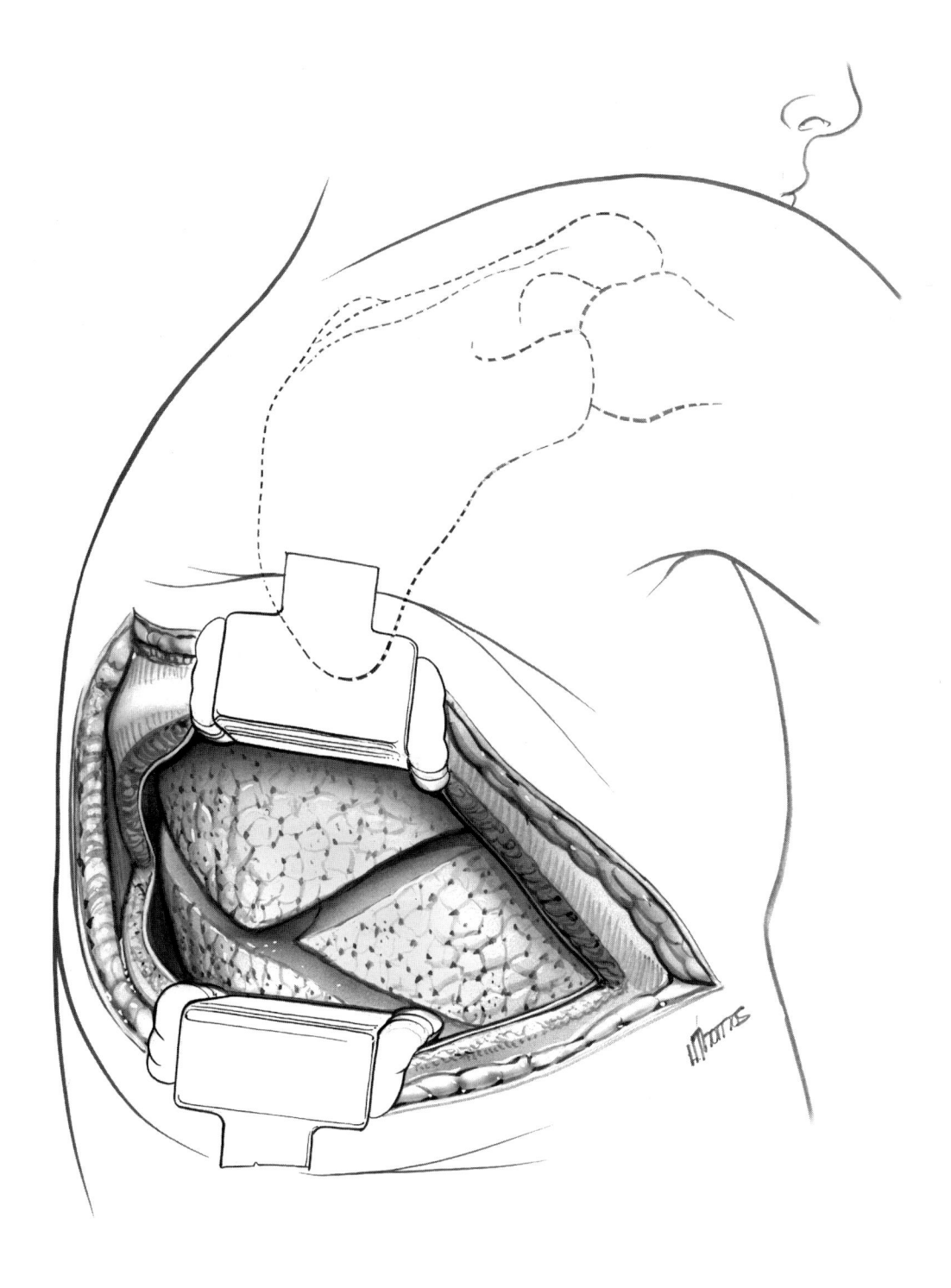

Figure 9–4 • The rib spreader is placed into the chest cavity and opened slowly to avoid fractures. Relaxation can be achieved by resecting the posterior portion of one rib.

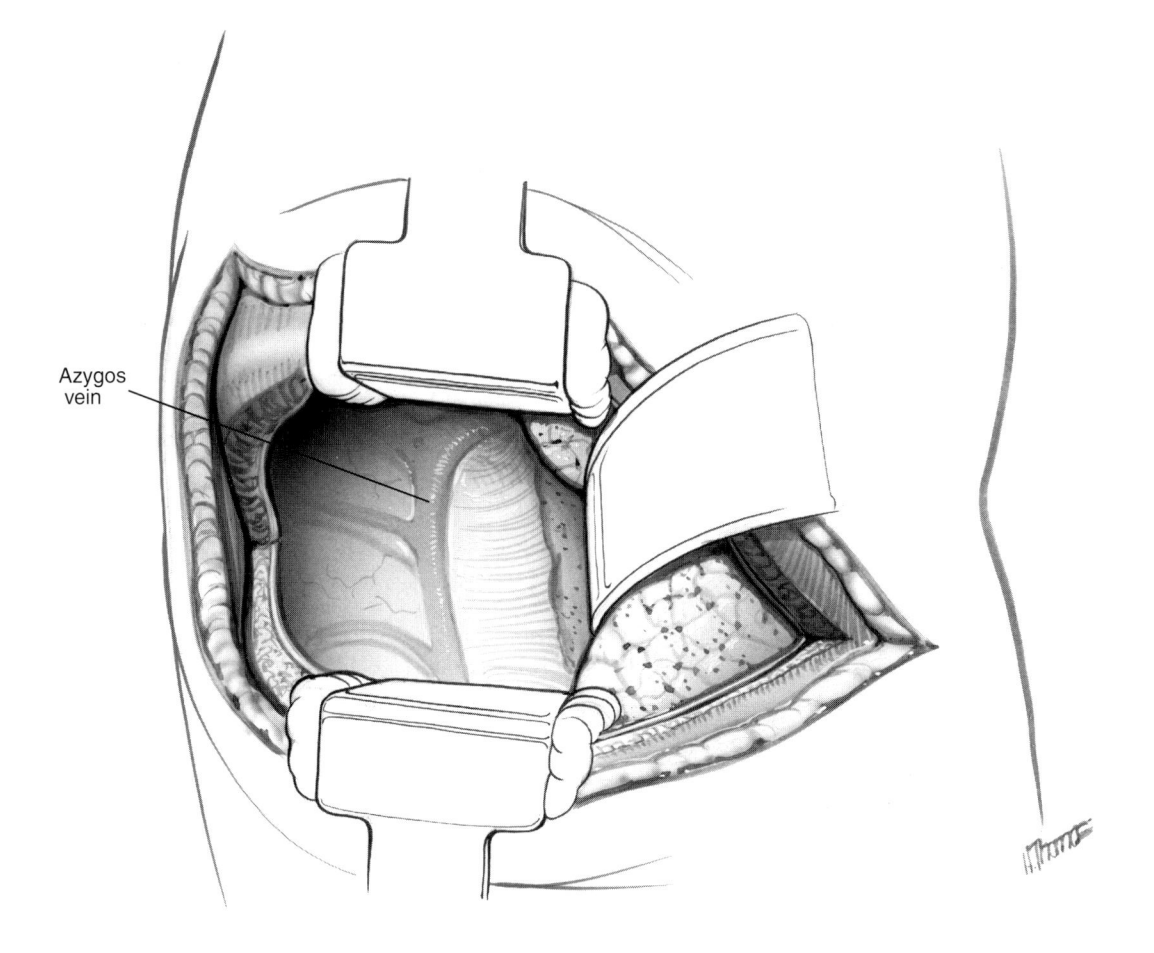

Figure 9–5 • With the lung retracted, the azygos vein is clearly demonstrated.

62 • Part II CHEST

Chapter 10
Right Upper Lobectomy

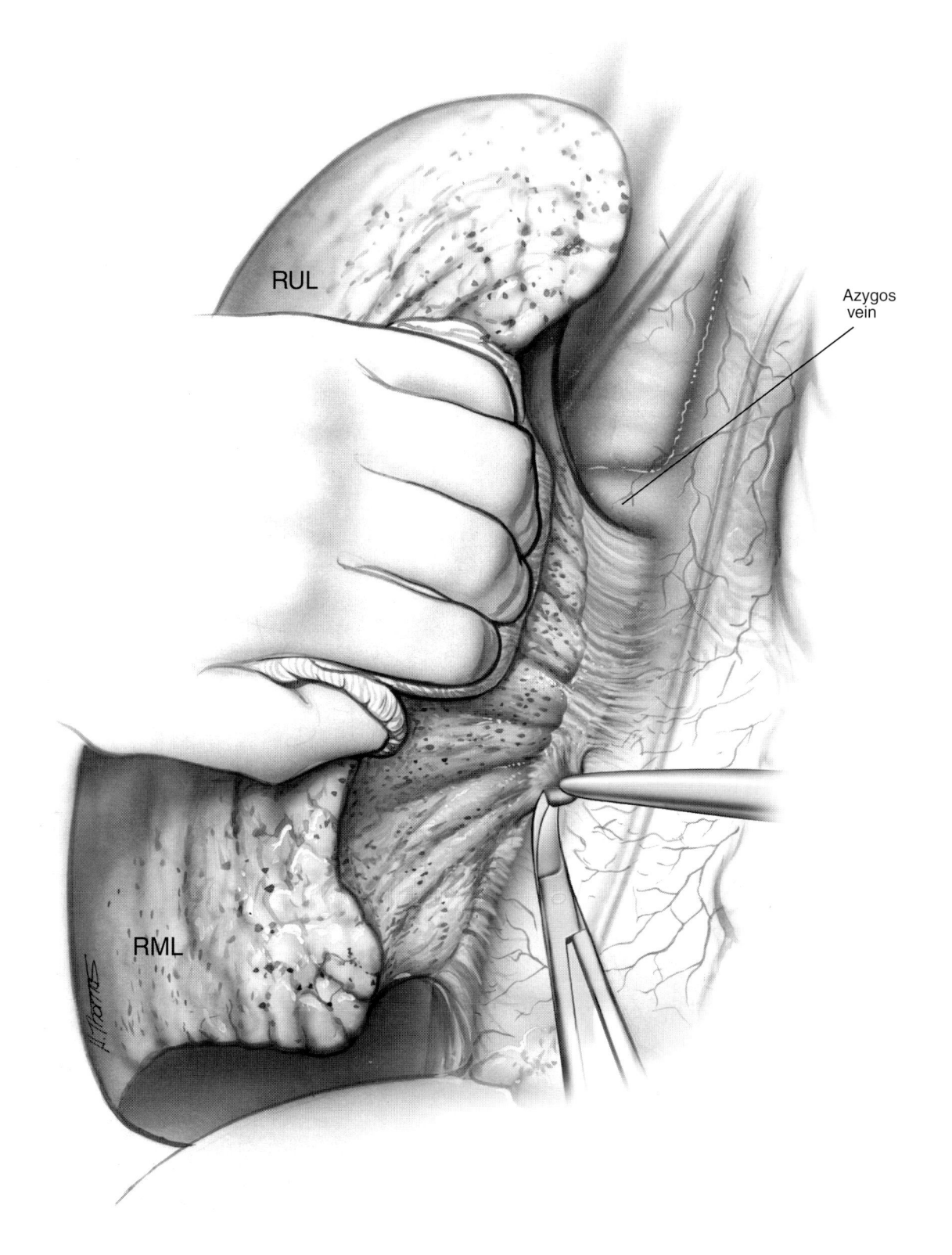

Figure 10–1 • The anterior mediastinal pleura is being incised to bring into view the hilar structures.

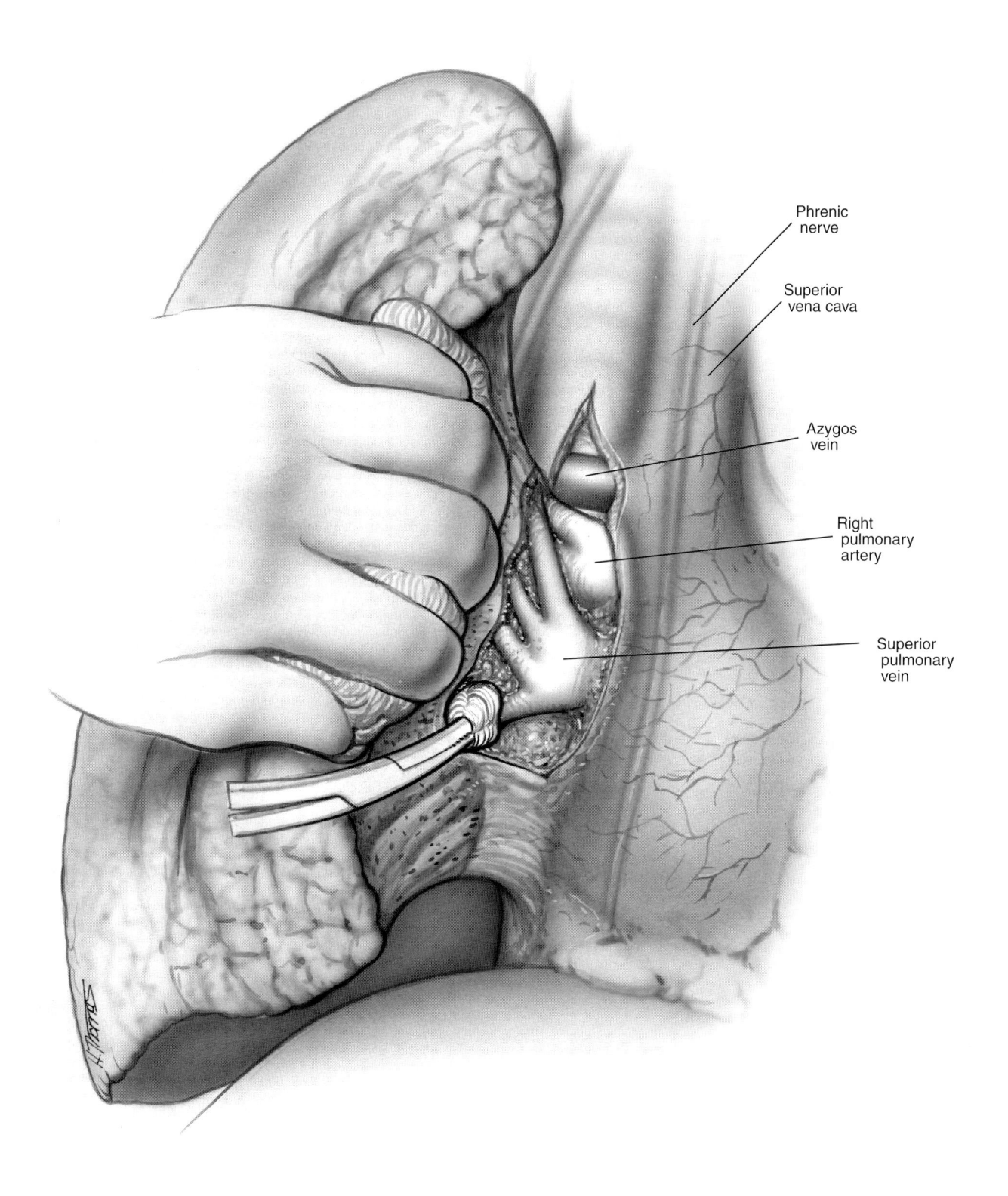

Figure 10–2 • From the cephalic aspect of the right hilum, a dissecting sponge is used to free the first branch of the pulmonary artery. If there is any question, the dissection should focus on the distal portion so that should tears occur they may be more safely controlled. Caudally, the dissection is completed exposing the branches of the superior pulmonary vein.

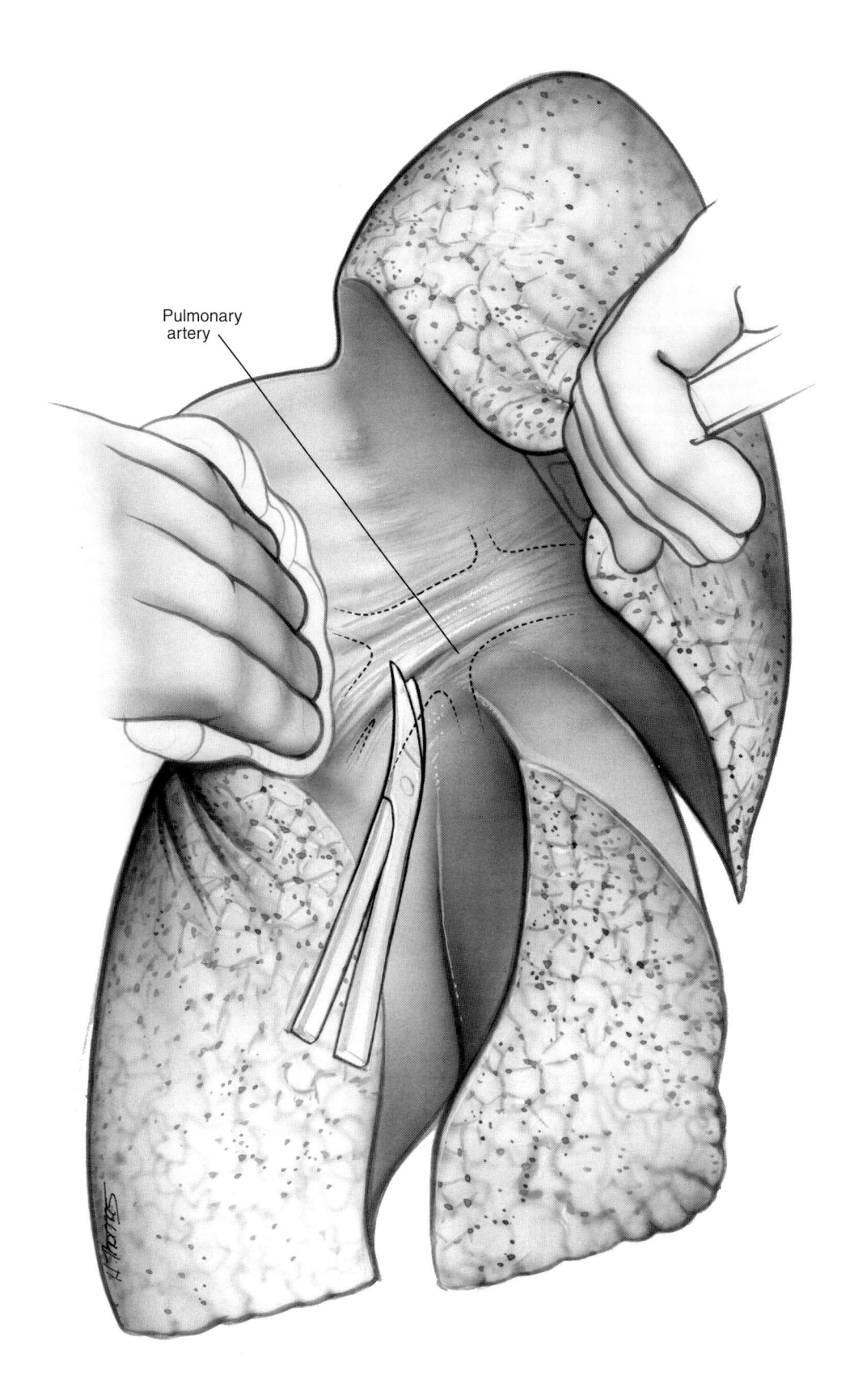

Figure 10-3 • Generally, by stretching at the confluence of the three lobes it is possible to dissect down to the pulmonary artery in the fissure. Once the artery branches have been identified, the fissure can be completed with a stapler.

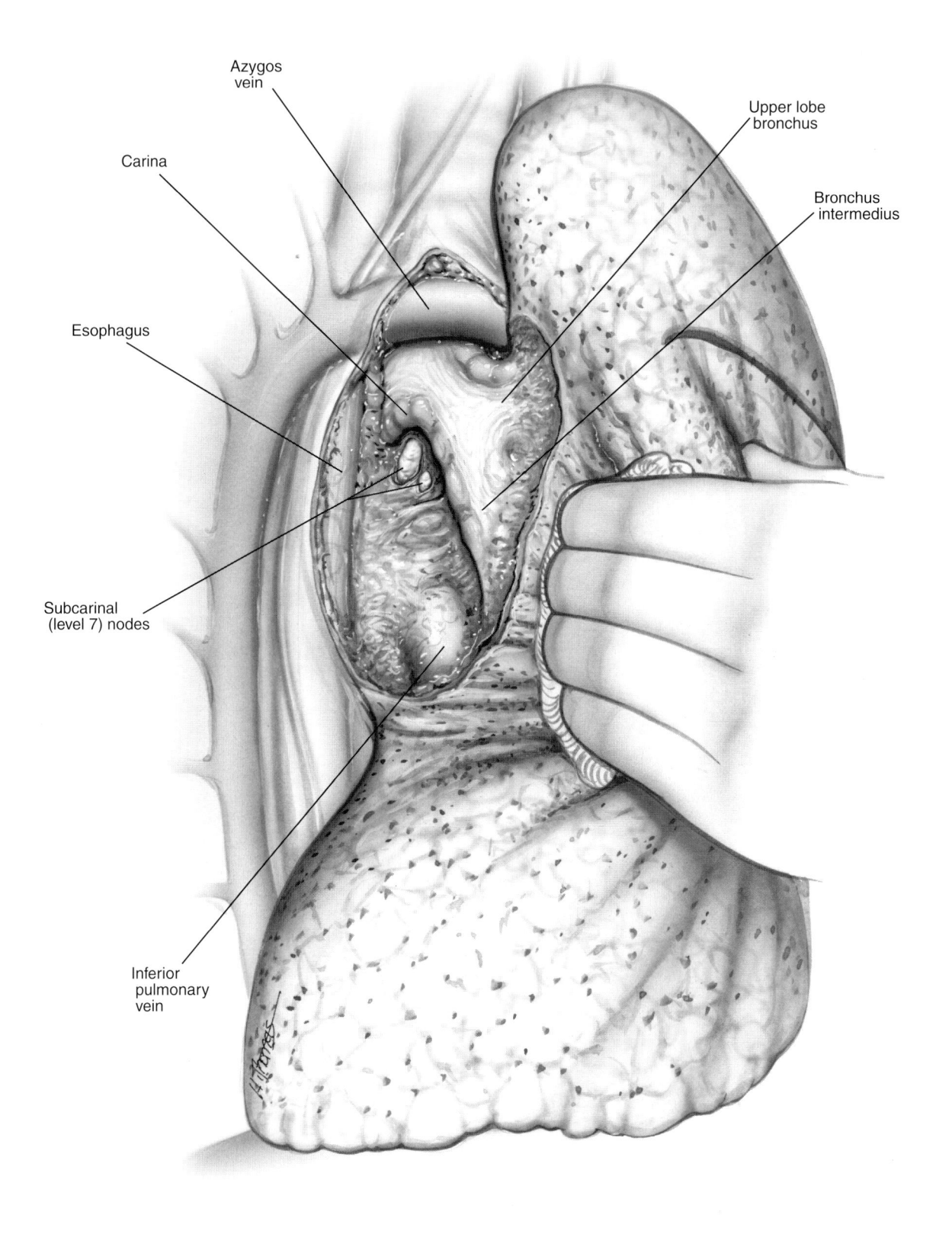

Figure 10–4 • The mediastinal pleura is incised posteriorly. With stretch on the lung parenchyma, the bifurcation of the right upper lobe bronchus with the bronchus intermedius is exposed.

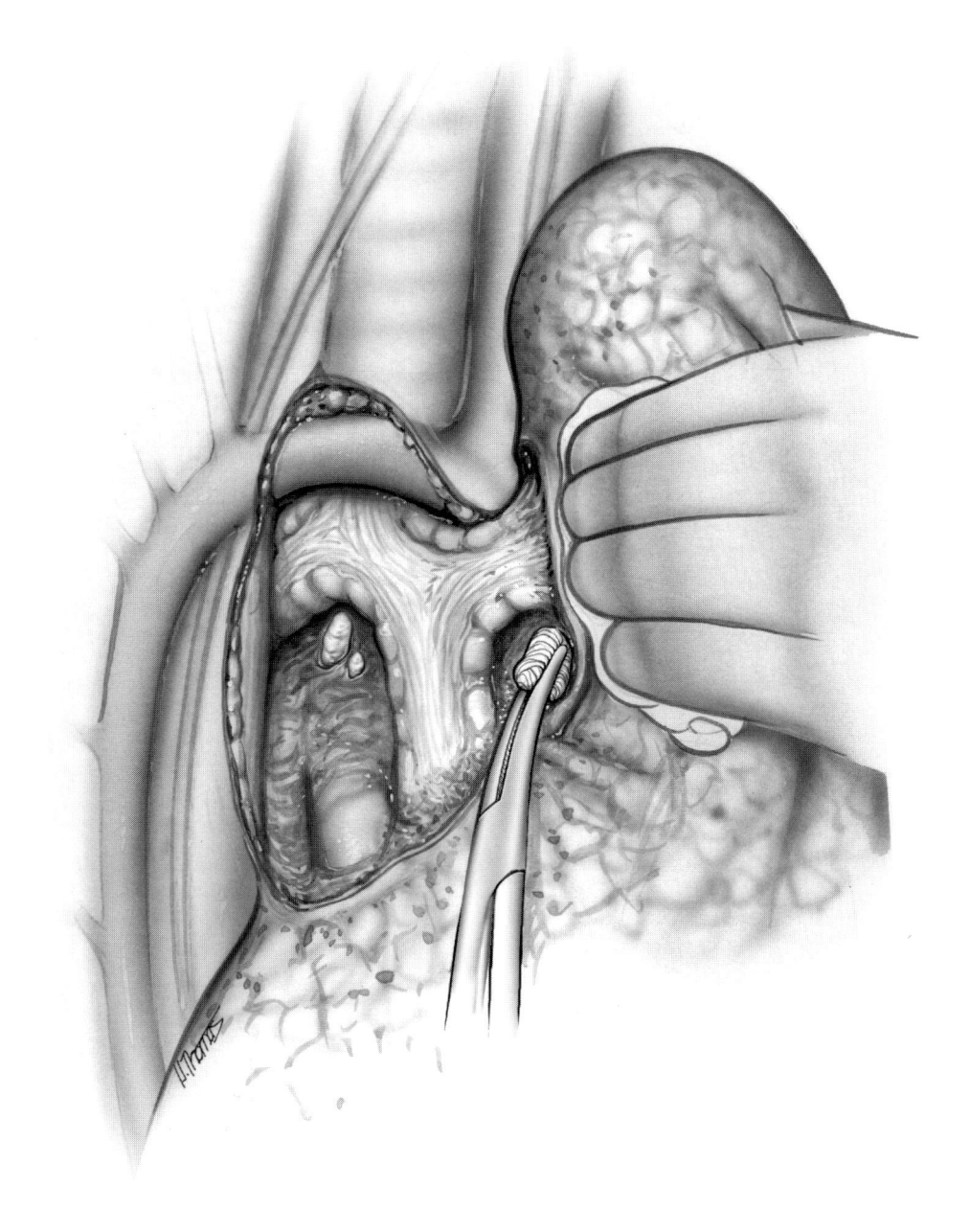

Figure 10-5 • The upper lobe bronchus can be further freed by use of the peanut dissector. Be aware that the main structure anterior to the bronchus at this point is the first branch of the pulmonary artery going to the apical segments of the right upper lobe. There also may be lymph nodes in this location.

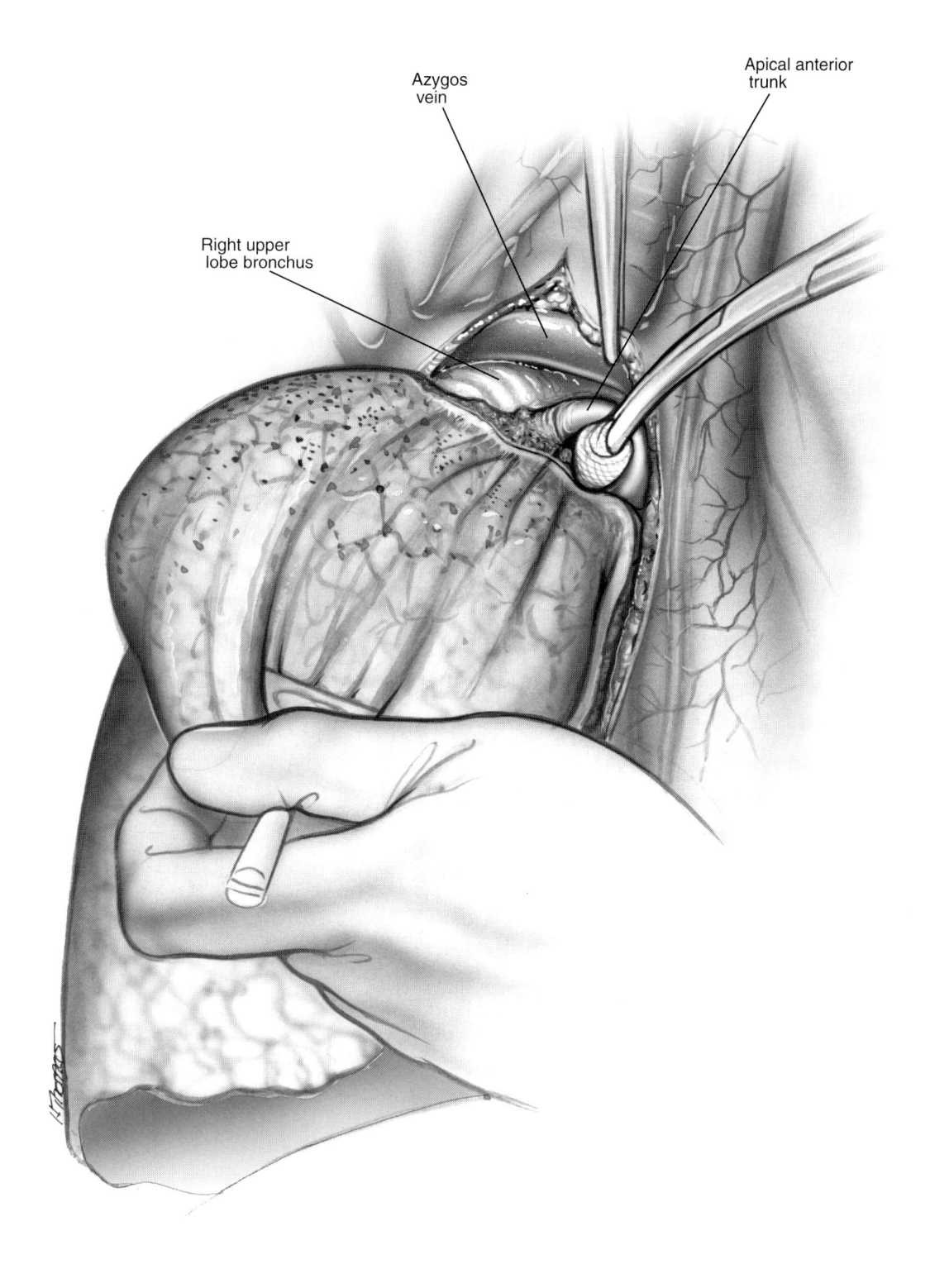

Figure 10–6 • With gentle retraction on the upper lobe caudally, dissection below the azygos vein allows exposure of the pulmonary artery.

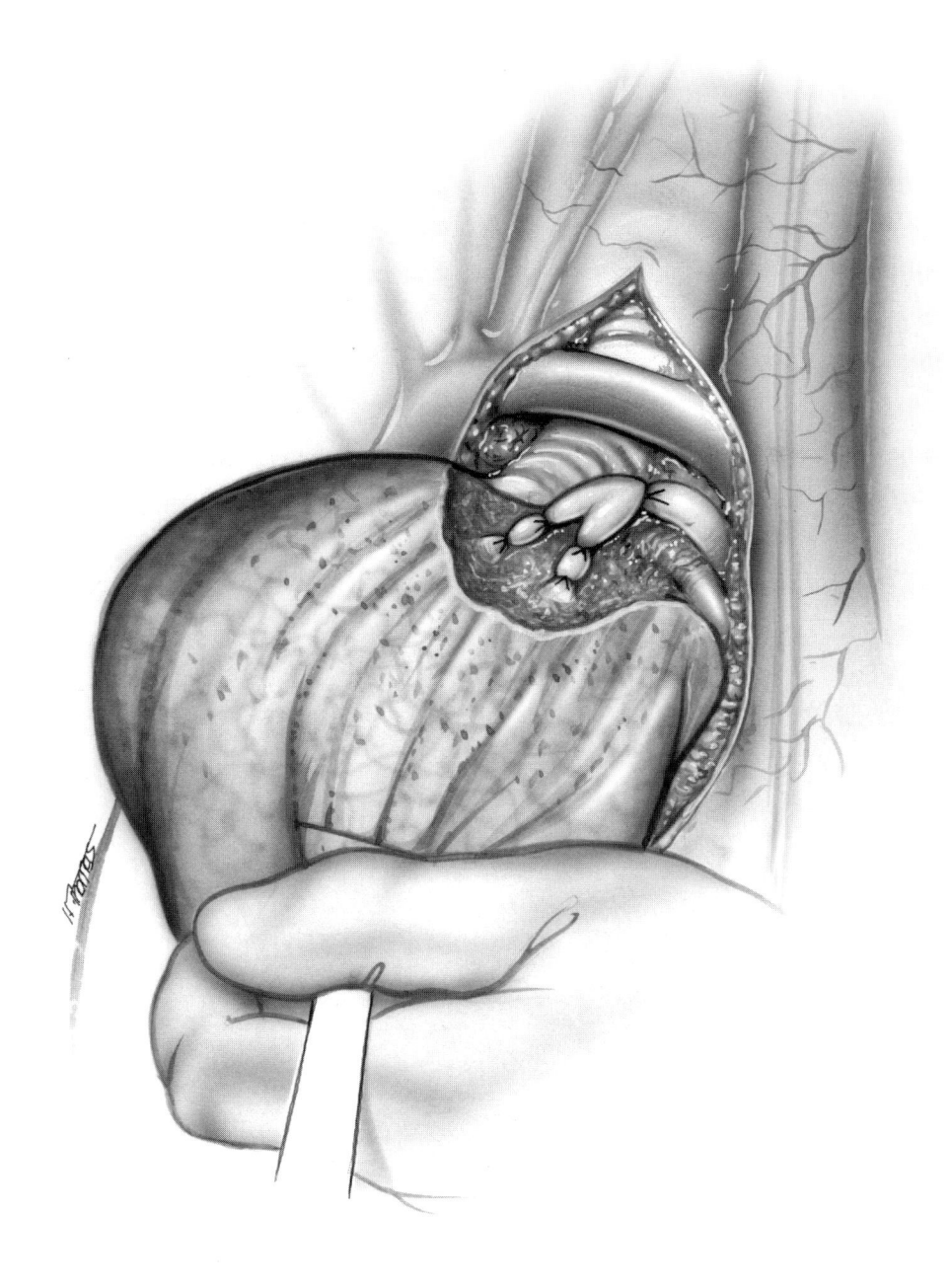

Figure 10–7 • In this view, the first branch of the main pulmonary artery has been proximally ligated with two sutures distal to the bifurcation. Distal sutures are placed as well. It is always good practice to ligate doubly the hilar vessels.

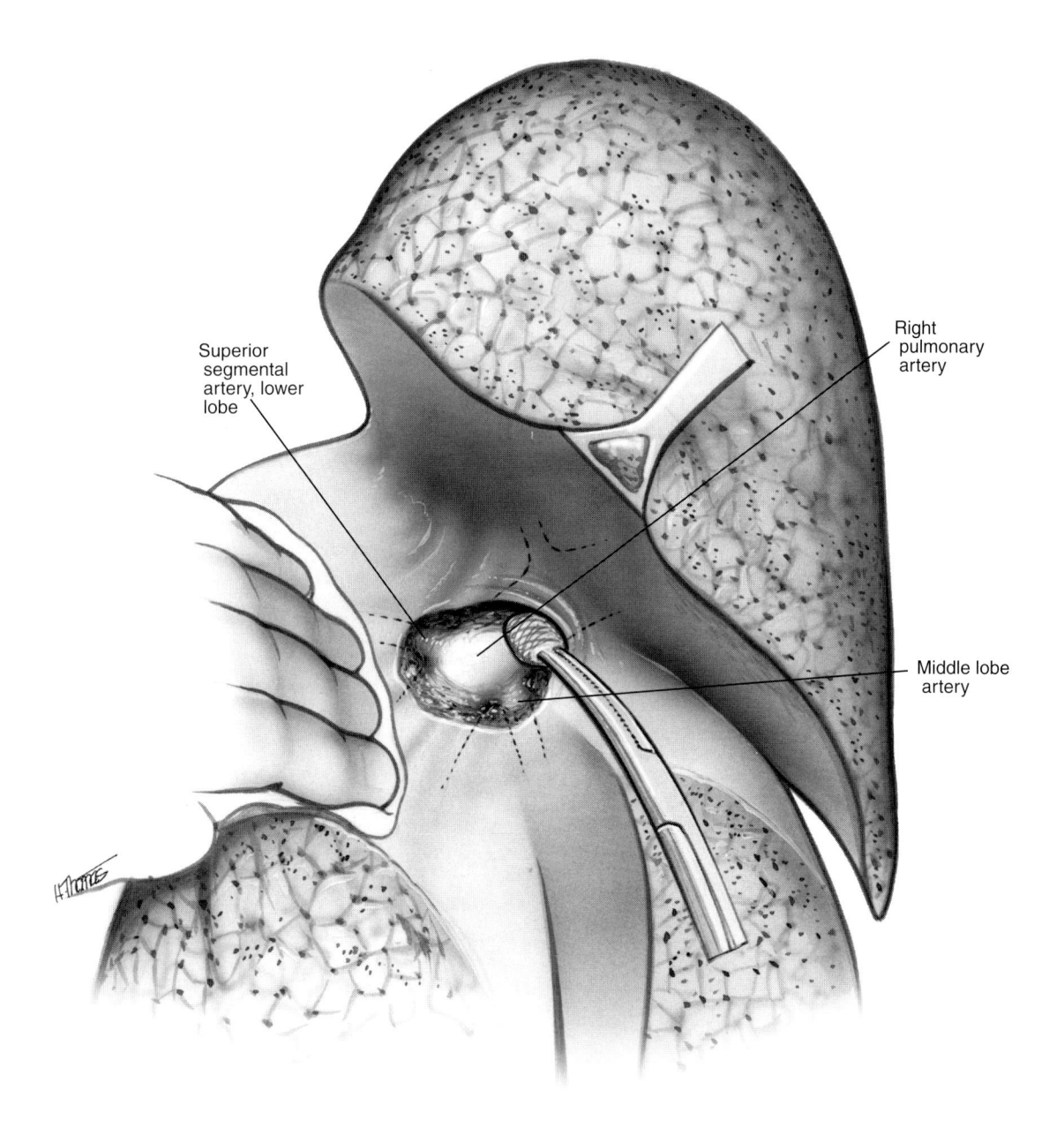

Figure 10-8 • After the visceral pleura in the longitudinal fissure are incised with traction on the lobes, it is generally possible to identify the pulmonary artery with all its segmental branches.

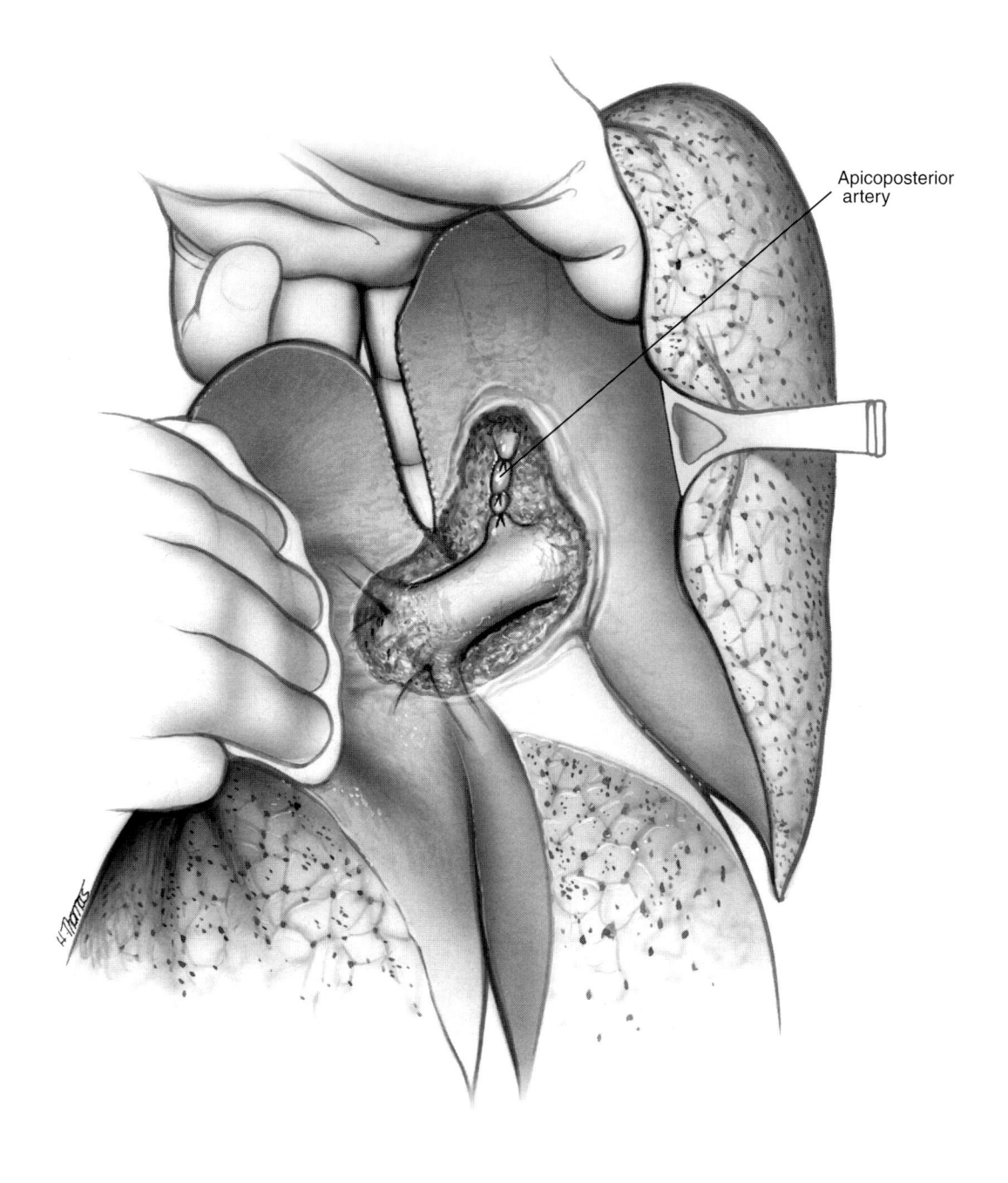

Figure 10-9 • After completing the fissure, usually with a stapling device, the posterior segmental branch of the upper lobe is doubly ligated and divided.

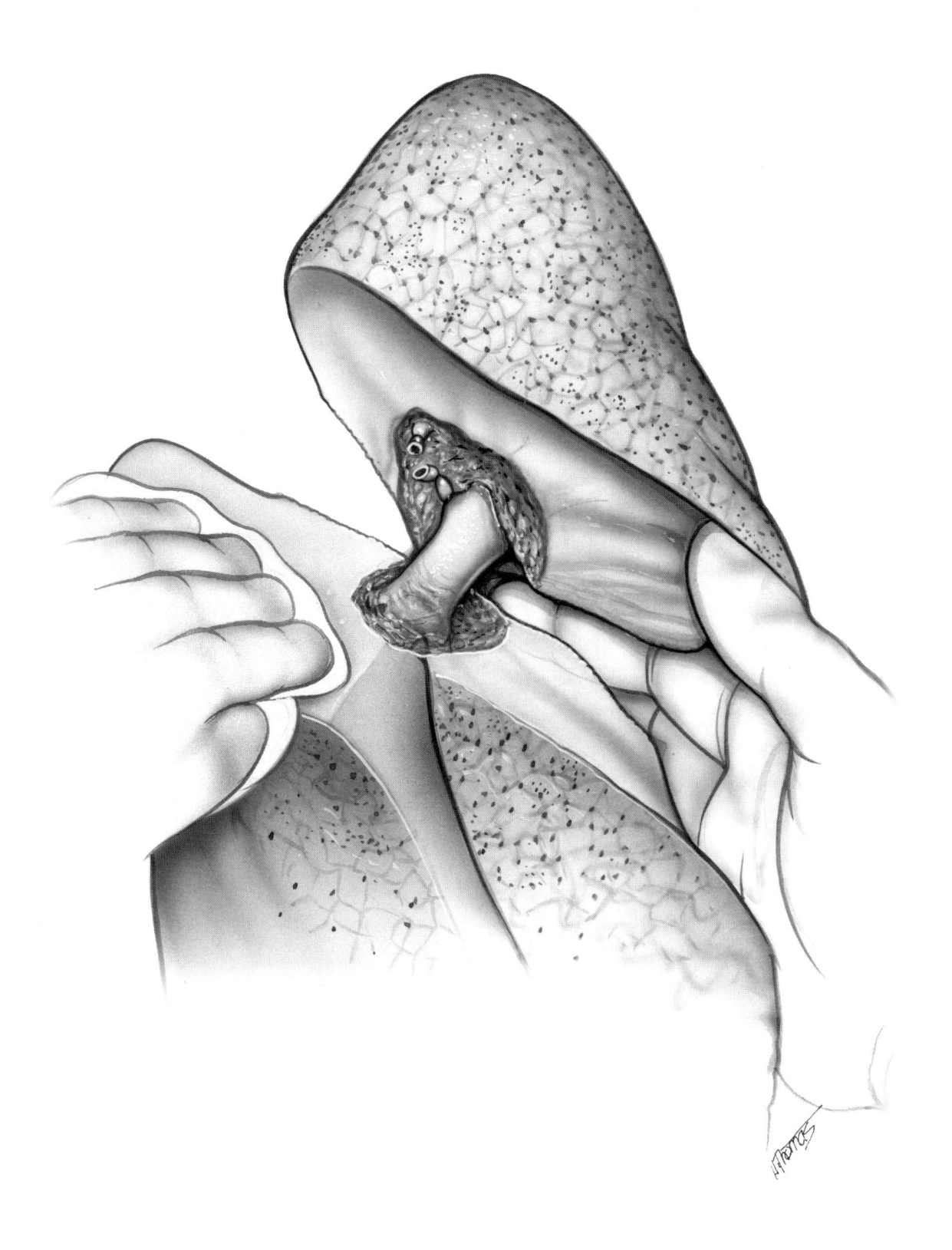

Figure 10–10 • After the arteries have been divided, other tissue around the hilum of the upper lobe may be dissected free and divided.

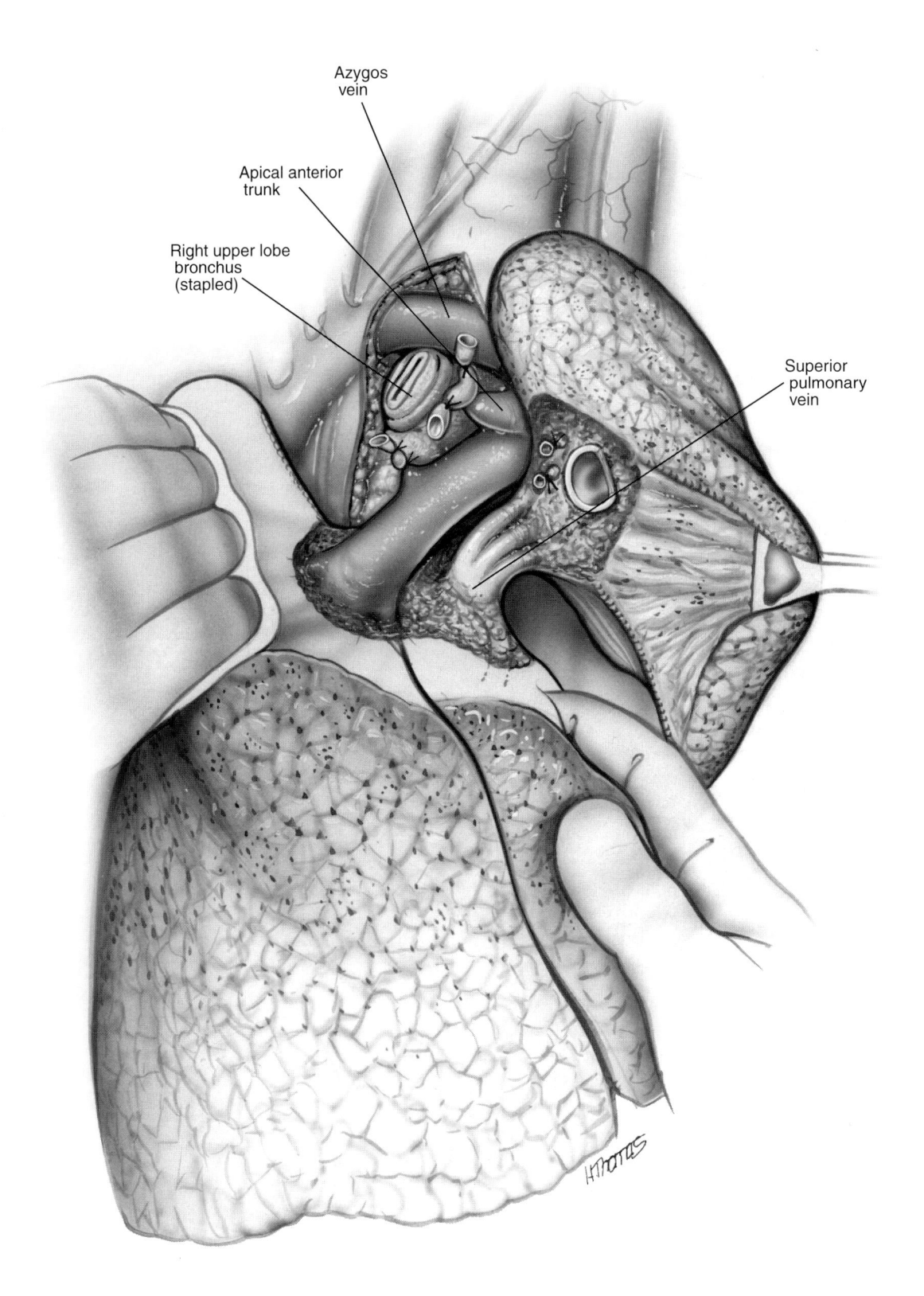

Figure 10–11 • After the arteries have been divided, the right upper lobe bronchus is stapled at its take-off. The stapler is applied and closed but not fired until it is ascertained that the anesthesiologist has aspirated and reinflated the right lung, demonstrating good inflation of the middle and lower lobes with no inflation of the upper lobe. The stapler is fired, and the lobe is shown attached to three branches of the superior pulmonary vein after the bronchus is divided.

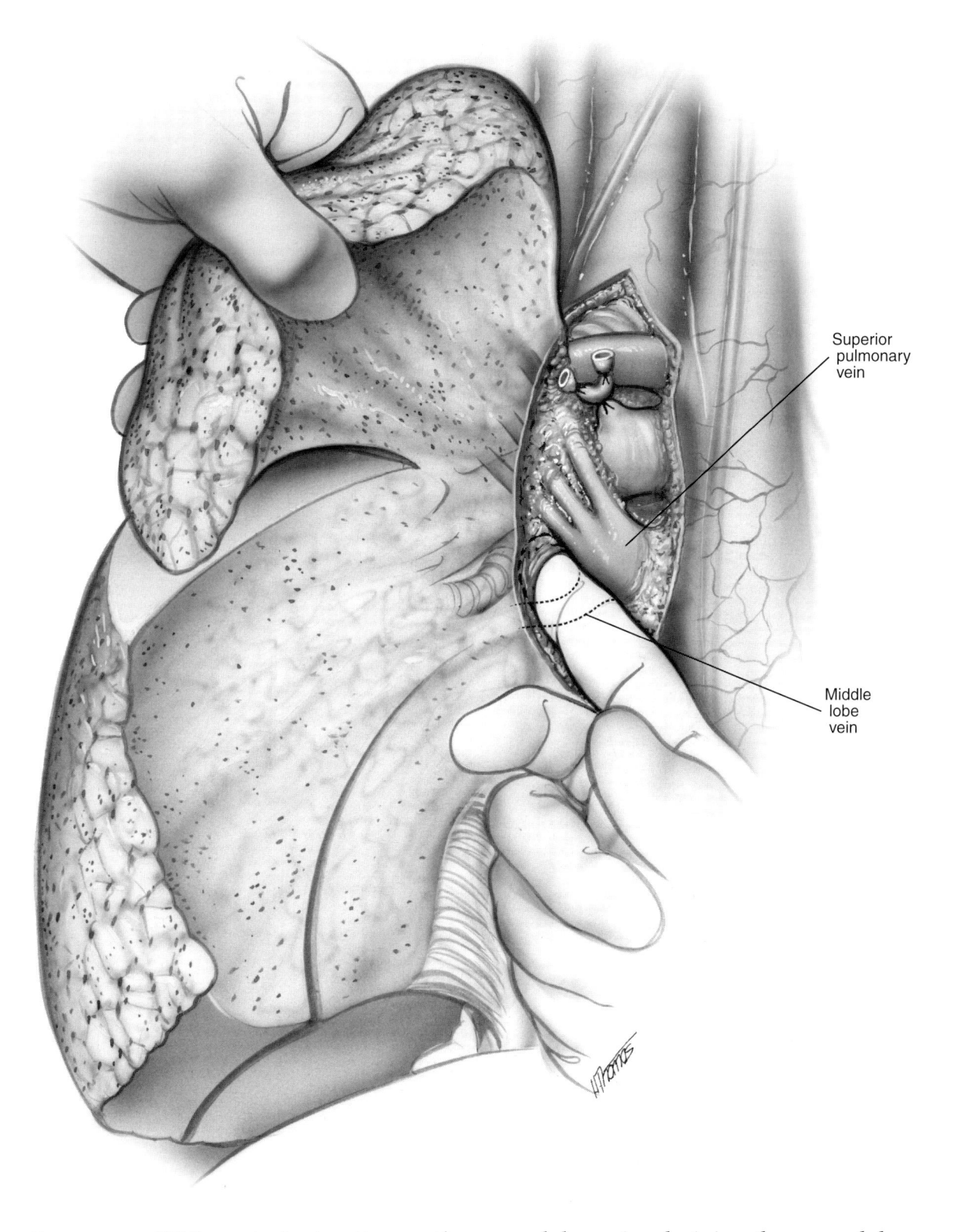

Figure 10–12 • With posterior traction on the upper lobe, veins draining the upper lobe are seen going into the superior pulmonary vein. Digital or pledget dissection helps free areolar tissue from the vessel. At this point, we must find the venous drainage from the middle lobe to the superior pulmonary vein before any ligation. Middle lobe drainage is not depicted but would be found inferior to the surgeon's index finger.

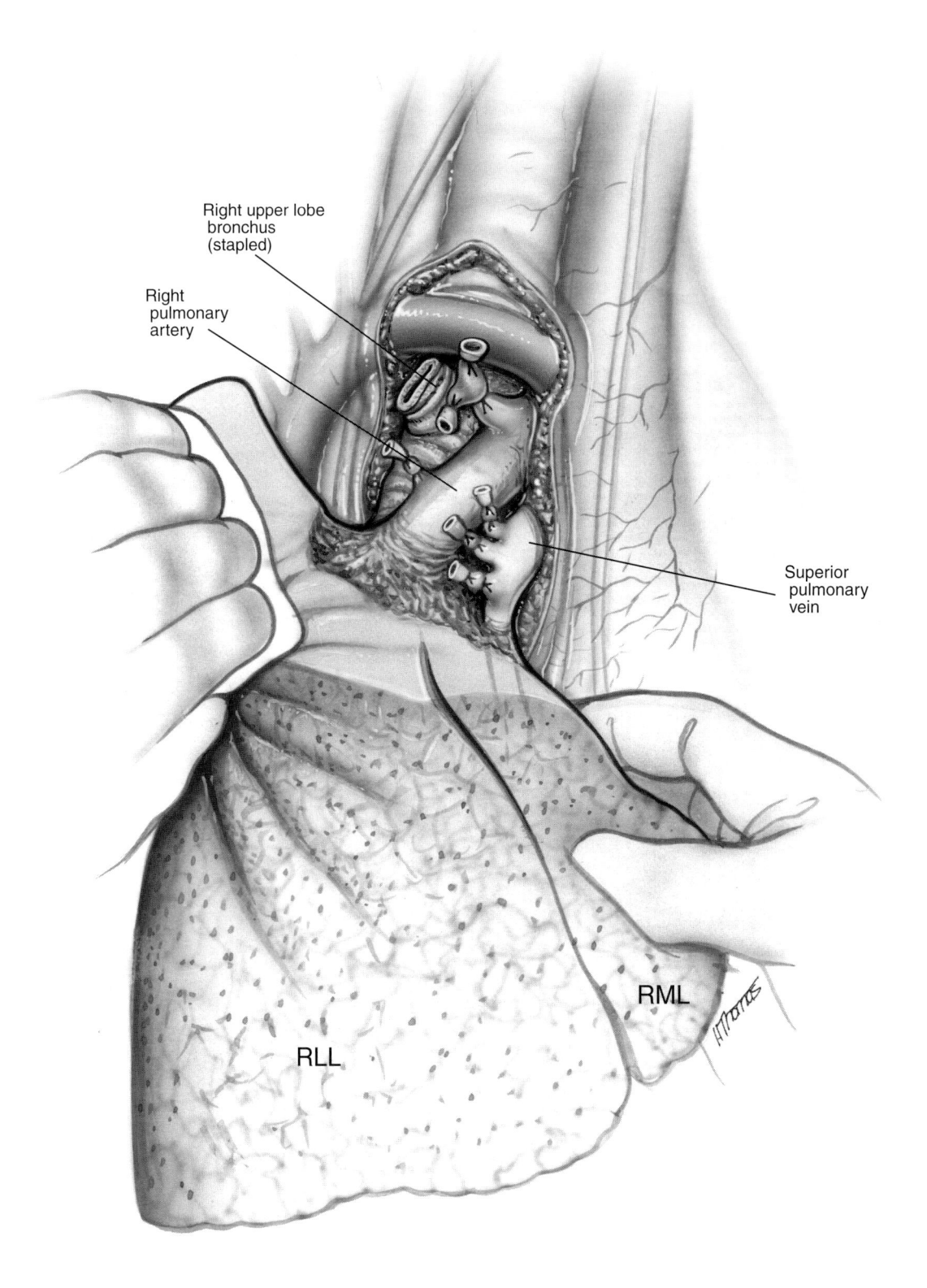

Figure 10–13 • The superior hilum is visualized with the three tributaries draining into the superior pulmonary vein ligated. We can see the middle lobe veins draining into the superior vein and the main pulmonary artery posterior to the vein. The bronchus intermedius is posterior to the pulmonary artery. The inferior pulmonary ligament must be divided to allow the remnant lobes to fill the chest cavity.

Chapter 11
Right Lower Lobectomy

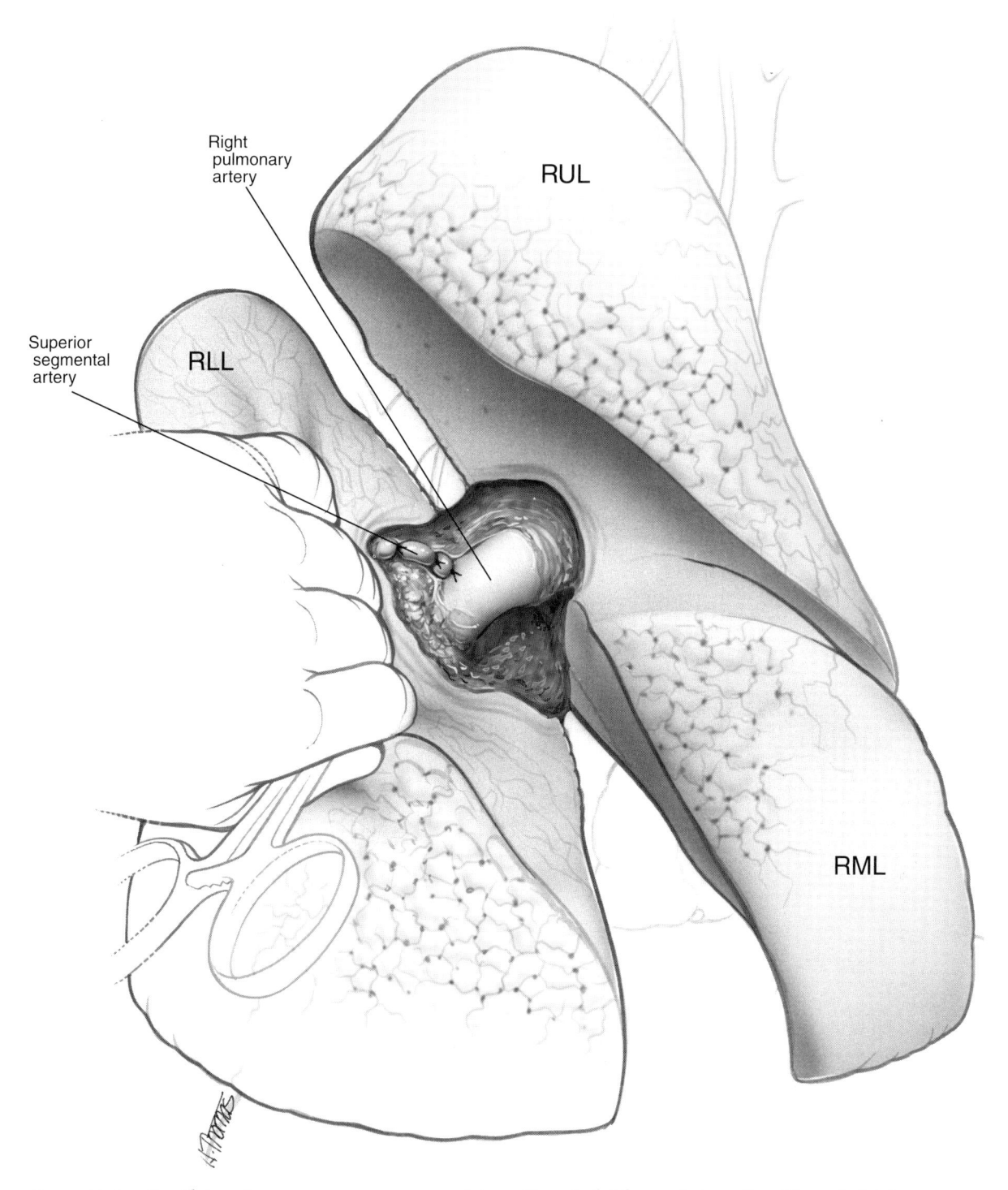

Figure 11–1 • In this view, we are approaching the right lung laterally. The right lower lobe is to the left; the right upper lobe and right middle lobe are to the right. The longitudinal fissure is almost completely open, and in the fissure we see the main pulmonary artery running from right to left. The sheath of the vessel has been opened. We have dissected out the lower lobe's superior segmental branch artery. There are a proximal ligature, a proximal suture ligature, and a distal tie.

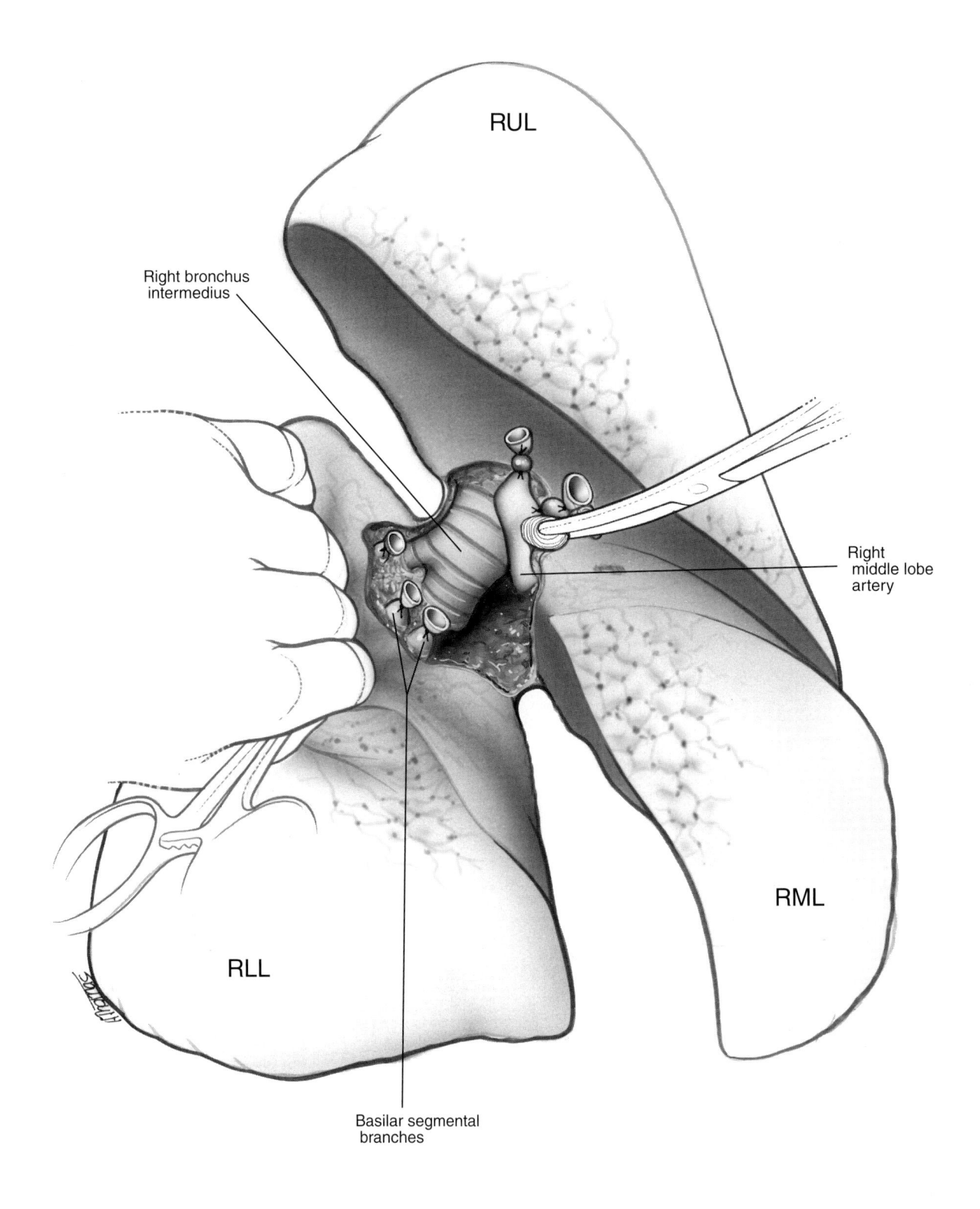

Figure 11–2 • The branches of the pulmonary artery are identified. They have been proximally suture ligated and divided. With very gentle displacement of this stump, one can see the right bronchus intermedius running to the right lower lobe. A branch to the superior segment is seen, and a major branch is running to the basal segment.

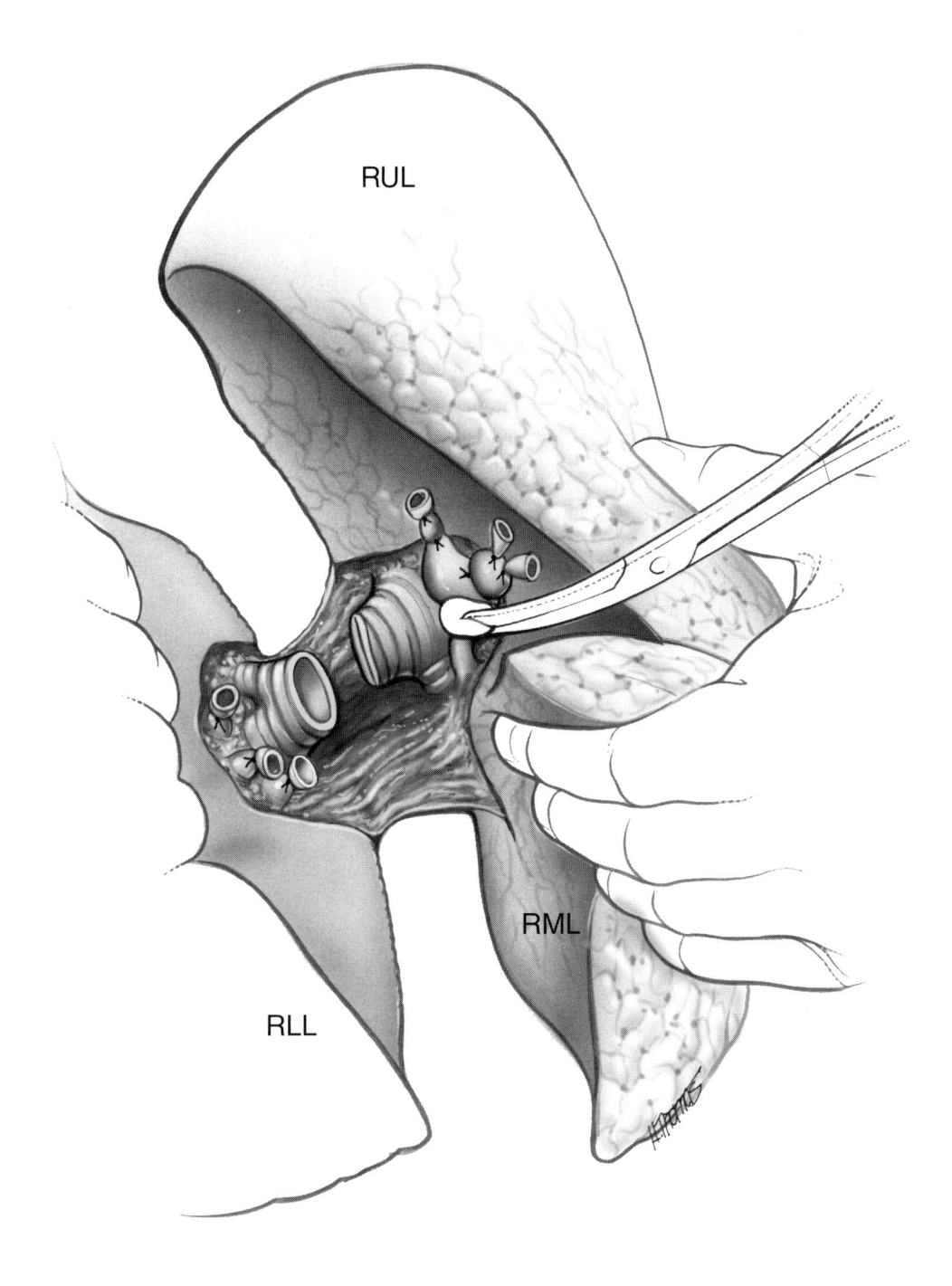

Figure 11–3 • The right lower lobe bronchus is stapled. If there is difficulty in doing this, the right lower lobe bronchus may have to be divided more distally at the superior and basal segmental levels if the tumor surgery permits.

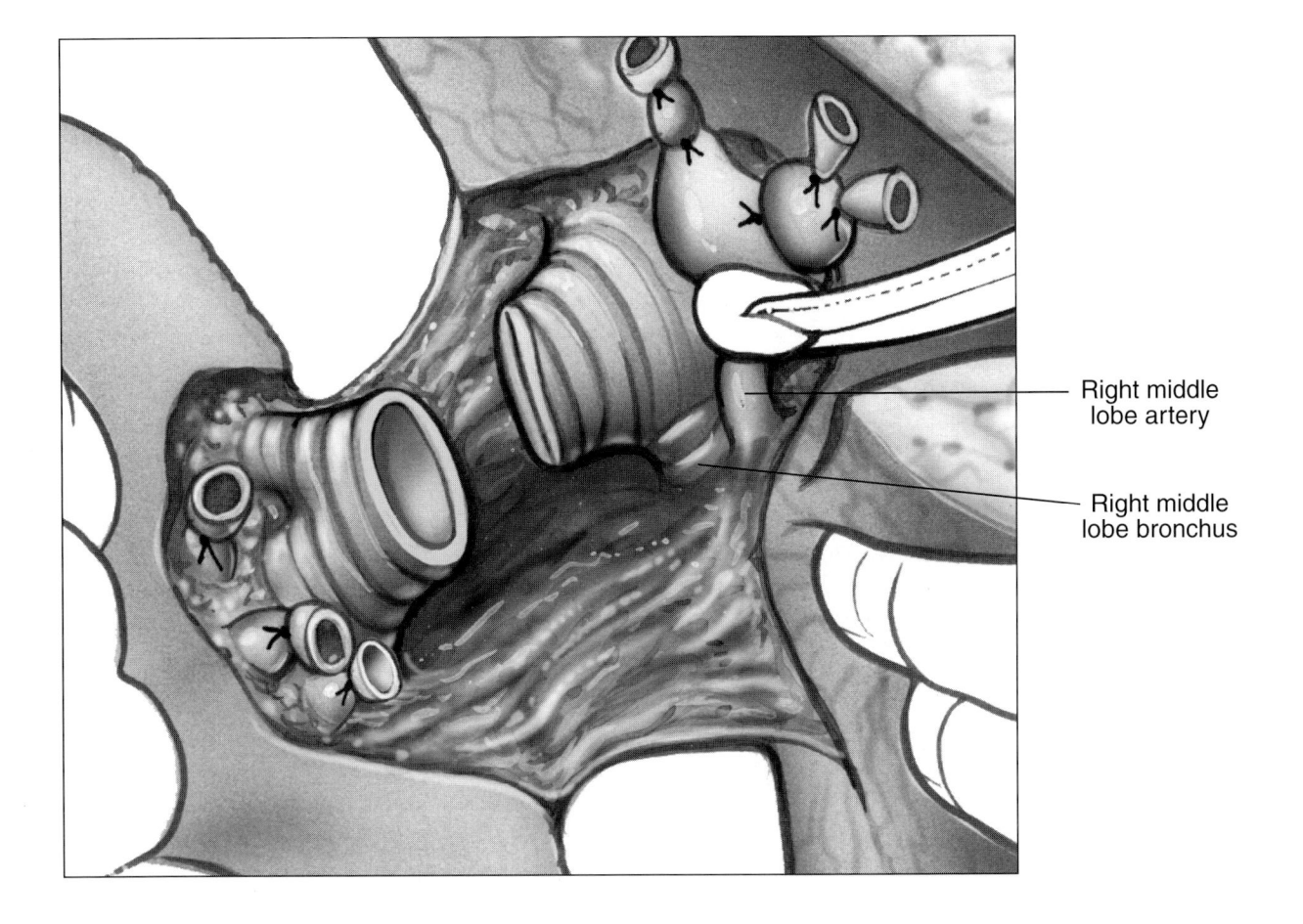

Figure 11–4 • To remove the middle lobe as well, the bronchus intermedius can be divided close to the upper lobe branches, and the stump length can be increased significantly by resecting the middle and lower lobes together. In this view one can see the right middle lobe artery branch. Although the dissecting sponge shows displacement of the vessel to make the anatomy clear, one must exercise caution in handling these pulmonary arteries, which are more the consistency of veins.

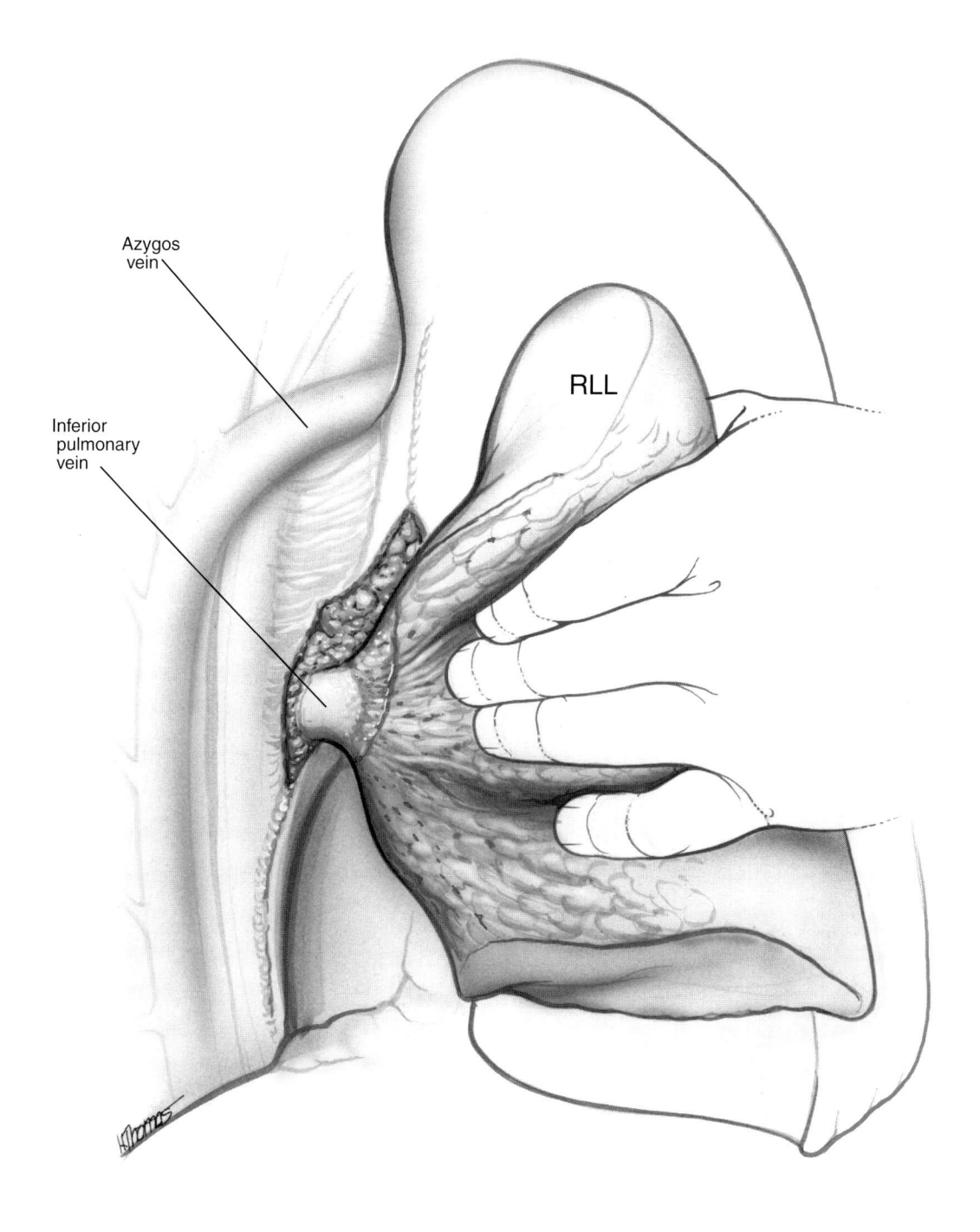

Figure 11–5 • In this view, the right lower lobe has been reflected anteriorly and is being lifted cephalad. The inferior pulmonary ligament has been opened, and we can see the inferior pulmonary vein. We should have looked for any venous drainage from the right middle lobe into this vein at the time we were exposing this area. There is no middle lobe venous drainage into this vein.

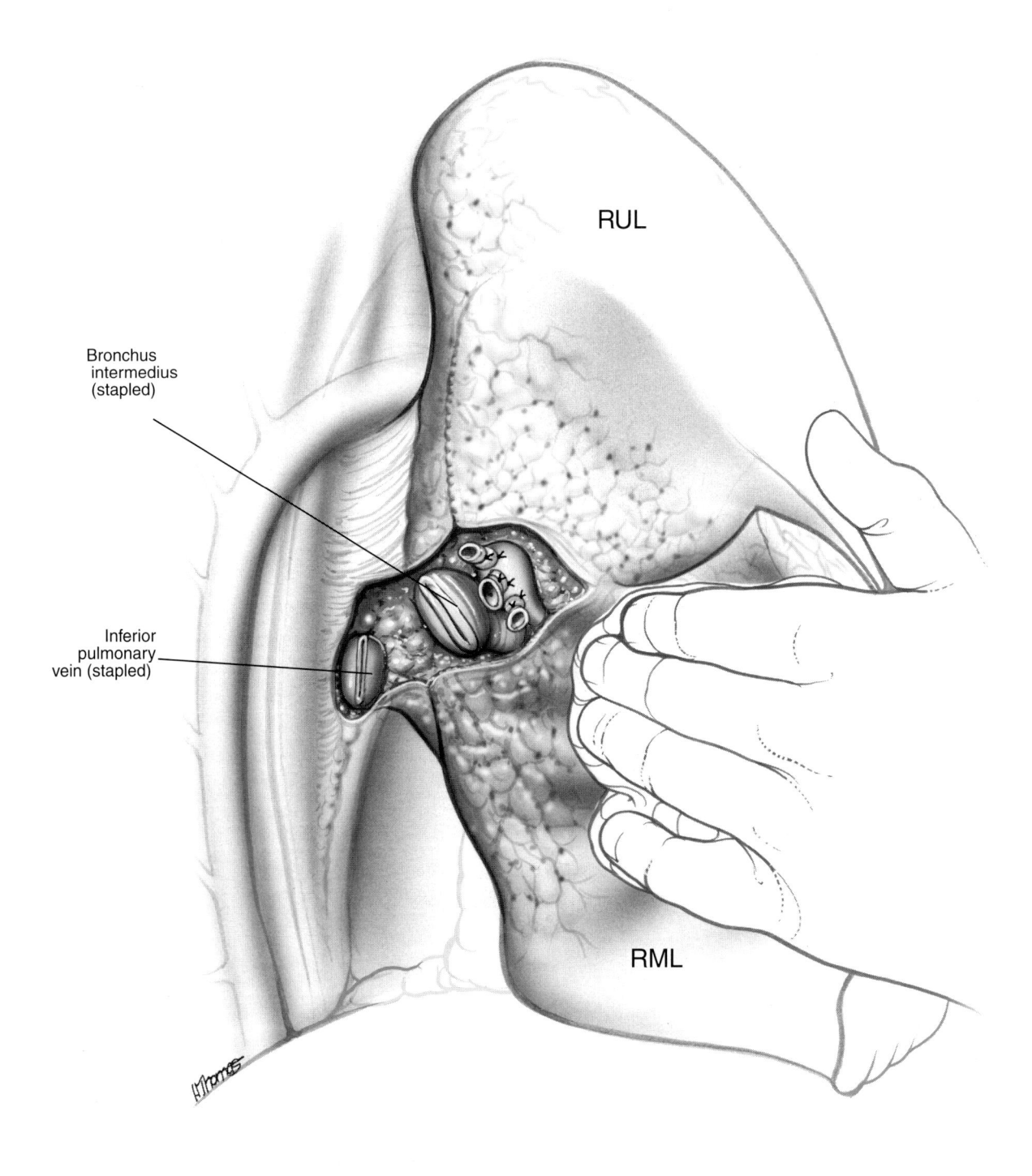

Figure 11–6 • This view depicts the right middle lobe being displaced anteriorly and upward. The right upper lobe is in the upper portion of the drawing. The right lower lobe has been removed. We are looking at the hilum of the right lower lobe, and in the posterior inferior portion we see the ligated inferior pulmonary vein.

Chapter 12
Surgical Anatomy of the Left Lung

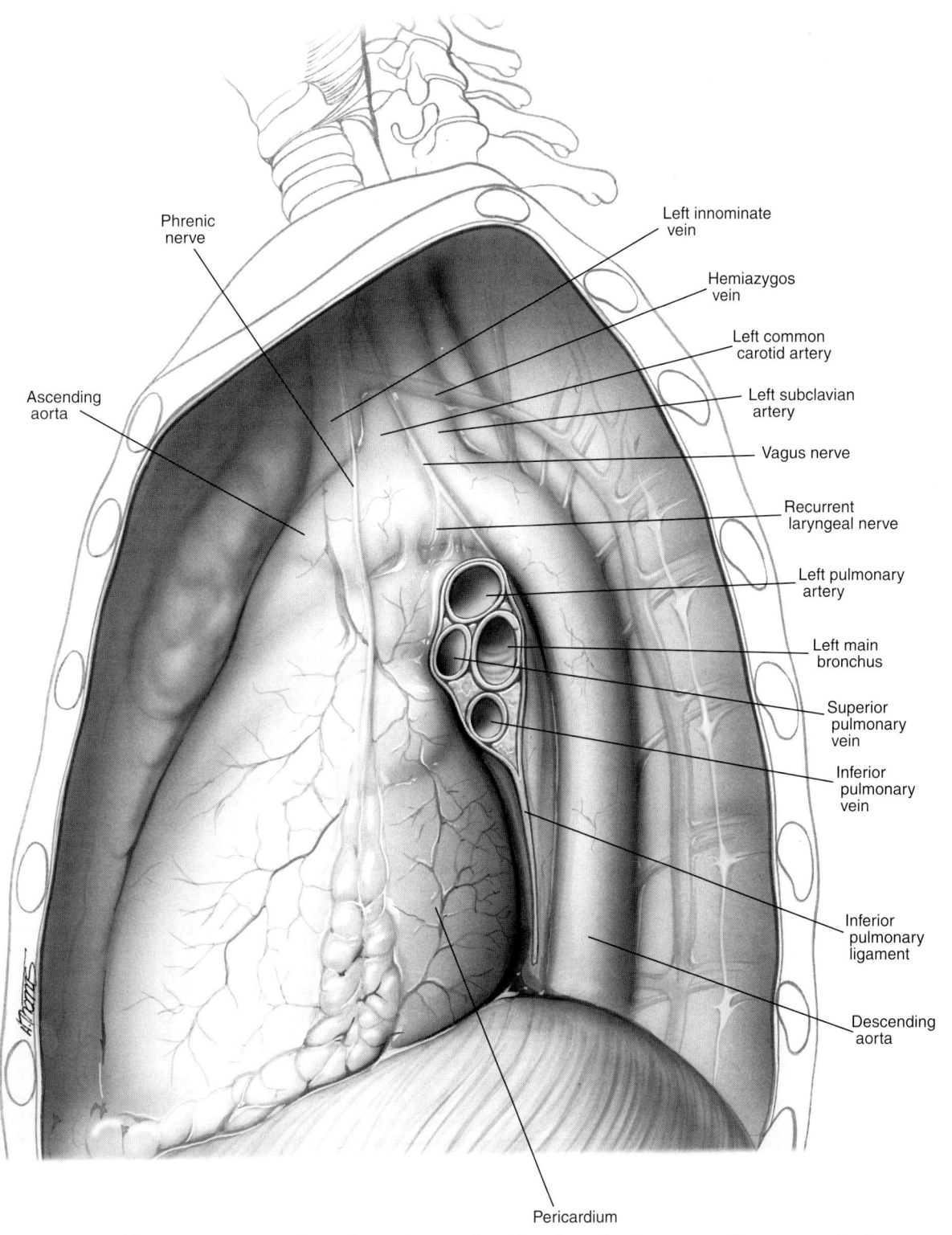

Figure 12–1 • Turning upward on the spine and collecting the intercostal venous drainage is the hemiazygos system. This system drains into the left innominate vein, which is anterior to the carotid artery. The subclavian artery arches out of the apex of the chest and crosses the first rib posterior to the scalene tubercle. The internal mammary artery runs down the anterior chest less than 1 cm lateral to the border of the sternum. The phrenic nerve can be seen entering the chest lateral to the innominate vein.

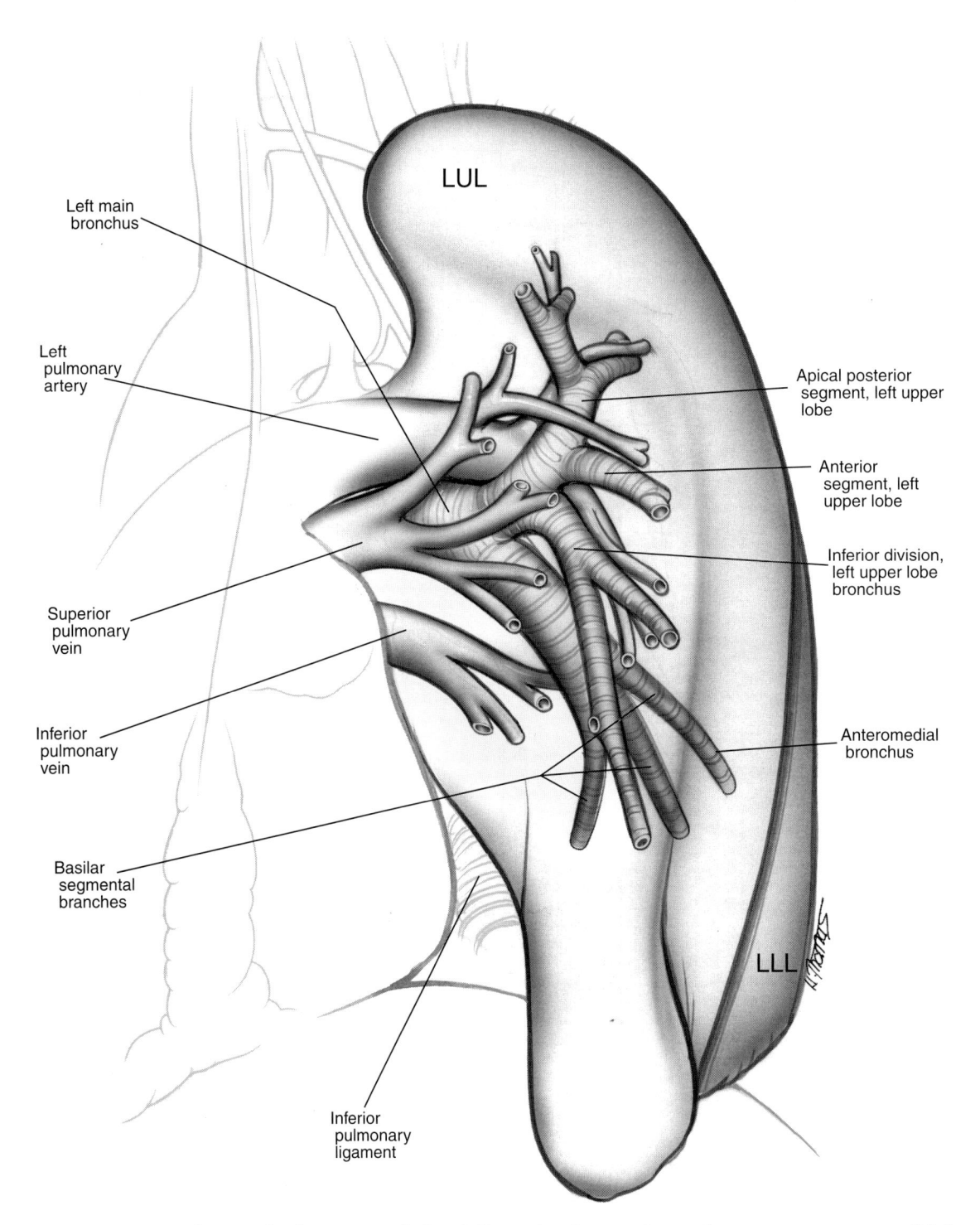

Figure 12-2 • In the cephalic part of the hilum is the main pulmonary artery, which comes out and swings around to descend in the longitudinal fissure between the upper and lower lobes. The artery gives off several branches to the left upper lobe before continuing down in the fissure to supply the lower lobe. The superior pulmonary vein is anterior to the artery. Posterior to the superior pulmonary vein and caudal to the pulmonary artery is the left mainstem bronchus, which branches into the left upper and lower lobes. The left upper lobe bronchus branches into the superior and inferior divisions. The inferior divisions supply the lingular while the superior branches supply the anterior and apical posterior segments. The lower lobe bronchus gives rise to three basal segmental bronchi, one of which is the antero-medial bronchus. The inferior pulmonary vein is in the caudal part of the hilum next to the main bronchus, and below that is the inferior pulmonary ligament.

Surgical Anatomy of the Left Lung • 83

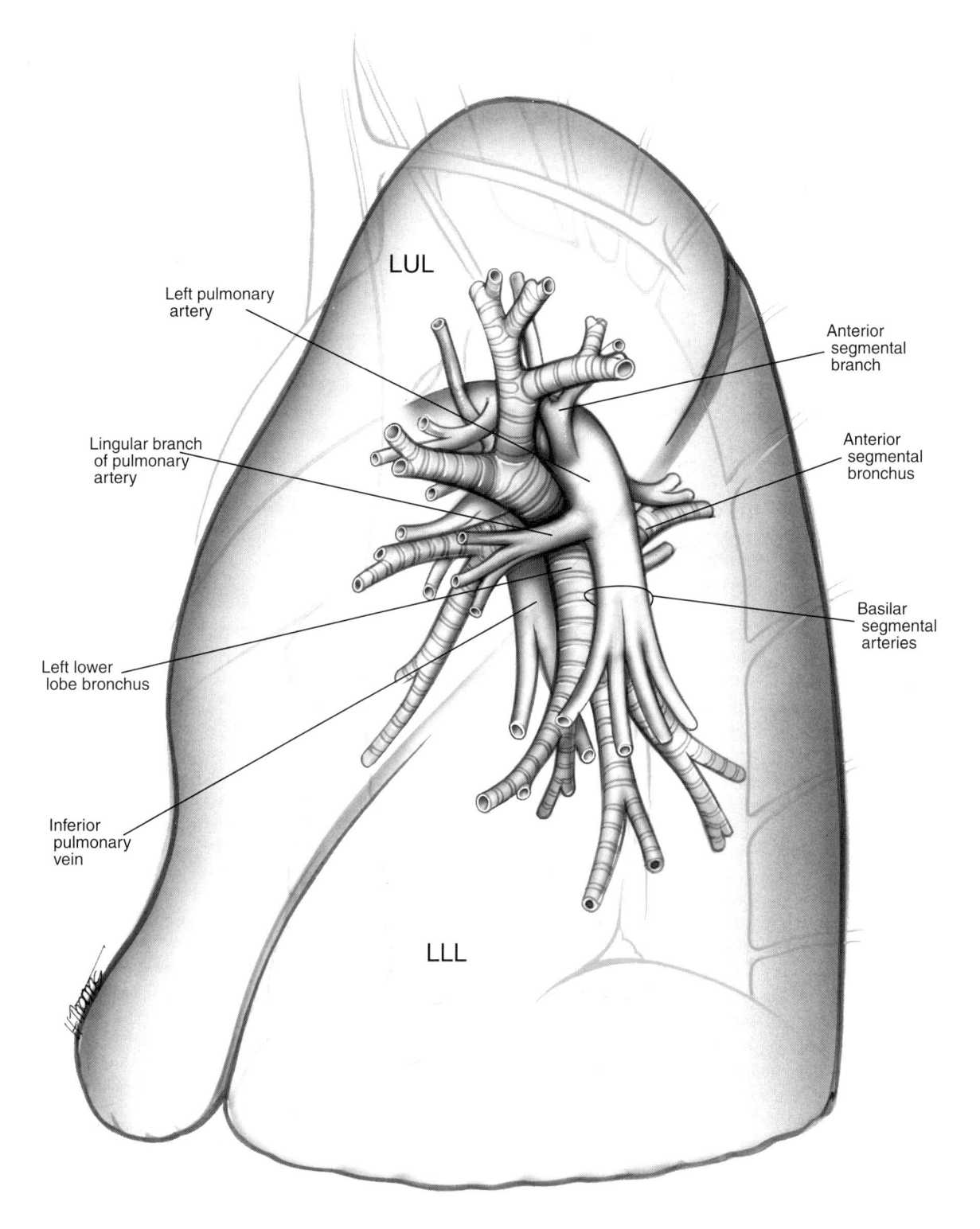

Figure 12–3 • The first structure seen in the longitudinal fissure is the main pulmonary artery. The lingular artery runs anteriorly in the lowest portion of the left upper lobe. There is a more proximal arterial branch going up to the anterior segment and a branch to the posterior segment. The bronchus is hard to expose until branches of the pulmonary artery are divided. The left upper lobe bronchus, with its inferior divisions to the lingula and superior divisions to the upper lobe segments, is seen. The remaining lower lobe segmental bronchi are seen as well. The inferior pulmonary vein is hidden and is not readily visible in this approach.

84 • Part II CHEST

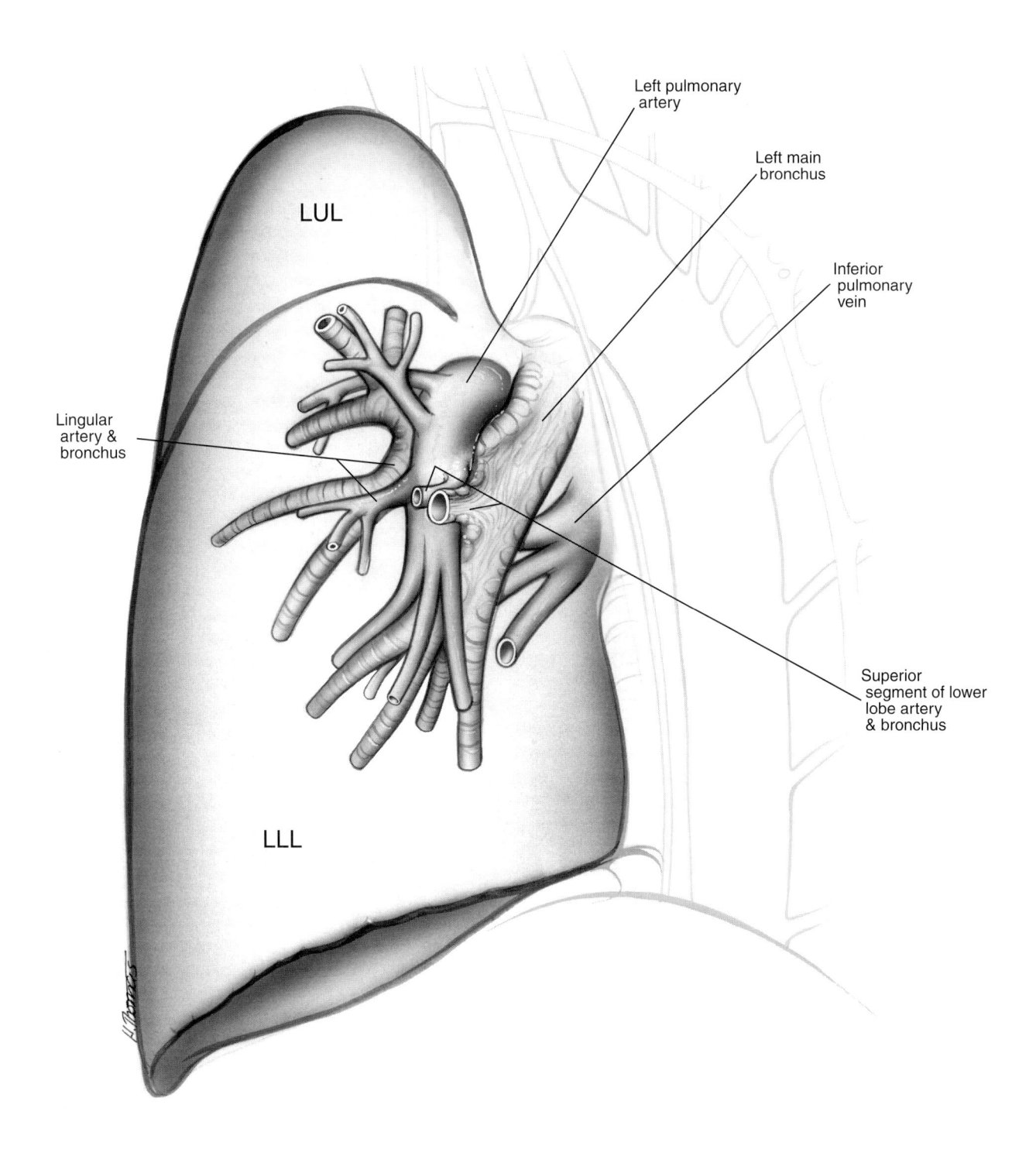

Figure 12–4 • In this view, we see the hilar anatomy from the rear. The pulmonary artery is in the highest portion of the hilum. Caudal to that is the left mainstem bronchus. The tracheal carina is high, near the aortic arch. The inferior pulmonary vein can be seen well since it is in the same plane as the bronchus and caudal to it. The various branches of the upper lobe and lower lobe bronchi are well depicted.

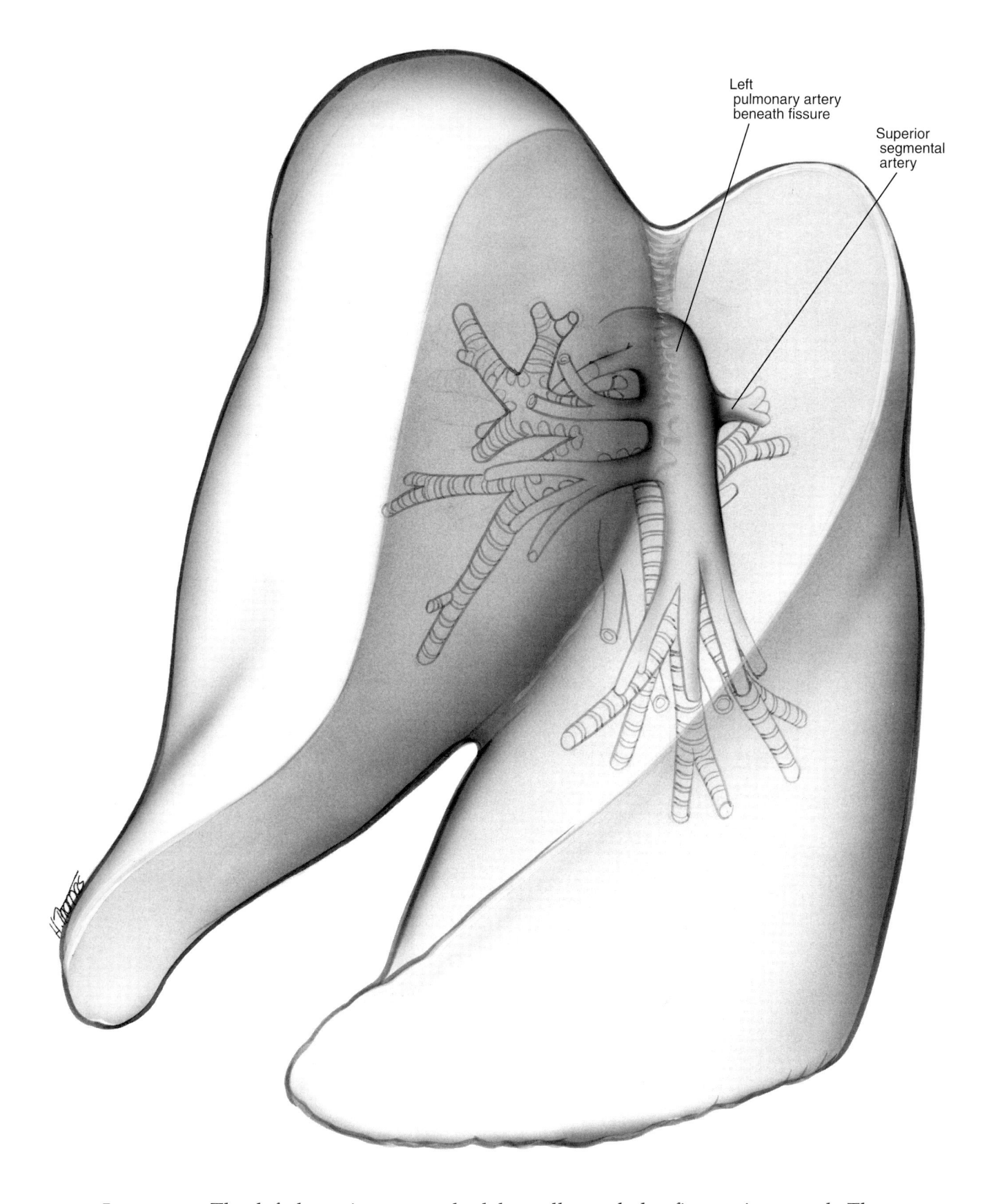

Figure 12–5 • The left lung is approached laterally, and the fissure is spread. The pulmonary artery runs down the fissure. The first posterior branch off the pulmonary artery is the superior segmental branch, which runs with the superior segmental bronchus. The bronchi are medial to the artery, and the venous drainage that comes from the intersegmental planes goes to the caudal and medial portions of the bronchial drainage.

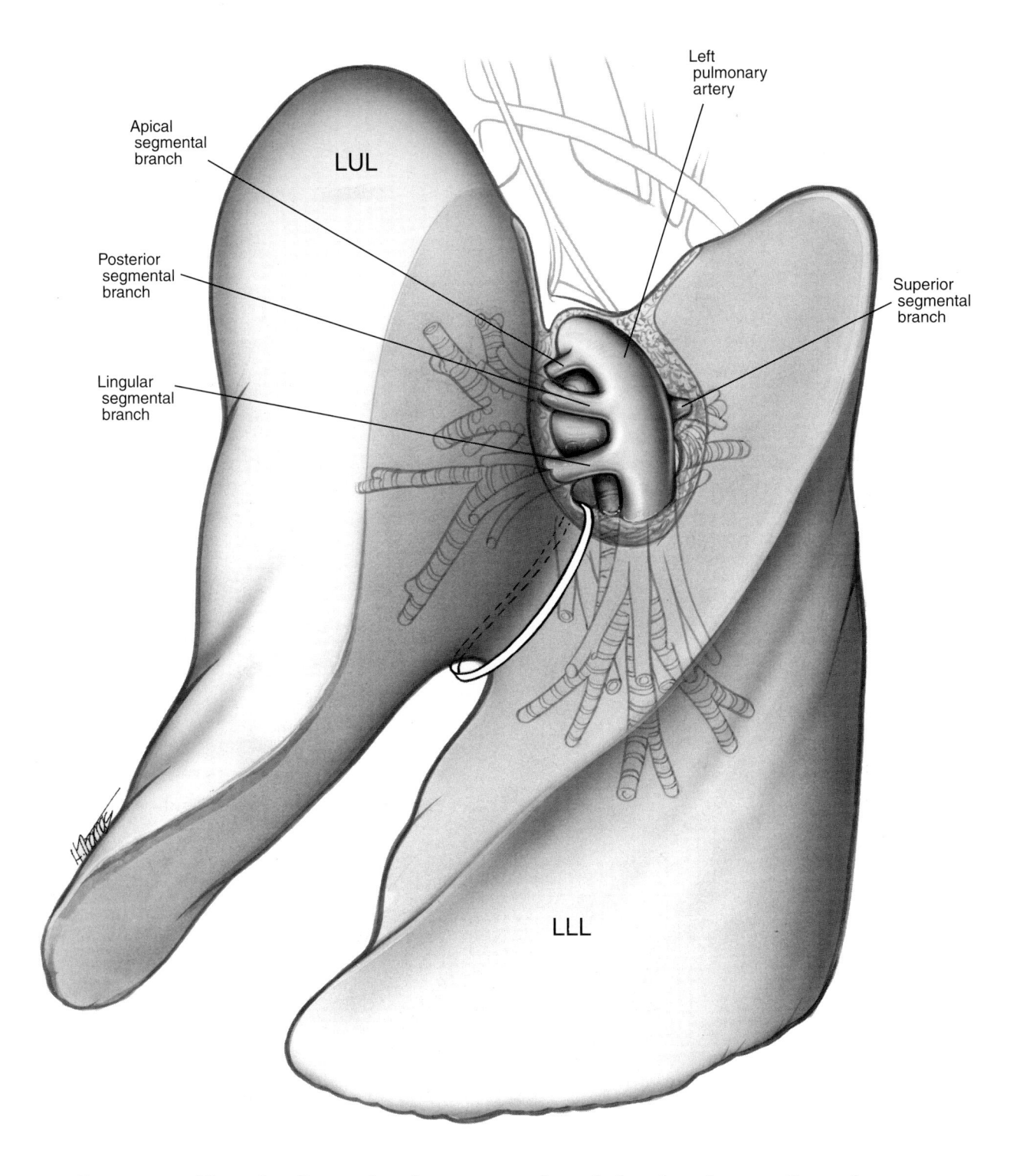

Figure 12-6 • Here the fissure has been opened, and the sheath over the pulmonary artery has been cut so that one can see the arterial branches to the left upper lobe. The inferior portion of the longitudinal fissure and the lung parenchyma between the left upper lobe and left lower lobe in the inferior portion of the hilum are still intact. The circle around this shows what has to be opened, but it can be seen that great care must be taken not to injure the lingular arterial branch and to watch out for the branches draining into the superior pulmonary vein and inferior pulmonary vein, since there may be vessels that cross this fissure.

Chapter 13
Left Upper Lobectomy

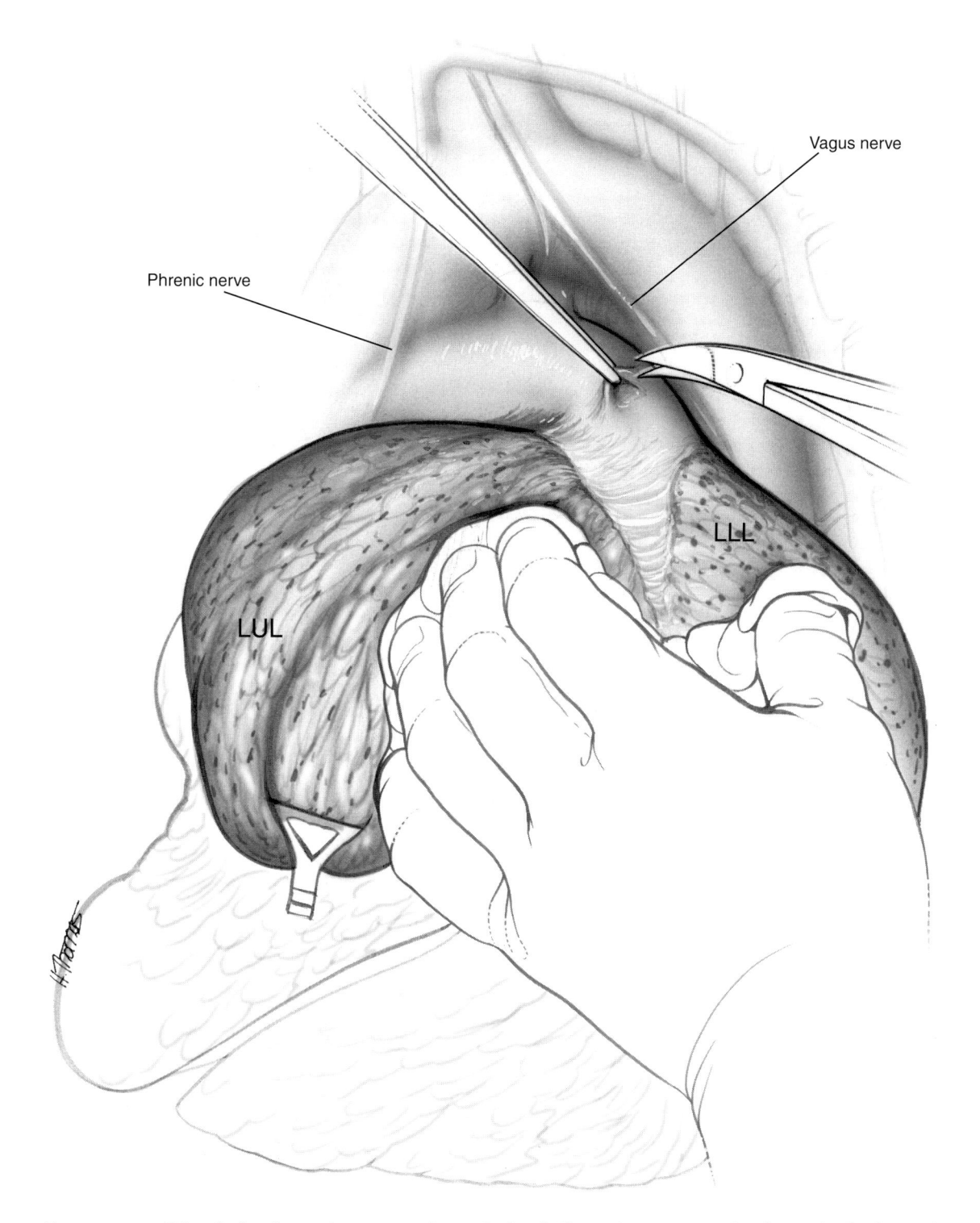

Figure 13–1 • The left chest is opened and the hilum is approached cephalad to the lung, with the left lung deflated. The mediastinal pleura over the main pulmonary artery is incised. The left upper lobe is to the operator's left and the left lower lobe to the right. The aortic arch is cephalad, the phrenic nerve is crossing anteriorly, and the vagus nerve is crossing toward the posterior portion of the hilum.

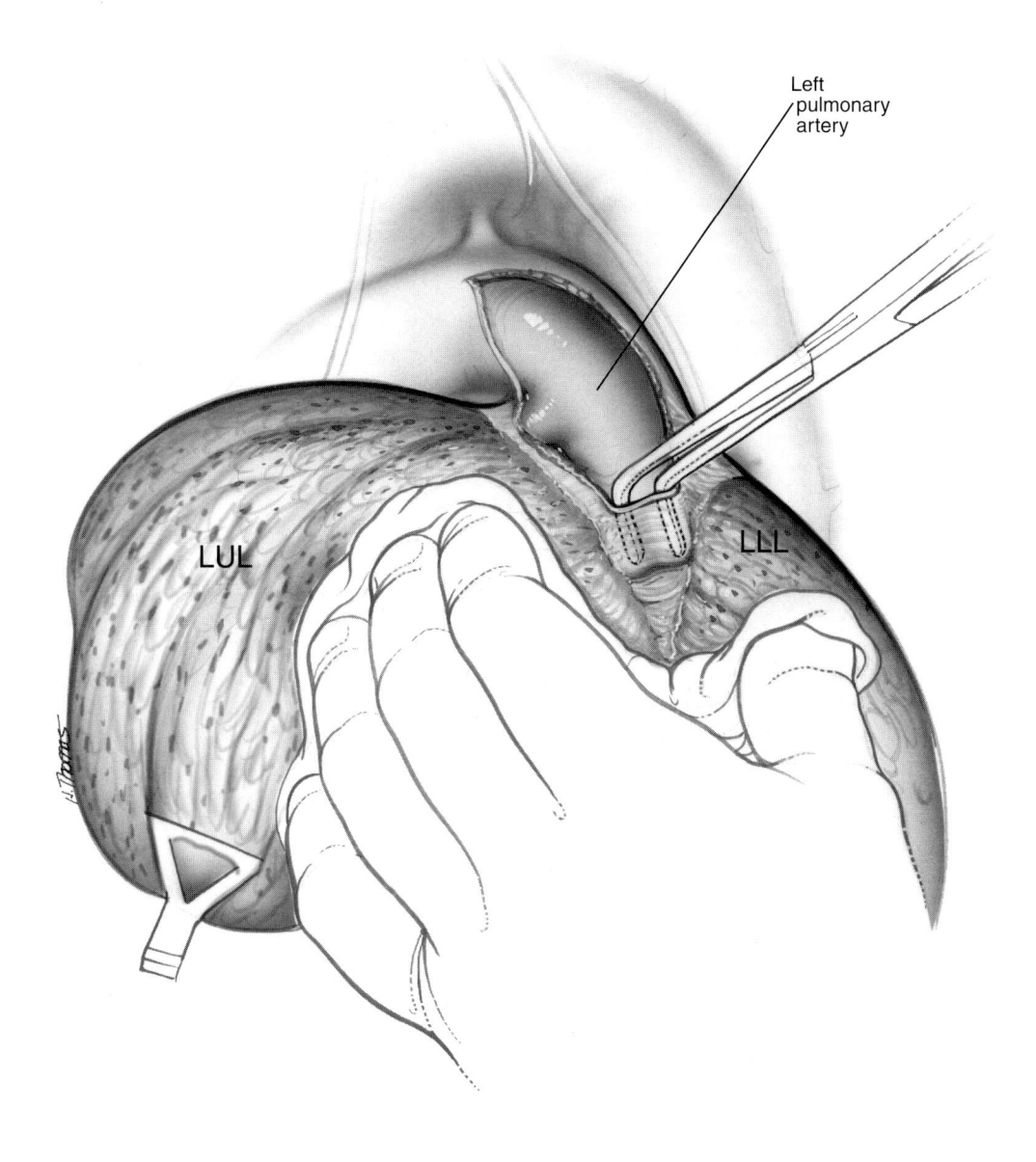

Figure 13–2 • The pleura and the sheath over the pulmonary artery have been opened using a Mixter clamp. When the patient has had preoperative chemotherapy or radiotherapy or both, this plane may be difficult to define and sometimes even dangerous. If it is potentially hazardous, one can better control this area by passing a Rumel tourniquet around the pulmonary artery in a safe proximal location so that this procedure can be done in a bloodless field.

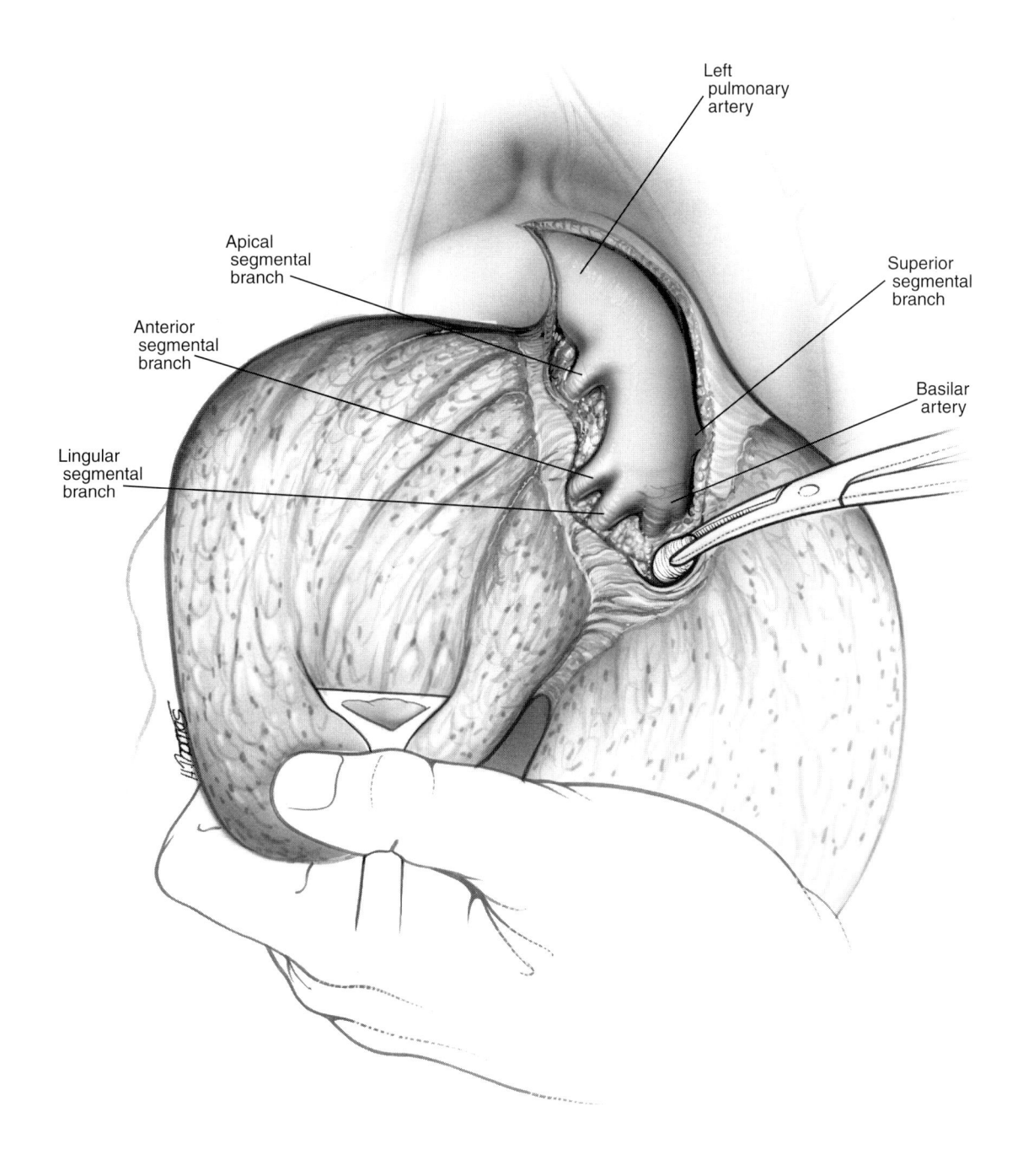

Figure 13–3 • The number of branches of the pulmonary artery to the left lobe is variable. Ordinarily there is one each to the apical segment, anterior segment, and lingula, but there may be more or fewer, and the surgeon must inspect carefully as the dissection continues to be certain that all these branches are found.

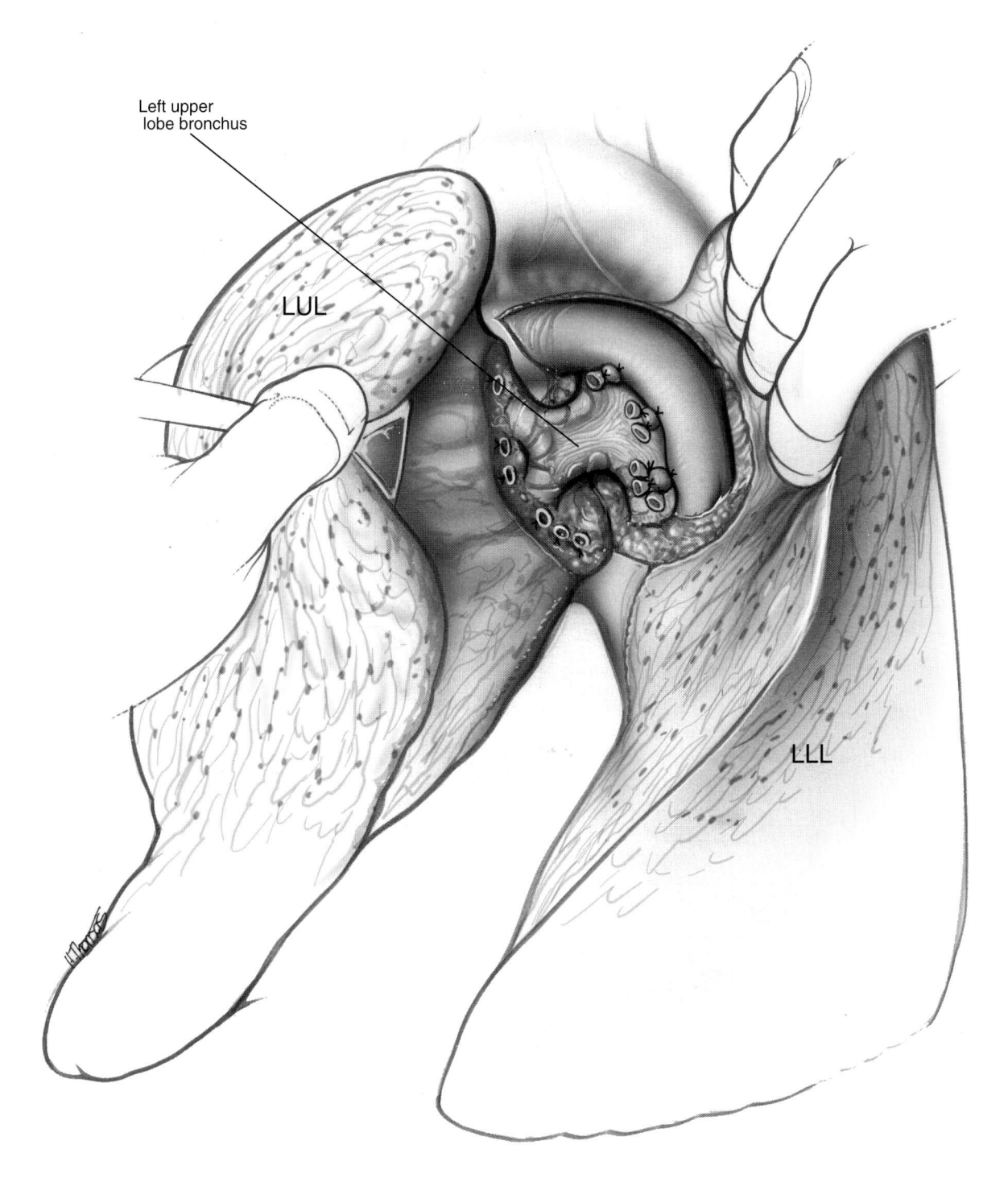

Figure 13–4 • In this view, the upper and lower lobes are separated, and one can see that there are three branches of the pulmonary artery to the left upper lobe that have been ligated. The first and highest branch is ligated, suture ligated, and distally ligated. Sometimes the highest branch of the superior pulmonary vein must be divided in order to expose the artery adequately. The second and third branches of the artery have been ligated proximal to the branches. Following division of the arterial branches, the left main bronchus is exposed where it is bifurcating into the left lower lobe bronchus and the left upper lobe bronchus. It soon branches into the superior division, which goes to the upper lobe, and the inferior or lingular branches.

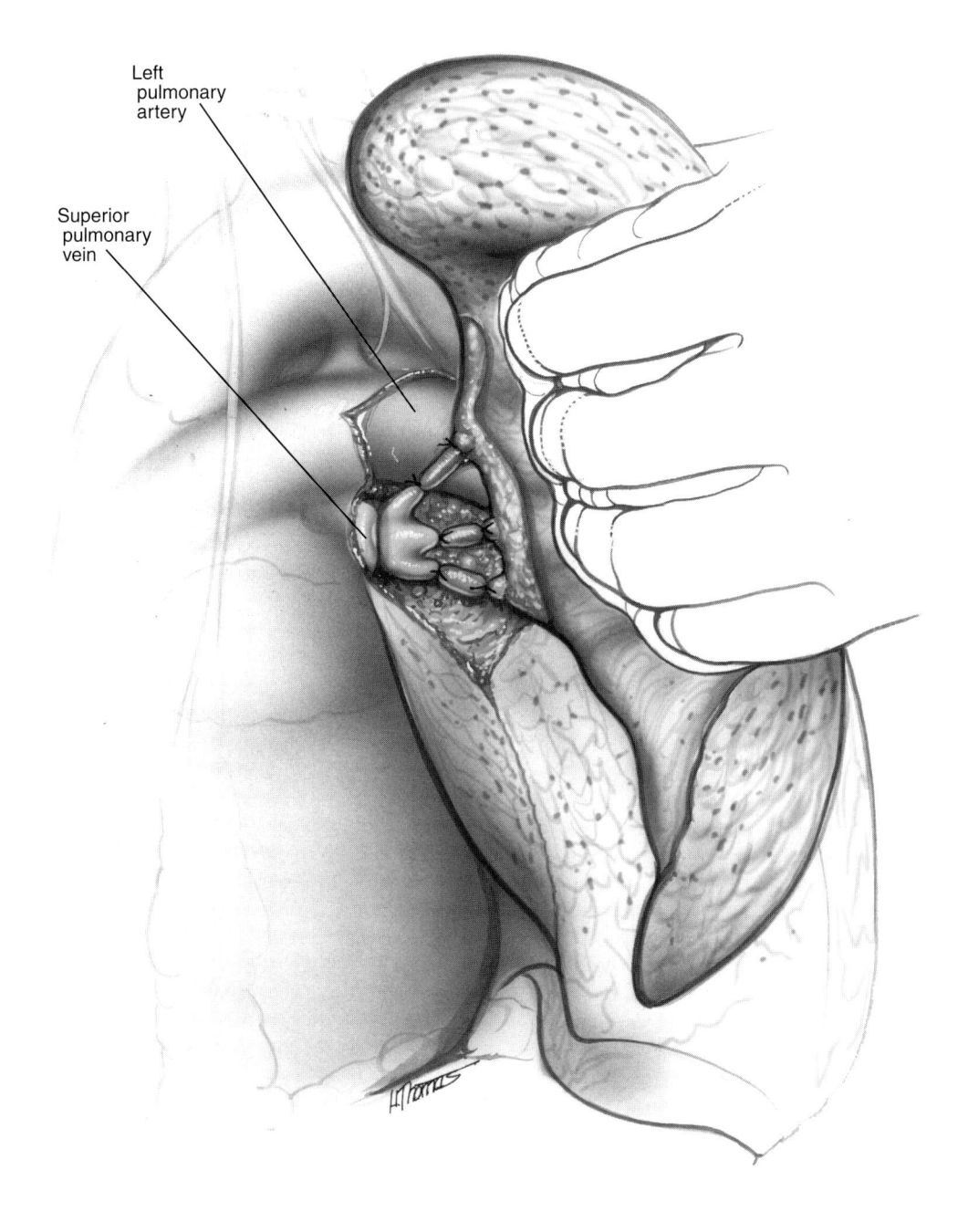

Figure 13–5 • Following reflection of the left upper lobe anteriorly, the superior pulmonary vein is identified and tied proximally. The suture ligatures on the branches are distal to the trifurcation, and there are additional ties to prevent backbleeding from the vein. An alternative to this technique would be to place the suture ligature distal to the first heavy tie and proximal to the trifurcation. A stapler can also be utilized.

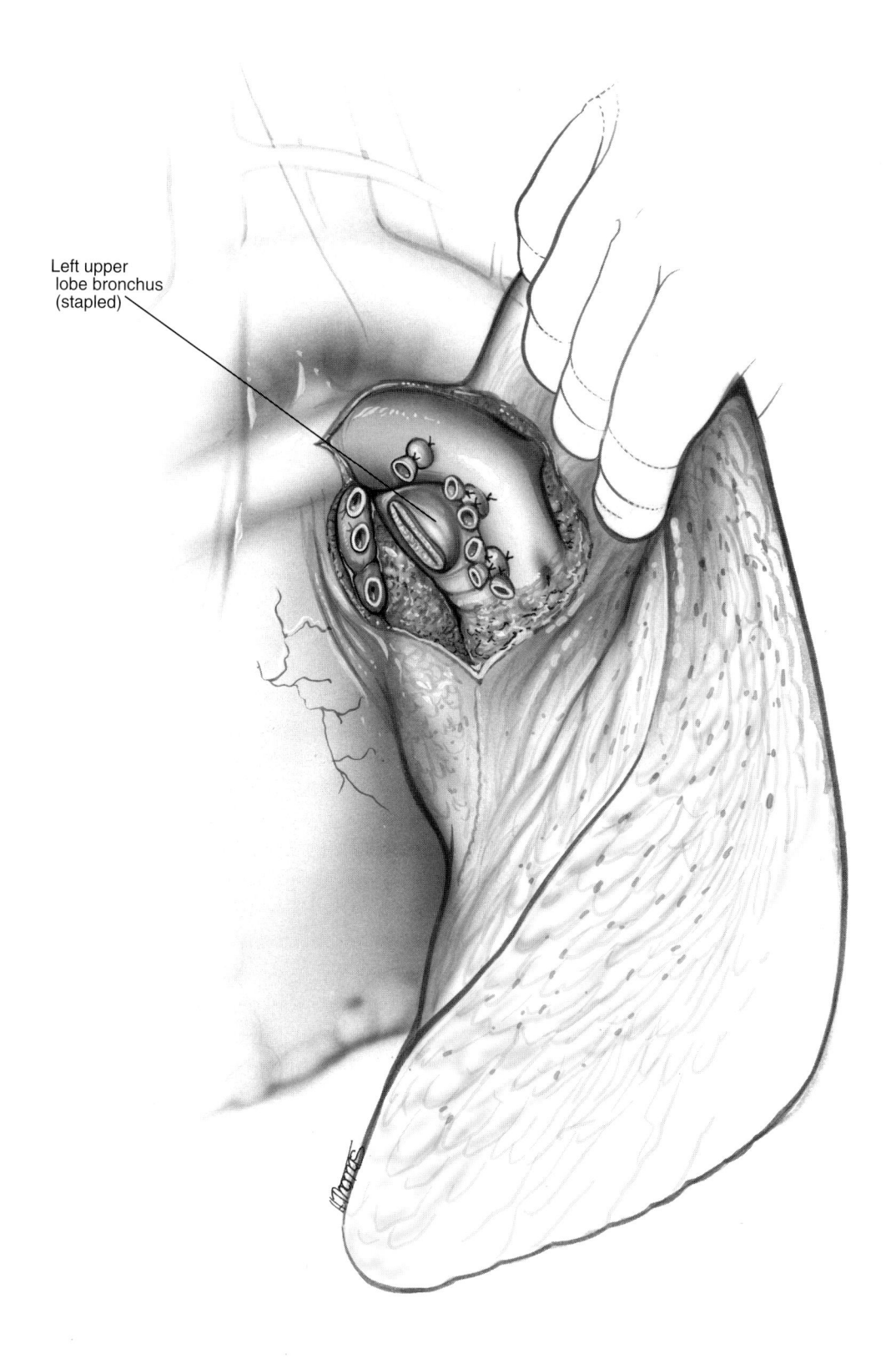

Figure 13-6 • The left upper lobe specimen is removed. The hilum of the left upper lobe is seen. Centrally is the stapled left upper lobe bronchial stump. Anteriorly is the ligated superior pulmonary vein with its three suture-ligated branches. The divided branches of the pulmonary artery are seen as well.

Chapter 14
Left Lower Lobectomy

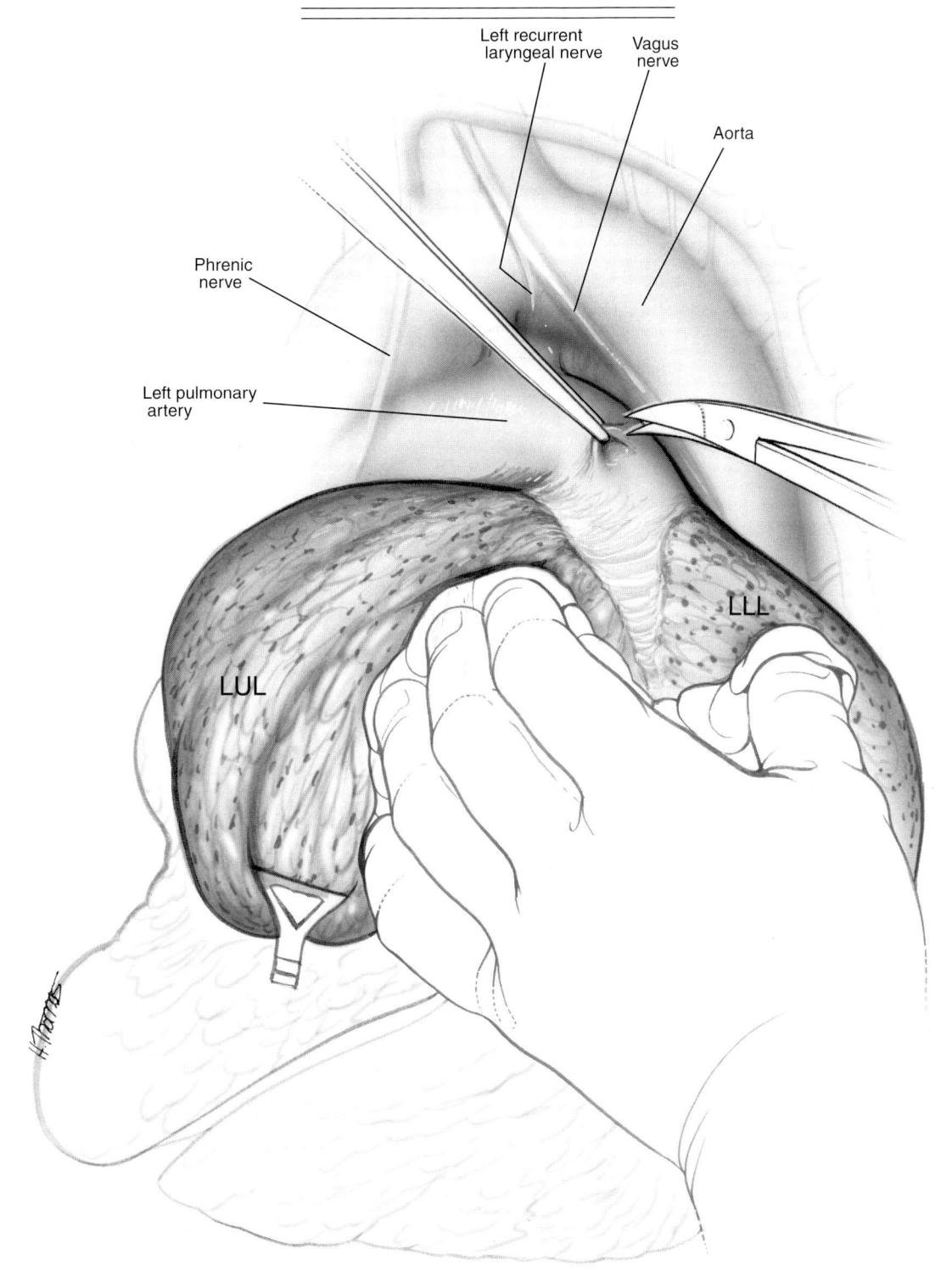

Figure 14–1 • The hilum of the lung is viewed with the left lung deflated. The mediastinal pleura over the main pulmonary artery is grasped with forceps and incised with scissors. The left upper lobe is in the operator's hand, and the left lower lobe is to the right. The aortic arch is seen with the phrenic nerve crossing anteriorly and the vagus nerve crossing posteriorly in the hilum. The left recurrent laryngeal nerve is labeled as it approaches the ligamentum arteriosum.

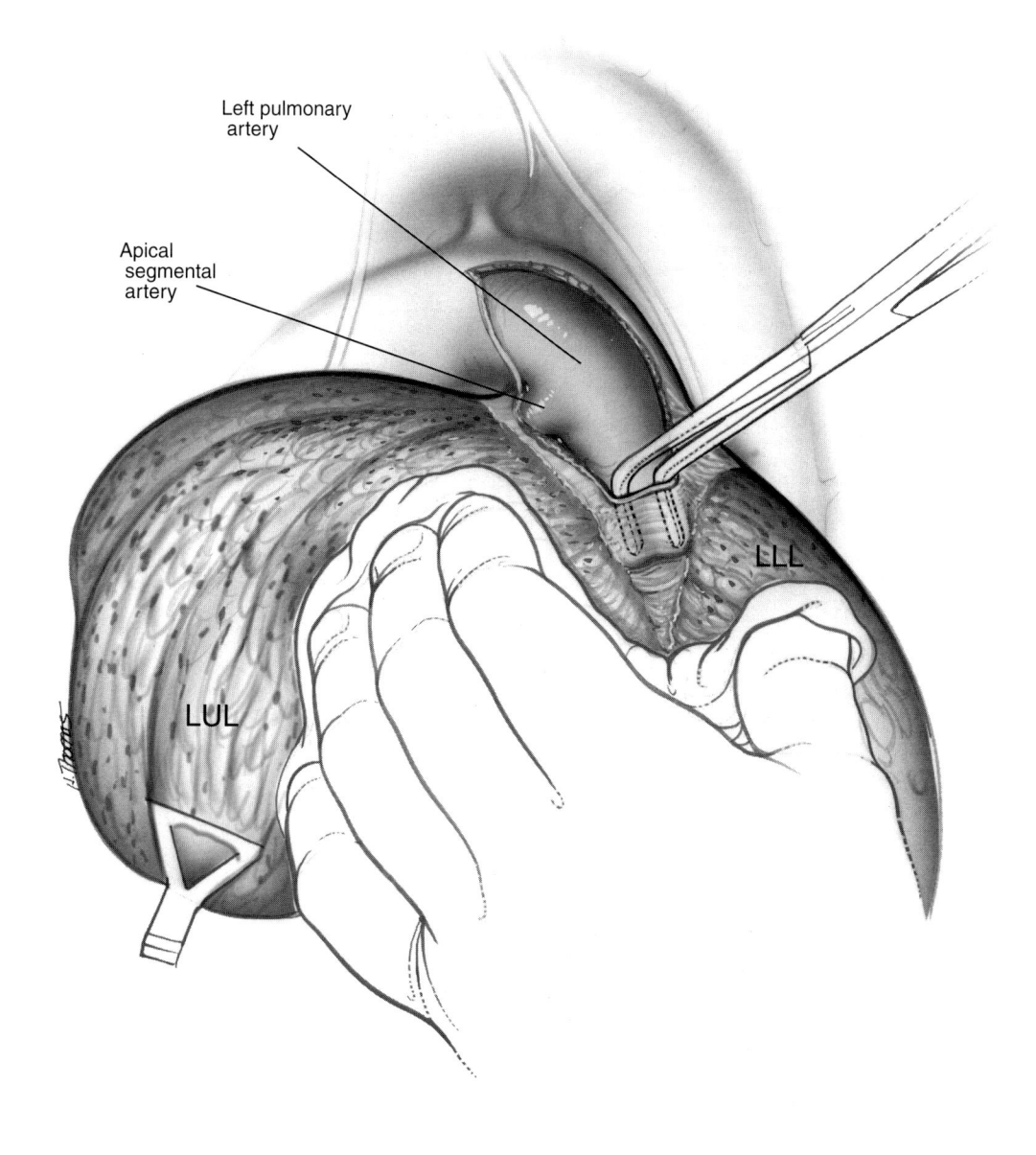

Figure 14–2 • The pleura and sheath over the pulmonary artery may be dissected free after incision. This is best done by grasping the perivascular tissue with a thumb forceps and using general blunt dissection to separate the pulmonary artery from its sheath.

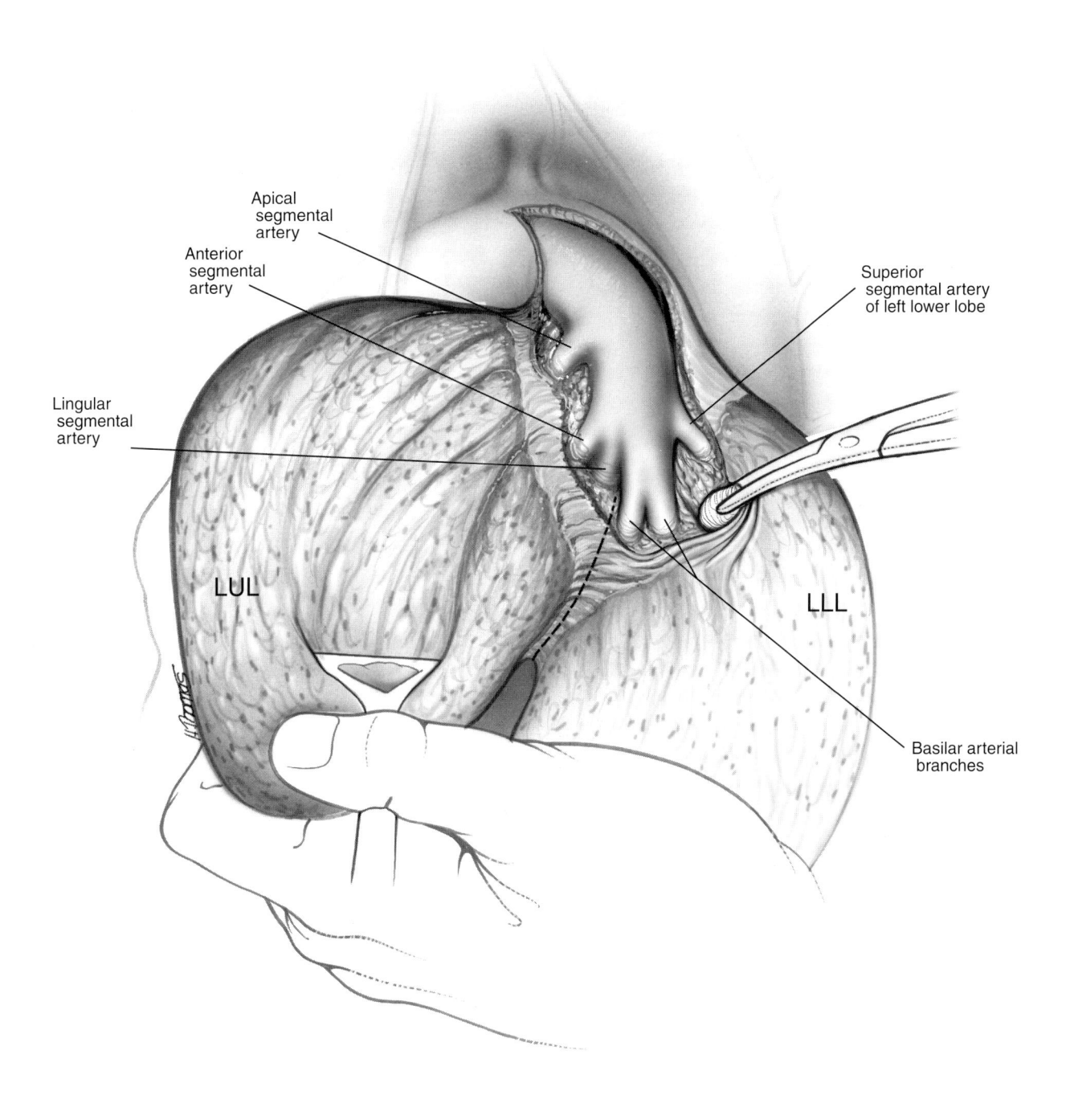

Figure 14–3 • The sheath over the main pulmonary artery is opened, and the branch to the superior segment of the lower lobe and the basilar segmental trunk are identified. At this point the fissure may be completely developed by dissecting a plane between the lingular branch of the pulmonary artery and the basilar trunk and stapling it through the fissure.

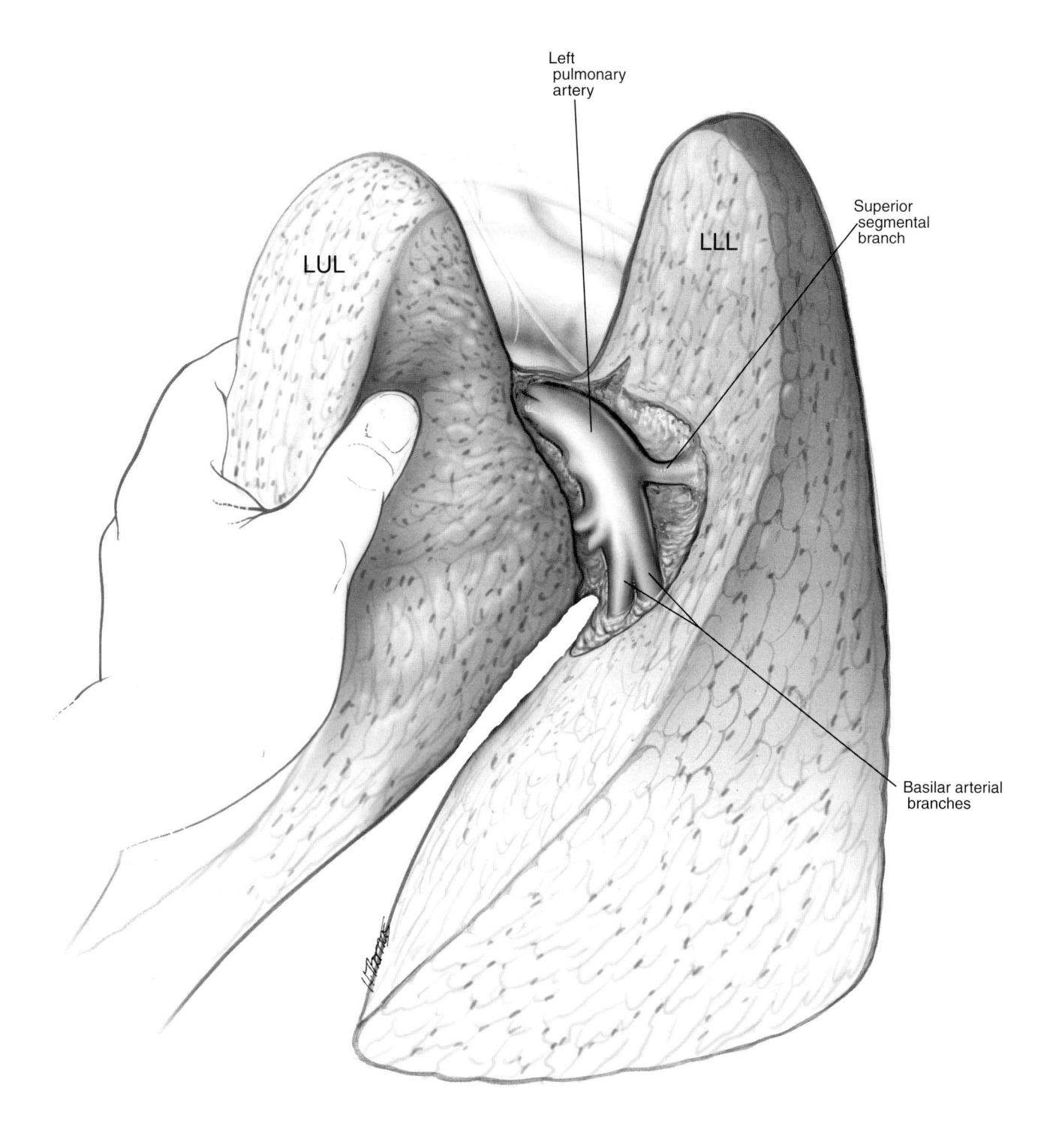

Figure 14–4 • Further dissection in the fissure exposes the arterial branches to be removed.

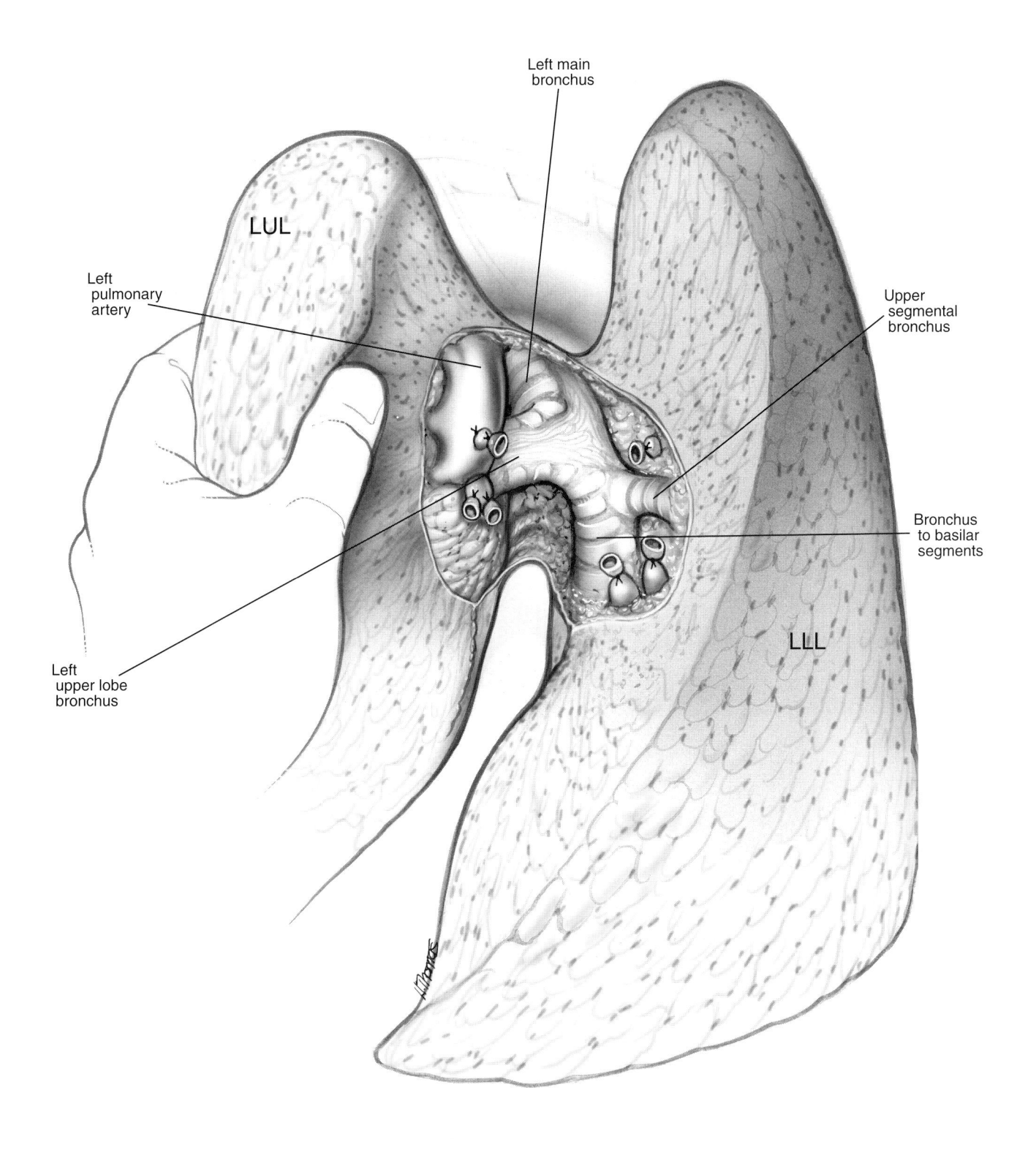

Figure 14–5 • The superior segmental and basilar segmental branches have been doubly ligated and divided, and we see their stumps on the main pulmonary artery.

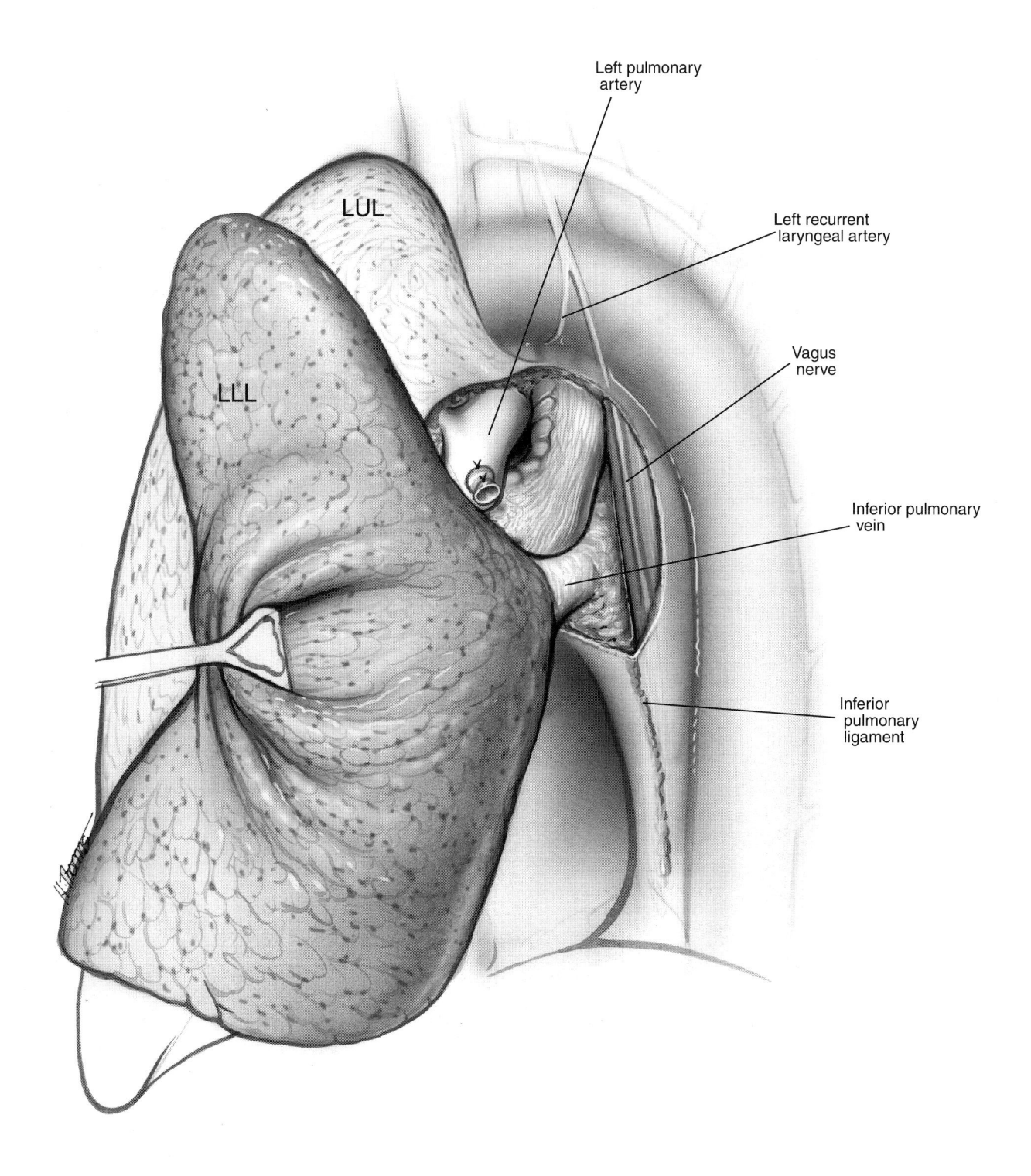

Figure 14-6 • The left lower lobe is retracted anteriorly, demonstrating the residual attachment of the inferior pulmonary vein just immediately inferior to and in the same plane as the mainstem bronchus. The inferior pulmonary ligament is divided. The esophagus is seen coursing anterior to the descending aorta. The vagus nerve accompanies the esophagus. The recurrent nerve is shown as it goes beneath the aortic arch.

Left Lower Lobectomy • 99

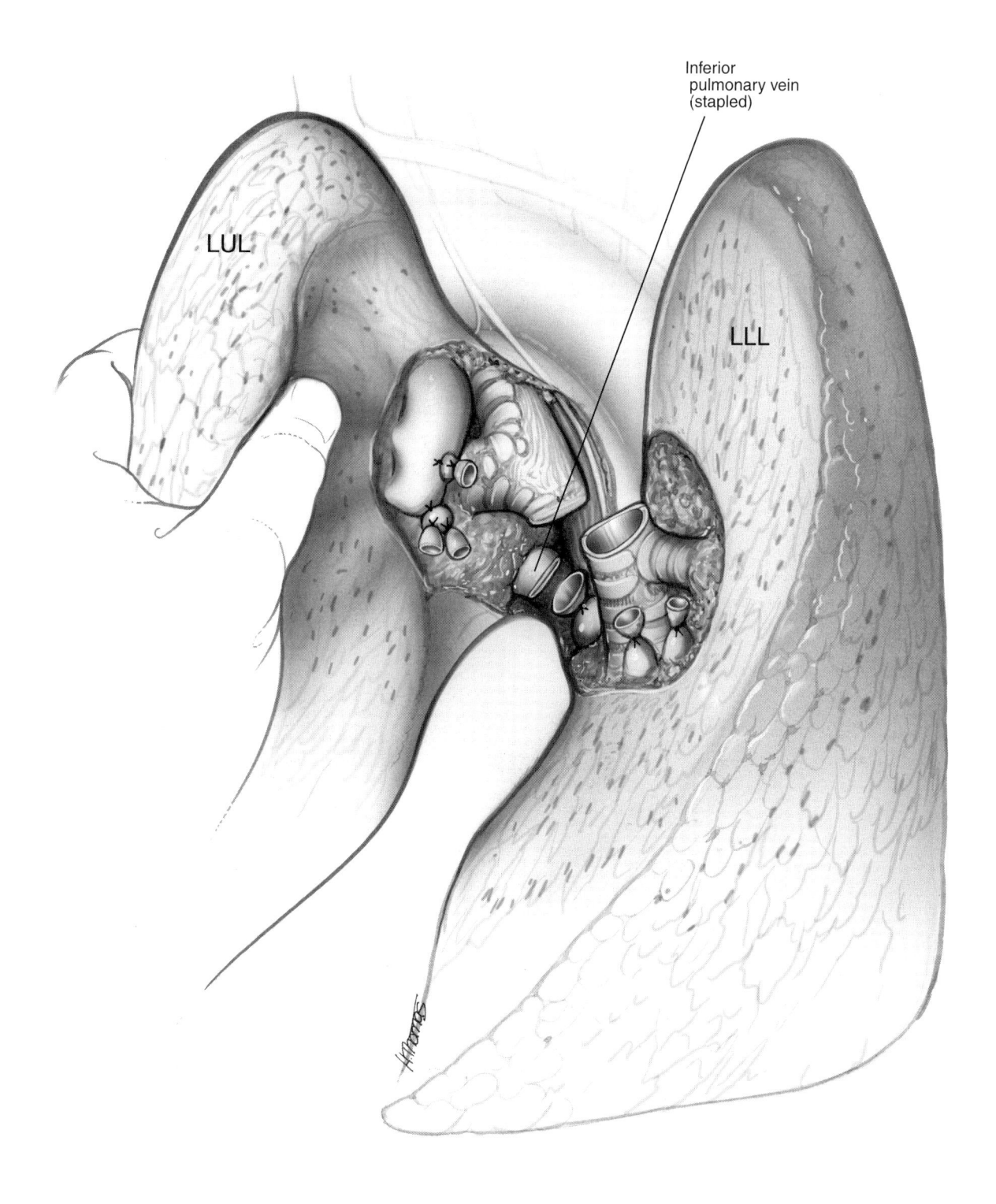

Figure 14–7 • We are viewing the lung laterally, looking directly into the fissure. The pulmonary vein and the bronchus have been stapled. Only a bit of areolar tissue and visceral pleura attach the lower lobe to the hilum.

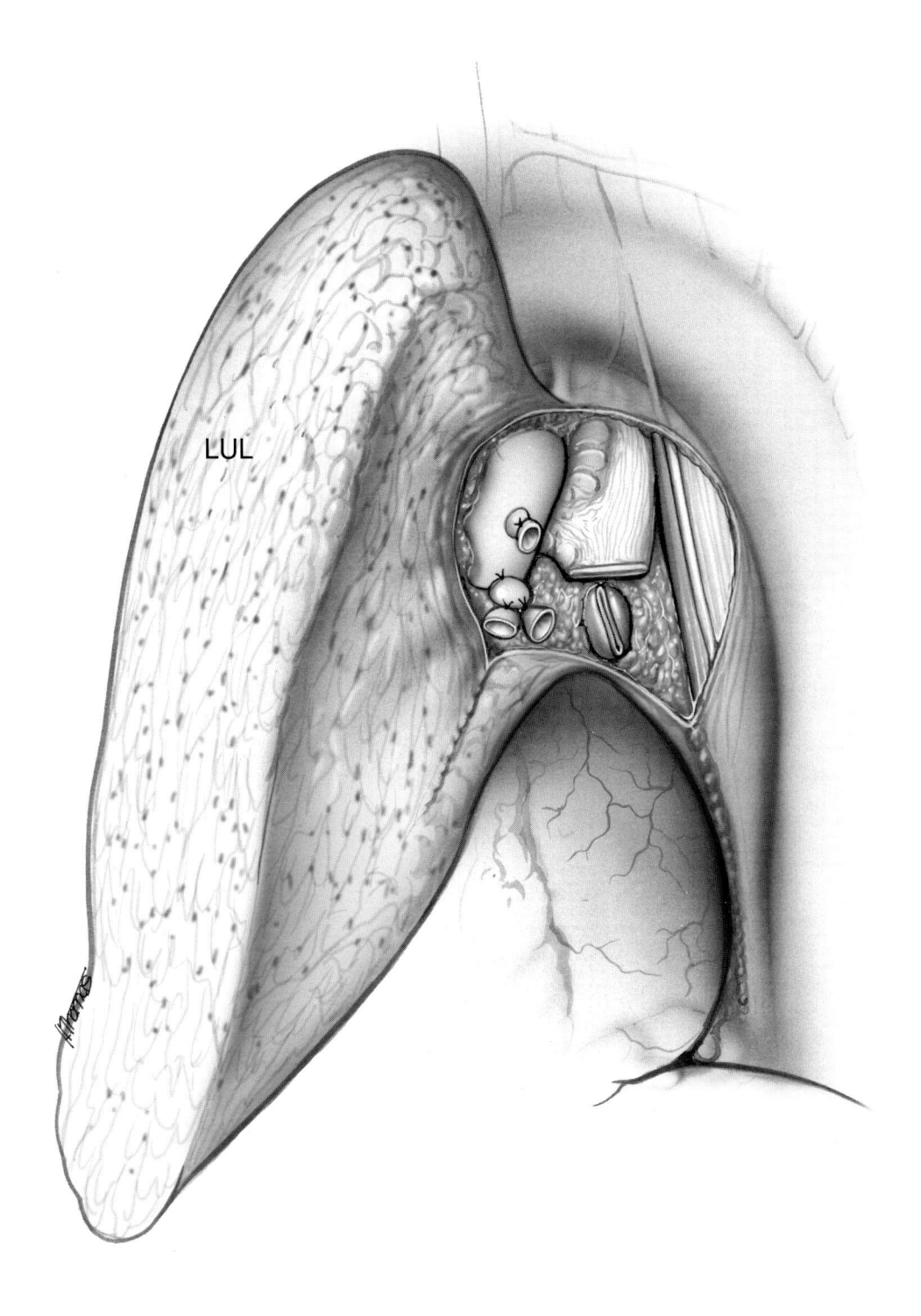

Figure 14–8 • The hilum is visualized following completion of the lower lobectomy.

Chapter 15
Clinical Case: Thymoma

Edward Beattie

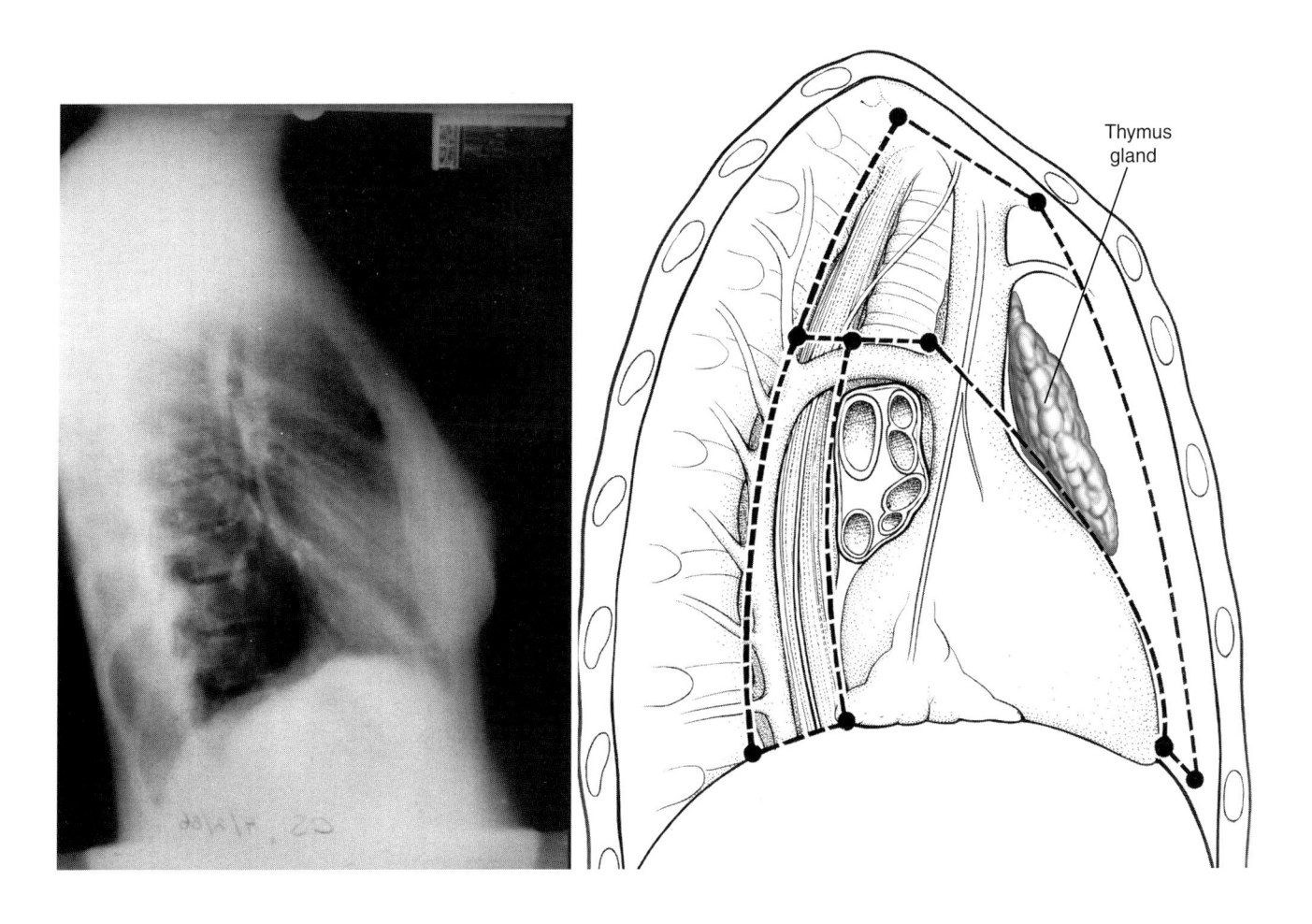

Figure 15–1 • A 31-year-old woman presented with an asymptomatic anterior mediastinal mass. Work-up revealed this mass to be consistent with a thymoma.

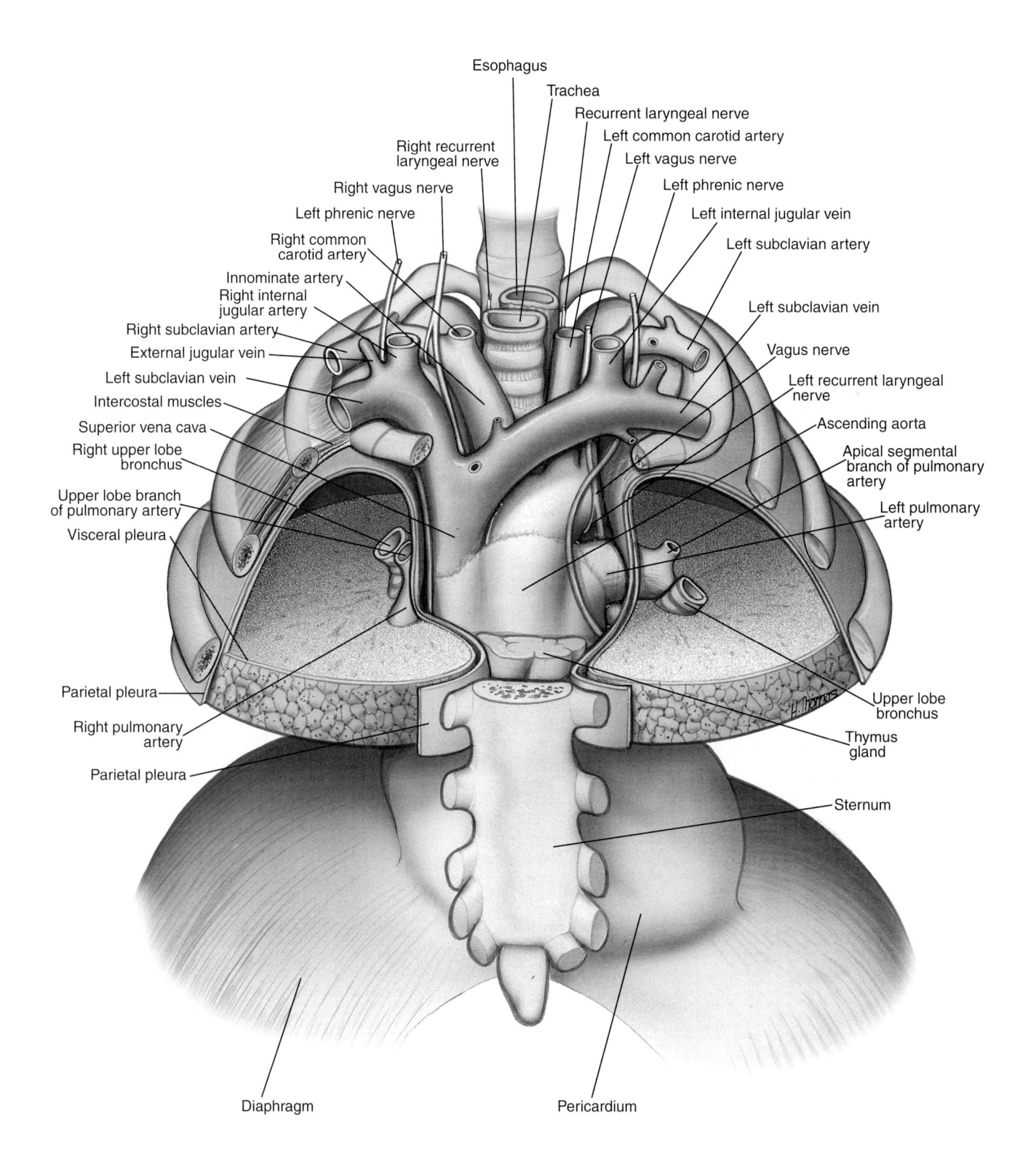

Figure 15–2 • A cross-sectional anatomic depiction of the anterior mediastinum.

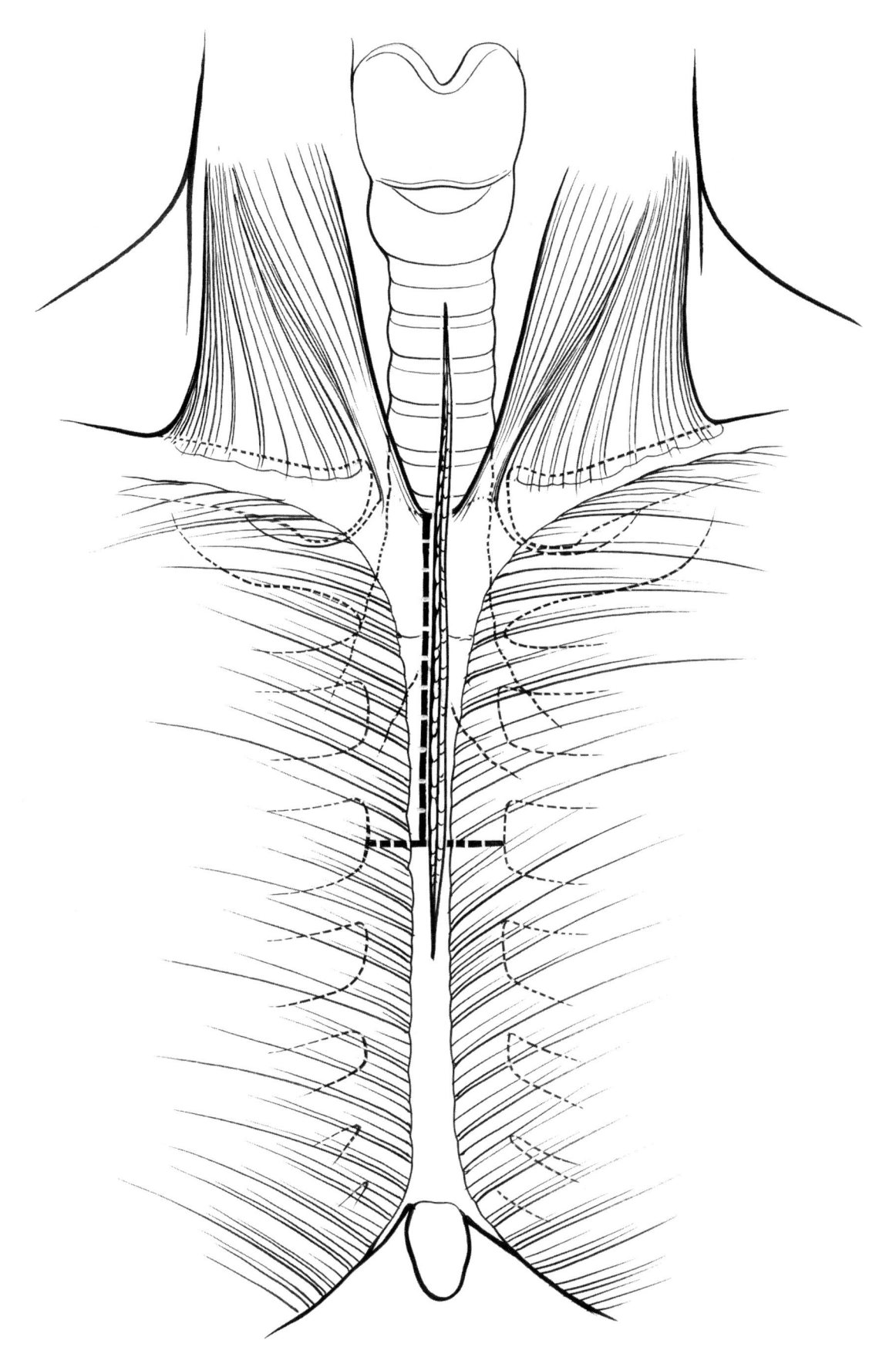

Figure 15–3 • In lieu of a complete mediasternotomy, a partial sternotomy to the level of the fifth rib is illustrated.

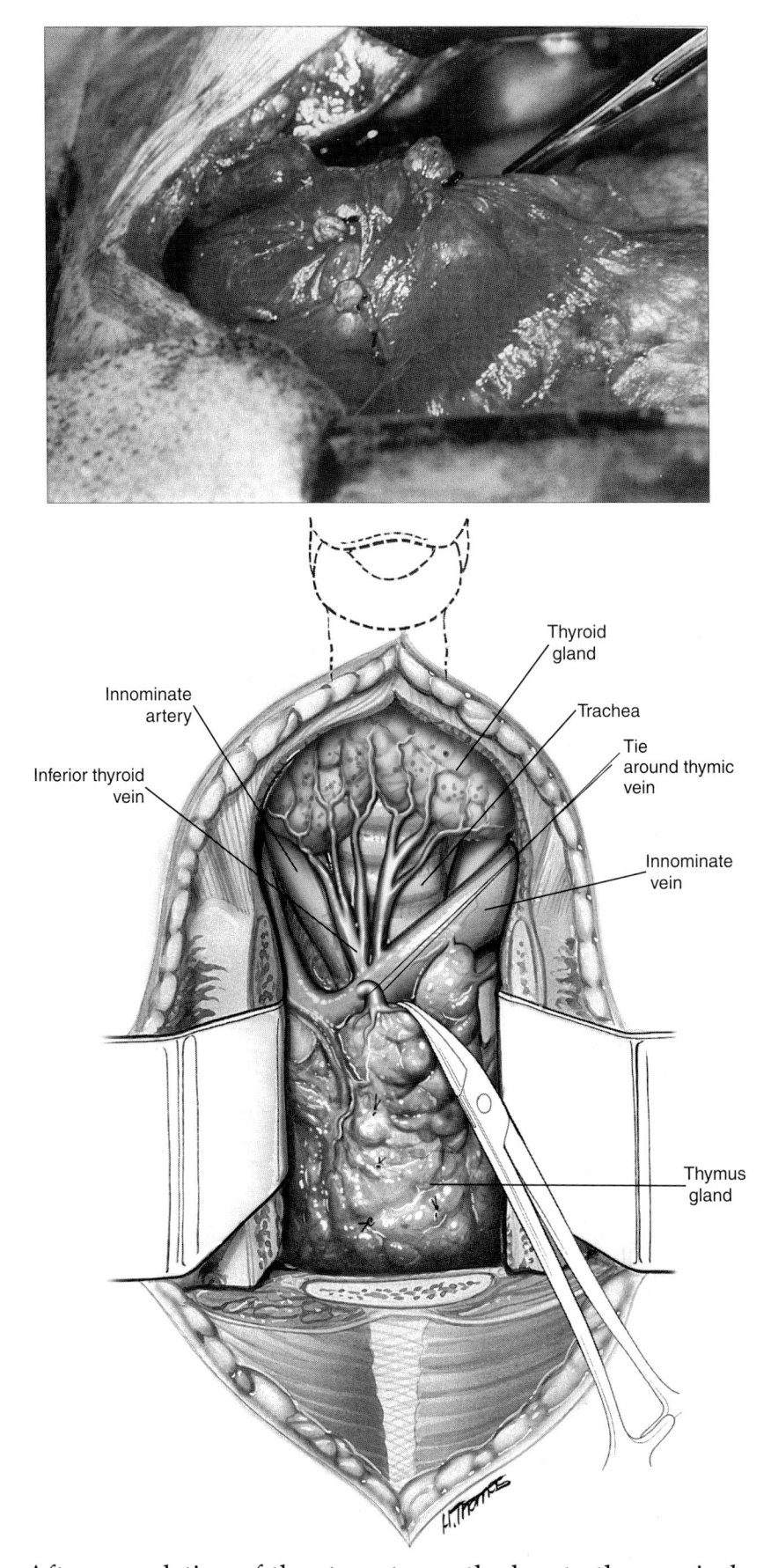

Figure 15–4 • After completion of the sternotomy, the key to the surgical resection of thymic tumors is identification and division of the thymic vein off the innominate.

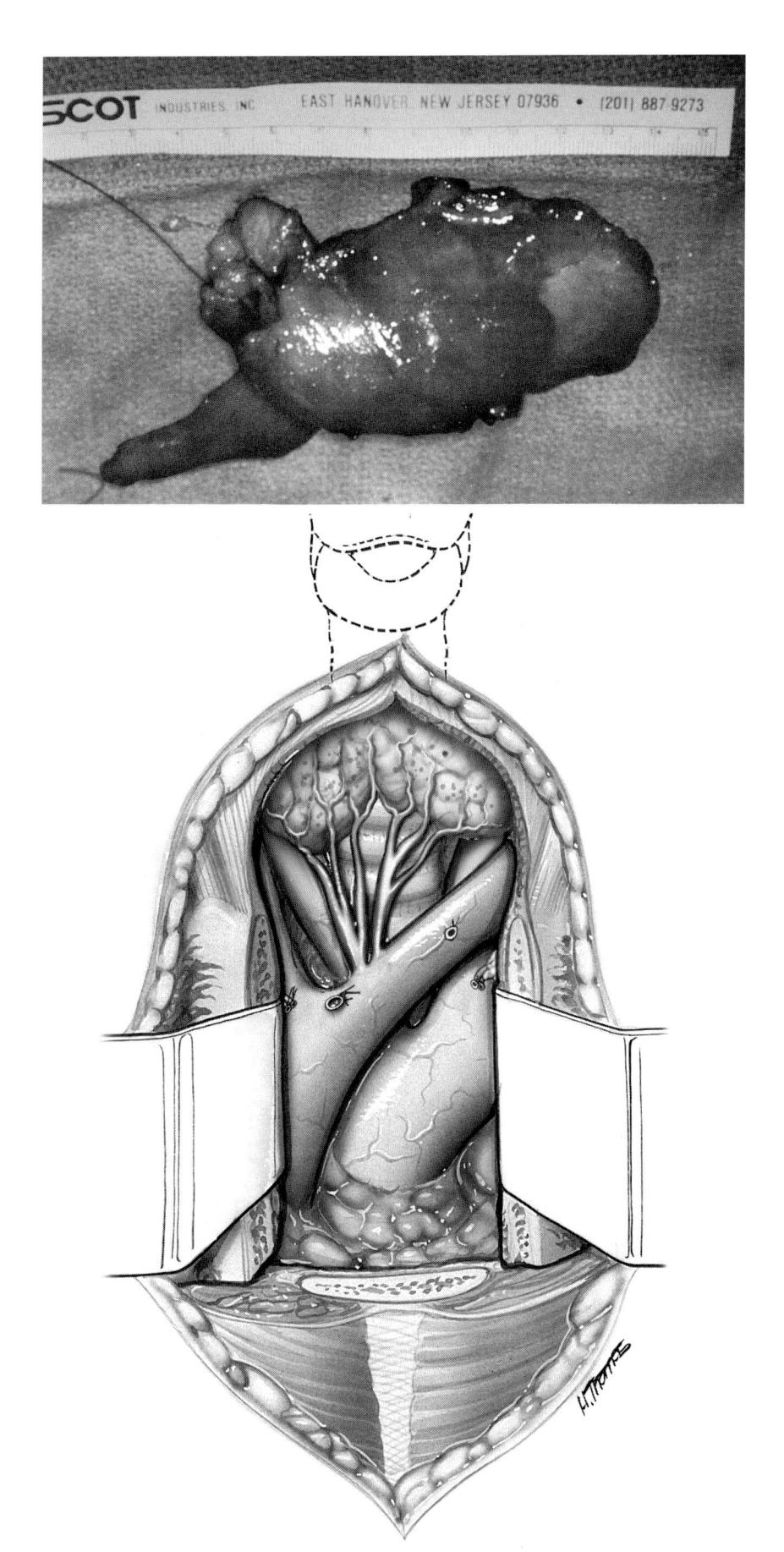

Figure 15–5 • The resected specimen and the resulting surgical defect are depicted.

Chapter 16
Clinical Case: Chondrosarcoma Sternum

James Harvey

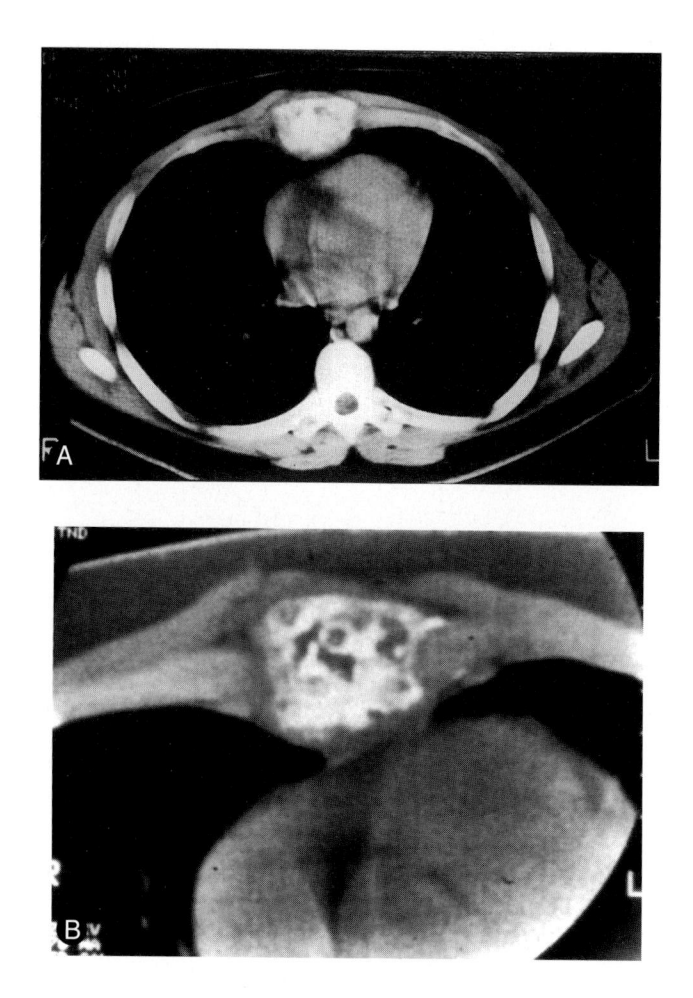

Figure 16–1 • **A,** A 36-year-old man presented with a history of intermittent chest pain for 3 years. Ultimately a soft tissue mass developed, and a computed tomography scan showed a destructive process involving the distal sternum.
B, This extended outside the sternum toward the pericardium.

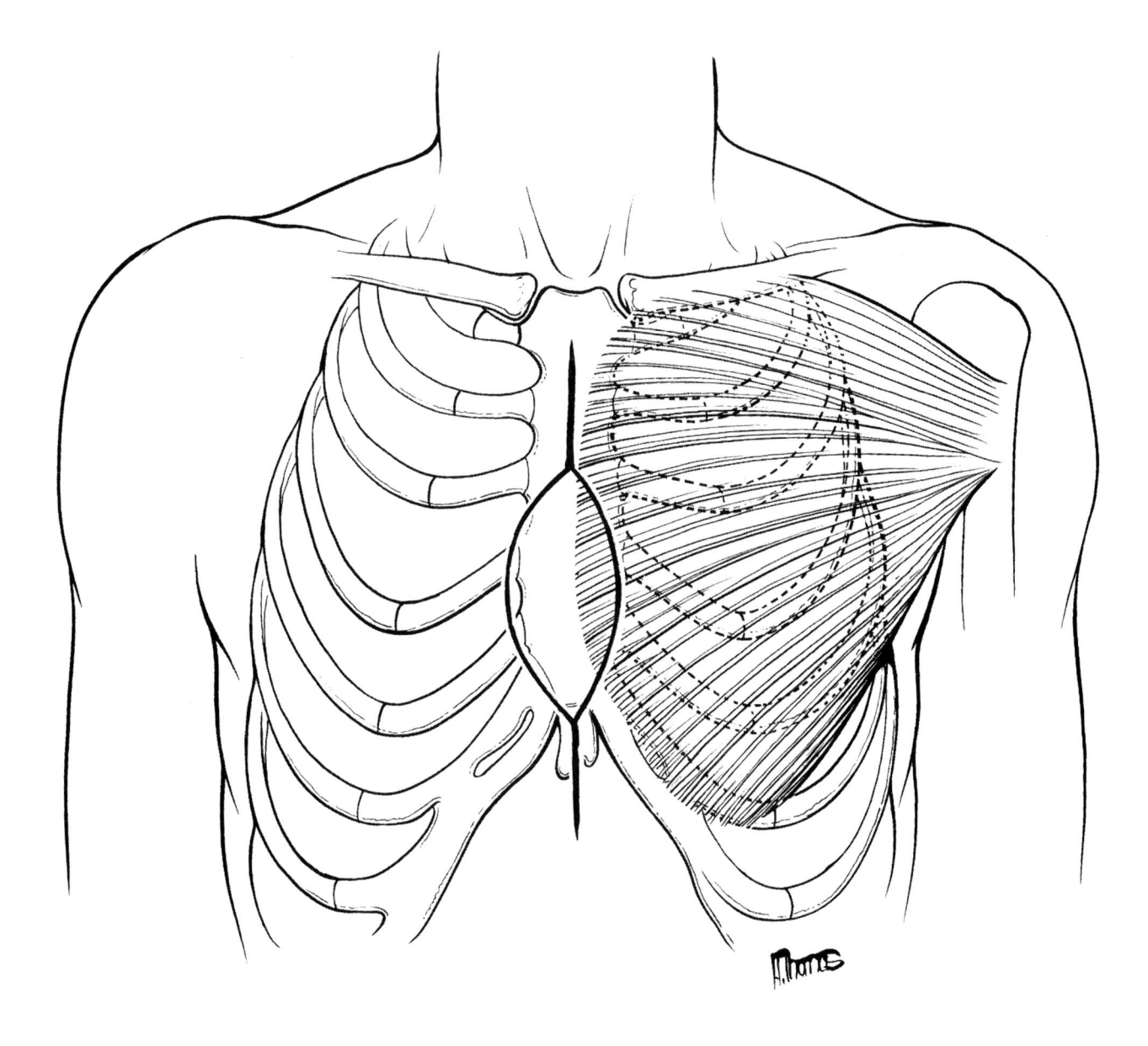

Figure 16–2 • An elliptical skin incision was made around the soft mass along the front of the sternum.

108 • Part II CHEST

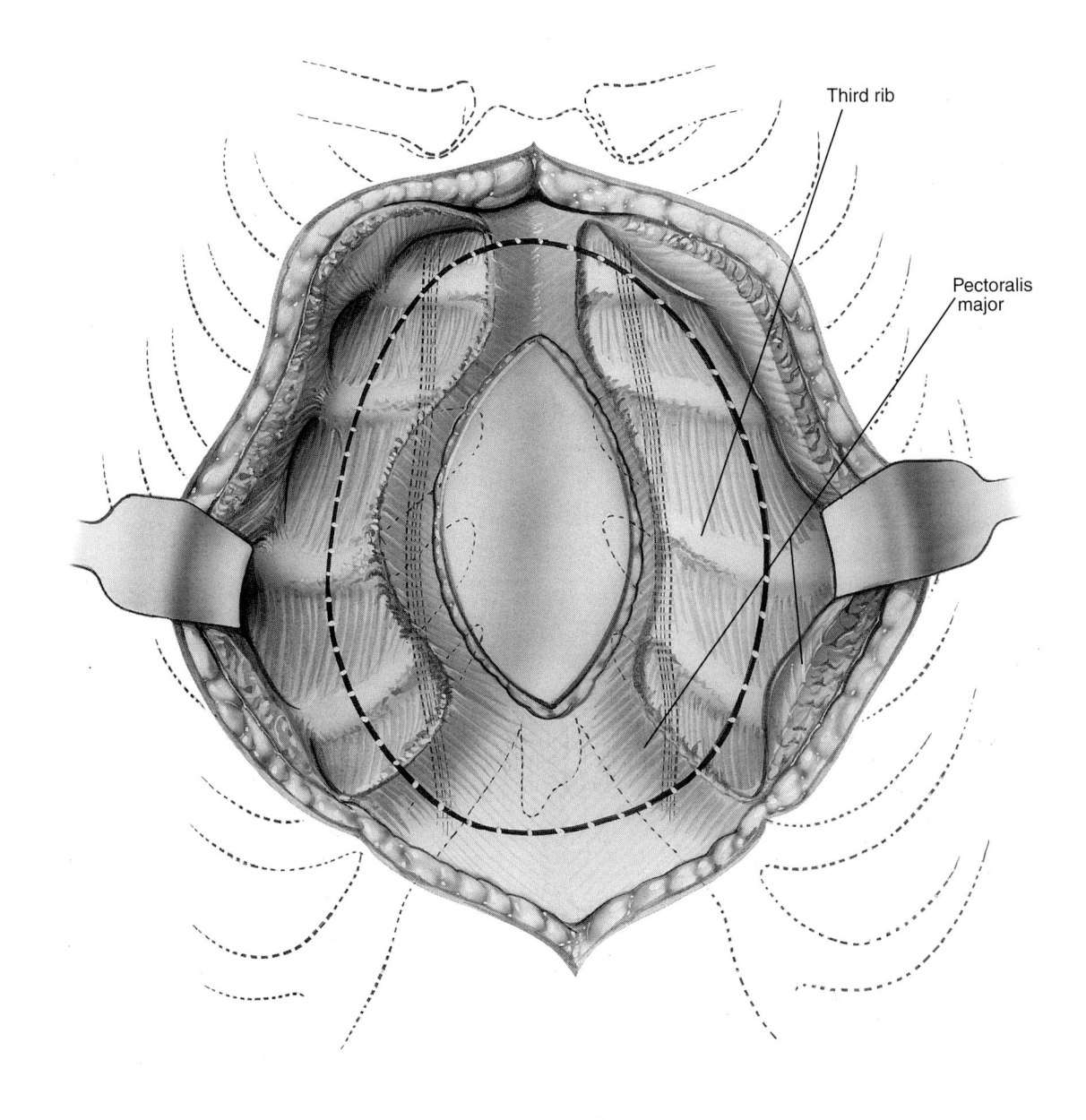

Figure 16–3 • After elevation of the skin flaps, the line of resection of the pectoralis major bilaterally is defined, as are the sections of the ribs to be removed.

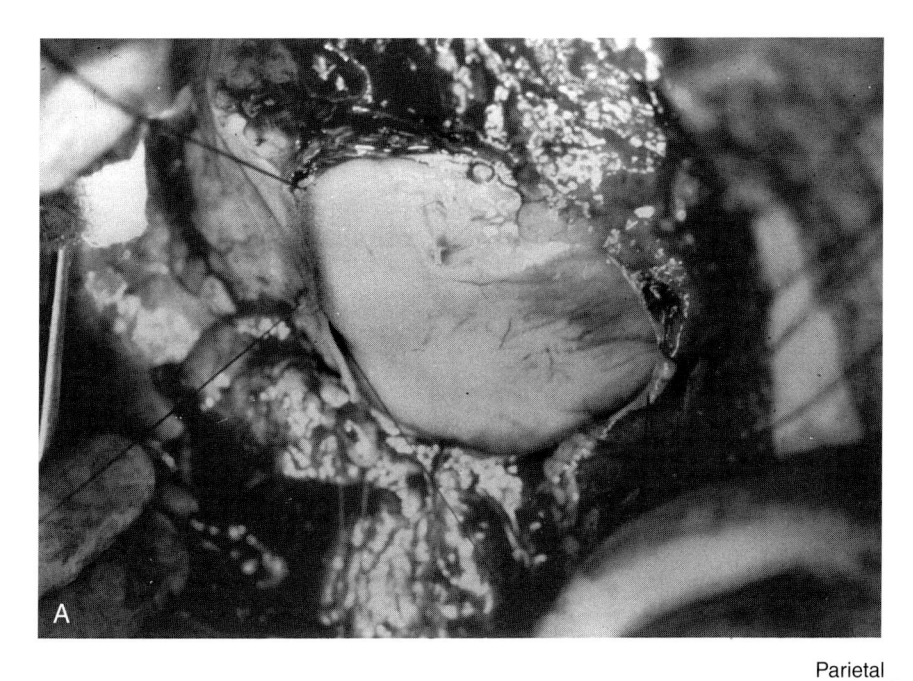

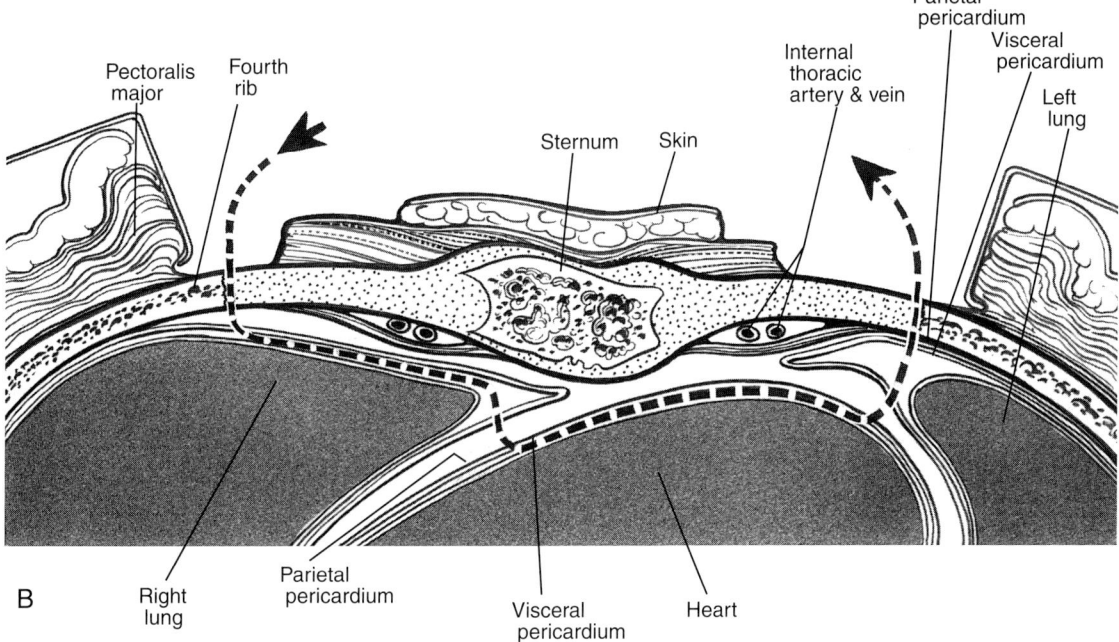

Figure 16–4 • **A,** The specimen is removed, and the resulting defect is depicted. A portion of the pericardium has been removed.
B, A cross-sectional view of the line of resection depicts the removal of a portion of the fourth rib, the parietal pleura, and pericardium, as well as both internal mammary vessels.

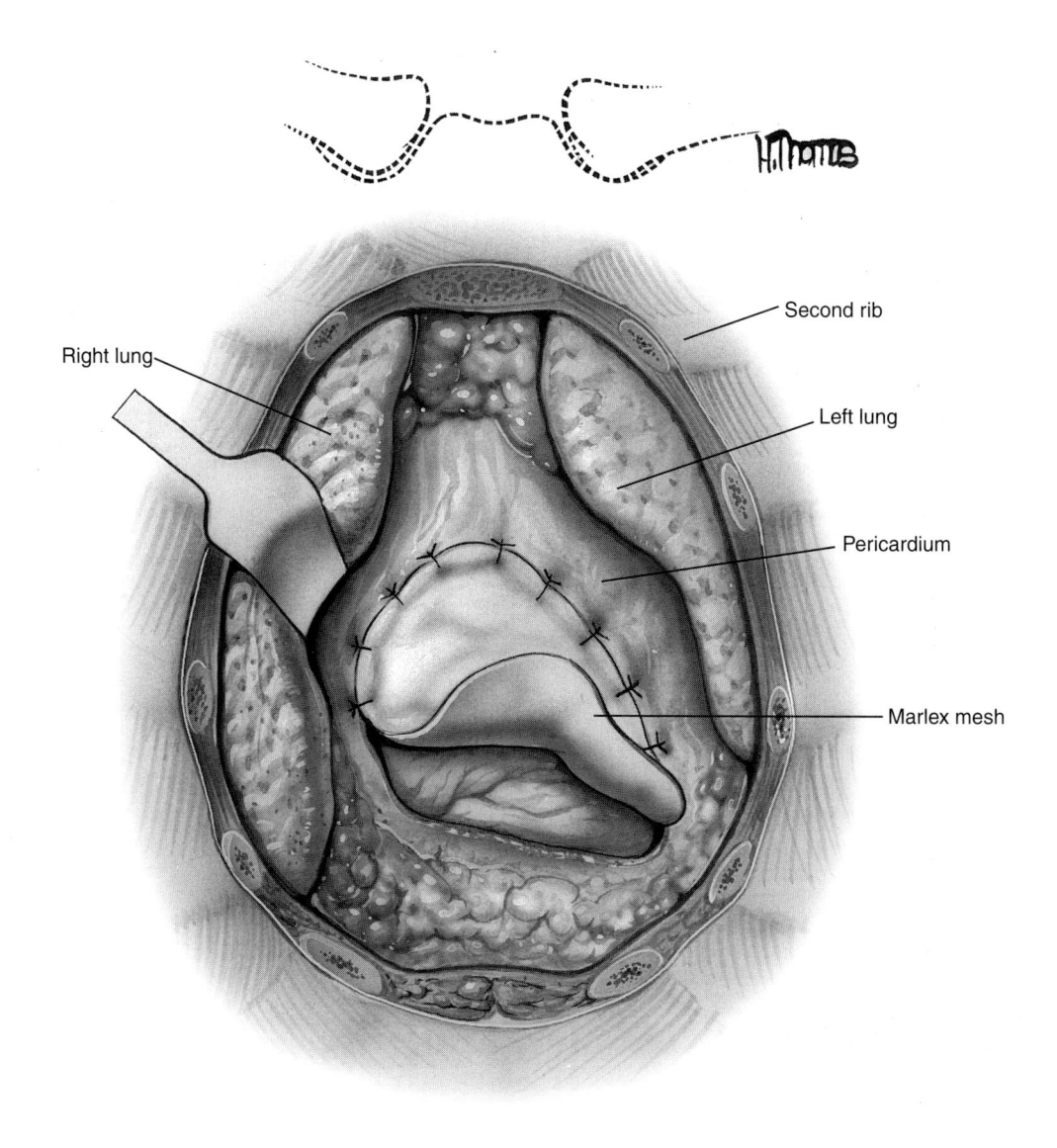

Figure 16–5 • Marlex mesh is used to reconstruct the pericardium.

Clinical Case: Chondrosarcoma Sternum • 111

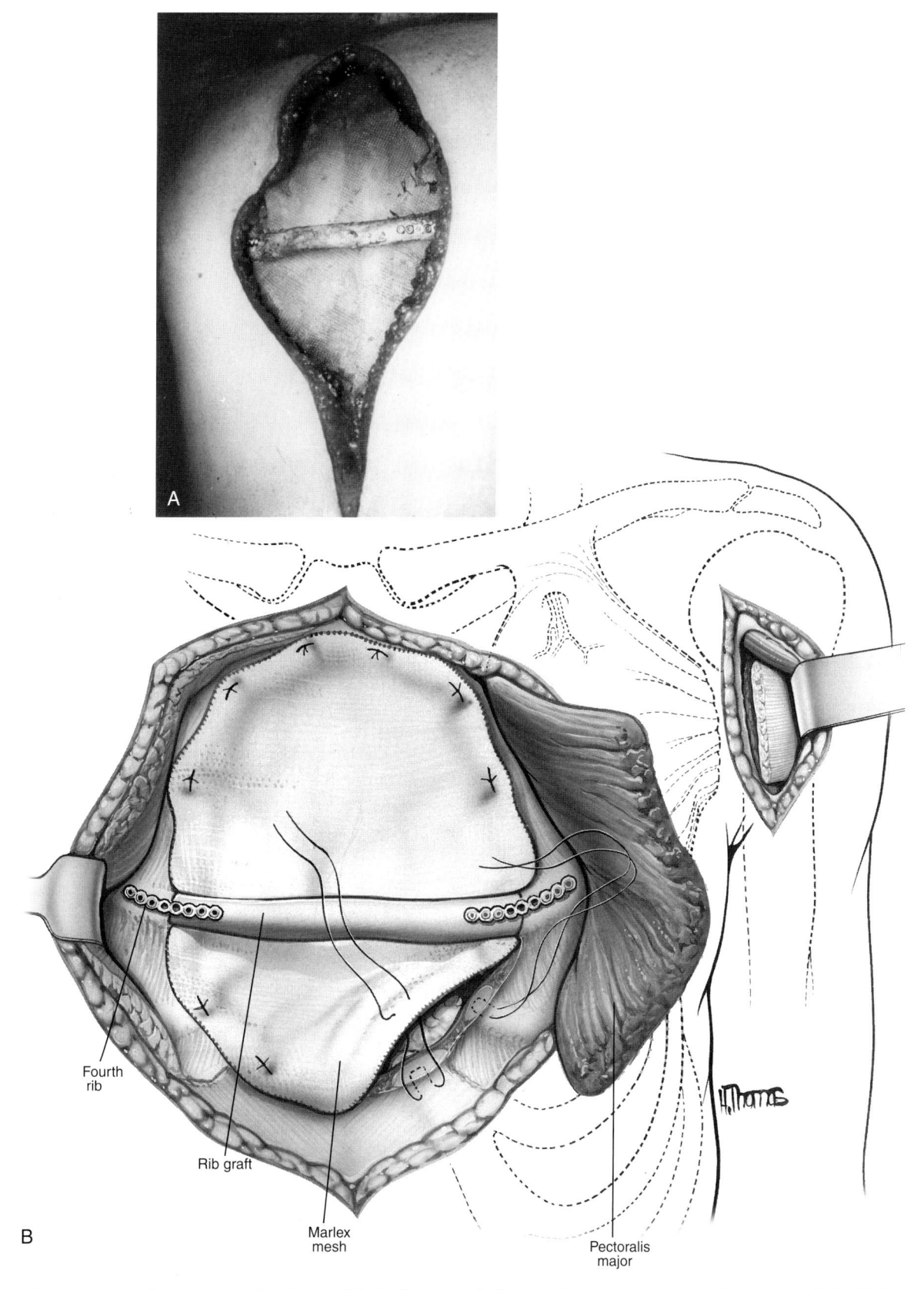

Figure 16–6 • **A,** A second piece of Marlex mesh is used to reconstruct the sternal deficit. A segment of rib is placed across the defect and secured with two small plates.
   B, In this illustration the pectoralis major head is cut to allow advancement of the pectoralis major muscle.

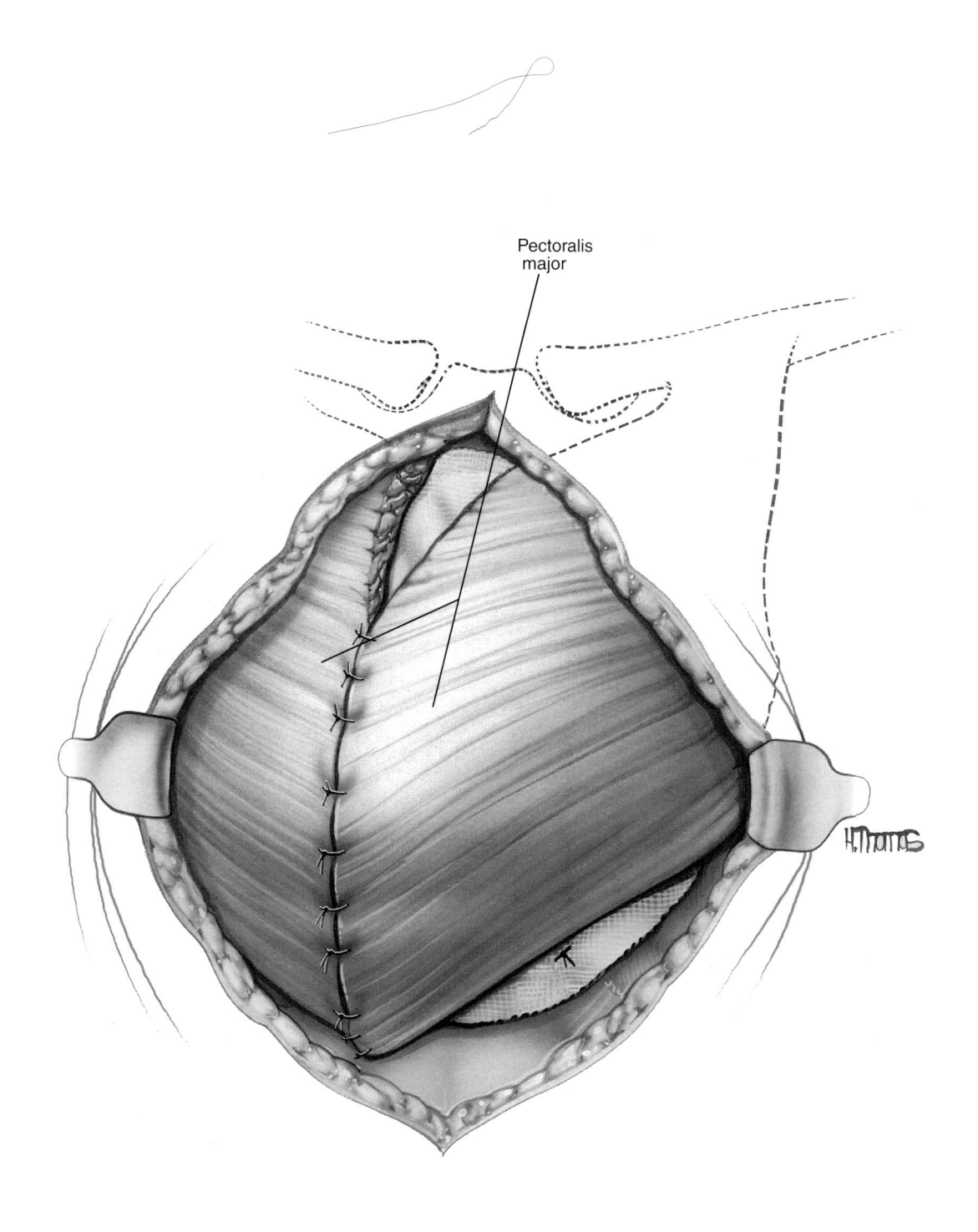

Figure 16–7 • The remaining pectoralis major muscles are advanced over the defect.

Chapter 17
Transhiatal Esophageal Resection and Gastric Pull-up

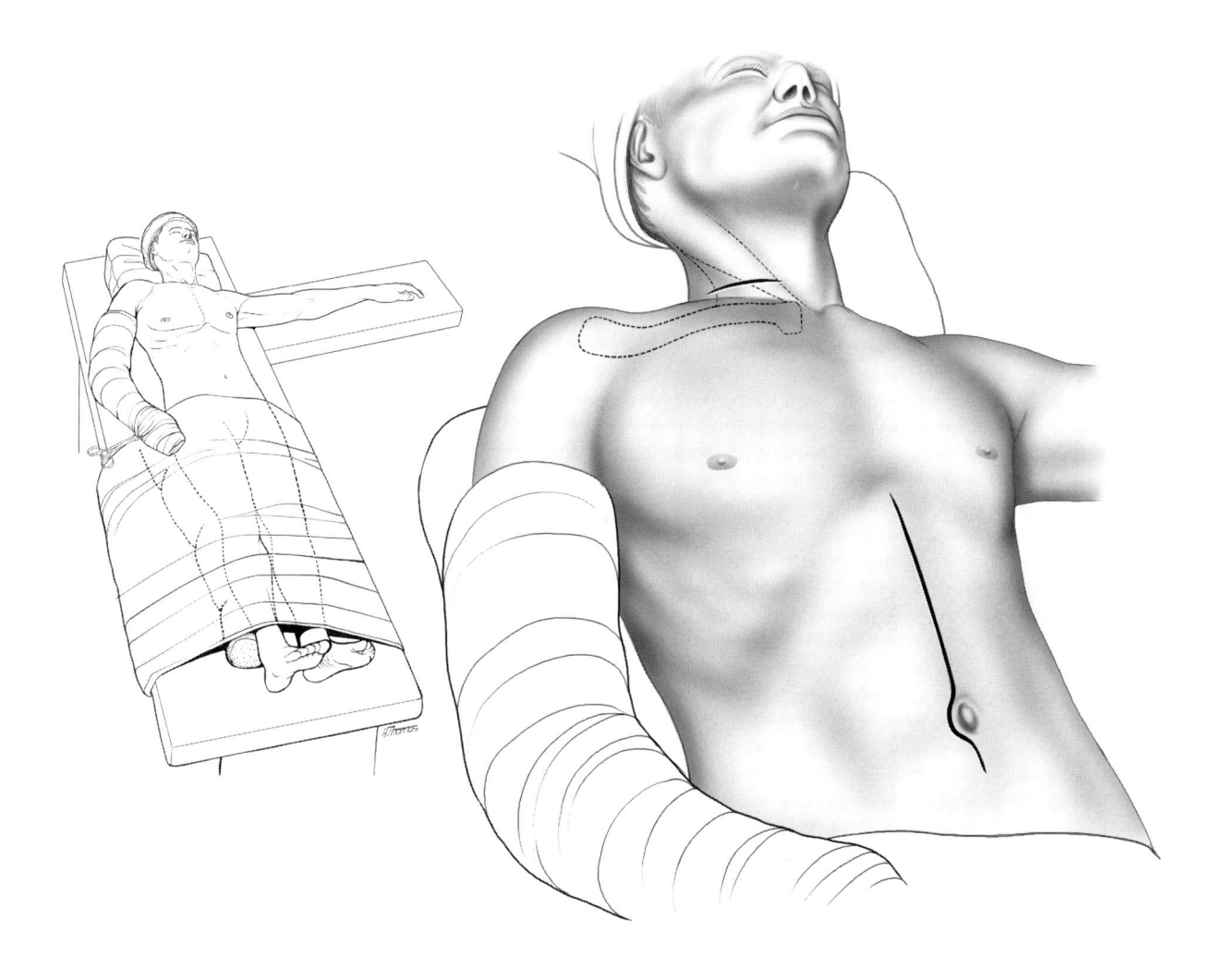

Figure 17–1 • The patient is placed on the operative table as indicated. This allows access to the right chest should a thoracotomy be necessary.

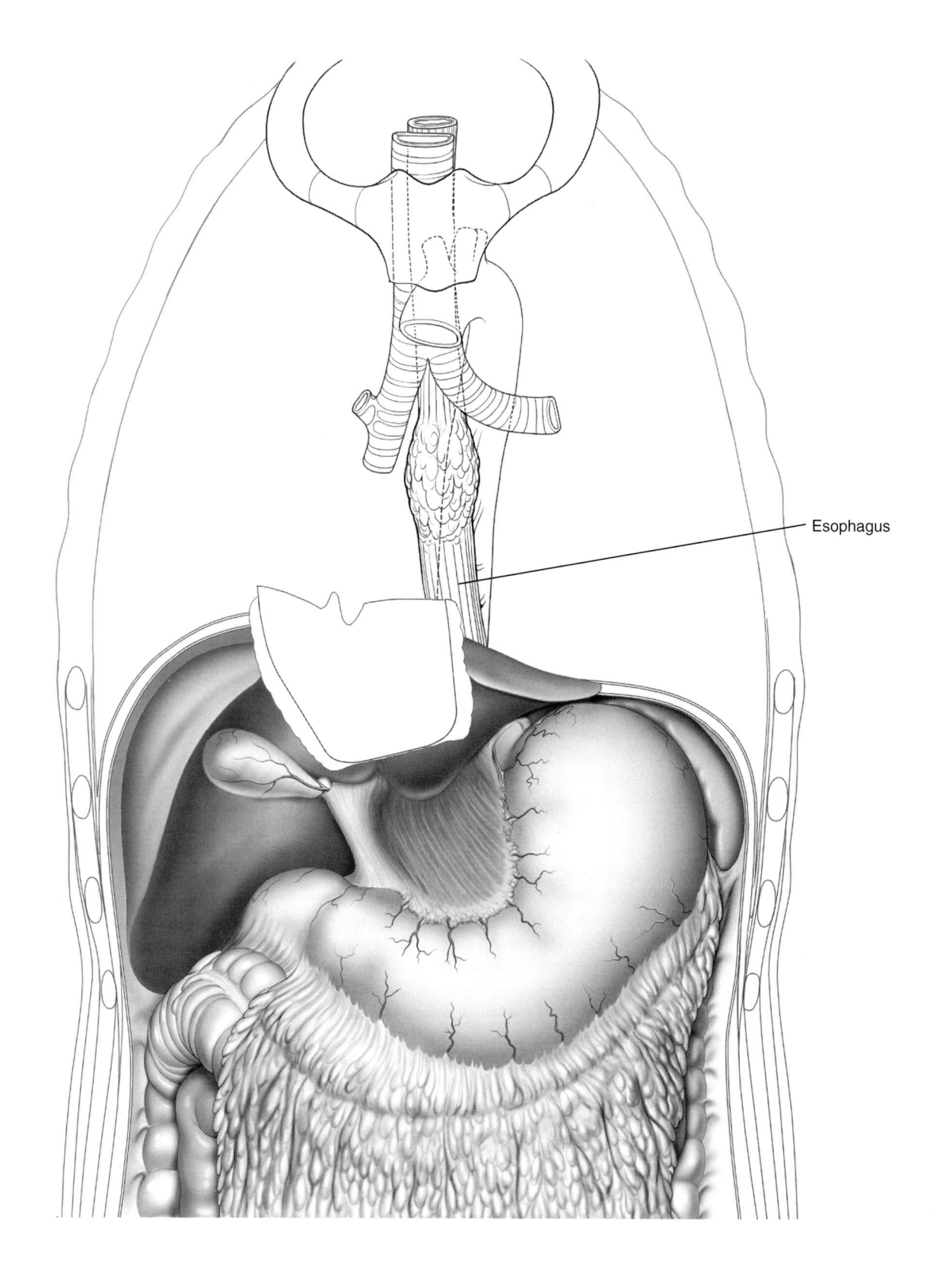

Figure 17–2 • A midline abdominal incision is performed.

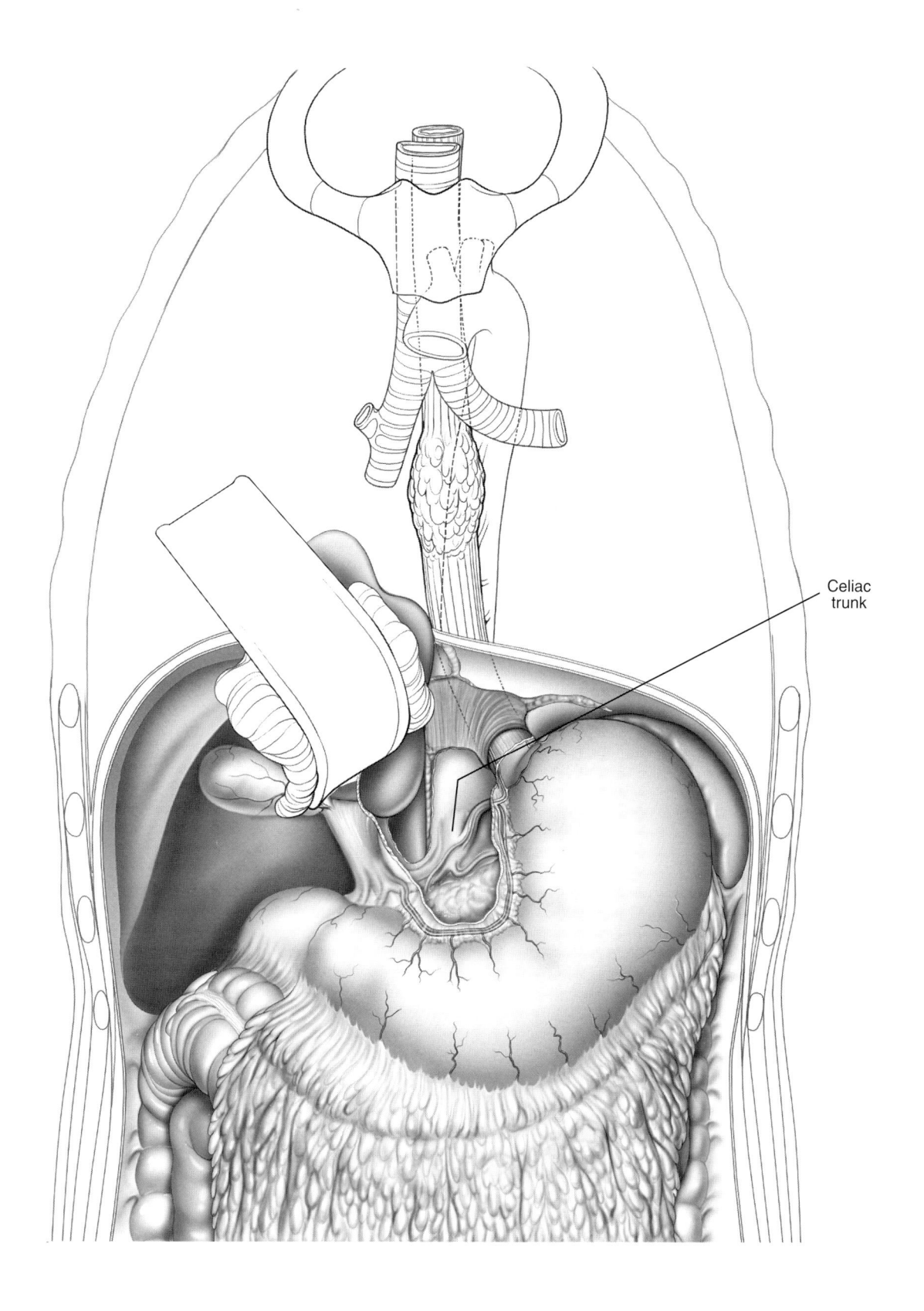

Figure 17–3 • The left triangular ligament is divided and the liver is reflected medially. The gastrohepatic ligament is incised.

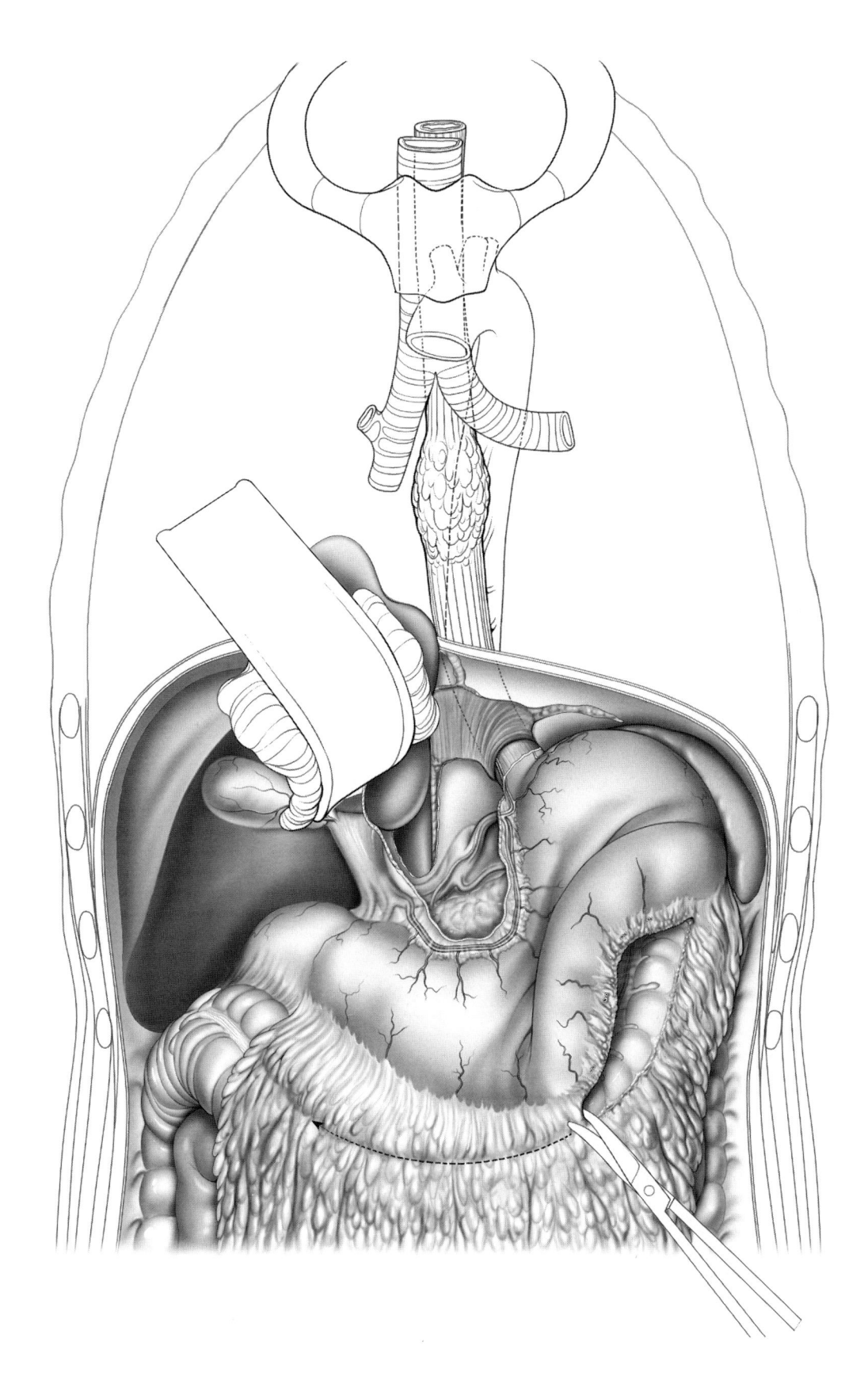

Figure 17–4 • The greater curvature of the stomach is mobilized by dividing the greater omentum distal to the vascular arcade of the gastroepiploics.

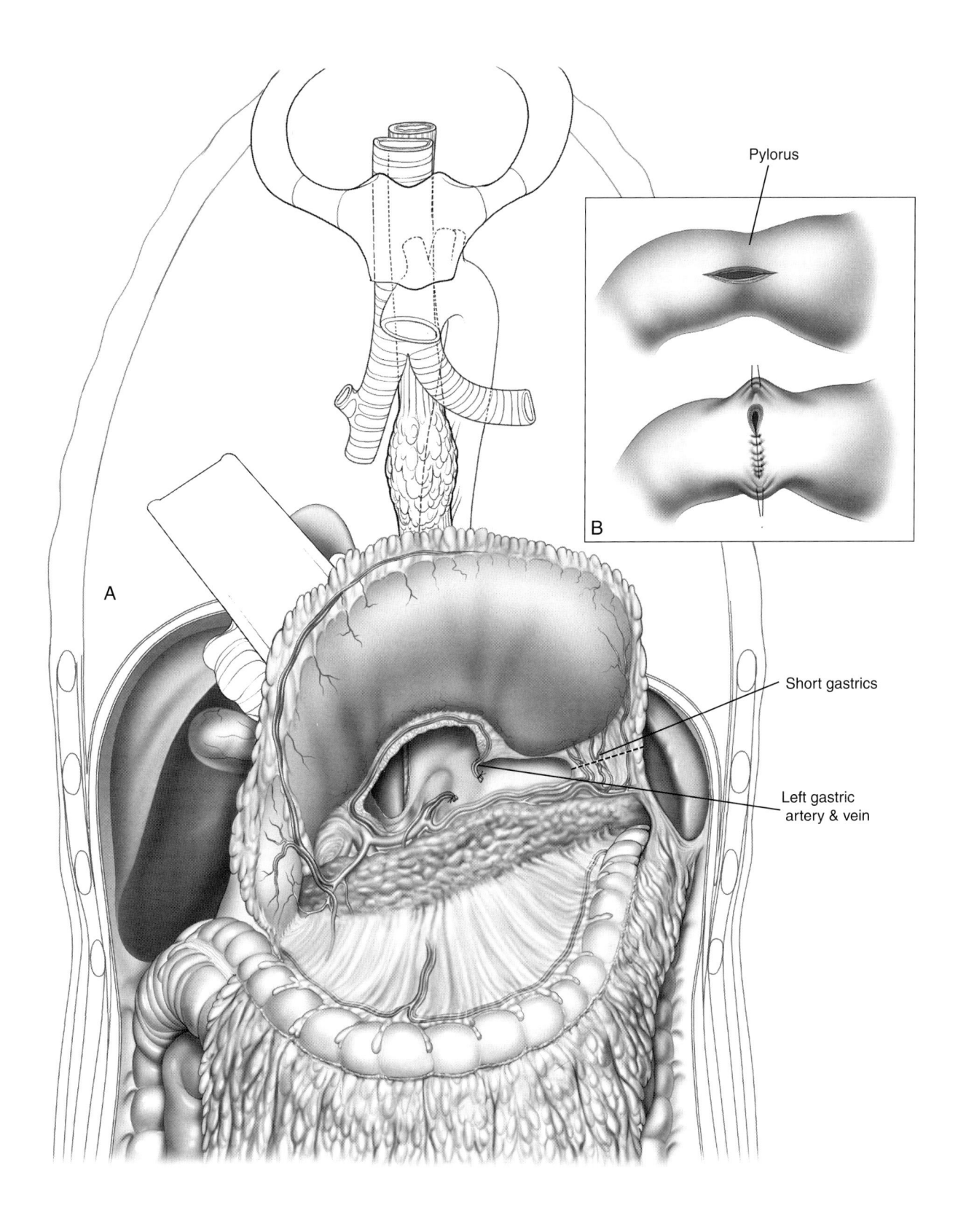

Figure 17–5 • **A,** The left gastric and short gastrics are divided.
B, A pyloroplasty is performed.

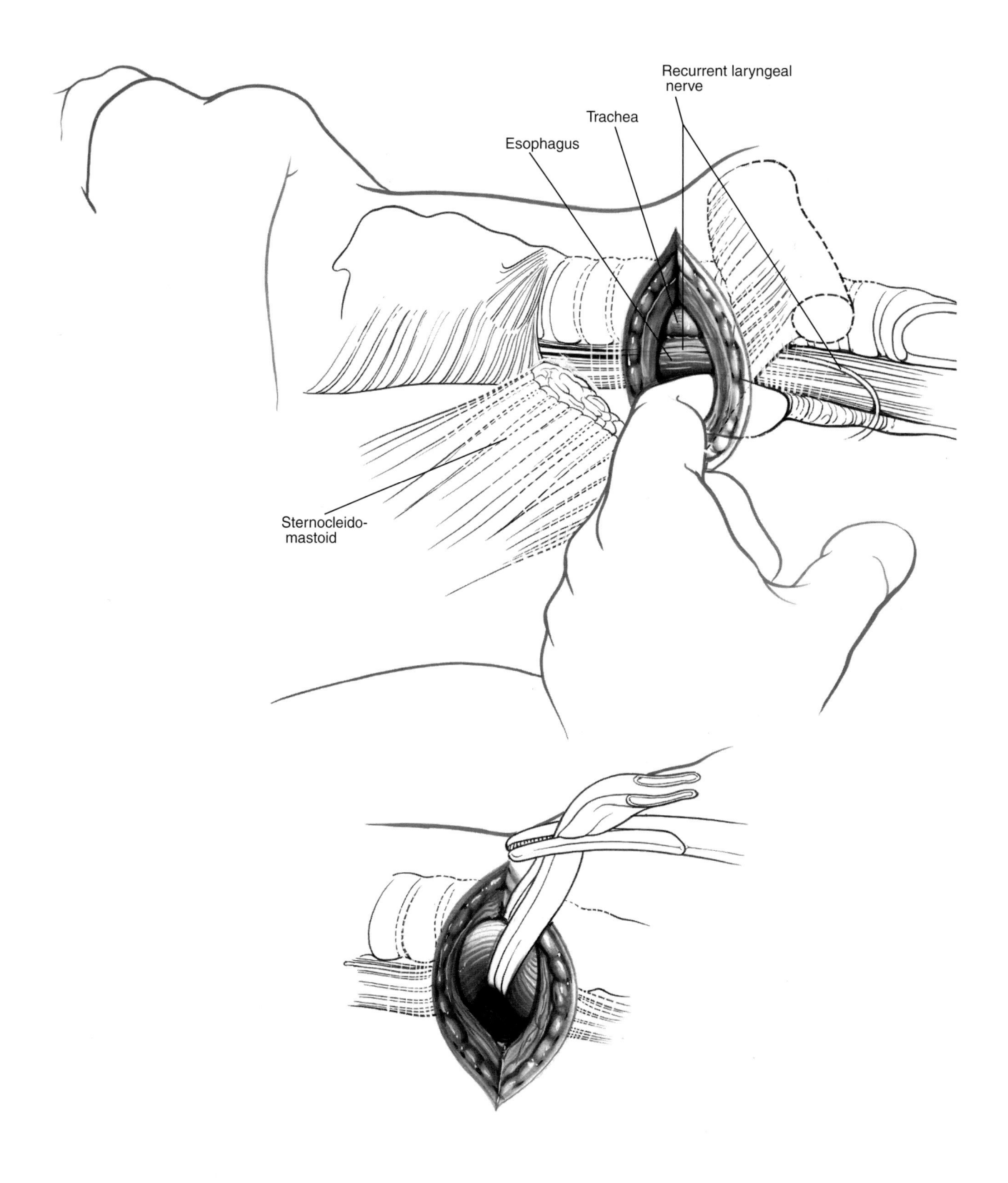

Figure 17–6 • An incision is made in the right neck, and the esophagus is initially mobilized off the prevertebral fascia.

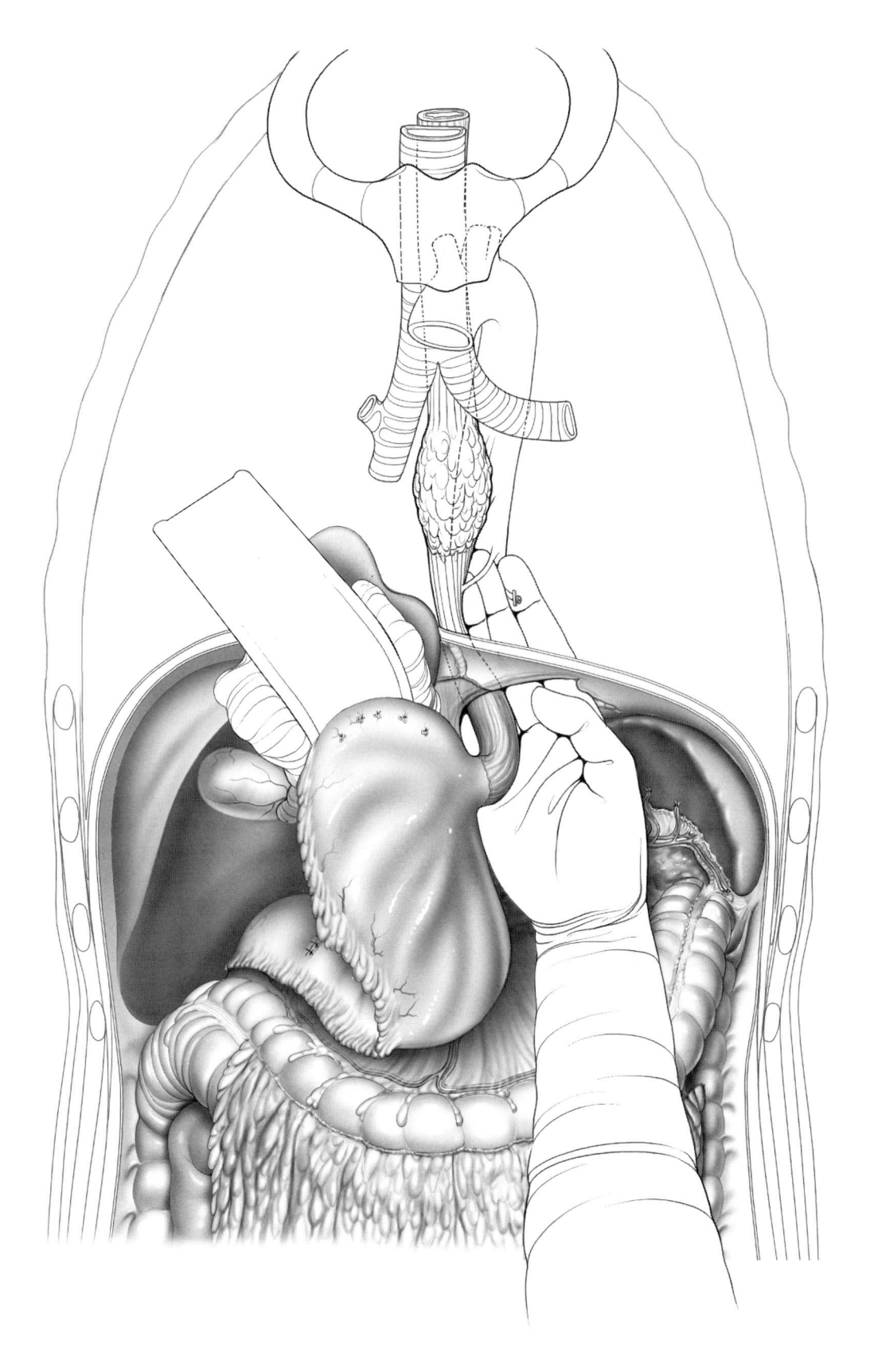

Figure 17–7 • Returning to the abdomen, the hiatus is widened and mobilization of the esophagus is commenced. Branches off the aorta are clipped and divided under direct vision initially through the hiatus.

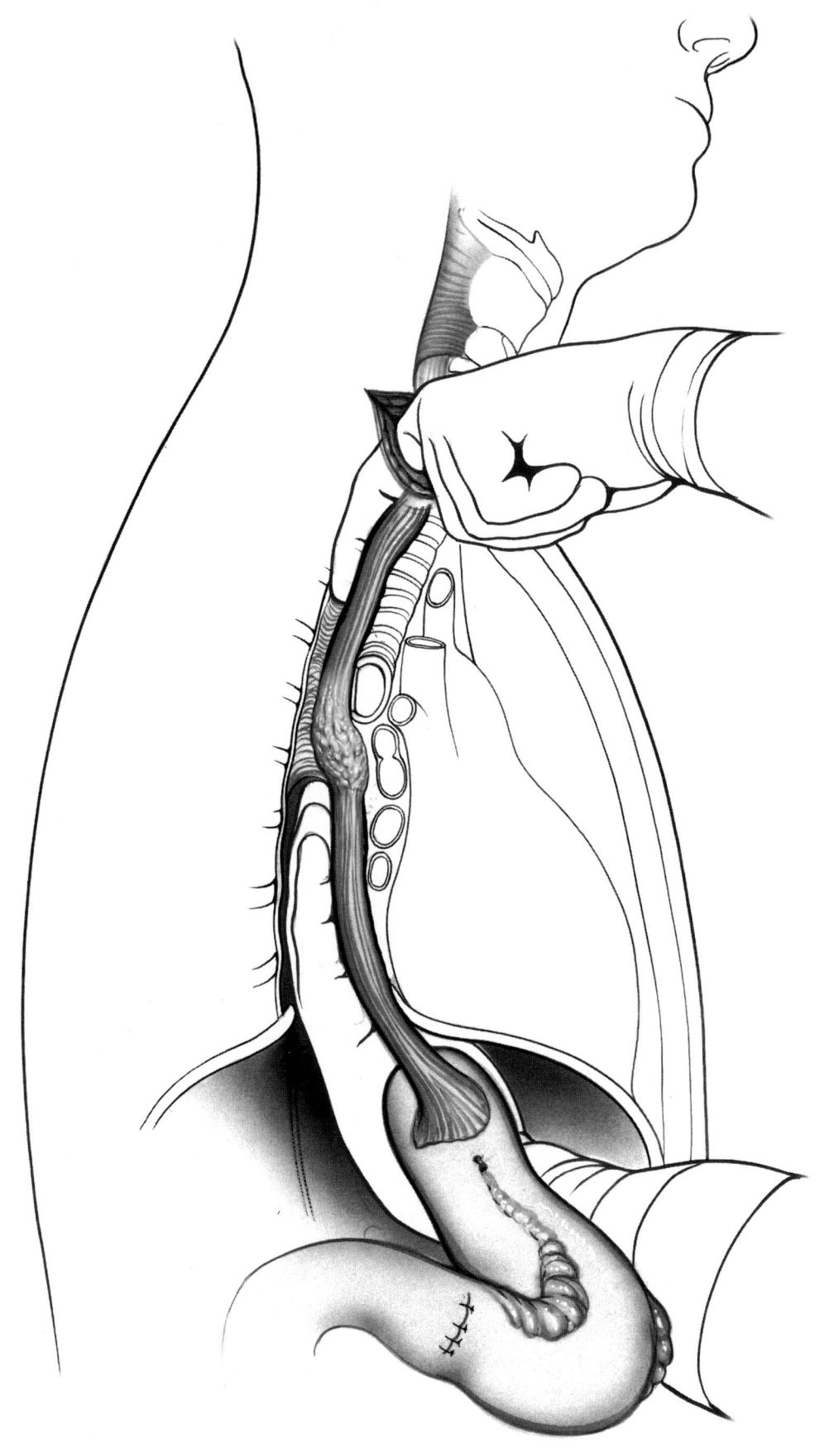

Figure 17–8 • The esophageal resection is completed bluntly from the neck and abdomen.

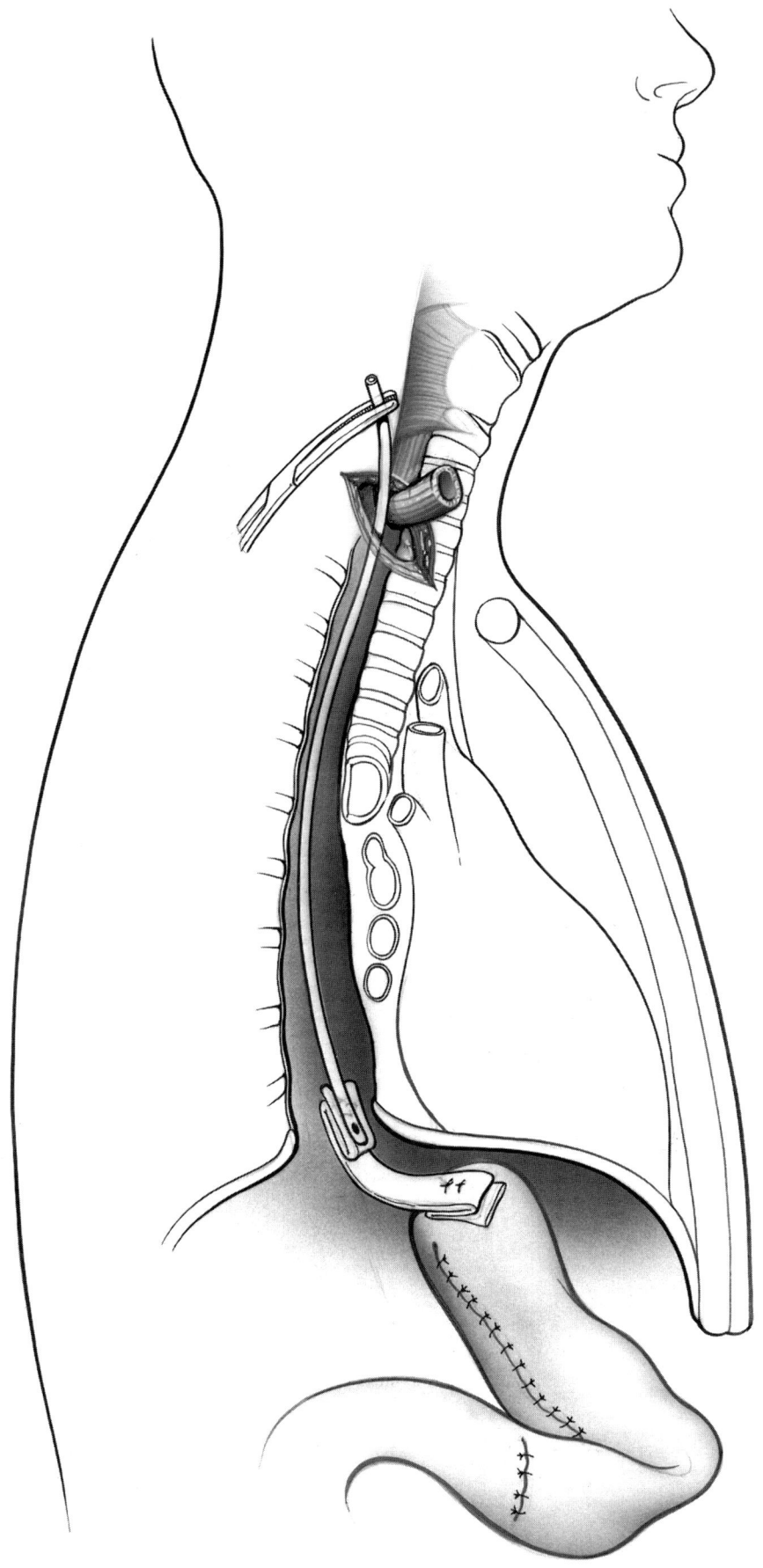

Figure 17–9 • The proximal esophagus is divided, and the specimen is delivered into the abdomen. The stomach is prepared, to bring it up through the resected bed of the esophagus.

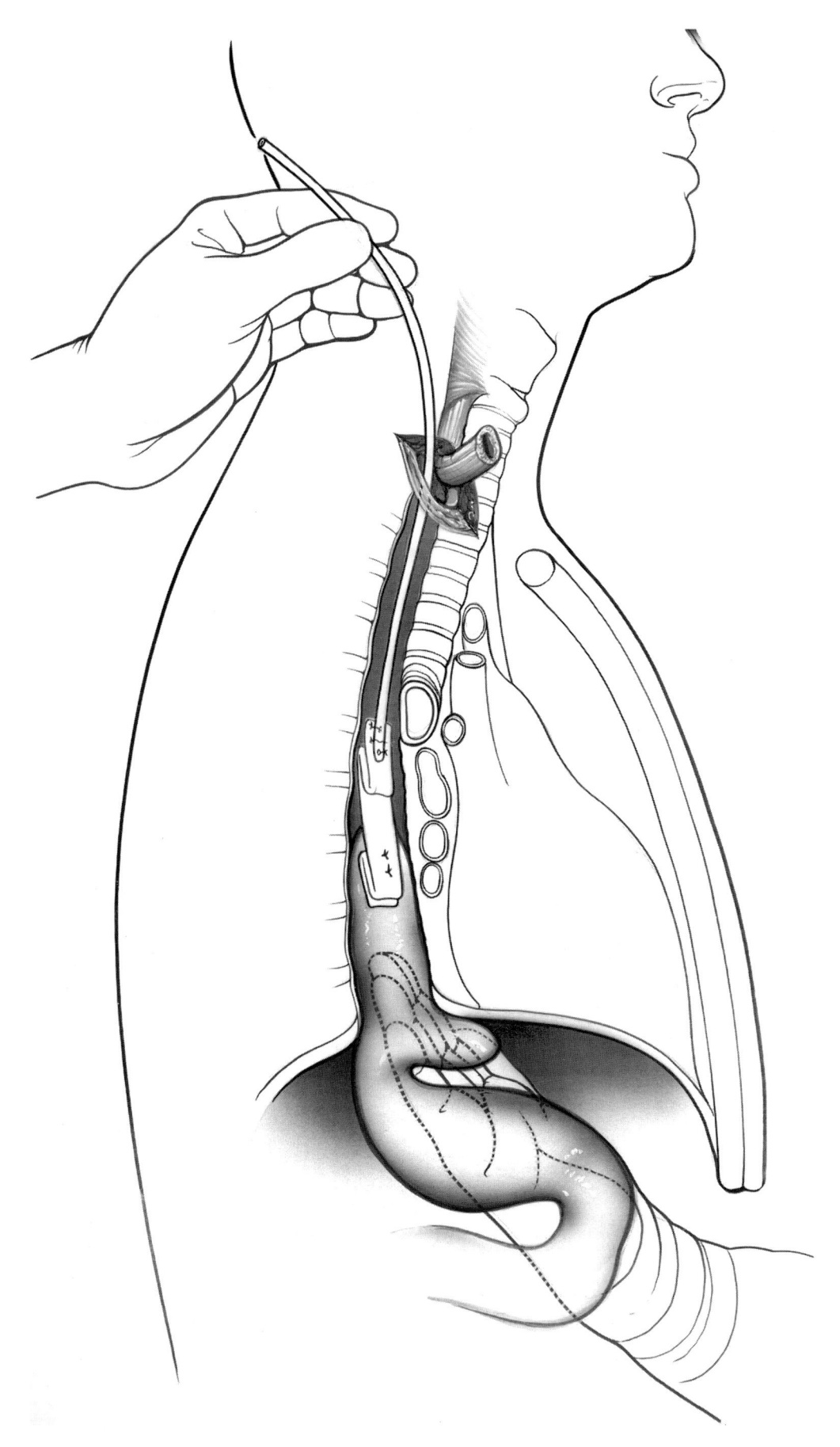

Figure 17–10 • Using gentle traction from above, the stomach is delivered into the neck.

Transhiatal Esophageal Resection and Gastric Pull-up • 123

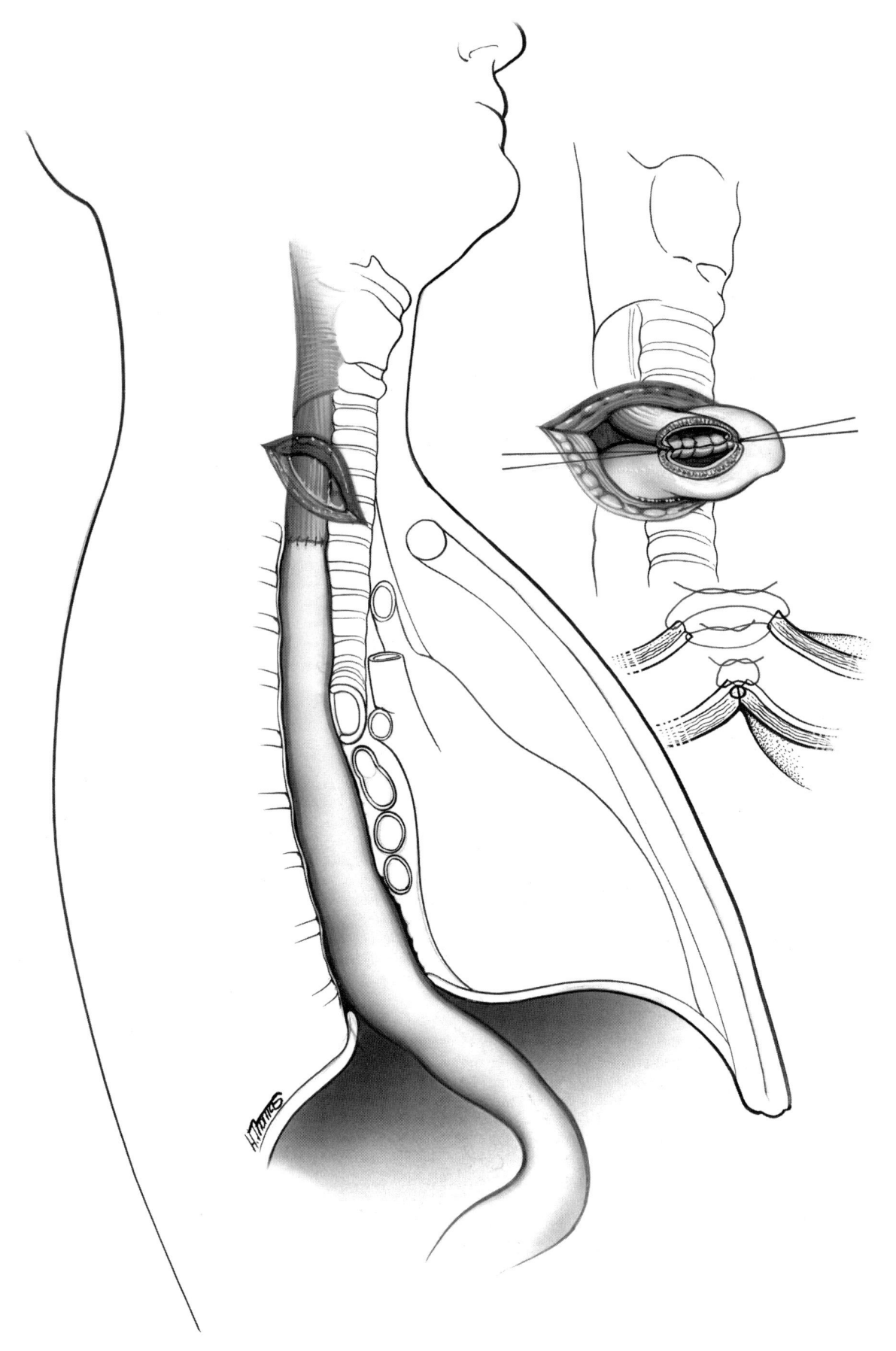

Figure 17–11 • An anastomosis is performed in the neck.

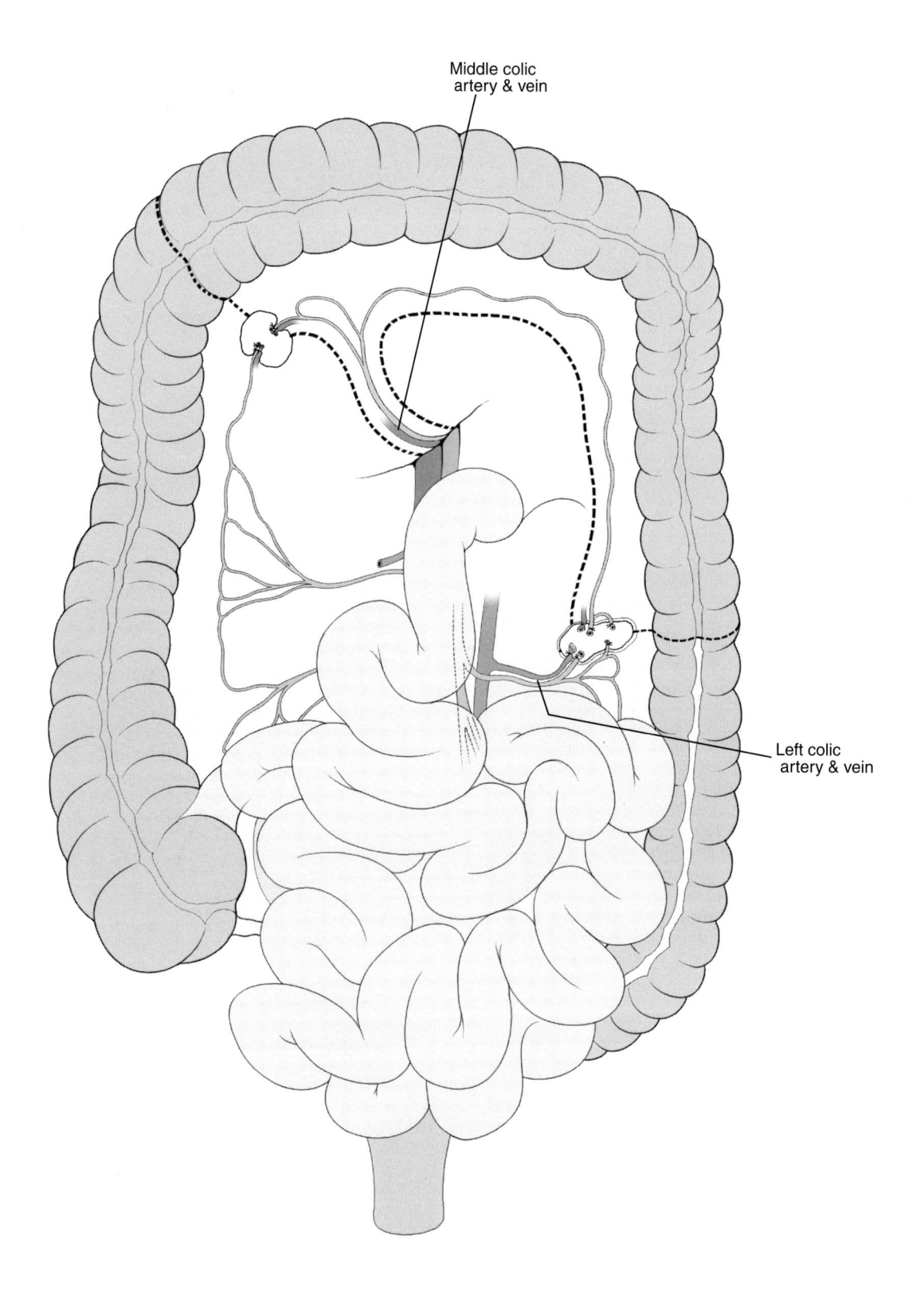

Figure 17–12 • As an alternative to a gastric interposition, a colonic segment such as the transverse colon can be utilized.

Transhiatal Esophageal Resection and Gastric Pull-up • 125

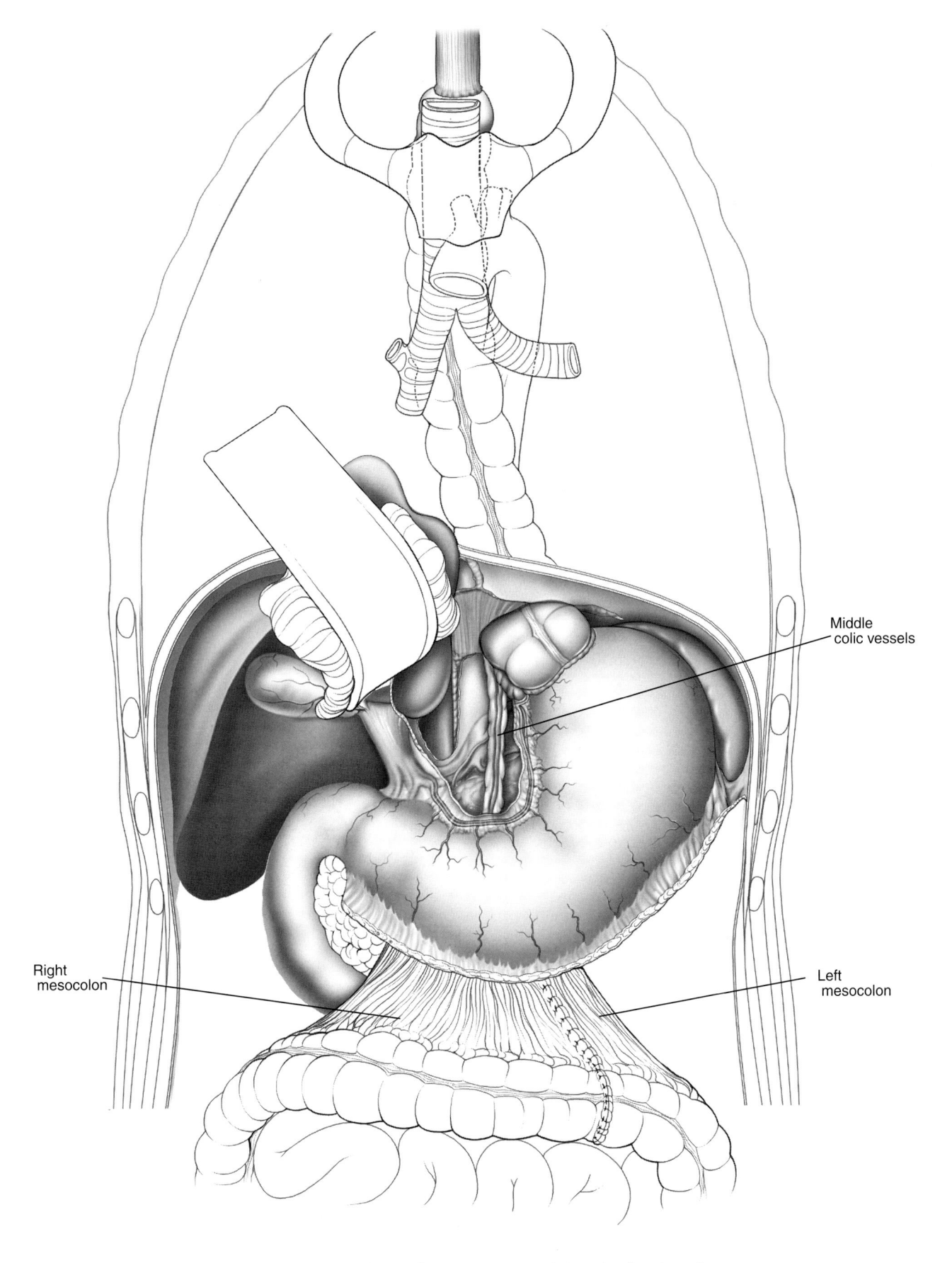

Figure 17–13 • The colonic interposition is depicted.

// Part II CHEST

Chapter 18
Thoracic Esophagectomy

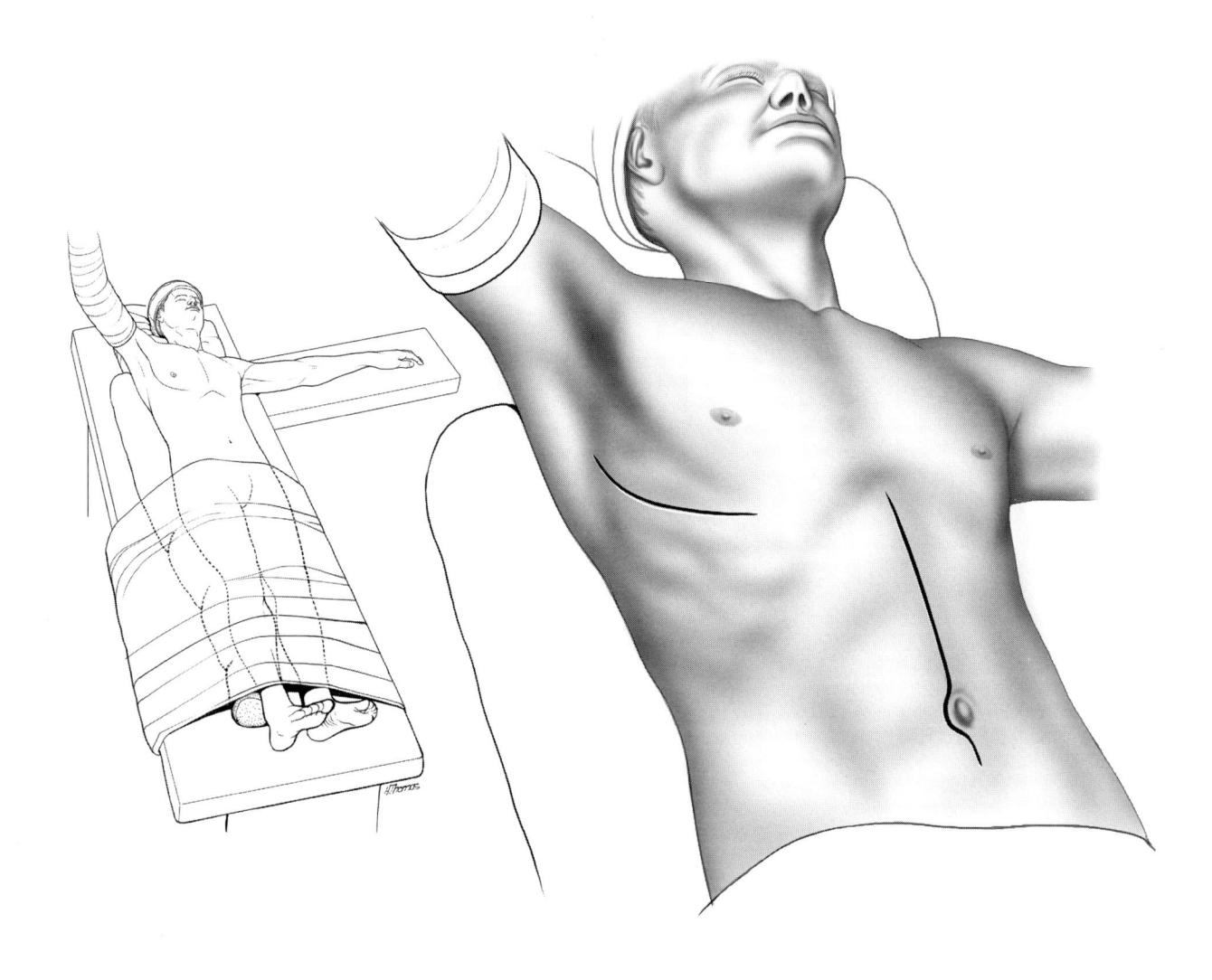

Figure 18–1 • The patient is placed on the operative table and positioned to allow a right thoracotomy incision and a midline abdominal incision.

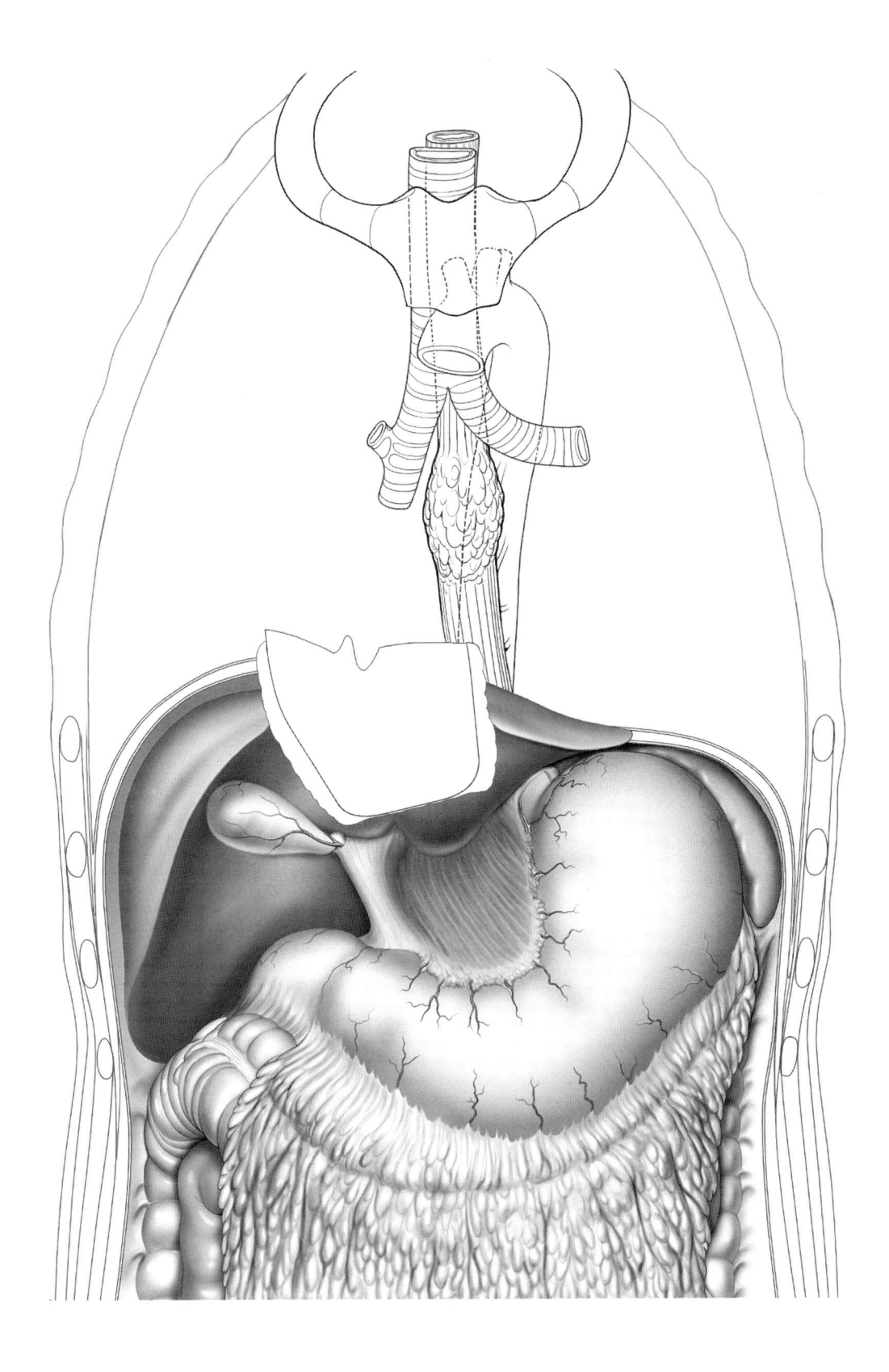

Figure 18–2 • A midline abdominal incision is performed.

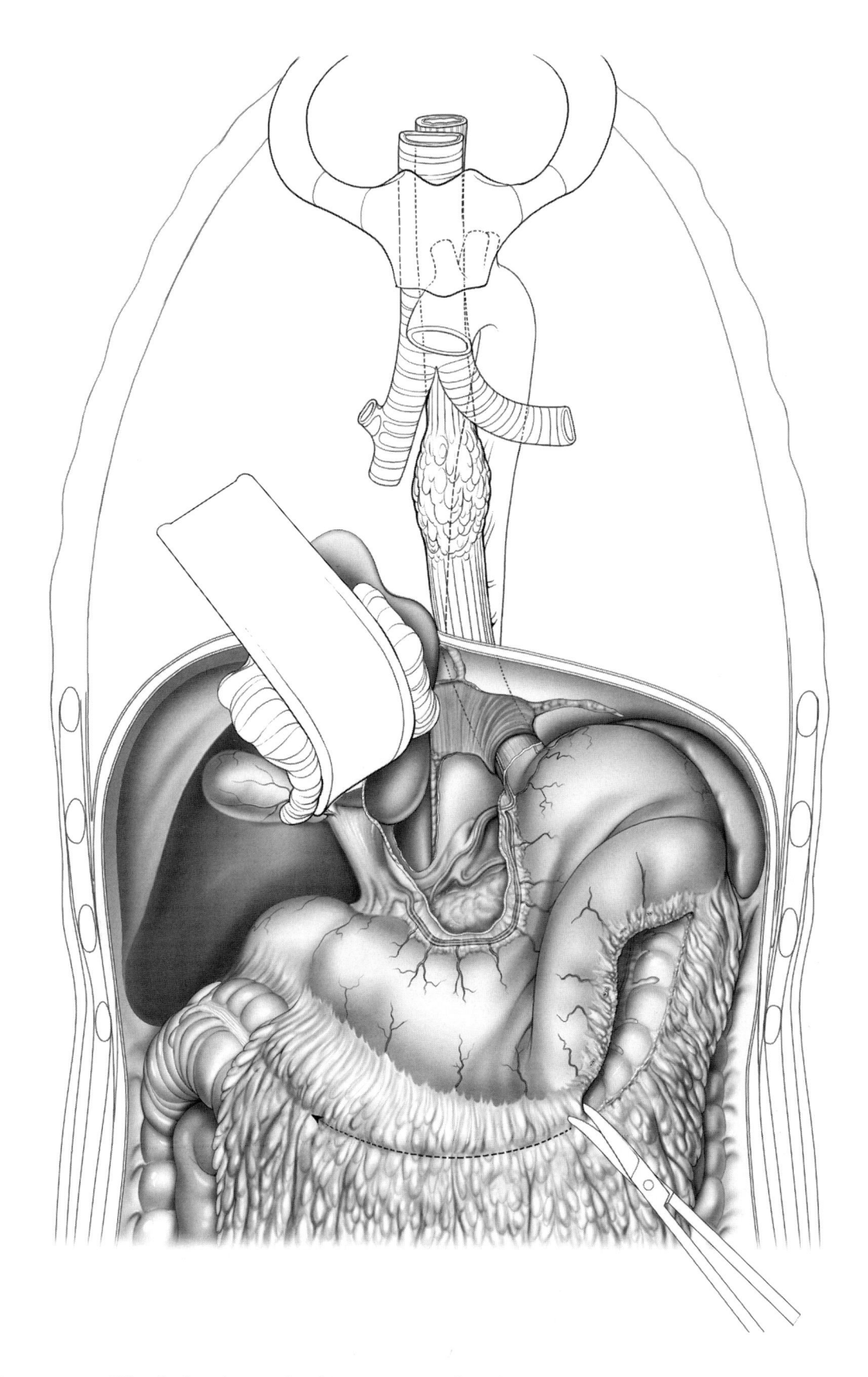

Figure 18-3 • The left triangular ligament is divided, and the liver is reflected medially. The gastrohepatic ligament is divided, and the greater curvature of the stomach is mobilized.

Thoracic Esophagectomy • 129

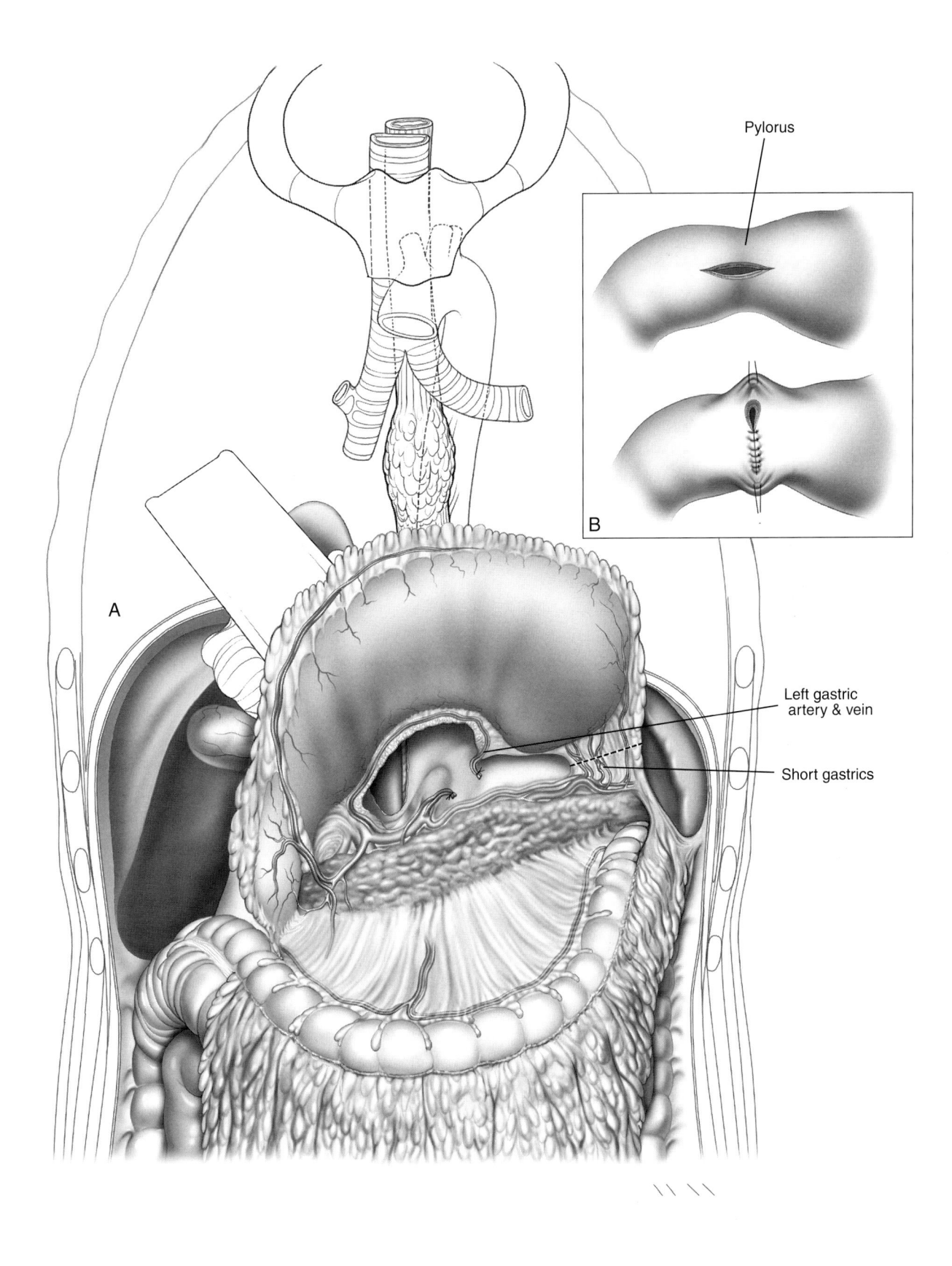

Figure 18–4 • **A,** The left gastric artery and vein are divided, as are the short gastrics. **B,** A pyloroplasty is performed.

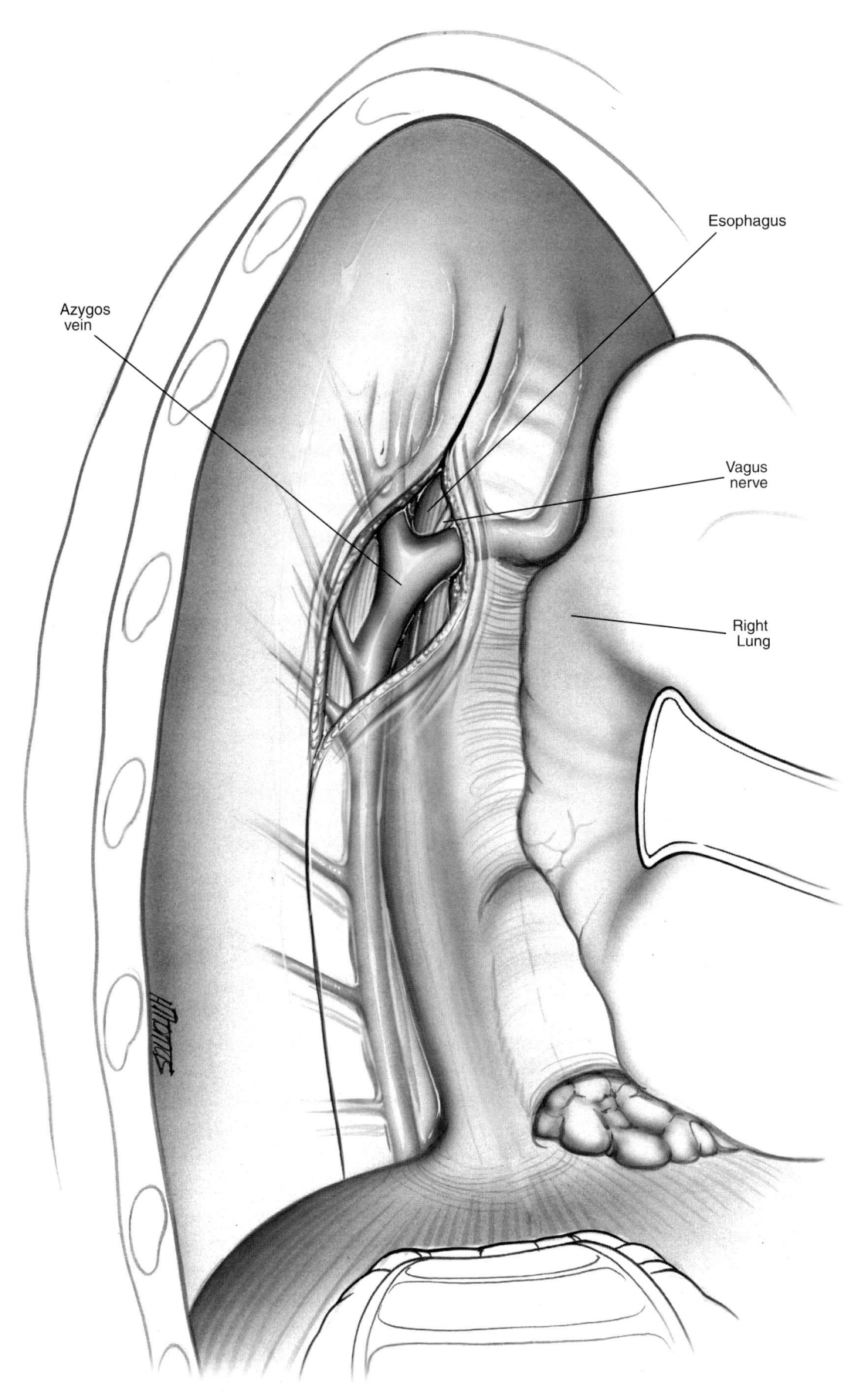

Figure 18–5 • Through a standard right thoracotomy incision the chest is entered, and the parietal pleura is incised at the level of the azygos vein. Single lung ventilation facilitates the exposure.

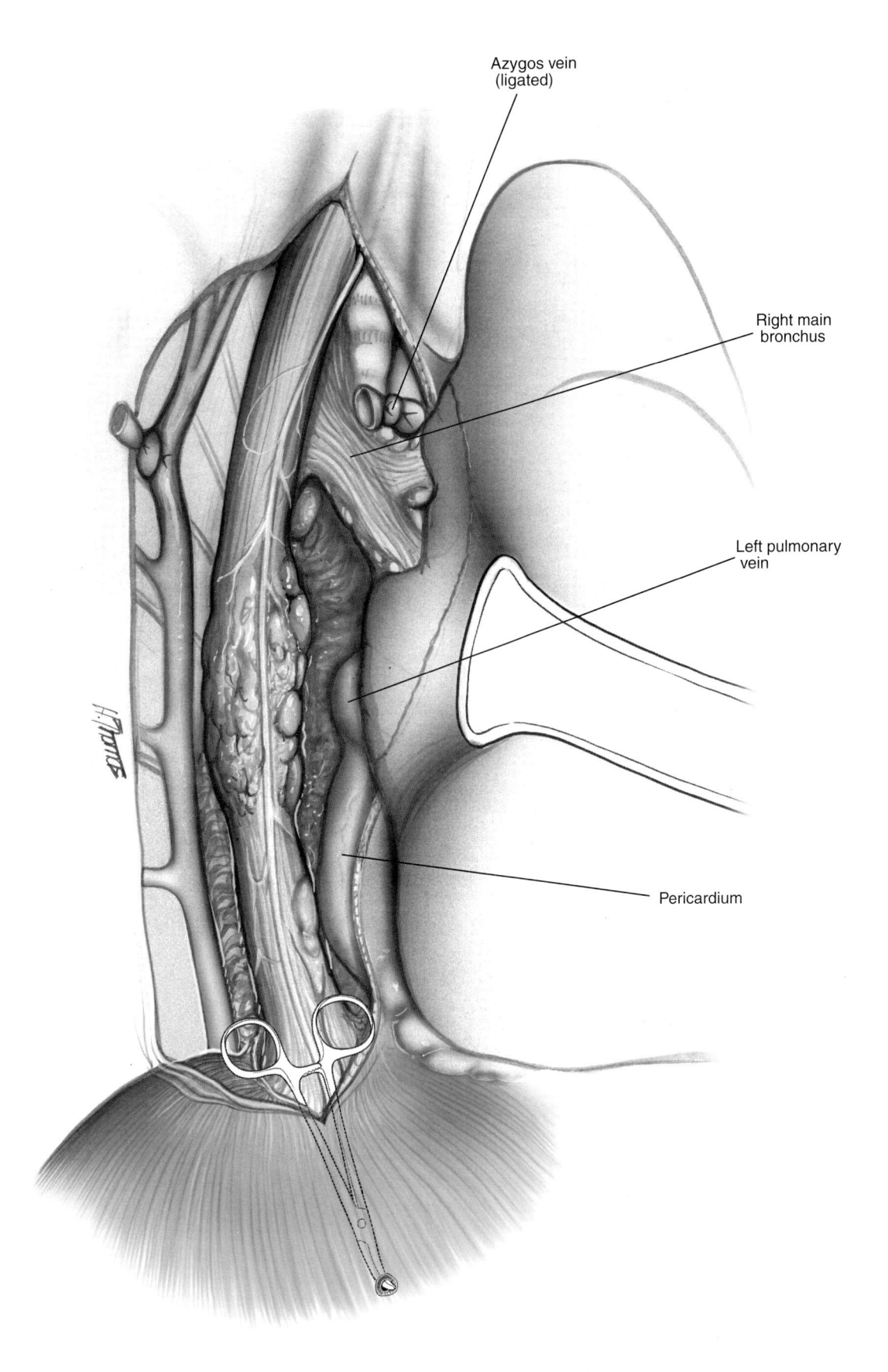

Figure 18–6 • The azygos vein is ligated and the parietal pleura along its entire length is incised. The hiatus is opened.

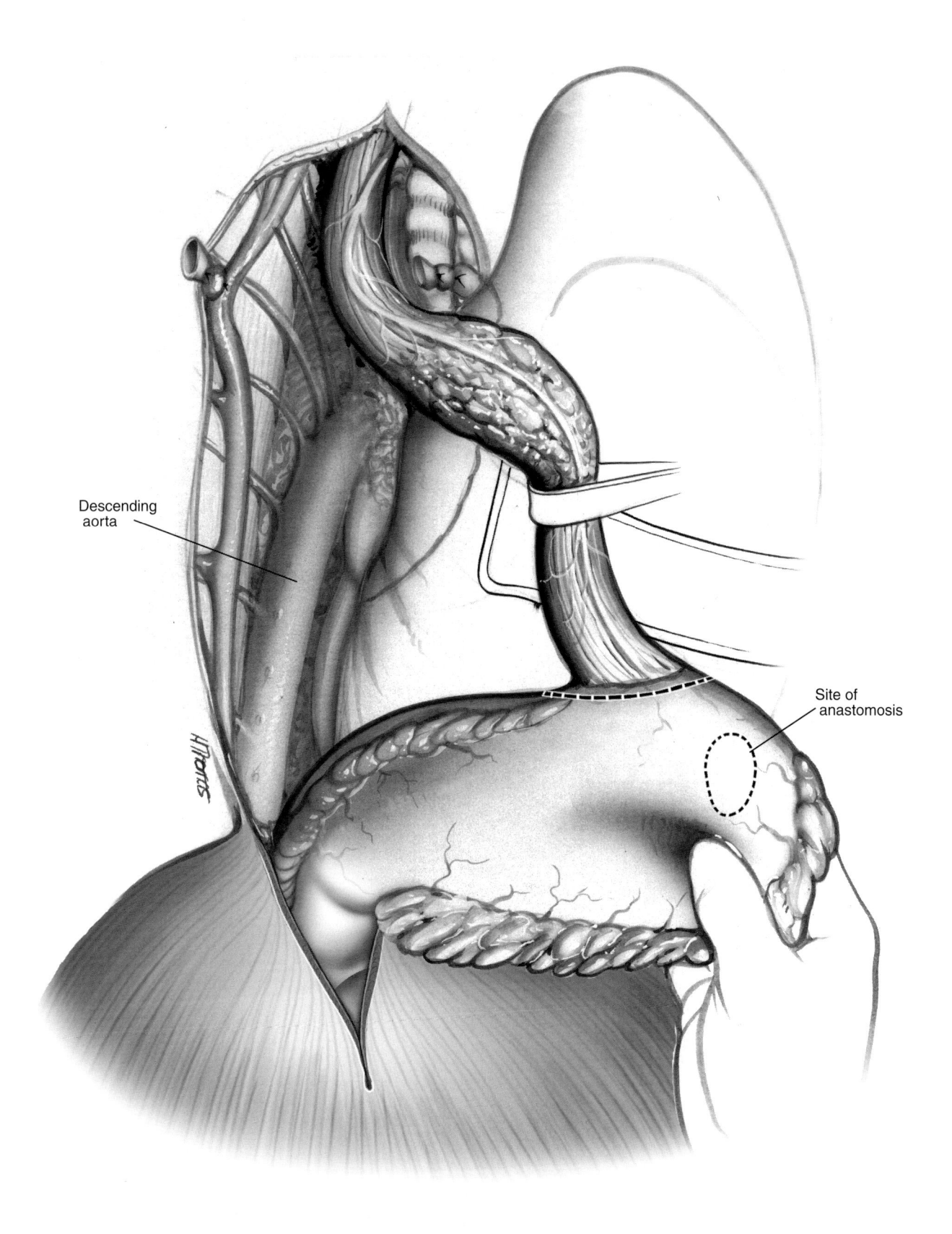

Figure 18–7 • The entire esophagus is mobilized and the stomach is delivered into the right chest.

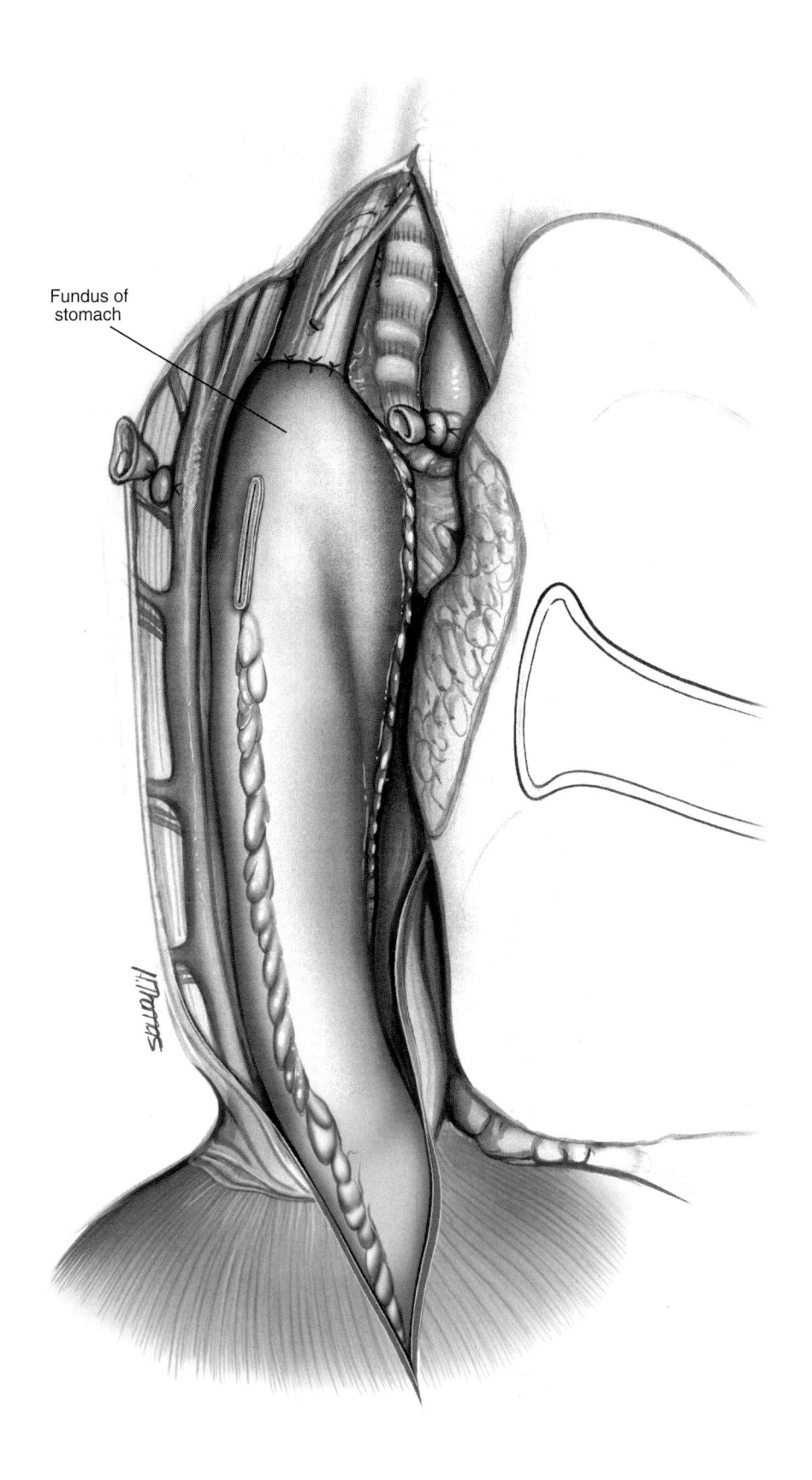

Figure 18–8 • The specimen is removed and a gastroesophageal anastomosis is performed.

Chapter 19
Esophagogastrectomy

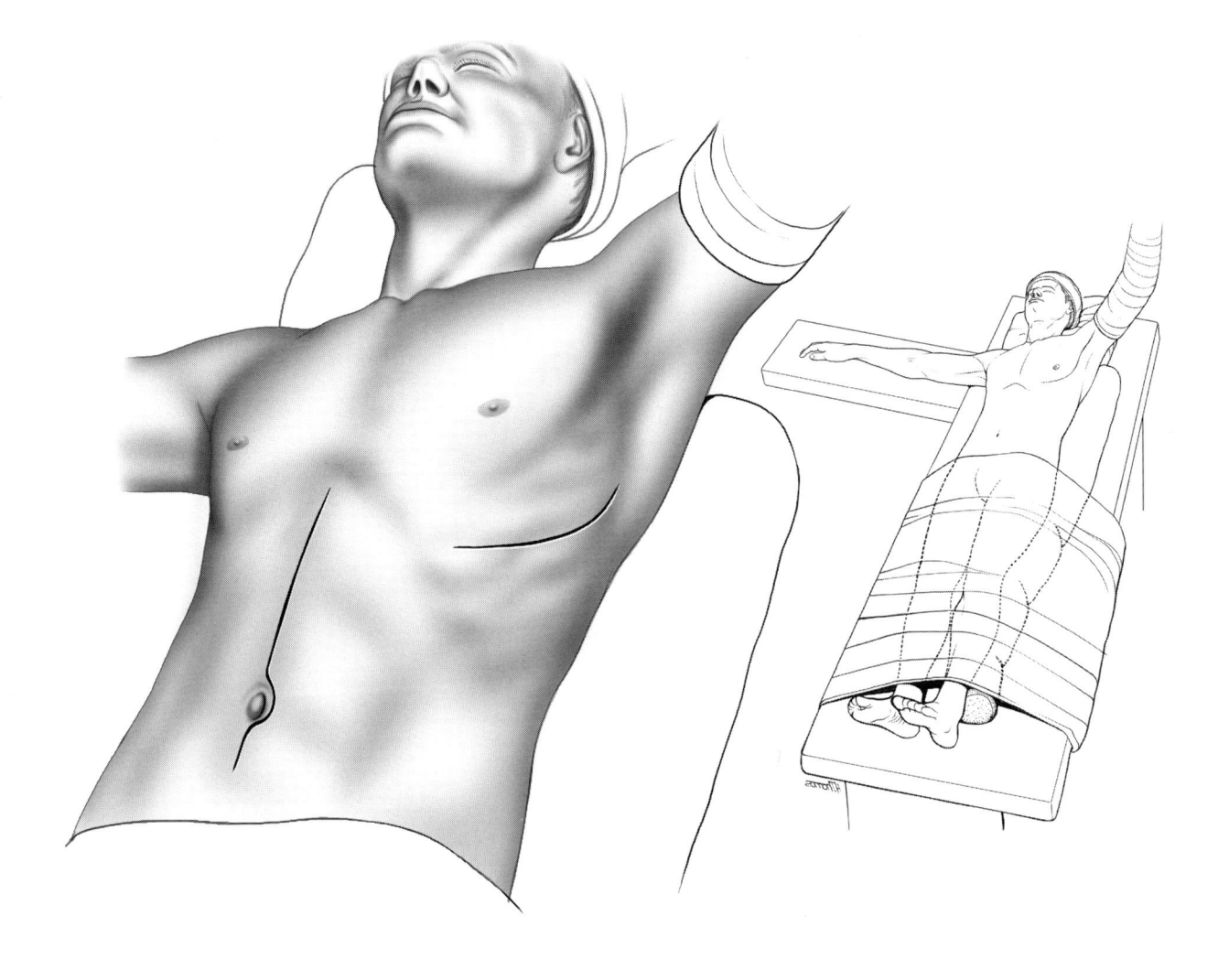

Figure 19–1 • The patient is positioned on the operating room table to allow for a midline abdominal incision and a left thoracotomy.

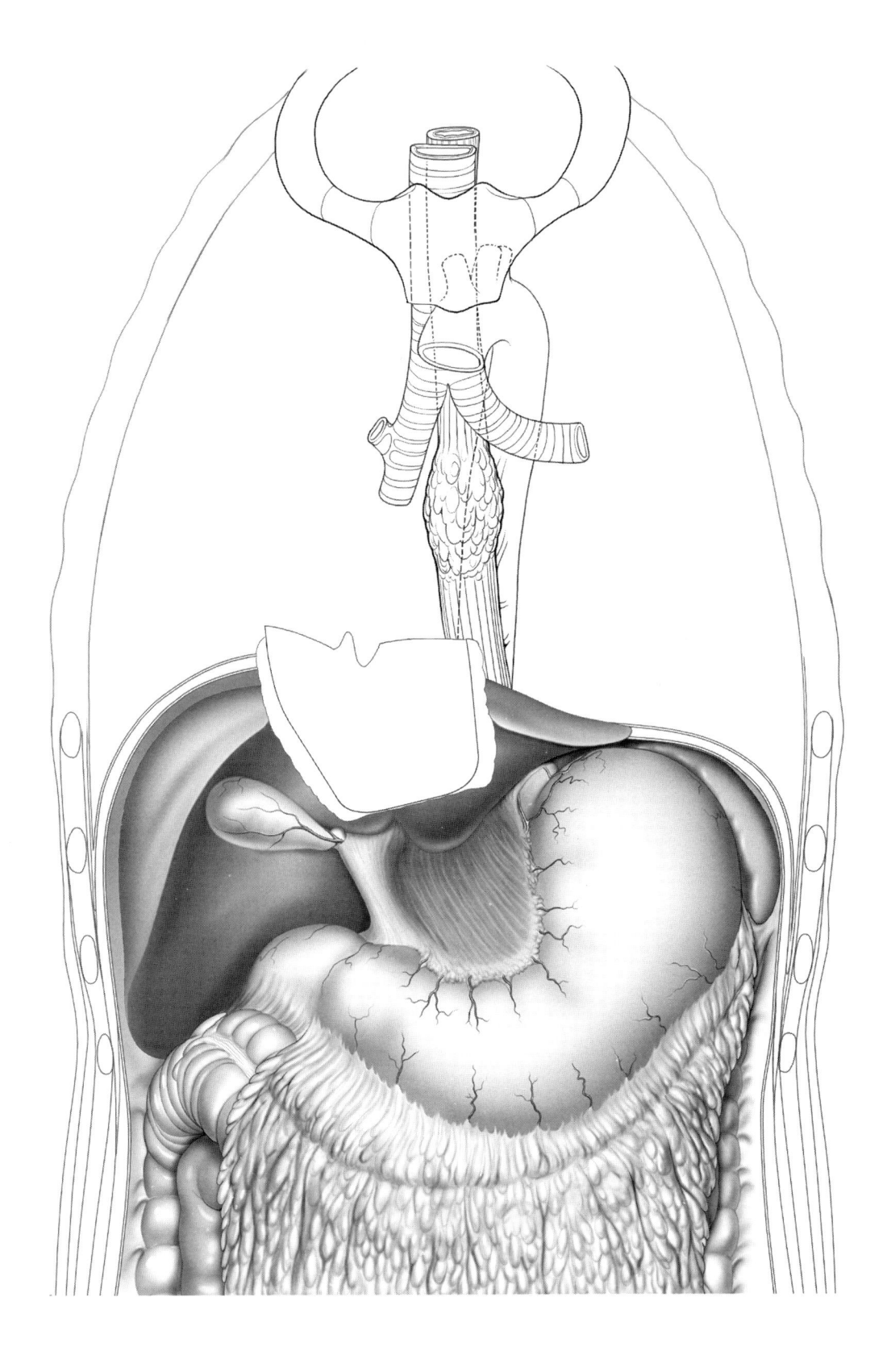

Figure 19–2 • A midline abdominal incision is performed.

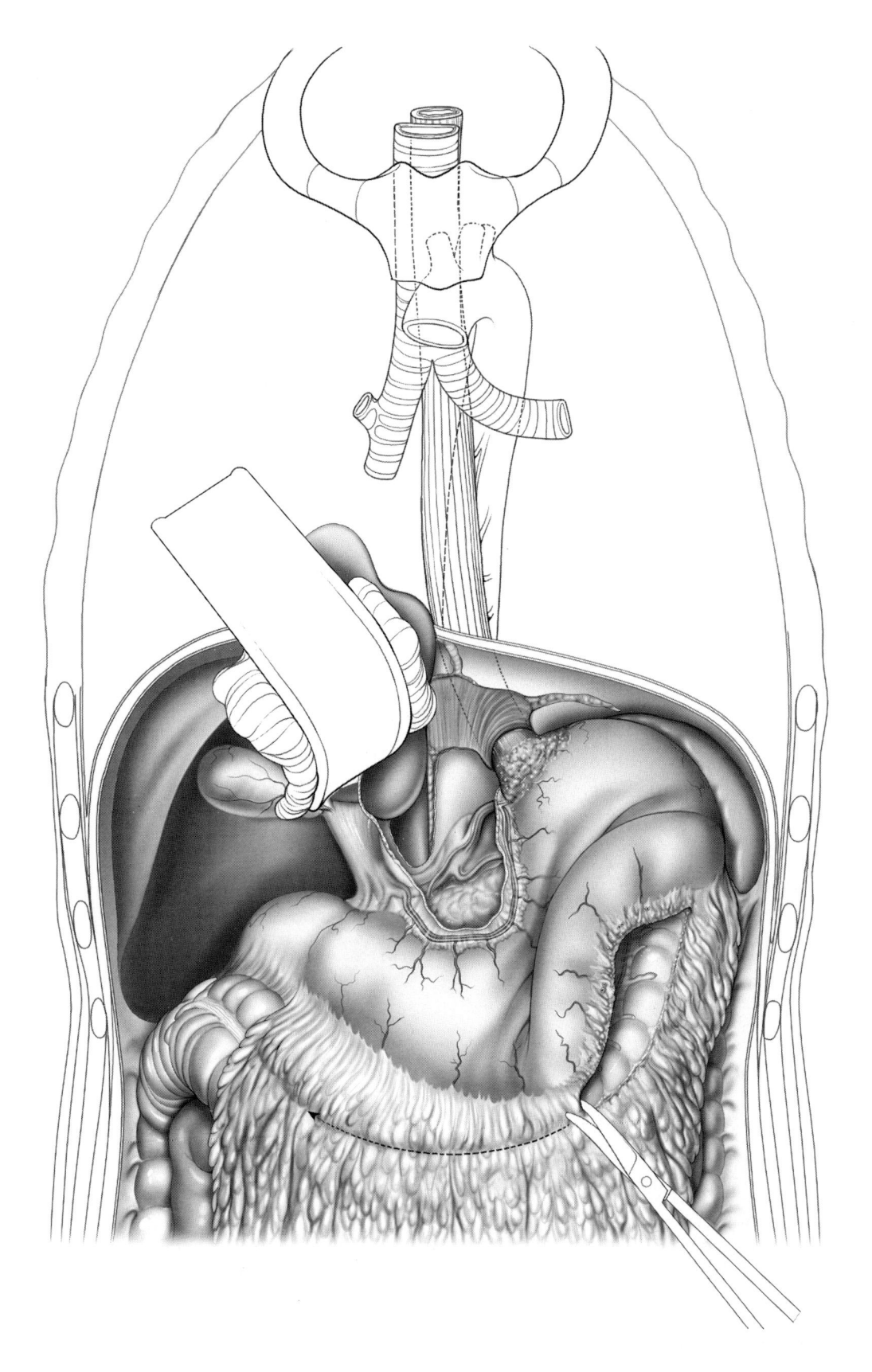

Figure 19–3 • The left triangular ligament is divided, and the liver is mobilized medially. The gastrohepatic ligament is divided, and the greater curvature of the stomach is mobilized.

Esophagogastrectomy • 137

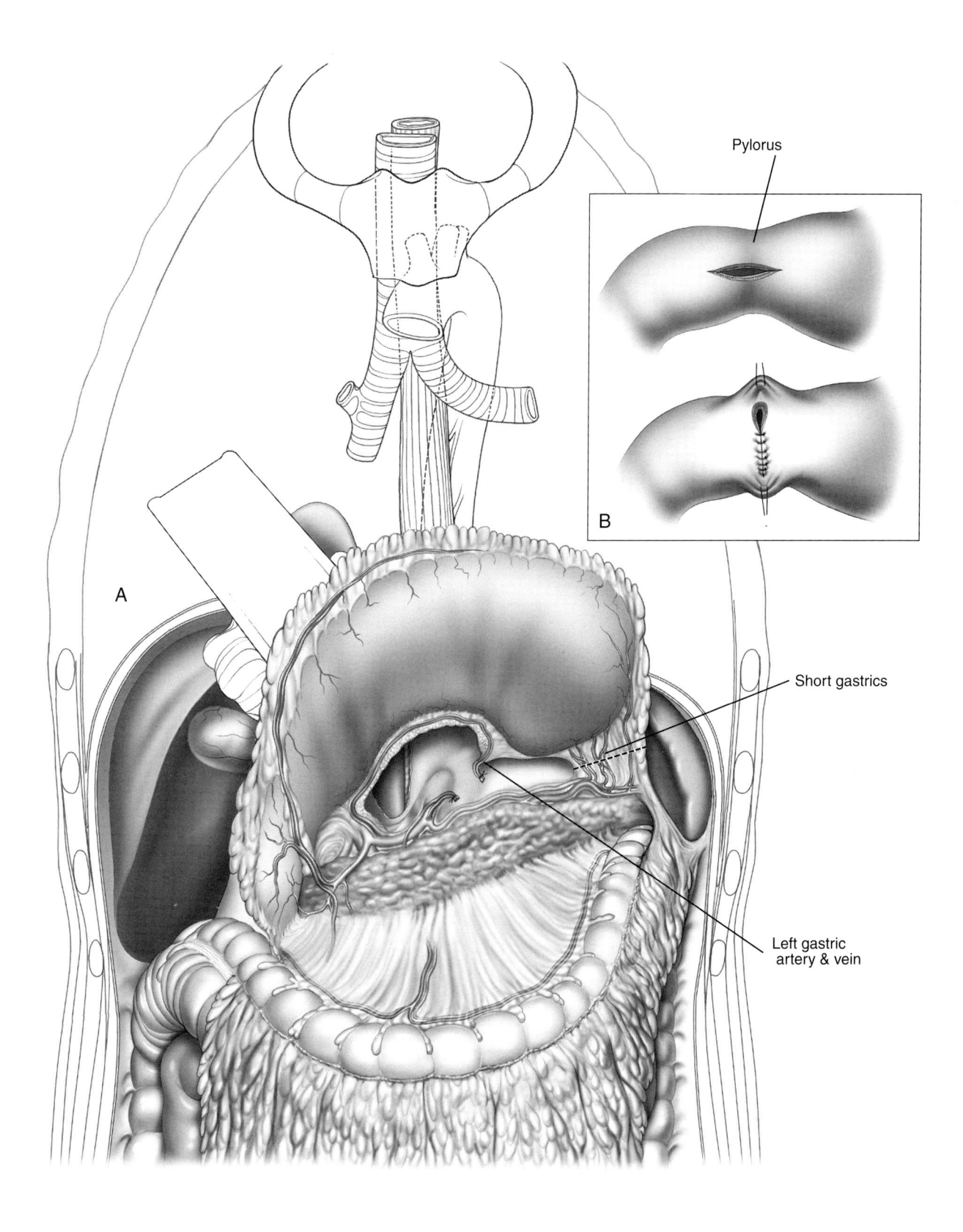

Figure 19–4 • **A,** The left gastric artery and vein are divided, as are the short gastrics. **B,** A pyloroplasty is performed.

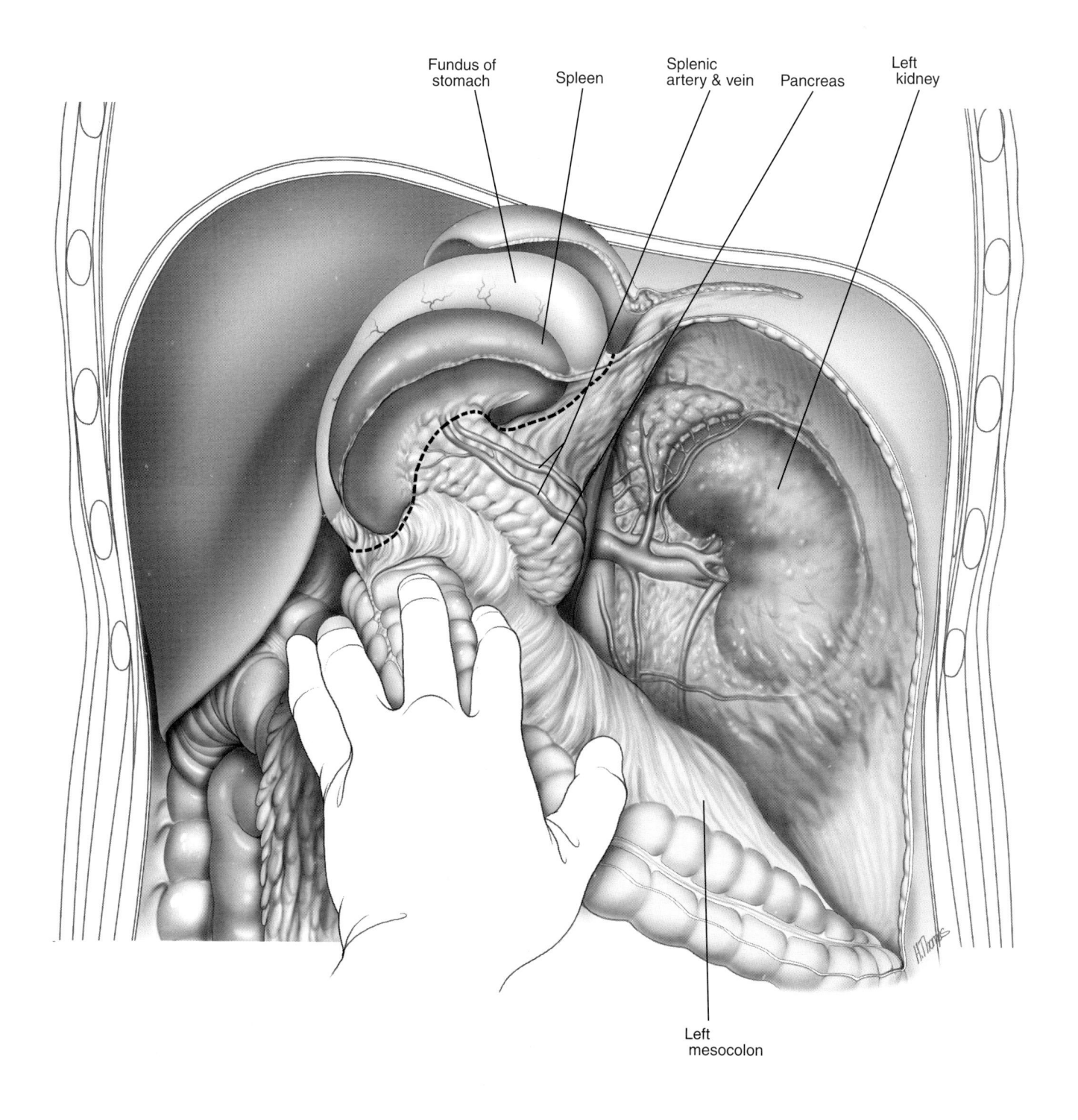

Figure 19-5 • If the spleen and short gastrics are to be included in the resected specimen, the spleen and tail of the pancreas are mobilized.

Esophagogastrectomy • 139

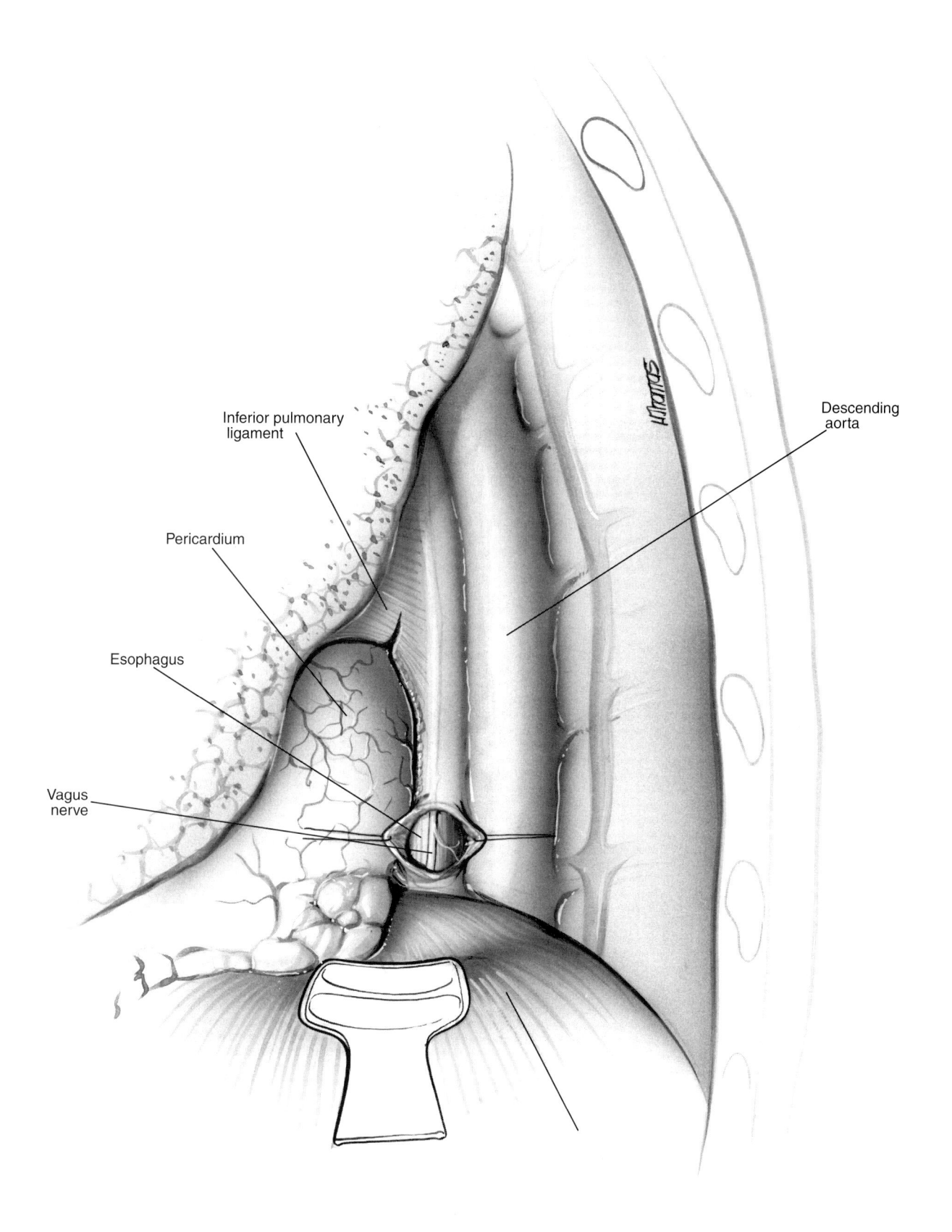

Figure 19–6 • The left chest is entered and the parietal pleura over the distal esophagus is incised. Single lung ventilation will facilitate this exposure.

140 • Part II CHEST

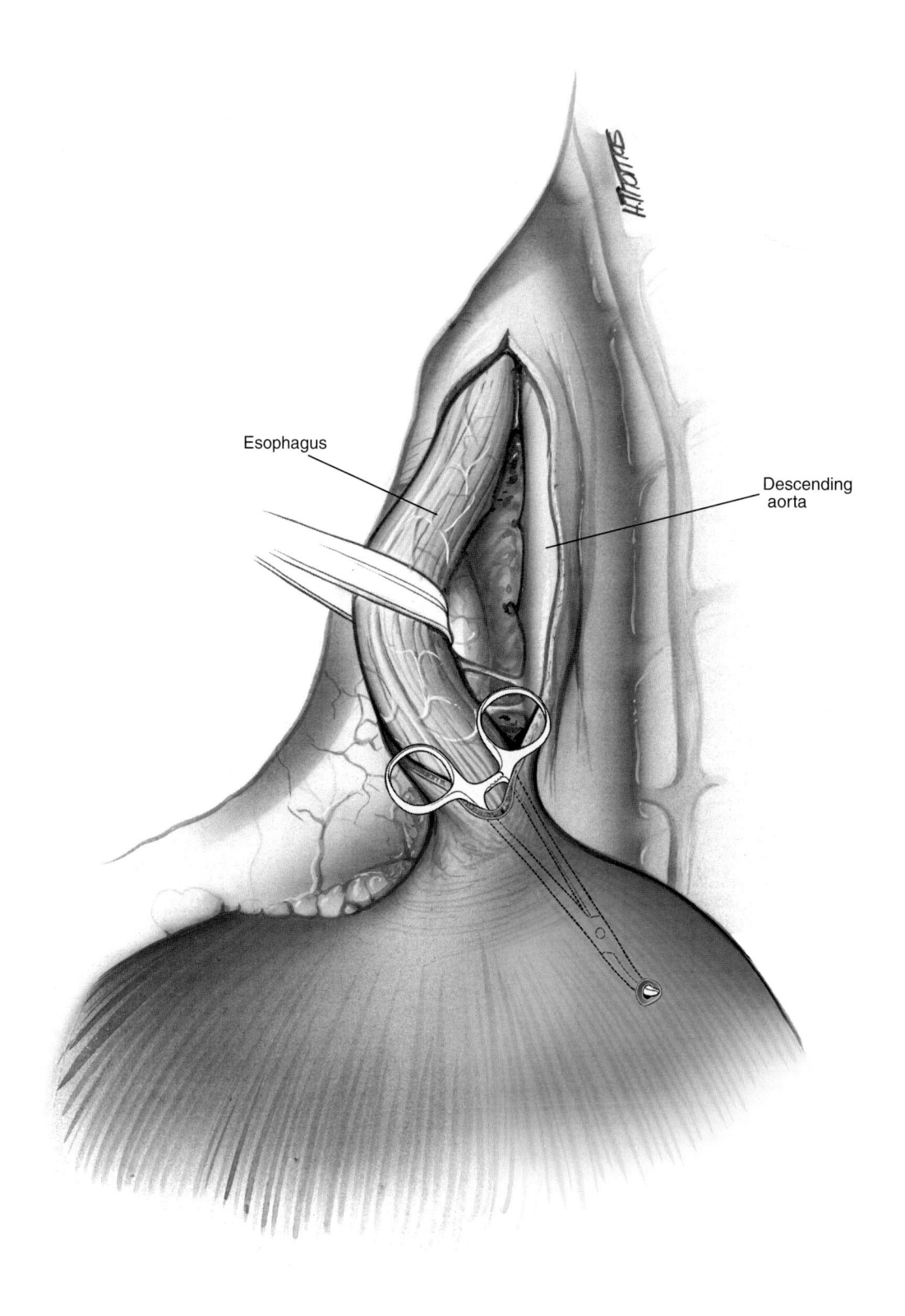

Figure 19–7 • The distal esophagus is mobilized and the hiatus is opened. Branches off the distal aorta are ligated and divided.

Esophagogastrectomy • 141

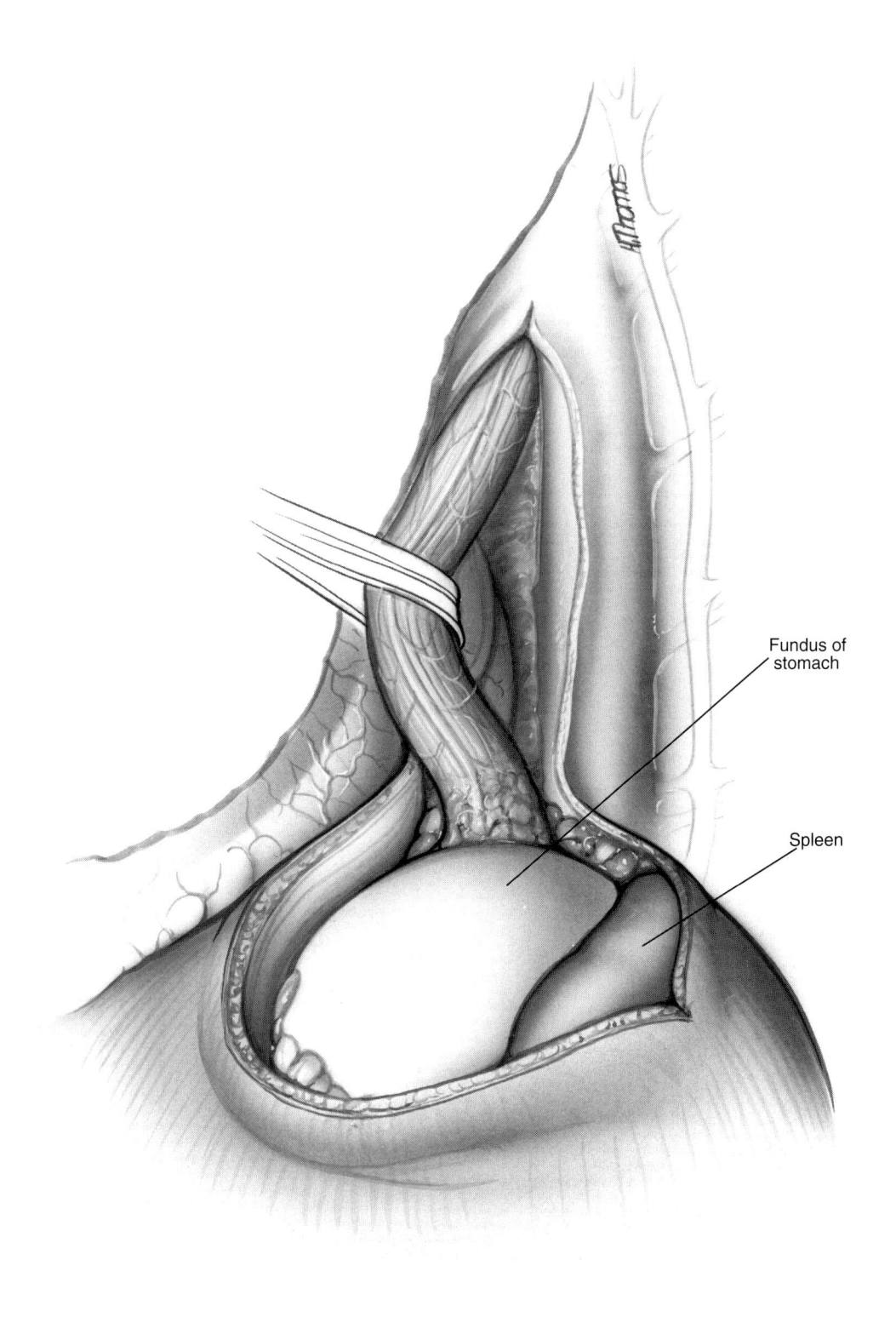

Figure 19–8 • The stomach is delivered into the left chest.

142 • Part II CHEST

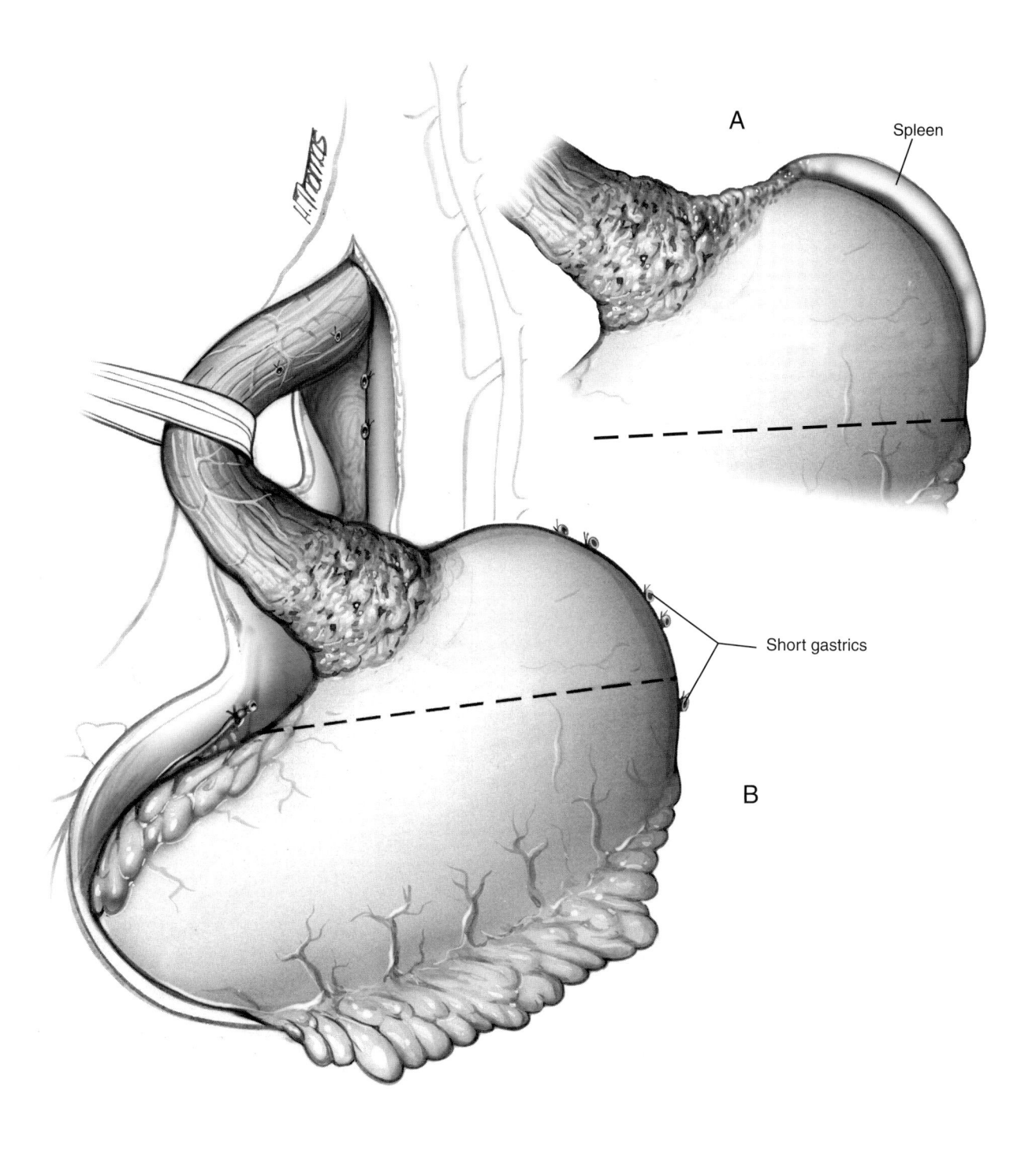

Figure 19–9 • **A,** The distal resection line is determined, with the spleen included in the specimen.
 B, The short gastrics have been divided, preserving the spleen.

Esophagogastrectomy • 143

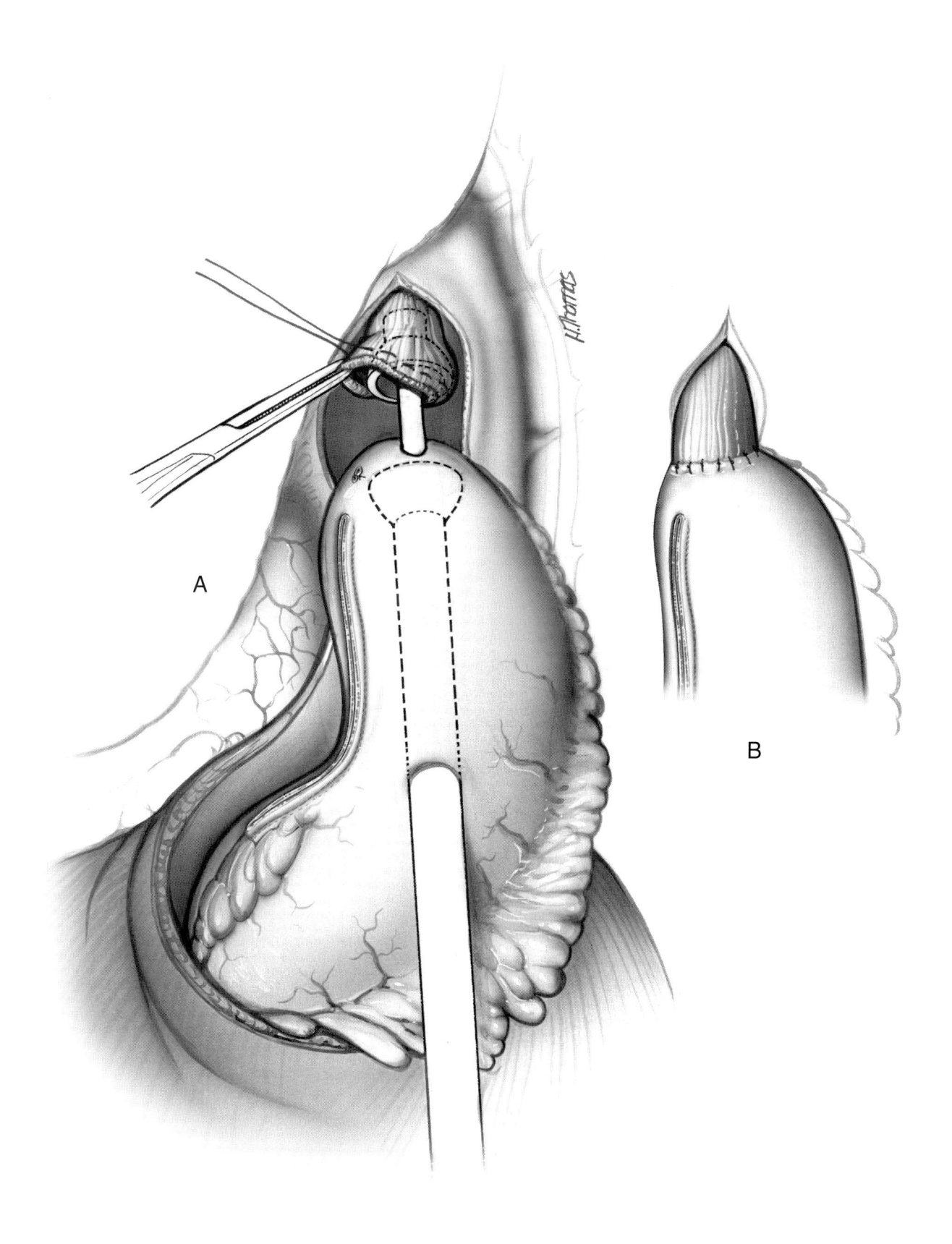

A

B

Figure 19–10 • A stapled anastomosis can be safely performed in the left chest.

Part III

UPPER ABDOMEN

146 • Part III UPPER ABDOMEN

Chapter 20
Upper Abdomen Anatomy

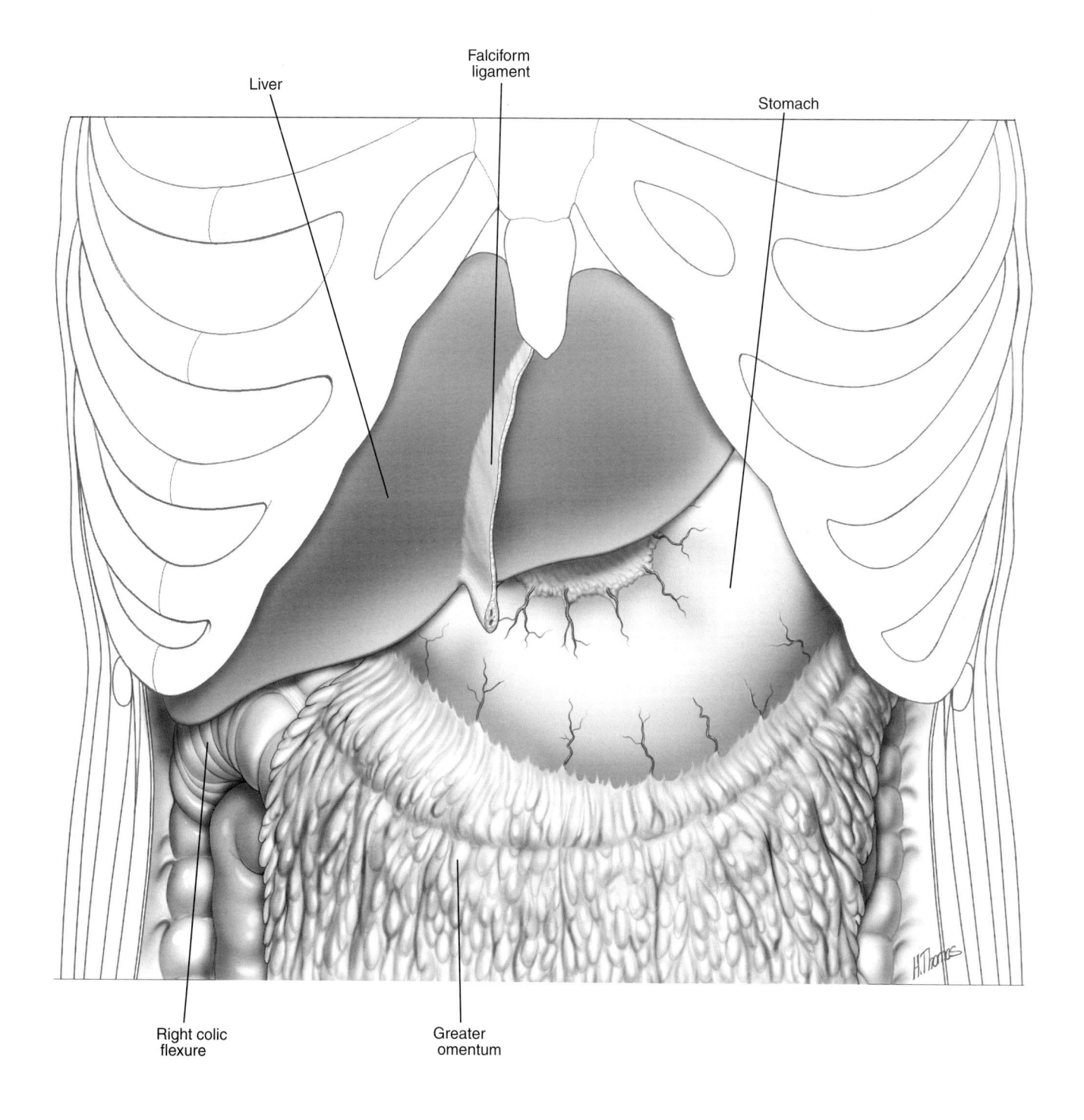

Figure 20–1 • The structures seen upon first opening the abdomen.

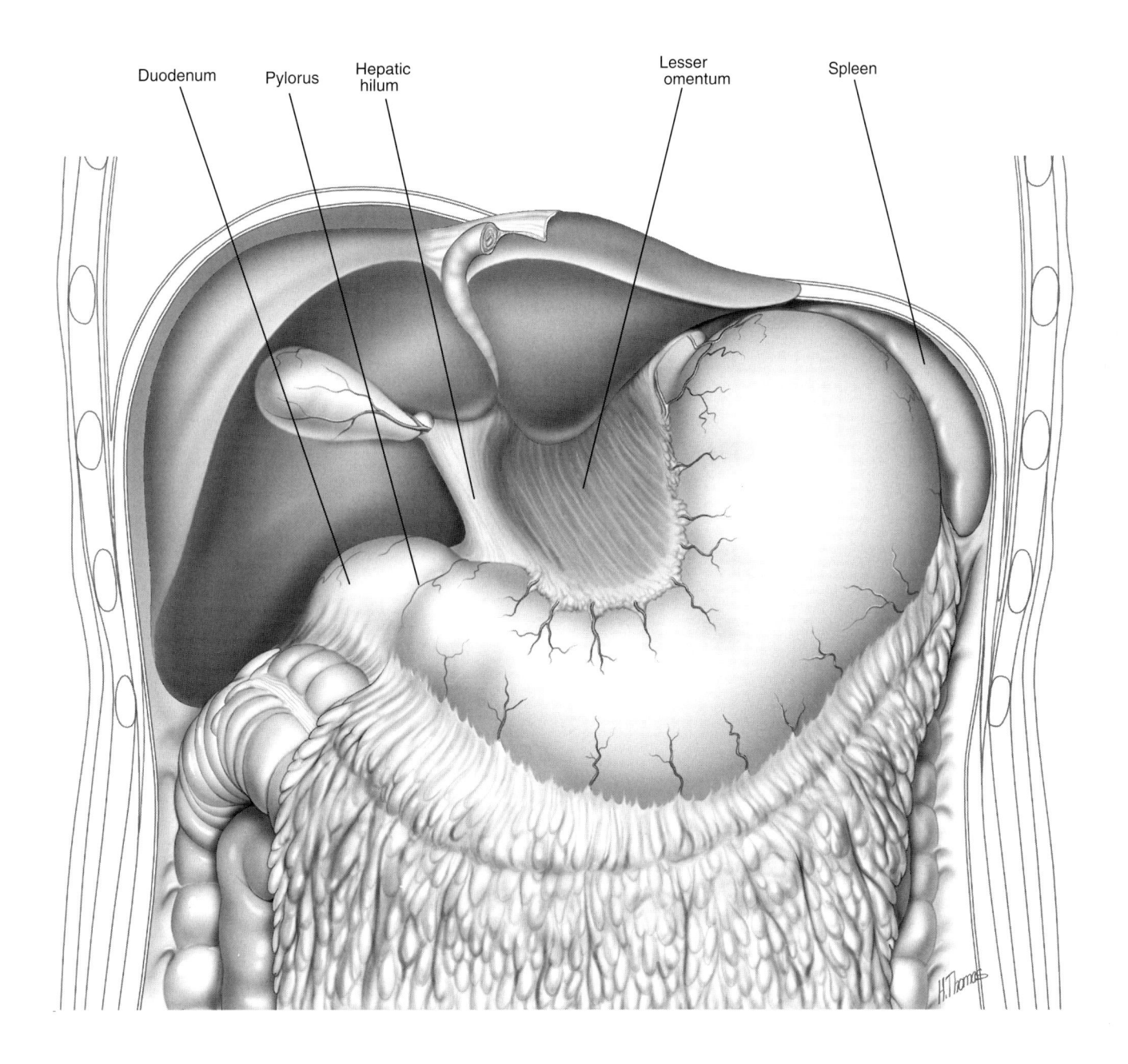

Figure 20-2 • The upper abdomen after division of the falciform ligament and elevation of the liver.

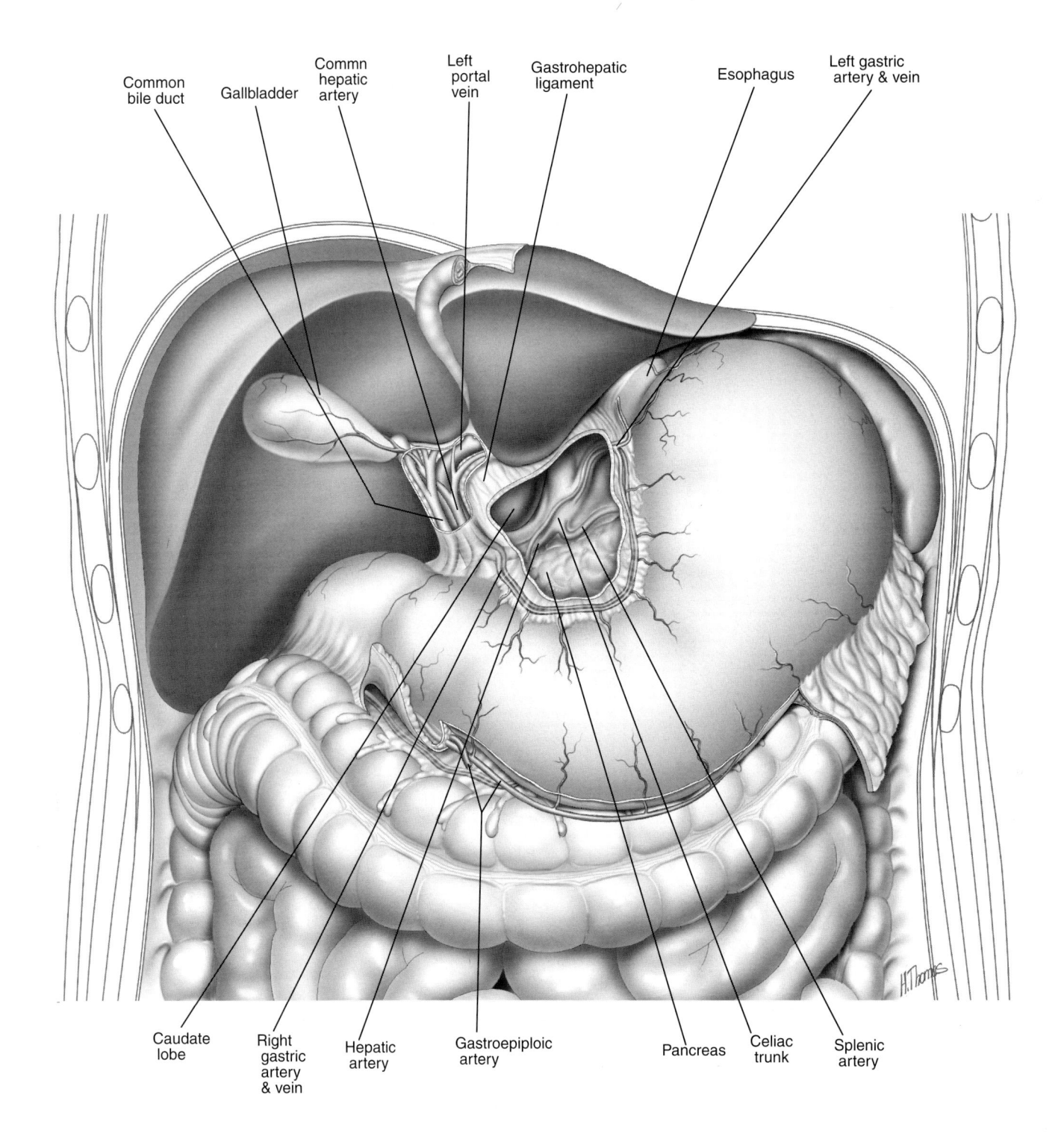

Figure 20–3 • The blood supply to the stomach is depicted by removing the gastrohepatic mesentery along the lesser curvature and the greater omentum off the transverse colon.

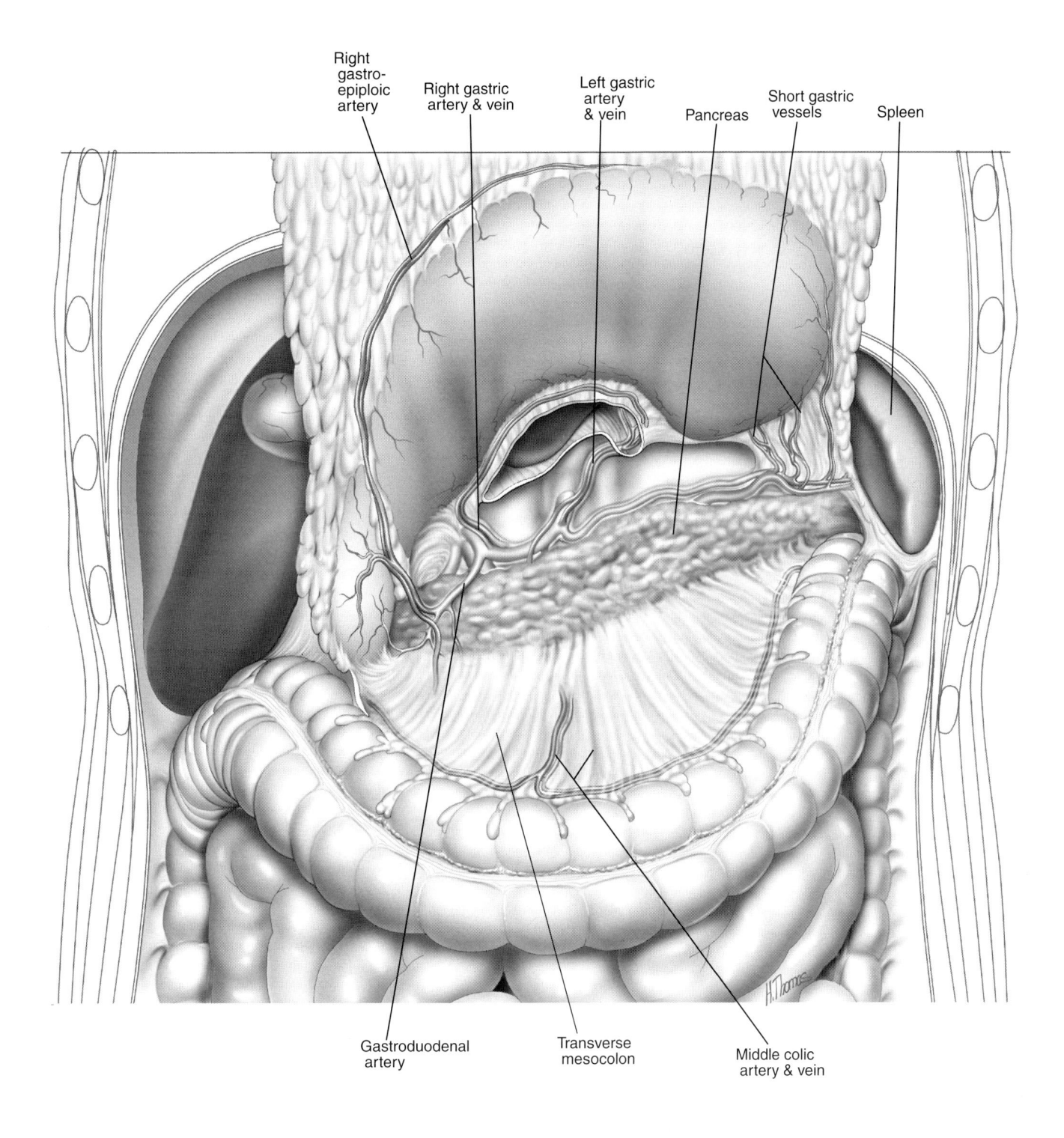

Figure 20–4 • The lesser sac is completely exposed by elevating the omentum and stomach superiorly.

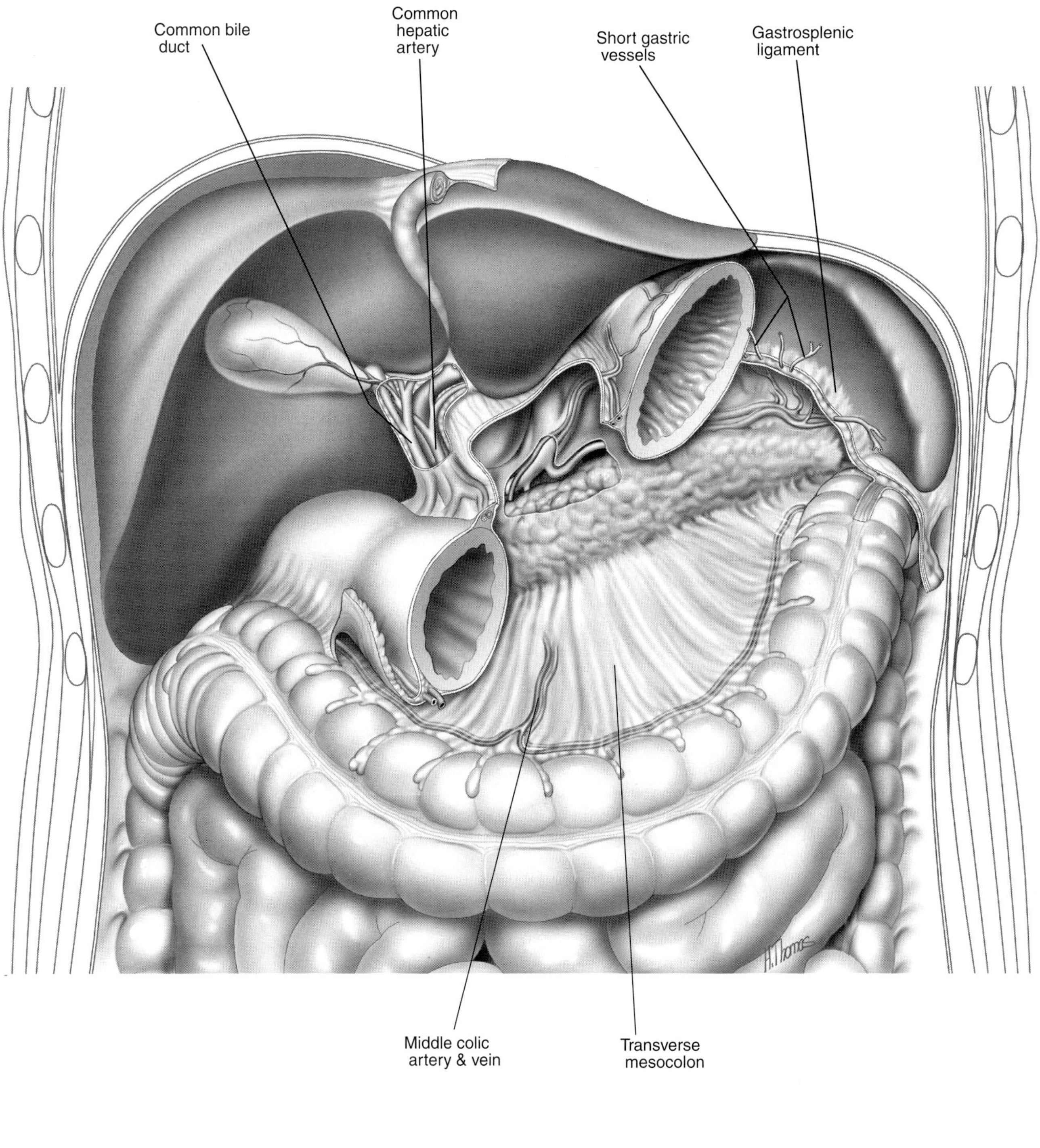

Figure 20-5 • The central portion of the stomach has been removed, along with its mesenteric attachments. The porta hepatis is defined, as are the body and tail of the pancreas.

Upper Abdomen Anatomy • 151

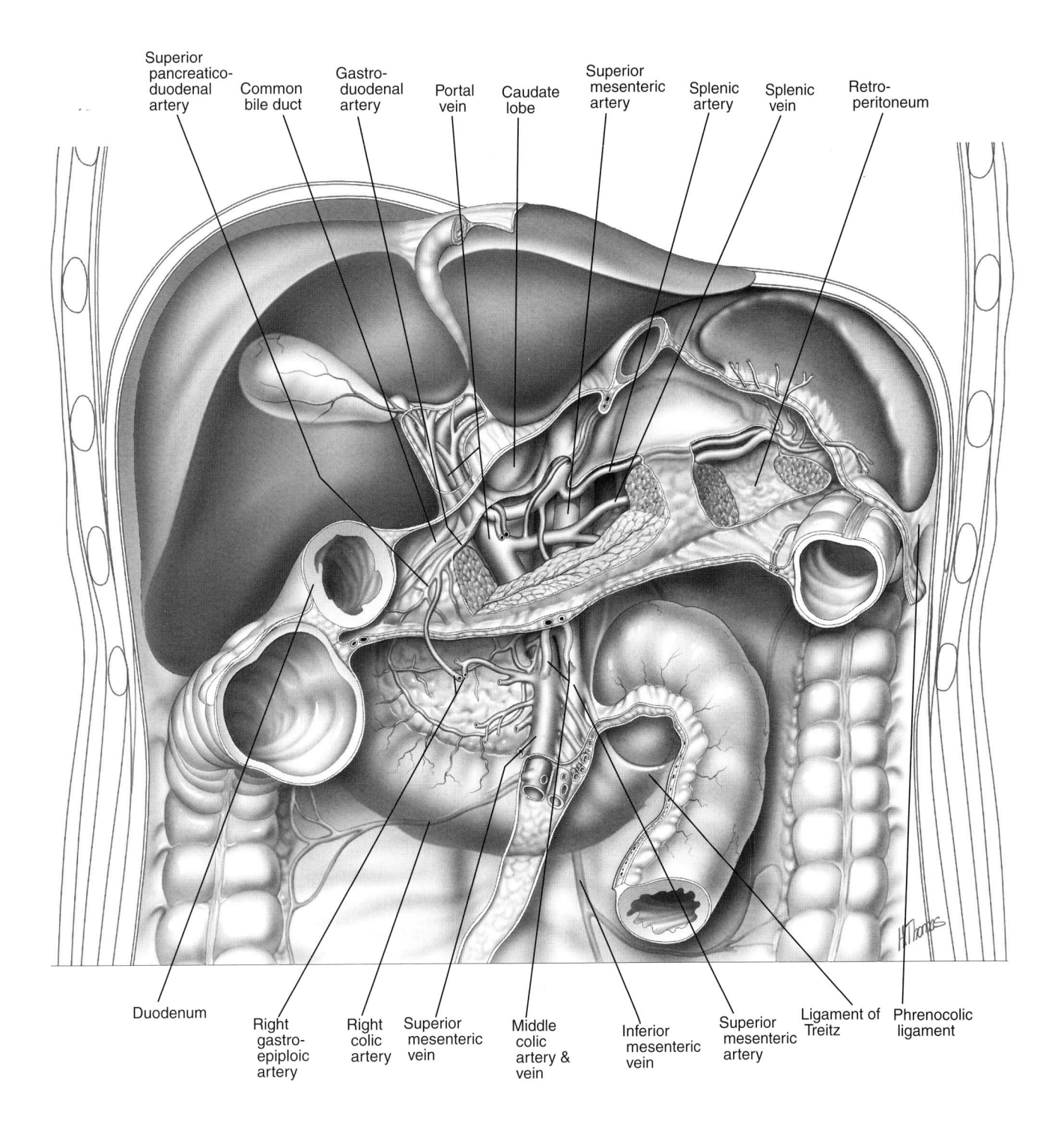

Figure 20–6 • The stomach and transverse colon and their mesenteric attachments have been completely removed, as well as the central portion of the pancreas. The complete vascular anatomy is depicted.

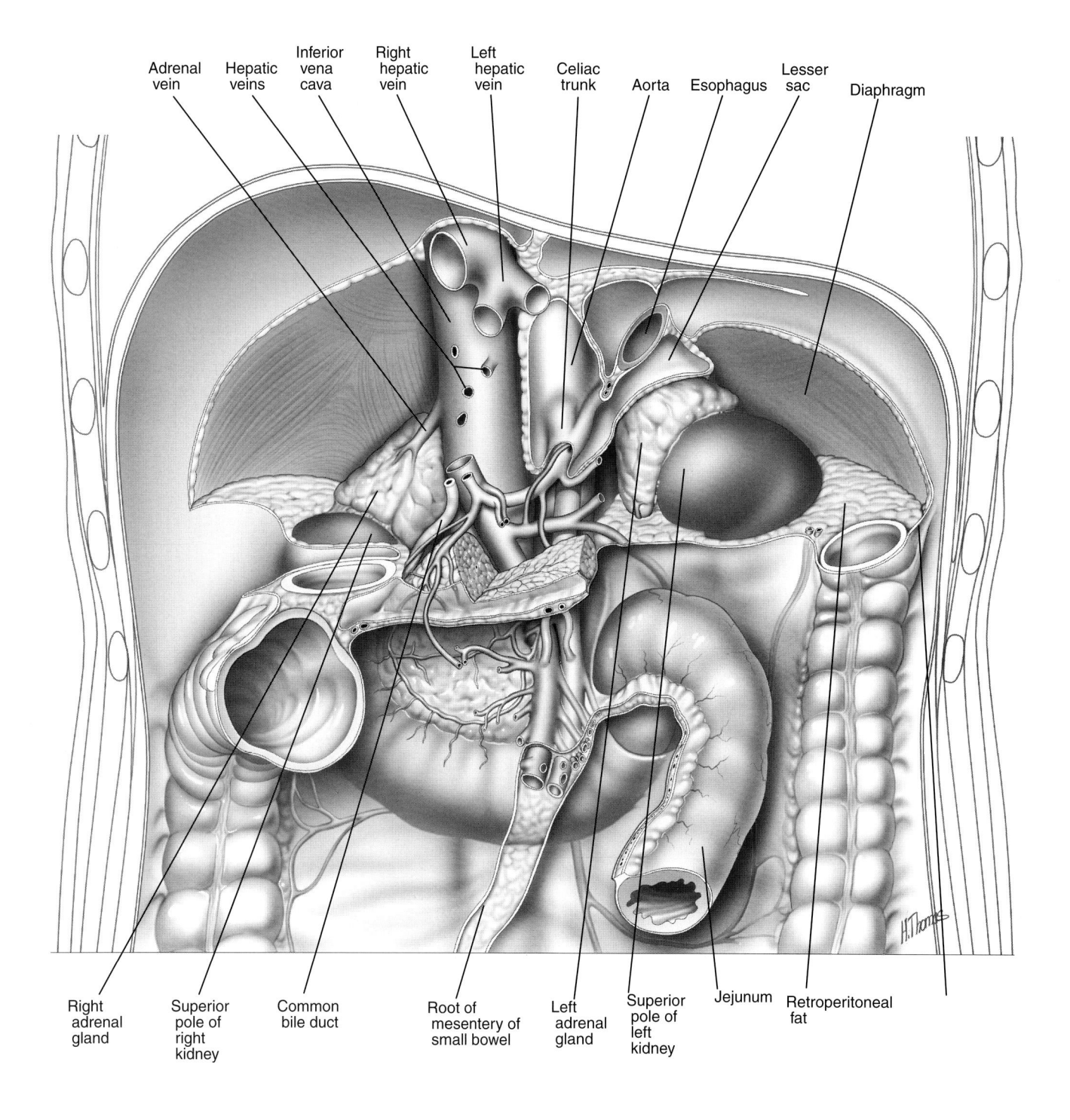

Figure 20-7 • The liver is removed, revealing the major branches off the vena cava.

Chapter 21
Gastric Surgery

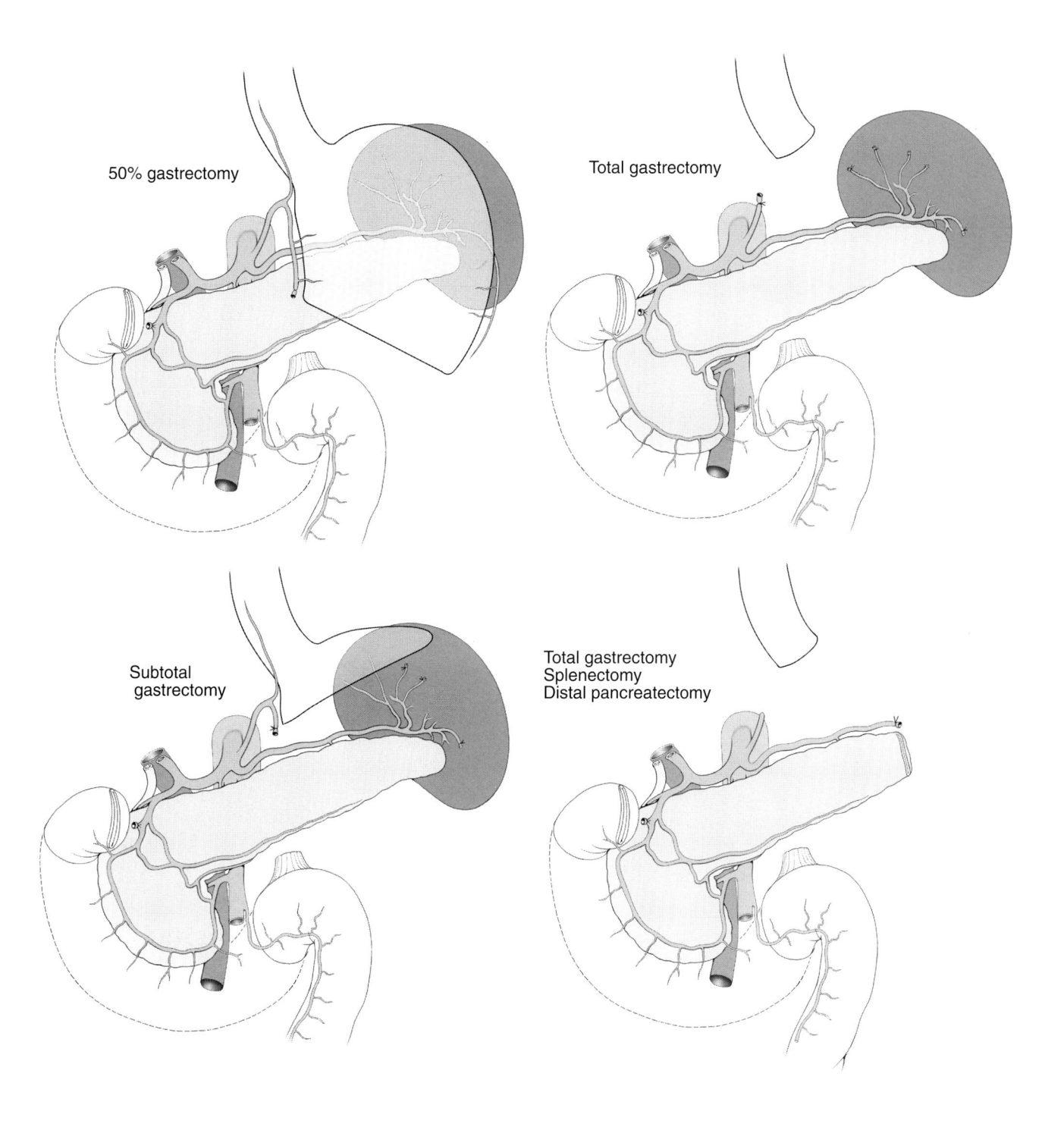

Figure 21–1 • These line drawings illustrate the various gastrectomies and the vascular structures to be ligated to facilitate these resections.

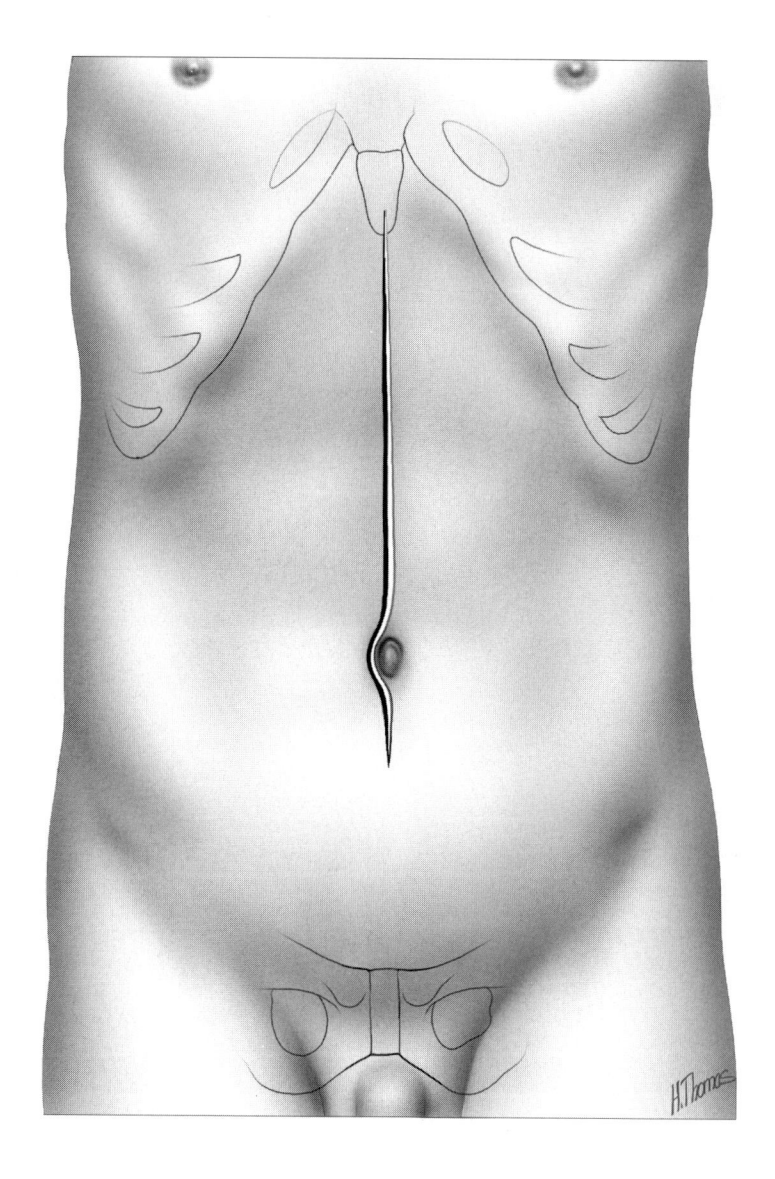

Figure 21–2 • A midline upper abdominal incision is performed.

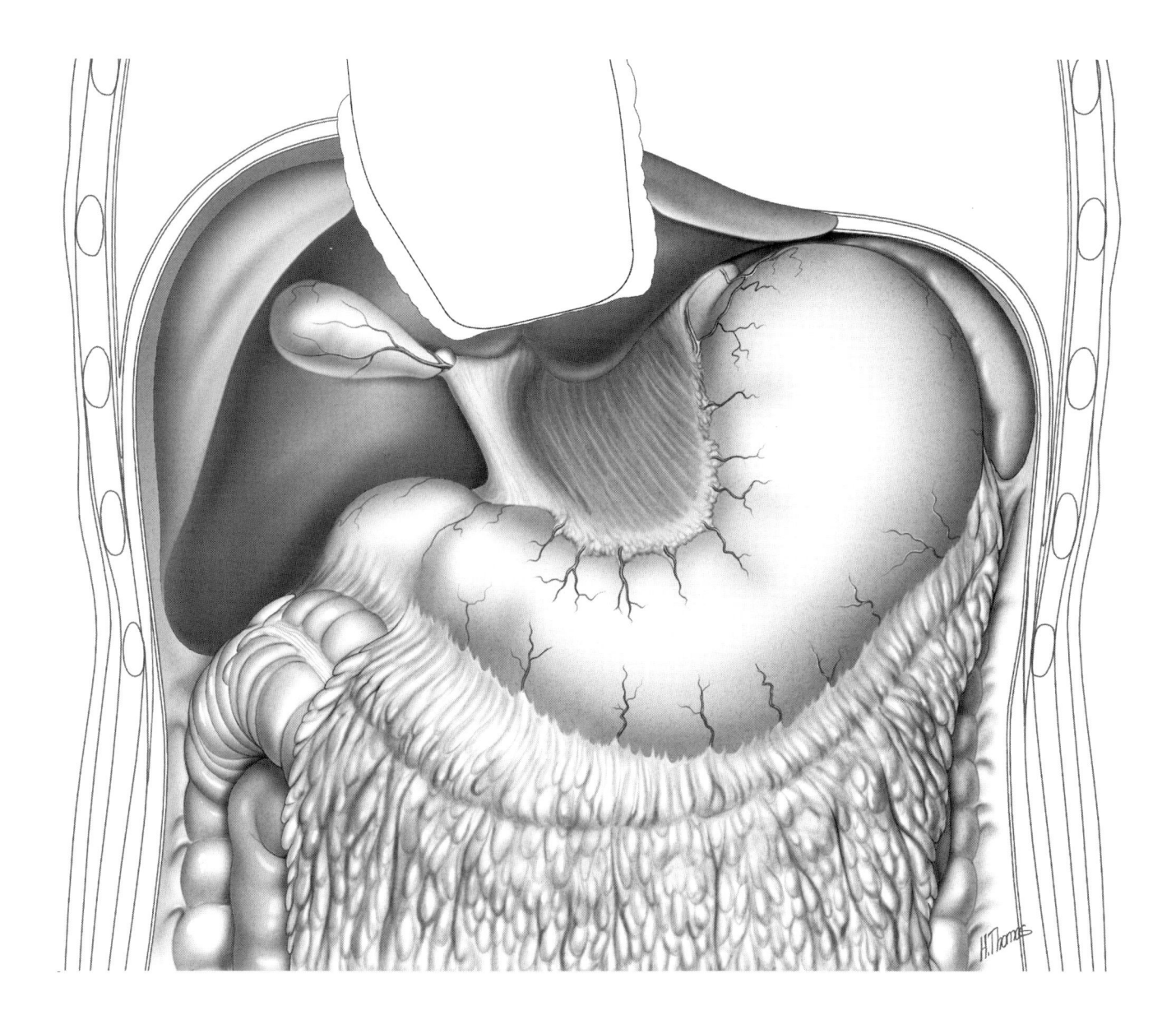

Figure 21–3 • The upper abdomen is exposed.

156 • Part III   UPPER ABDOMEN

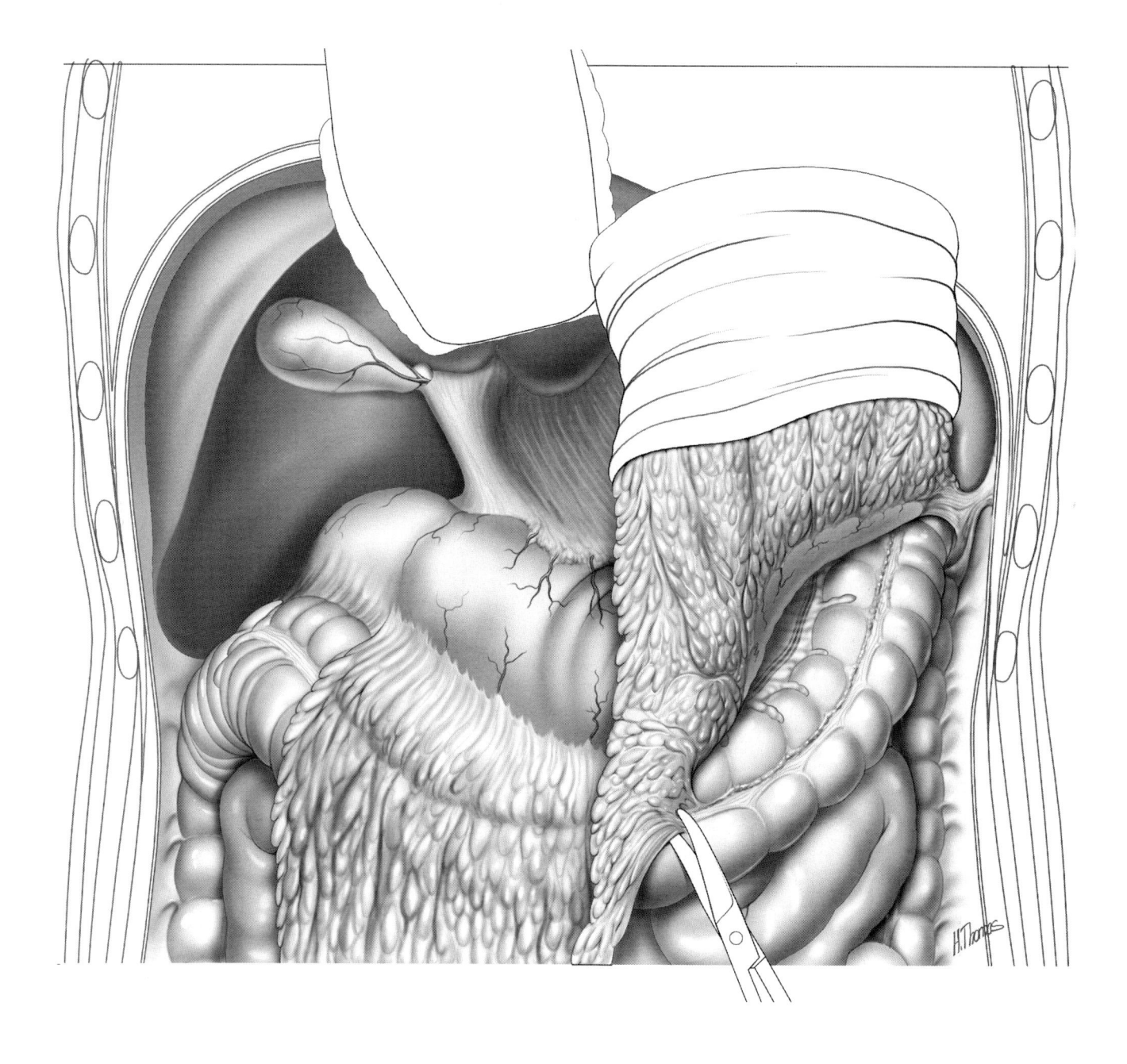

Figure 21–4 • The greater omentum is detached from the transverse colon along an avascular plane, utilizing a Metzenbaum or cautery.

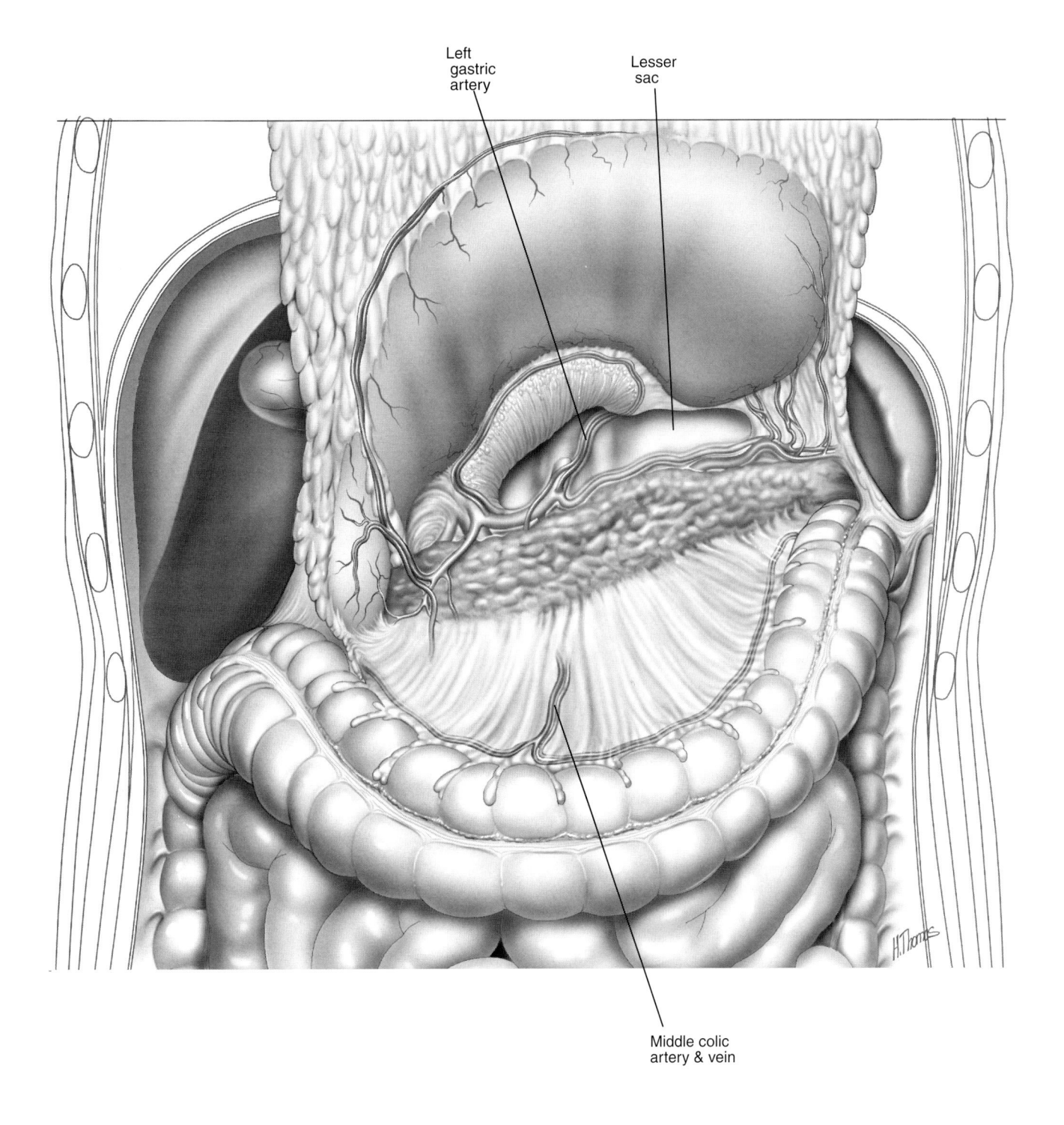

Figure 21–5 • Complete mobilization of the greater omentum allows elevation of the stomach and complete exposure of the lesser sac.

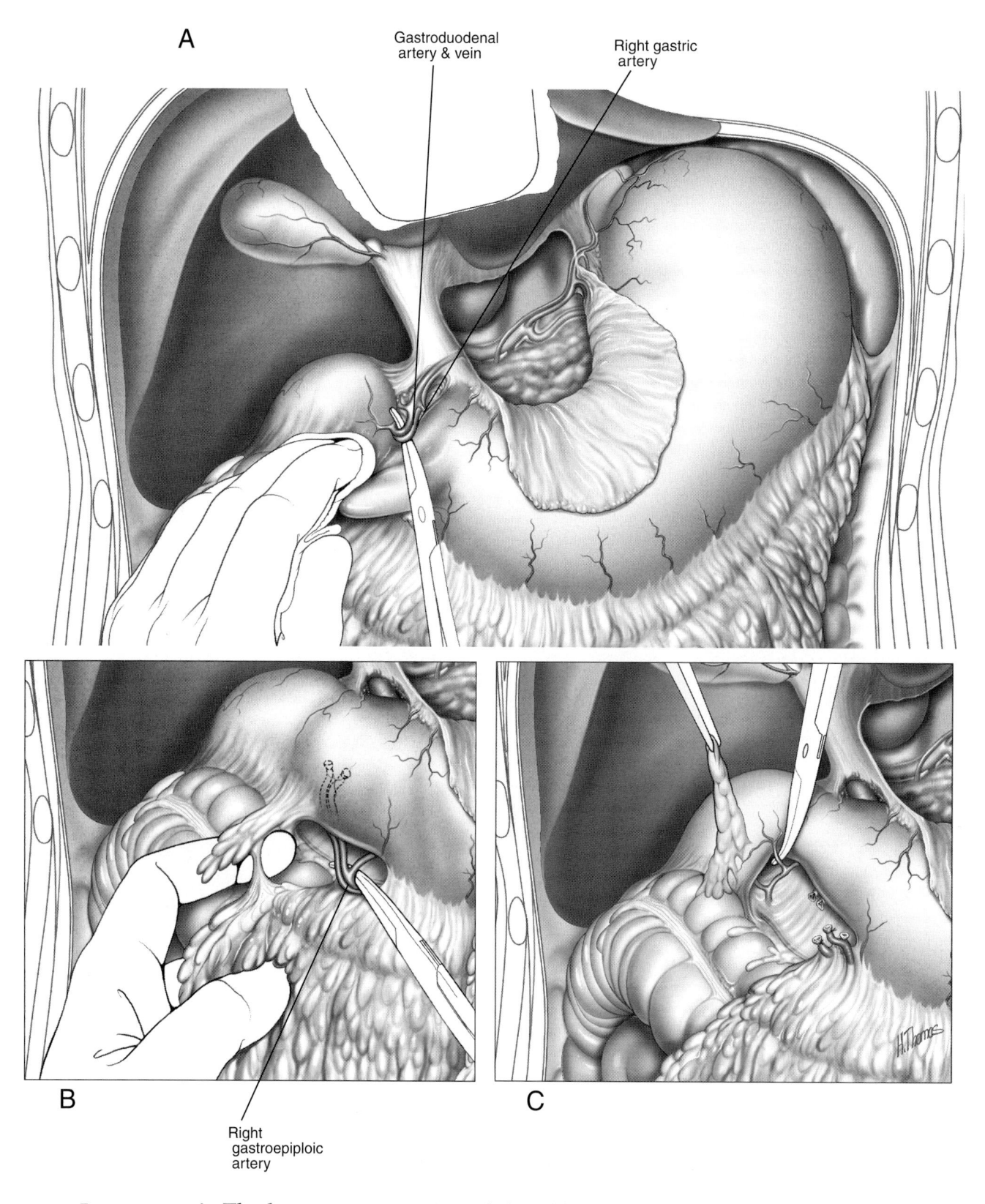

Figure 21-6 • **A,** The lesser curvature is mobilized by incising the gastrohepatic ligament. Division of the right gastroduodenal artery and vein is illustrated.
B, The right gastroepiploic vessels are identified.
C, Small branches off the superior pancreaticoduodenal artery to the proximal duodenum are ligated.

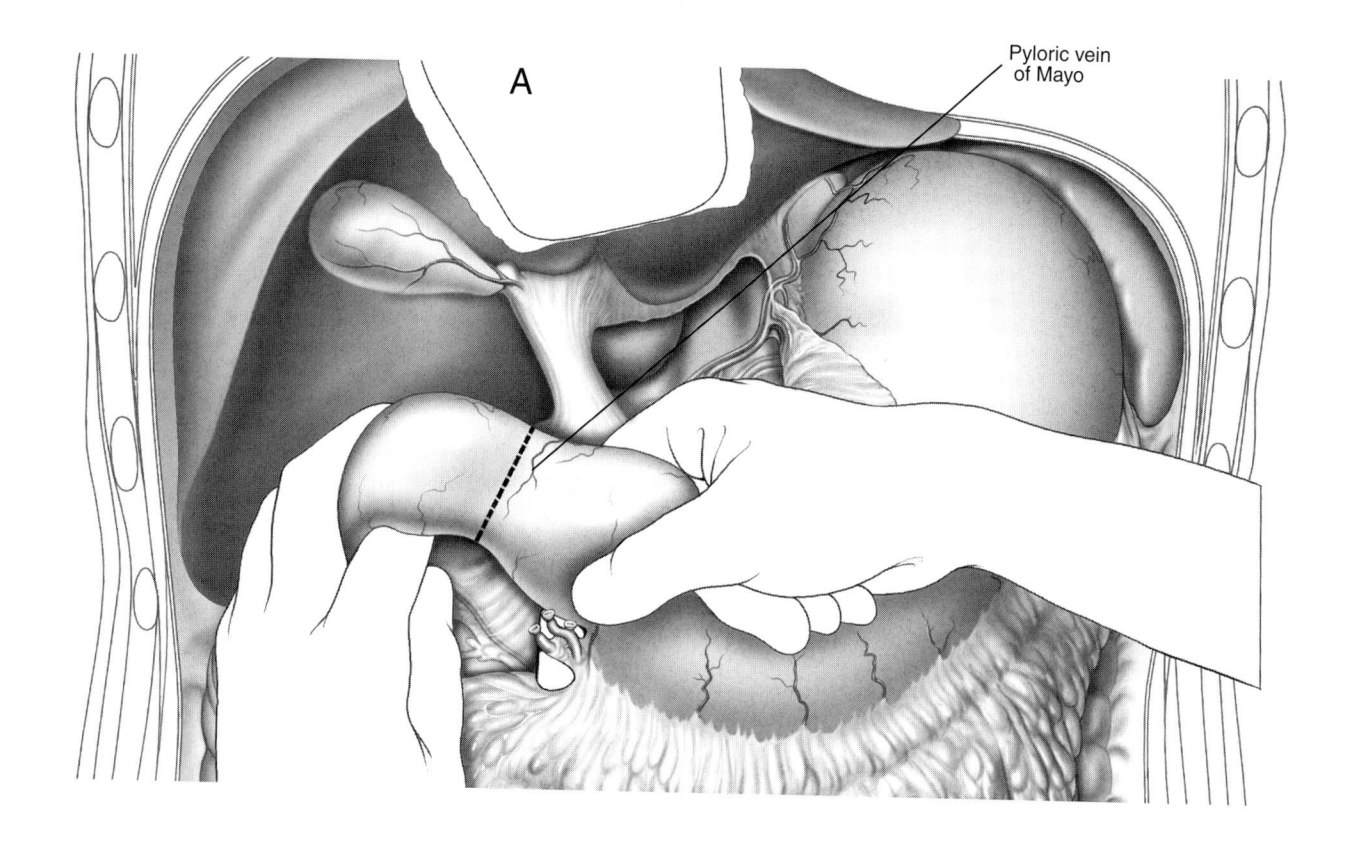

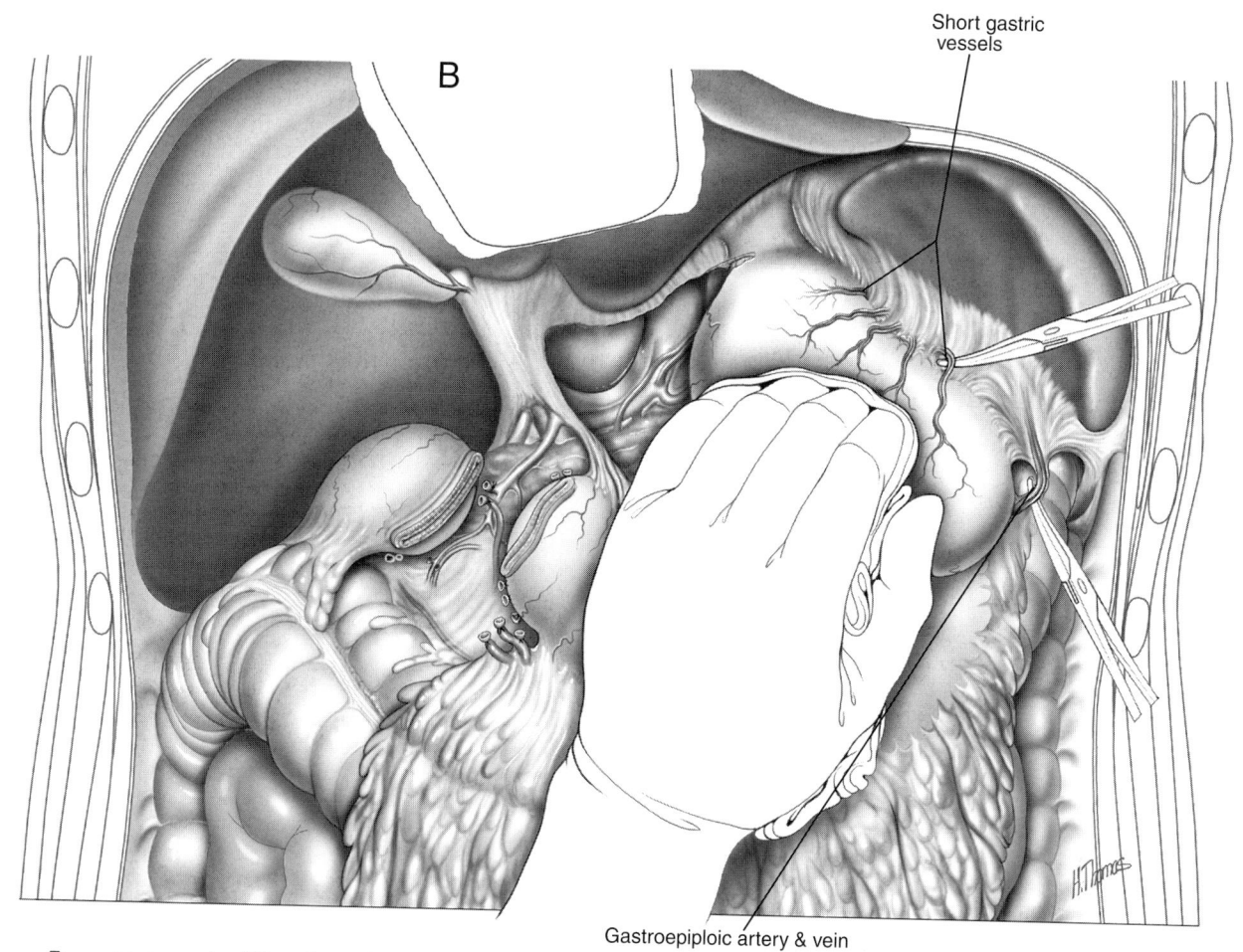

Figure 21–7 • **A,** The duodenum is divided distal to the pyloric vein of Mayo.
B, For a subtotal or total gastrectomy, the short gastric vessels and the gastroepiploic artery and vein are divided.

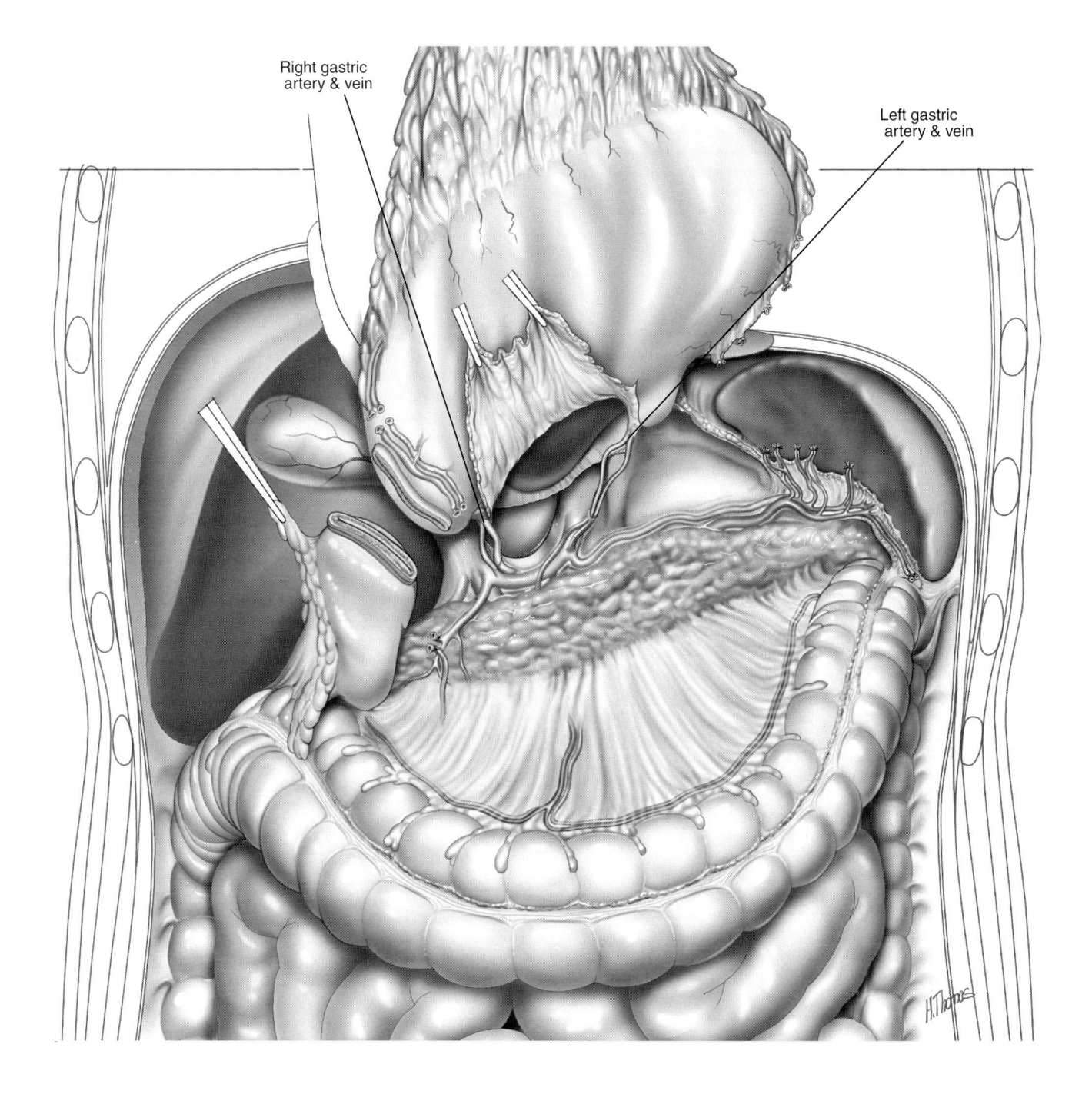

Figure 21–8 • The right and left gastric arteries are identified and divided if necessary.

Gastric Surgery • 161

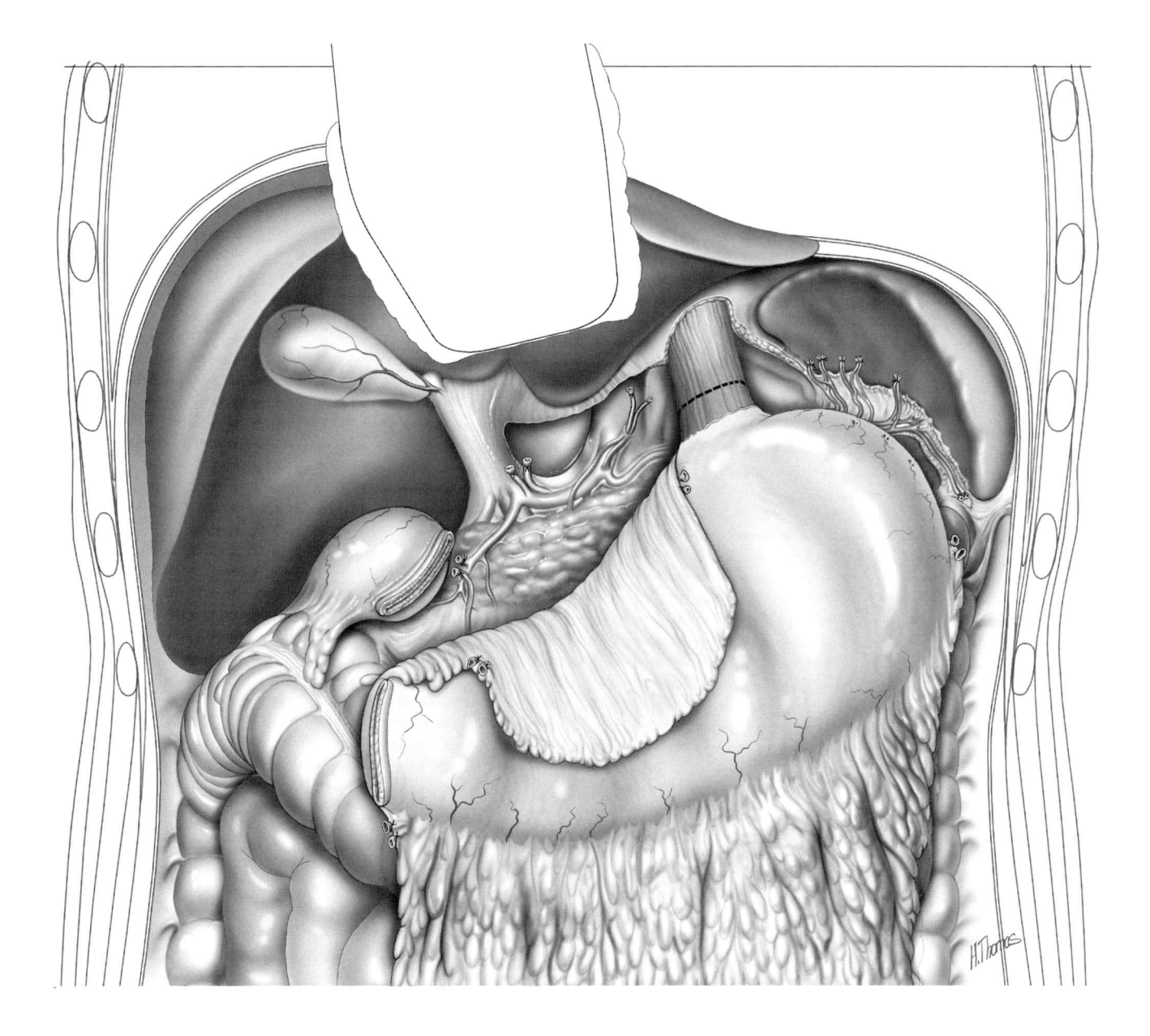

Figure 21-9 • For a total gastrectomy, the esophageal resection line is defined.

162 • Part III UPPER ABDOMEN

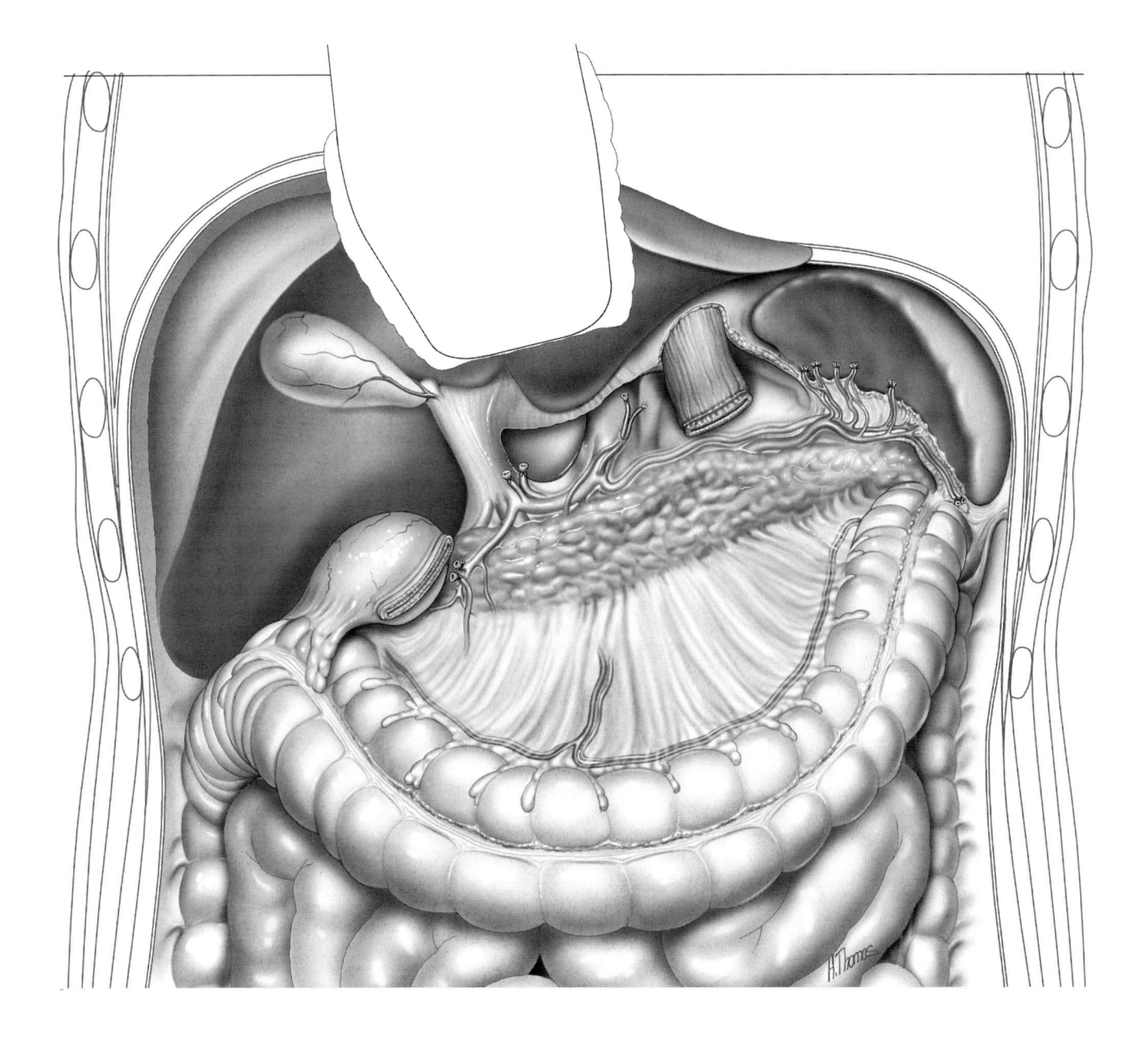

Figure 21–10 • The resulting defect is illustrated if a total gastrectomy without splenectomy is performed.

Gastric Surgery • 163

Left colic gutter

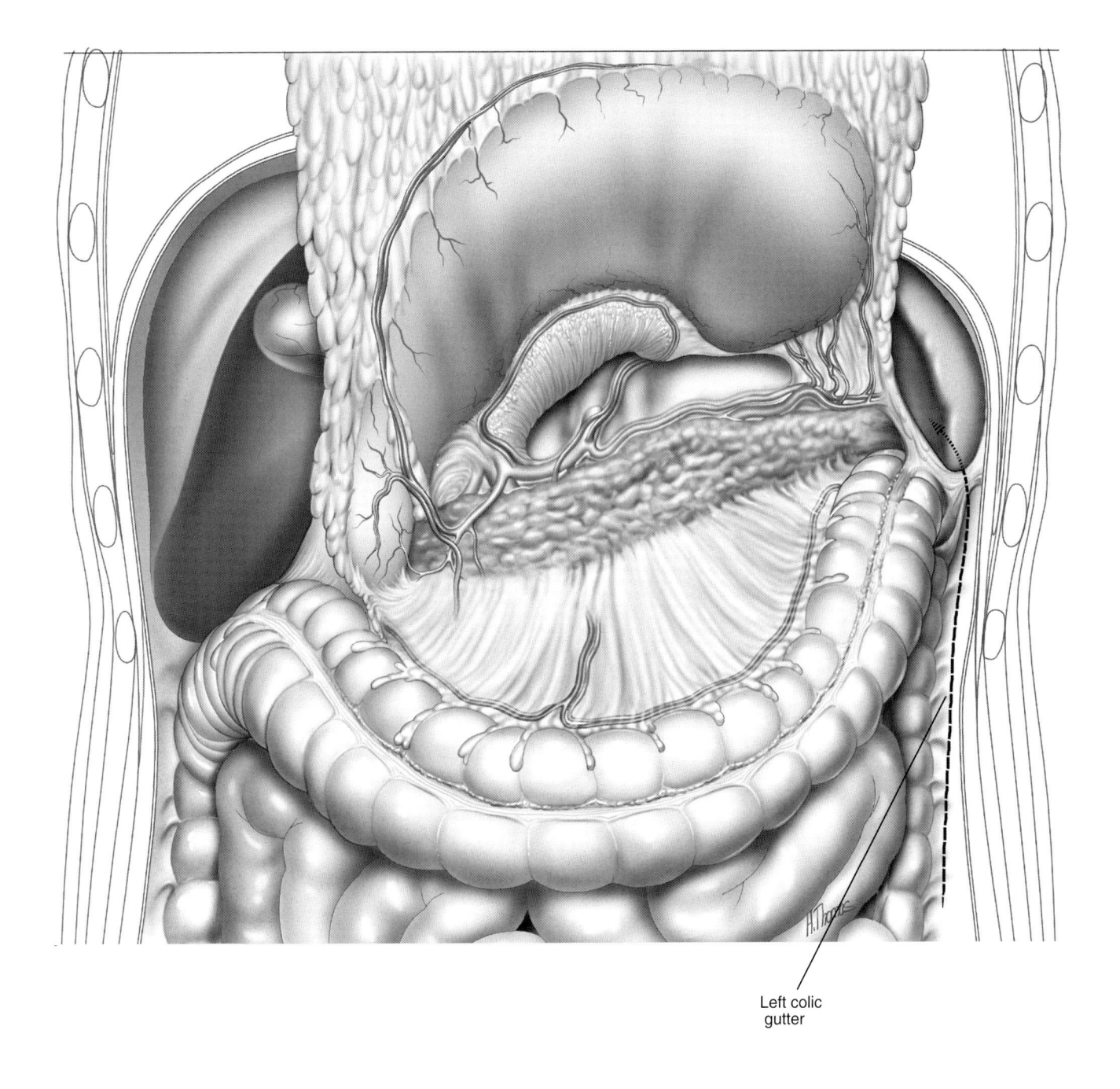

Figure 21–11 • If a total gastrectomy and splenectomy are to be performed, the left colic gutter is mobilized and the colosplenic ligament is divided.

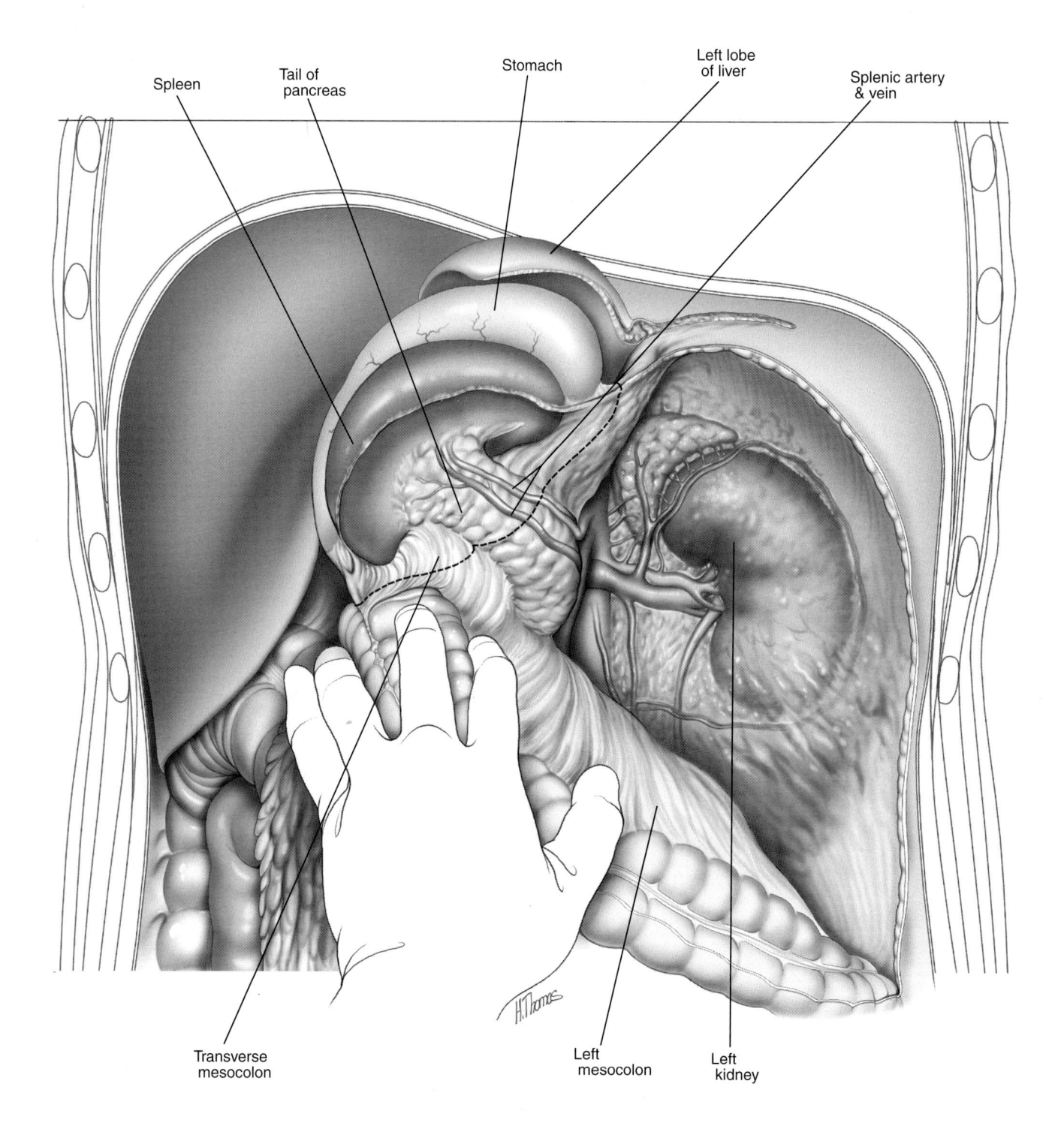

Figure 21–12 • The spleen and tail of the pancreas are mobilized by dividing the splenic attachments to the retroperitoneum.

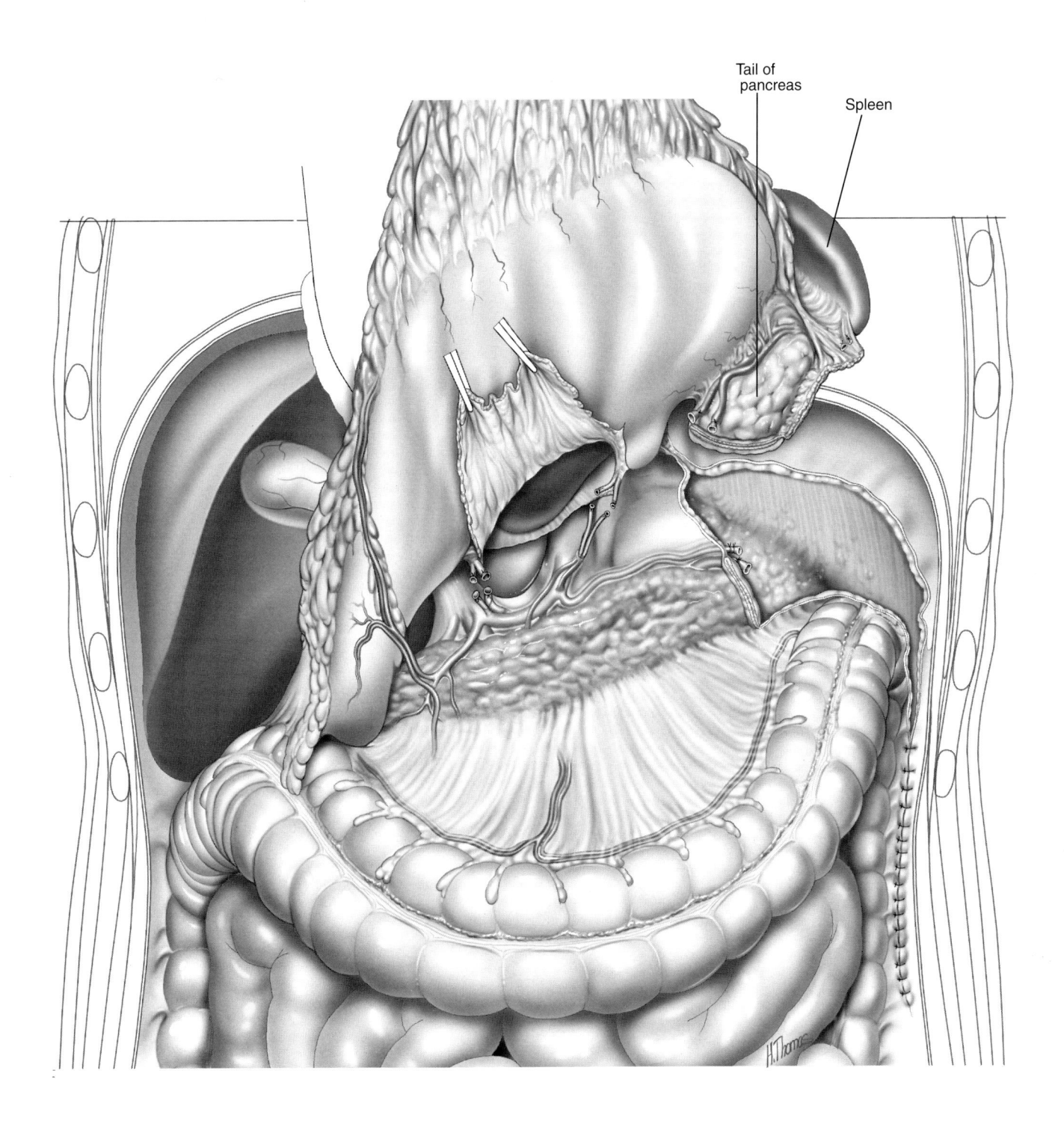

Figure 21–13 • The splenic artery and vein are divided, as well as the tail of the pancreas.

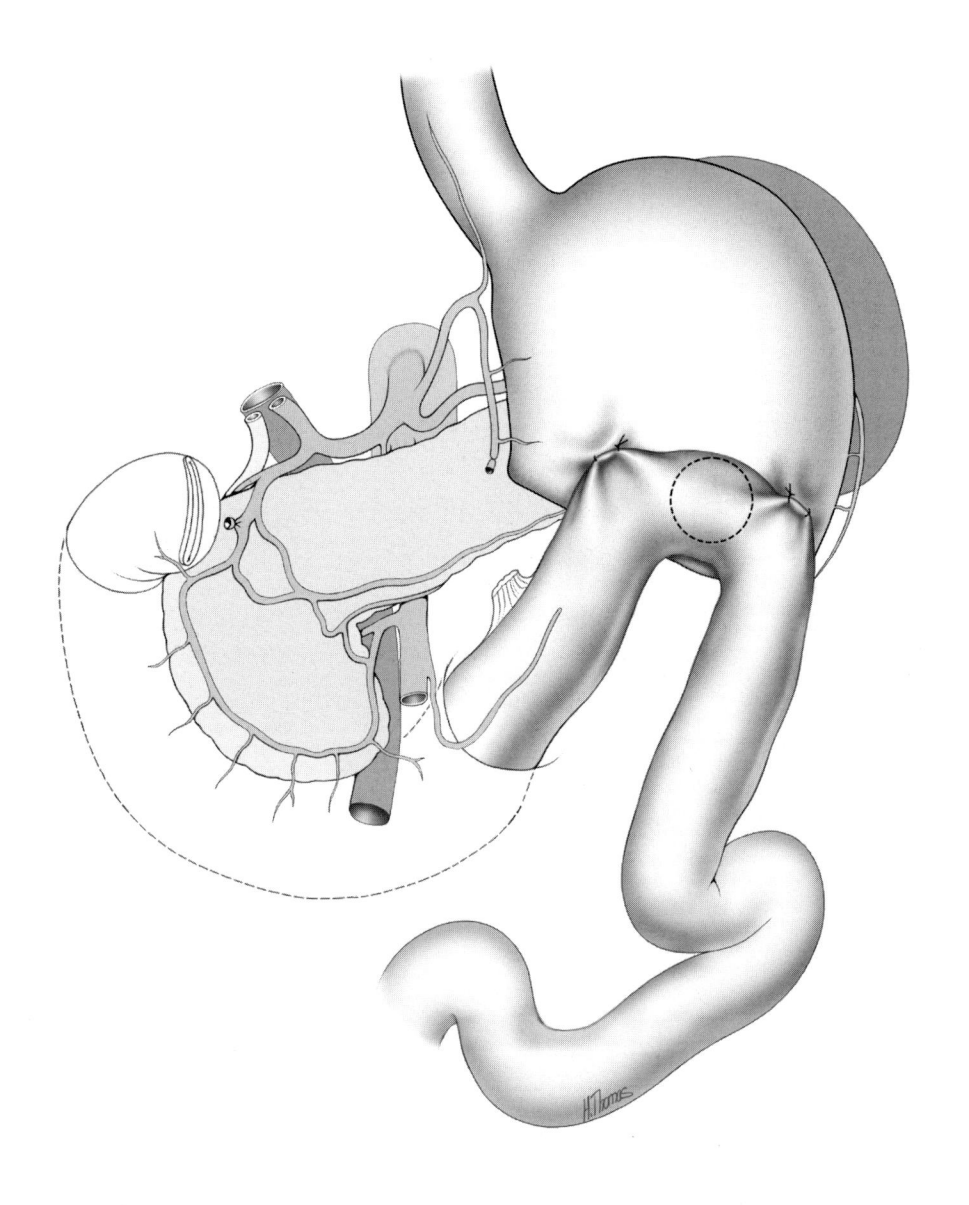

Figure 21–14 • An antecolic gastrojejunostomy is illustrated.

Gastric Surgery • 167

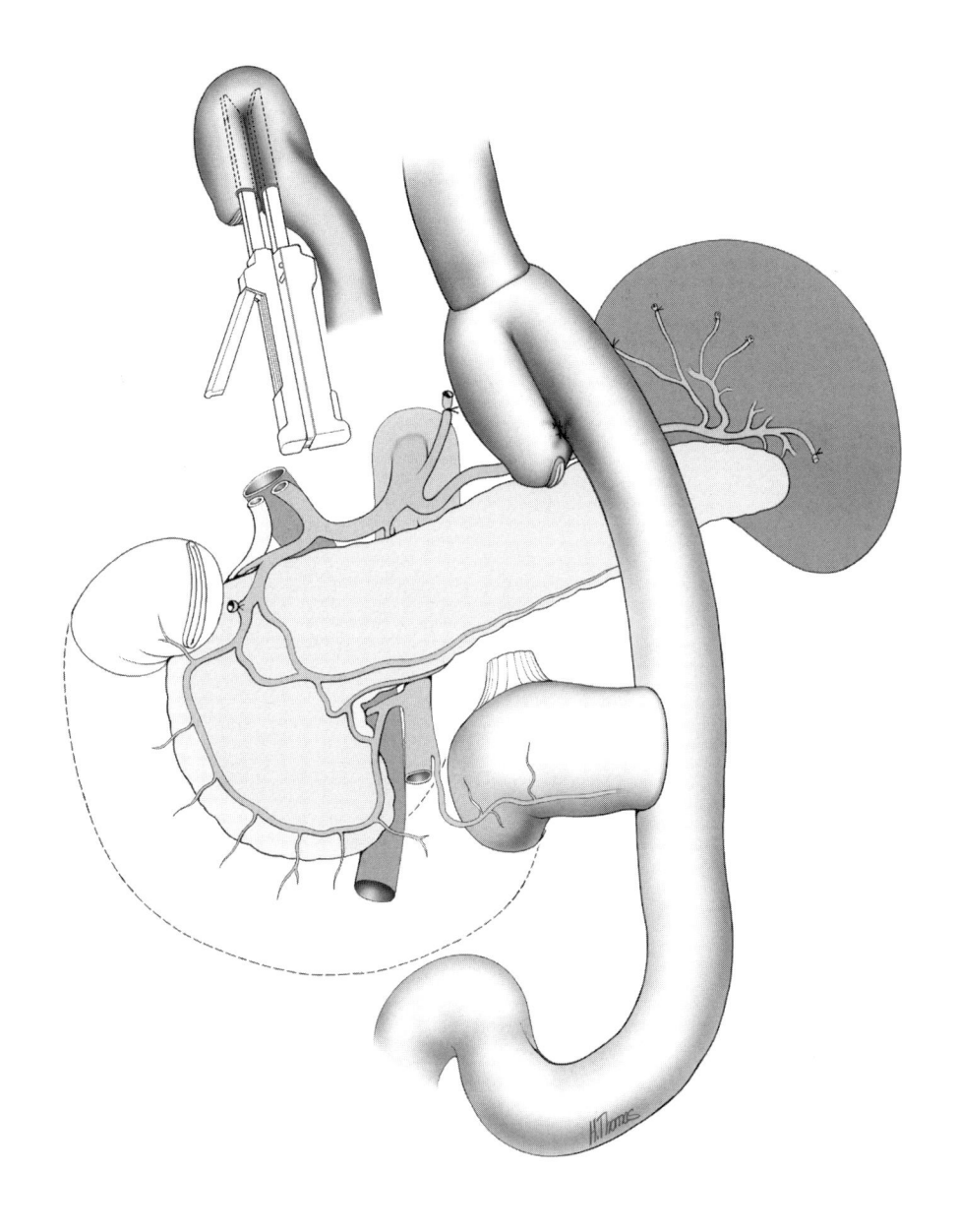

Figure 21–15 • An esophagojejunostomy following a total gastrectomy is illustrated.

Chapter 22
Clinical Case: Extended Gastrectomy With Radical Lymphadenectomy

Takashi Takaohashi

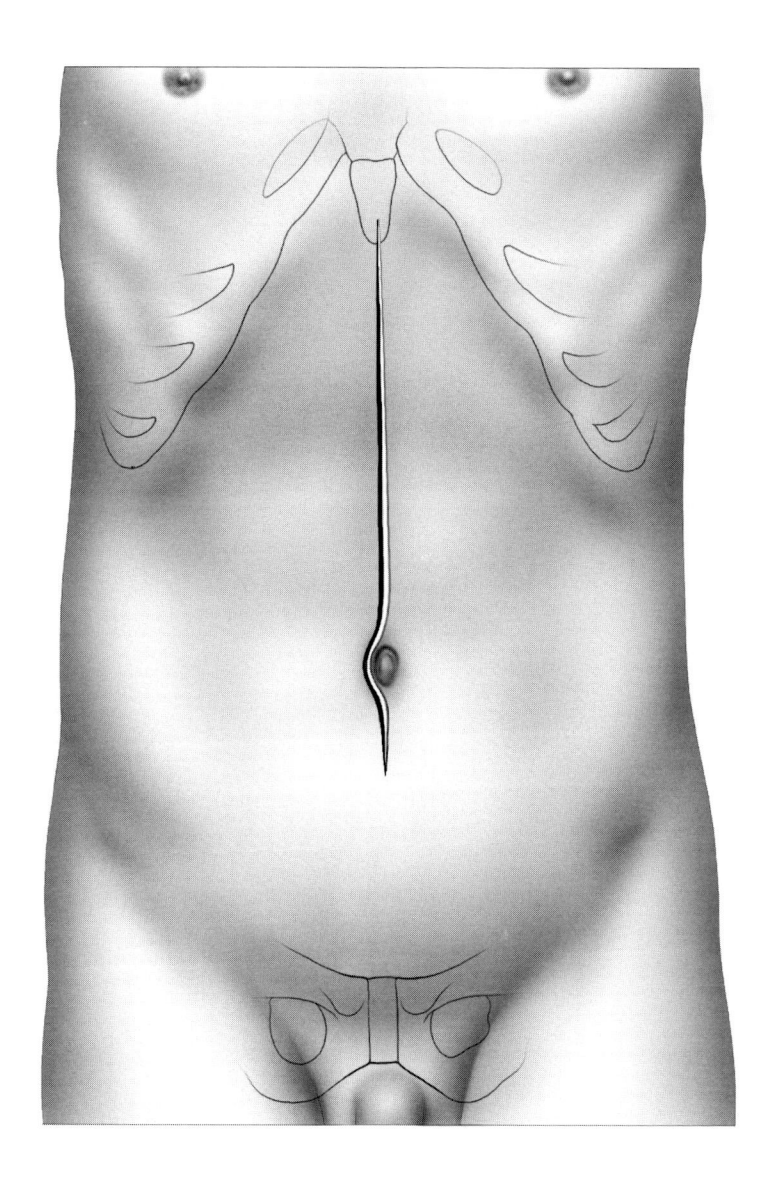

Figure 22–1 • A generous midline abdominal incision is employed.

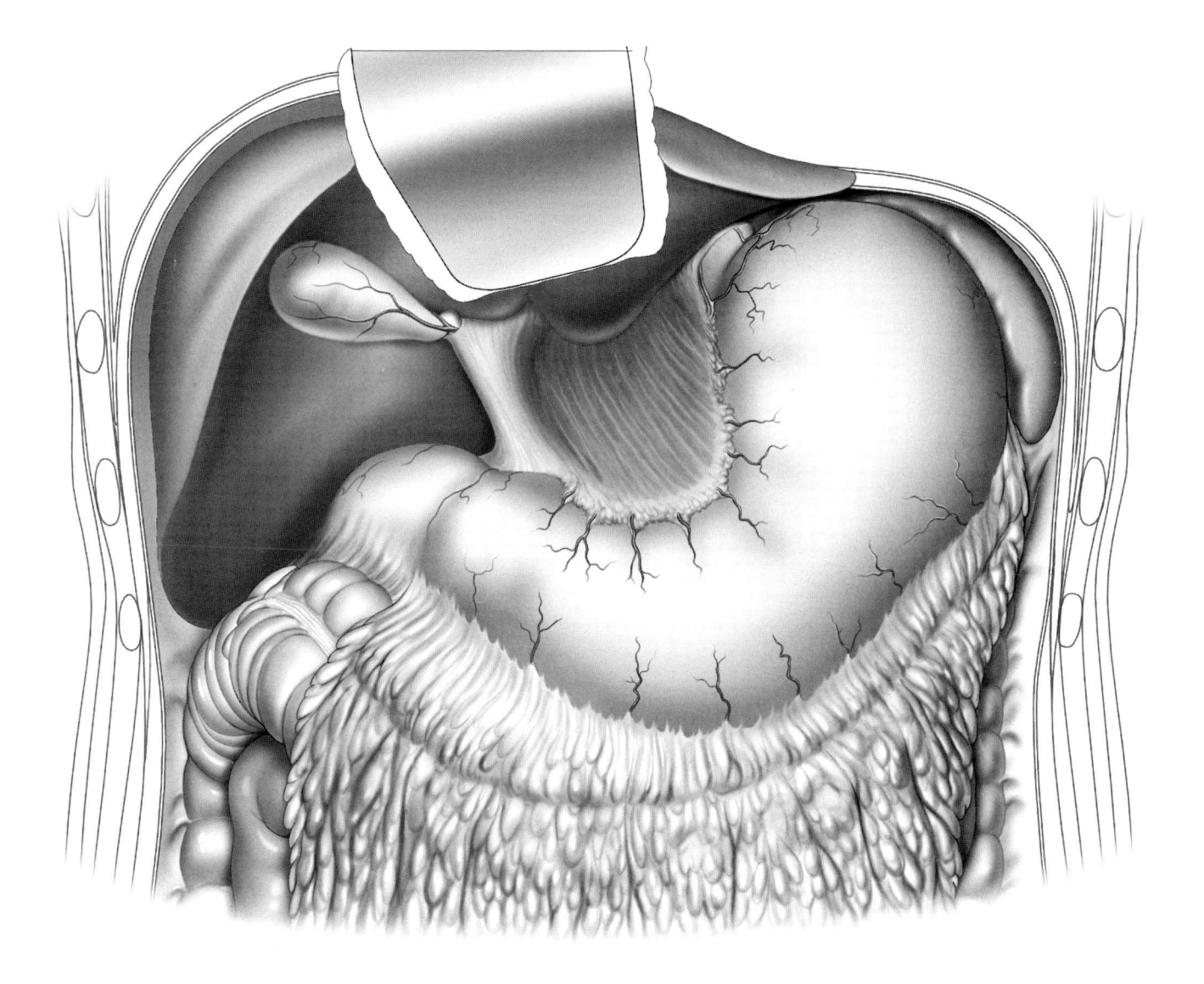

Figure 22–2 • The upper intraabdominal organs are exposed.

170 • Part III UPPER ABDOMEN

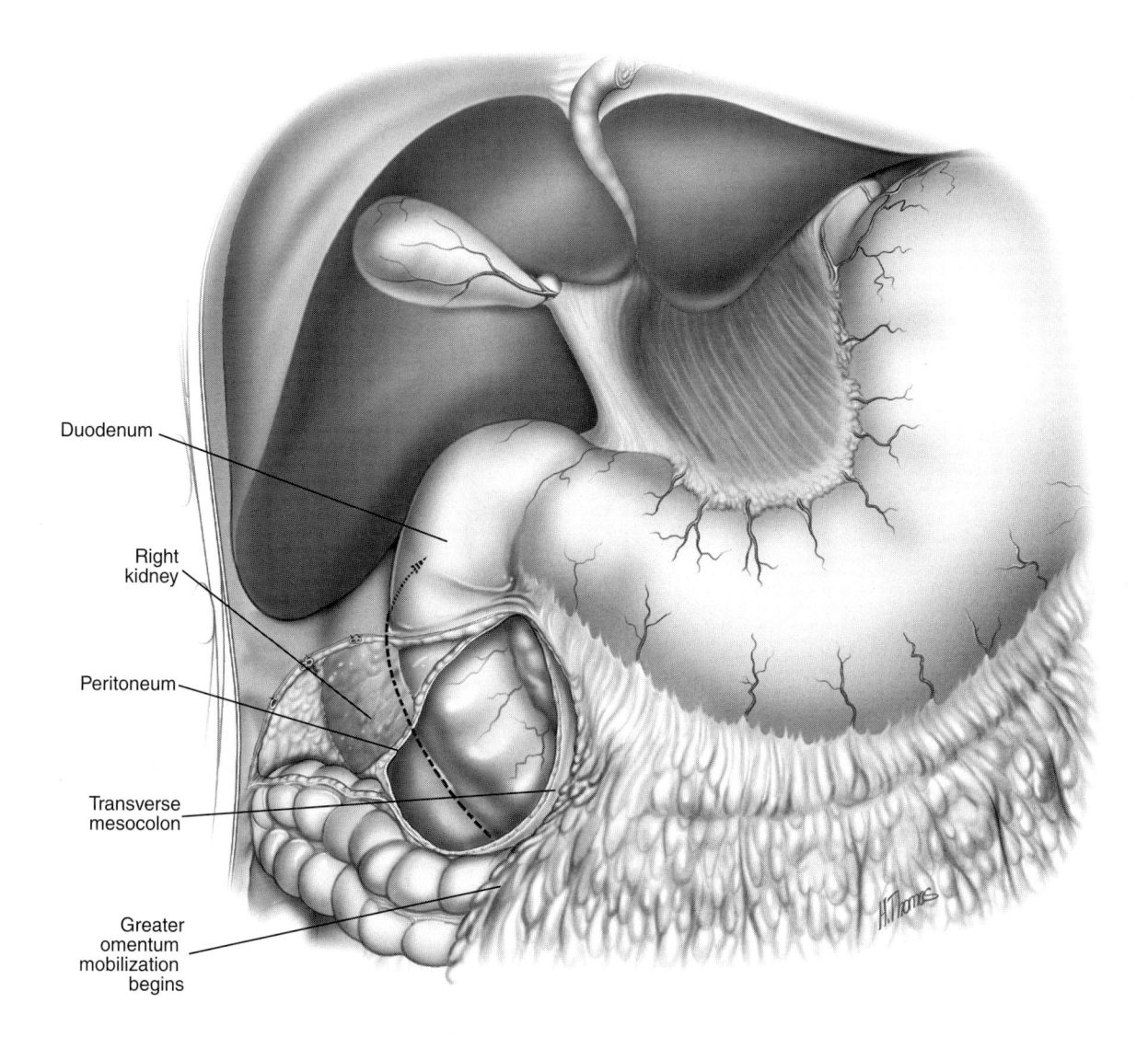

Figure 22–3 • The right hepatic flexure is mobilized. The duodenum is kocherized, and mobilization of the greater omentum off the transverse colon is commenced.

Clinical Case: Extended Gastrectomy with Radical Lymphadenectomy • 171

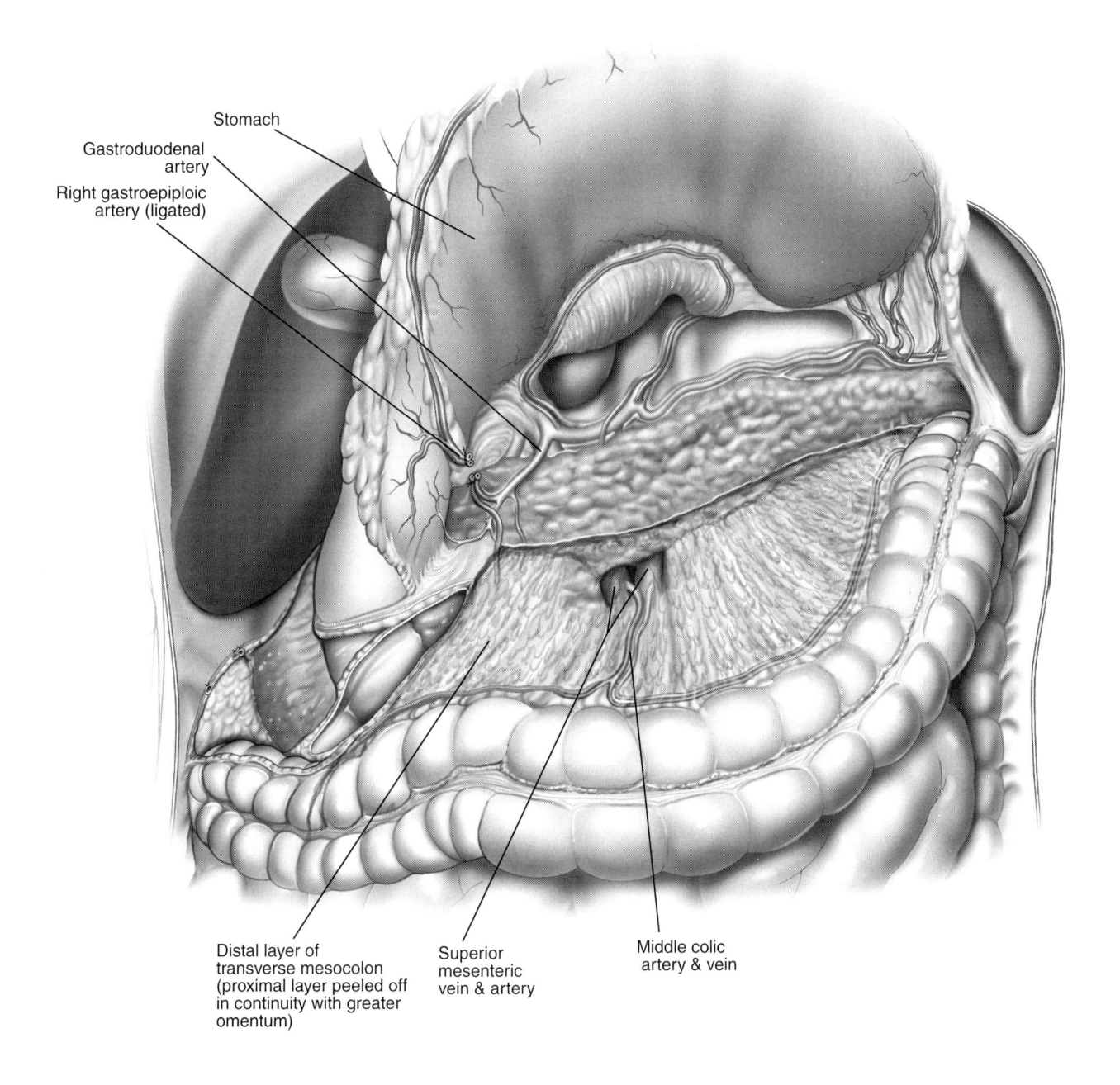

Figure 22–4 • Mobilization of the greater omentum is completed. The superior mesenteric artery and vein are identified at the base of the transverse mesocolon. The right gastroepiploic artery is identified.

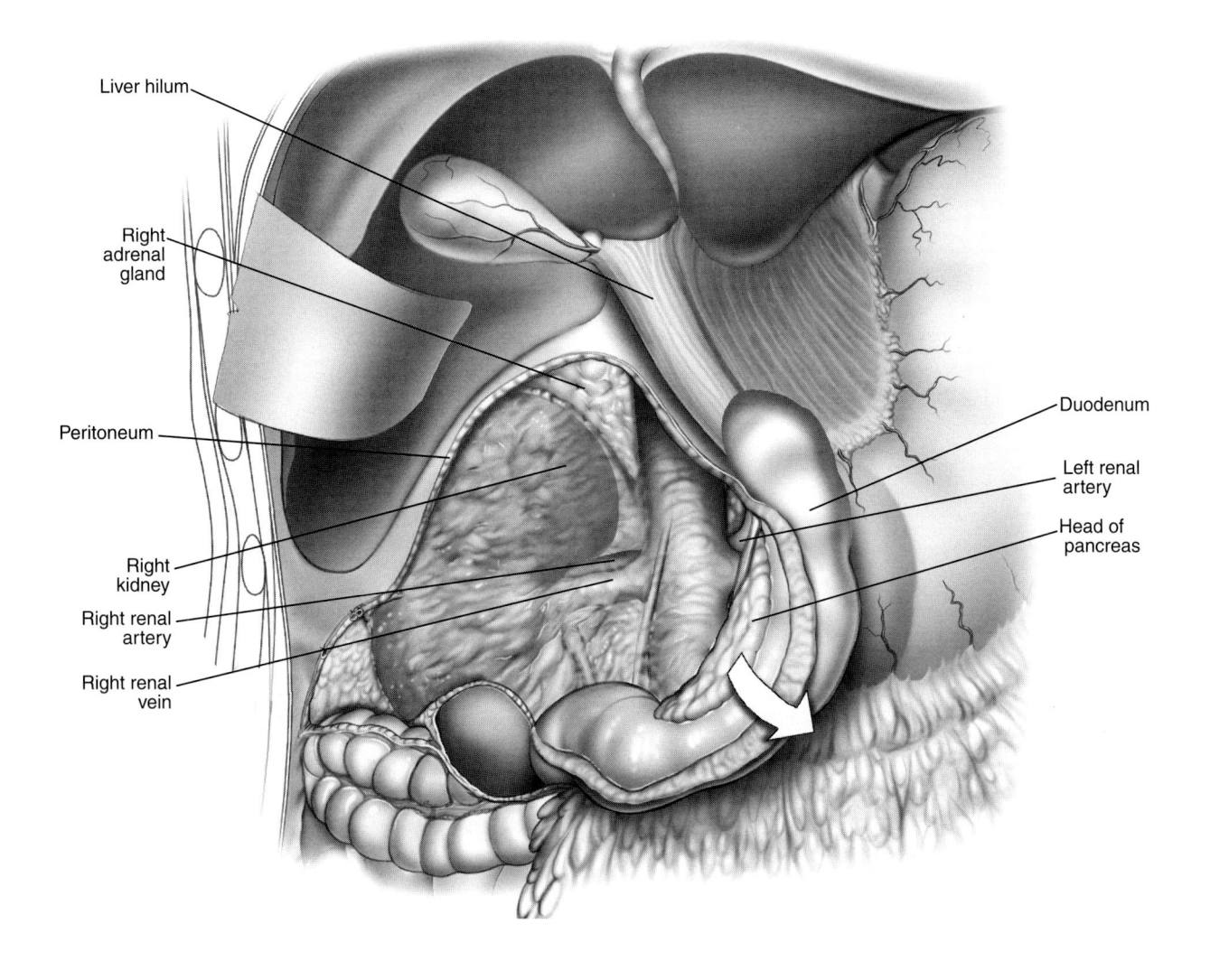

Figure 22-5 • The kocherization of the duodenum and head of the pancreas is completed, identifying the renal arteries.

Clinical Case: Extended Gastrectomy with Radical Lymphadenectomy • 173

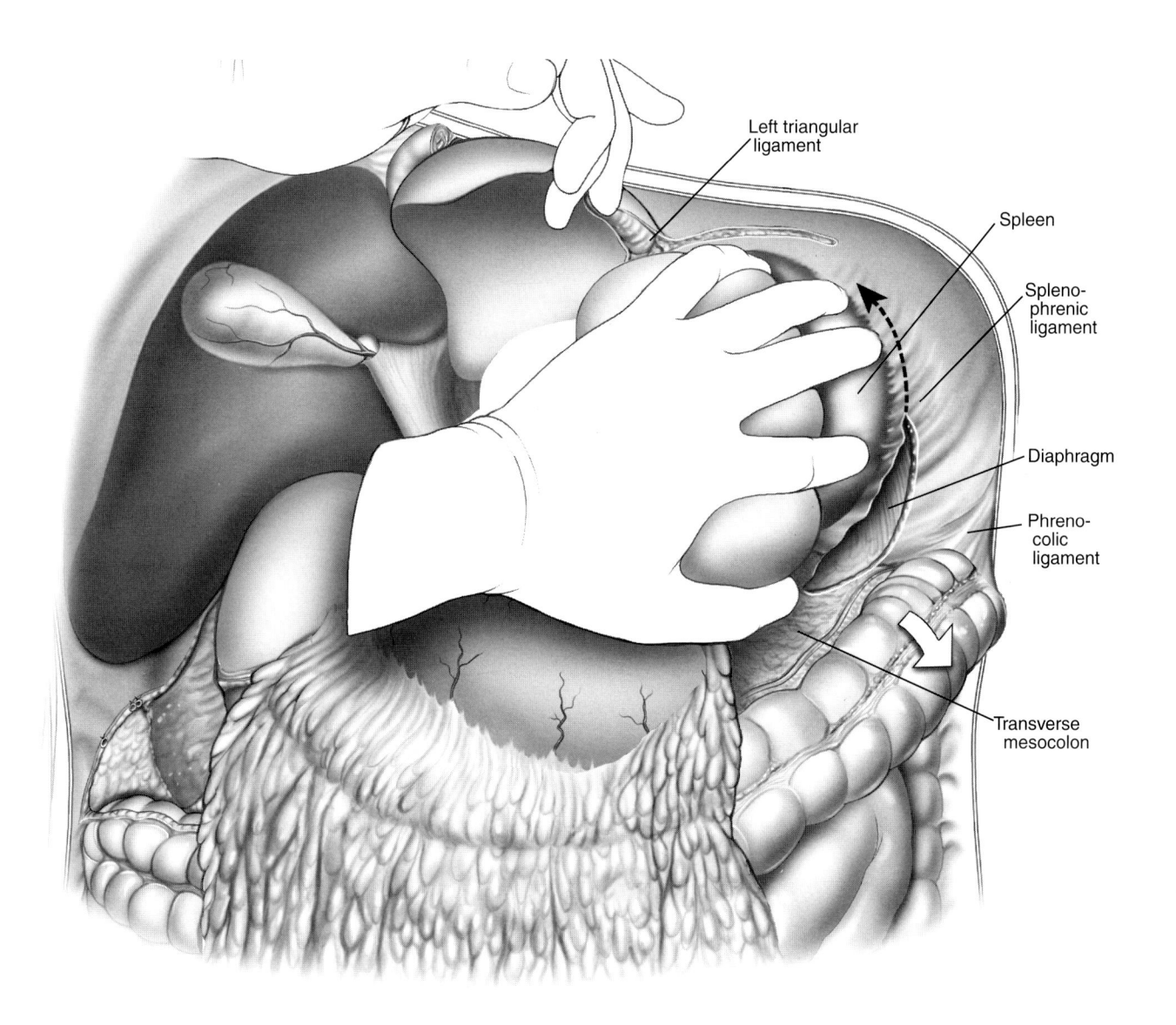

Figure 22–6 • The left triangular ligament is cut. The splenophrenic ligament is mobilized, and the splenic flexure of the colon is displaced downward.

174 • Part III UPPER ABDOMEN

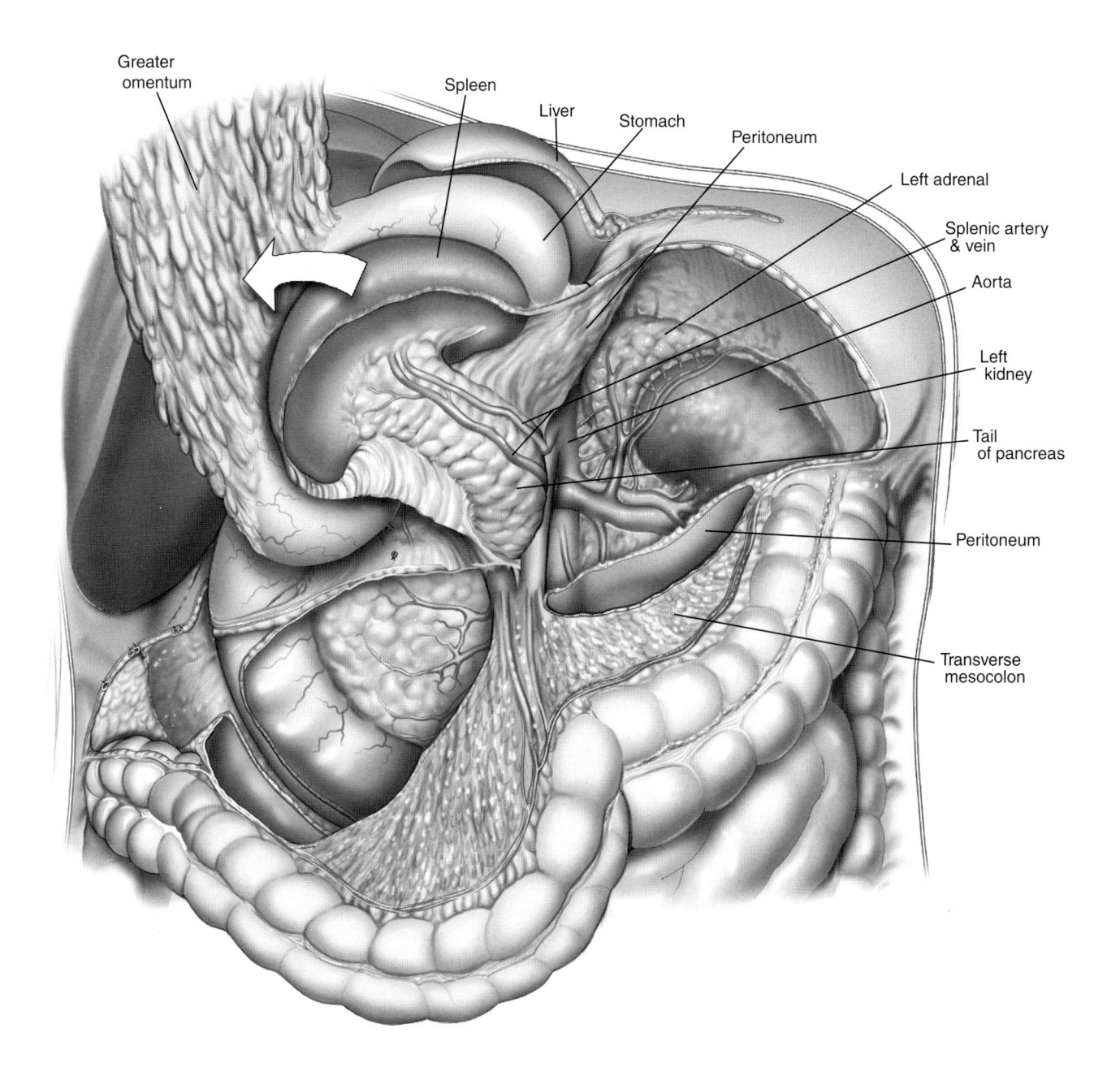

Figure 22–7 • The completed mobilization of the spleen and pancreas allows for dissection of the nodal tissue around the left renal vessels. The mesentery of the transverse colon is incised to the superior mesenteric vessels, which are skeletonized.

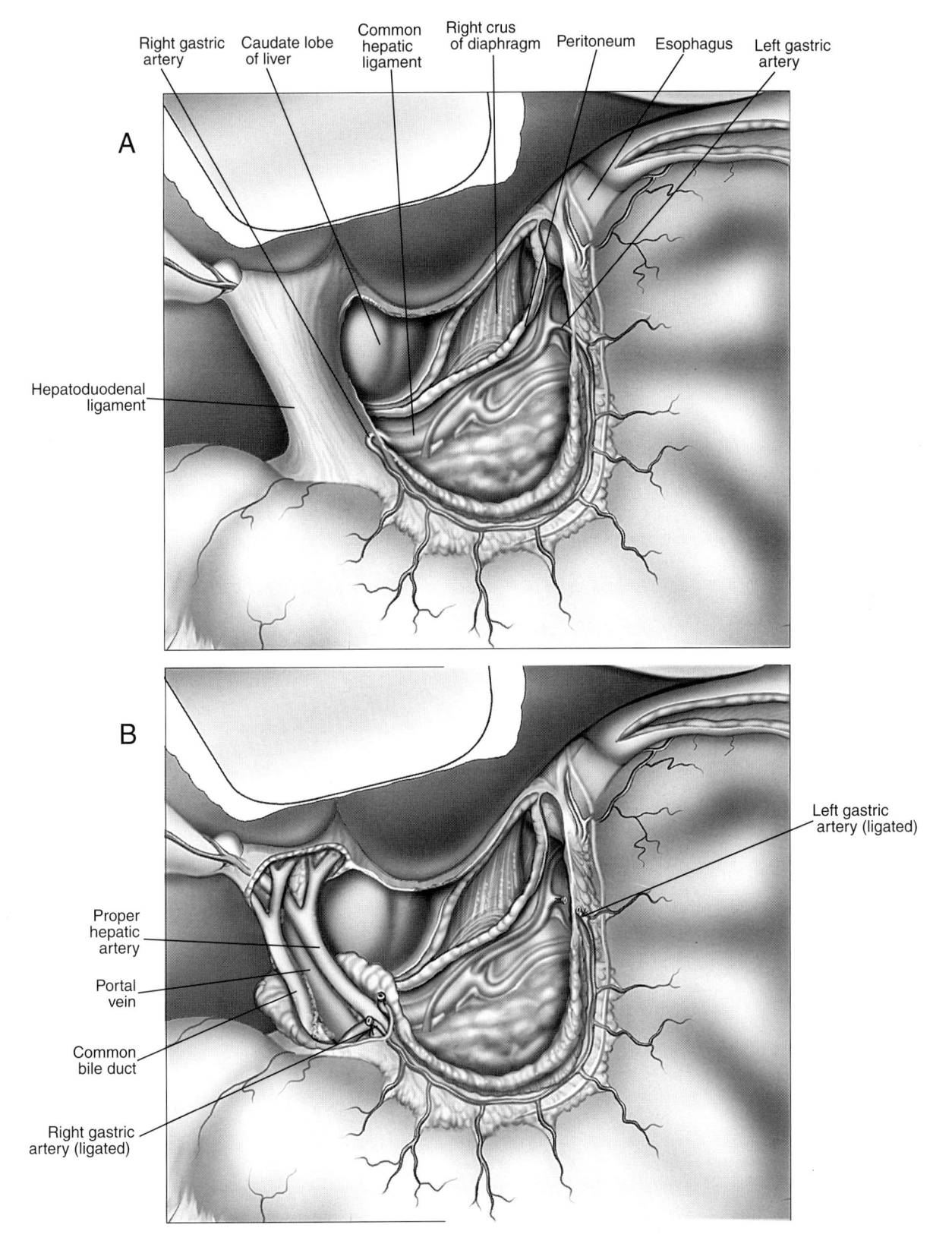

Clinical Case: Extended Gastrectomy with Radical Lymphadenectomy • 175

Figure 22–8 • **A,** The gastrohepatic ligament is divided. The investing fascia of the retroperitoneal space is peeled off the right crus of the diaphragm inferiorly to expose the celiac axis.

B, The hepatoduodenal ligament is dissected, skeletonizing the hepatic artery, portal vein, and common bile duct. The right gastric artery is divided.

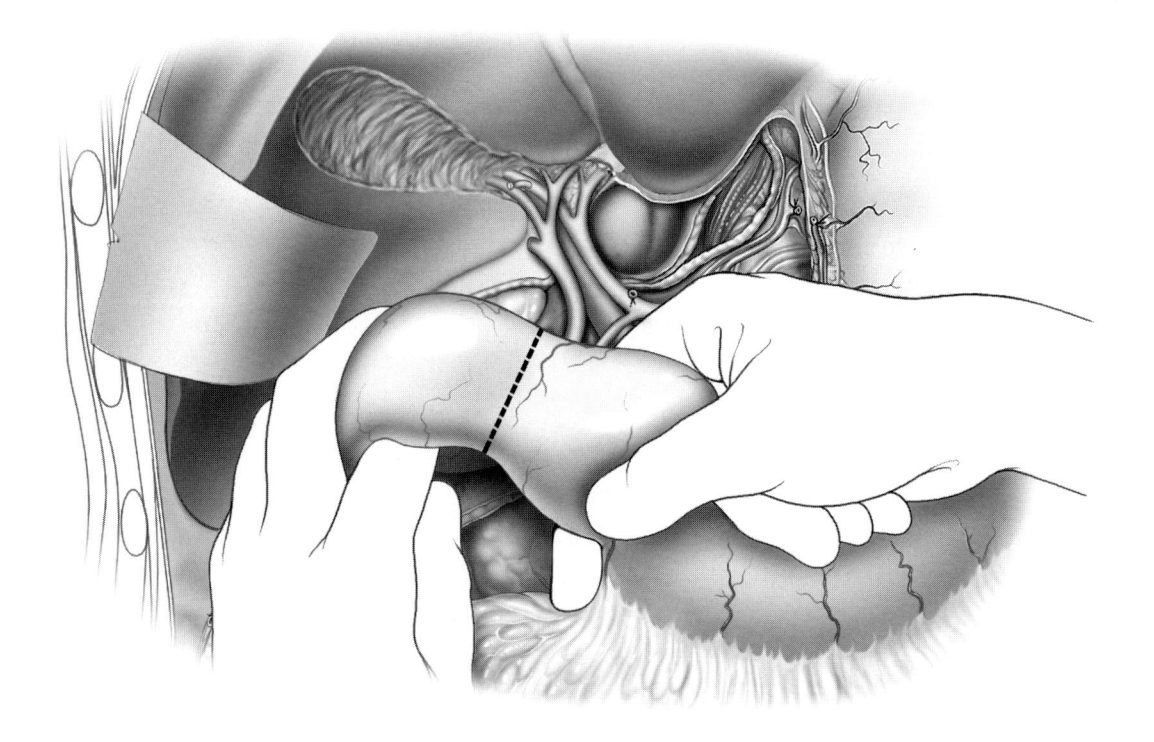

Figure 22-9 • The pylorus is divided and the gallbladder is removed.

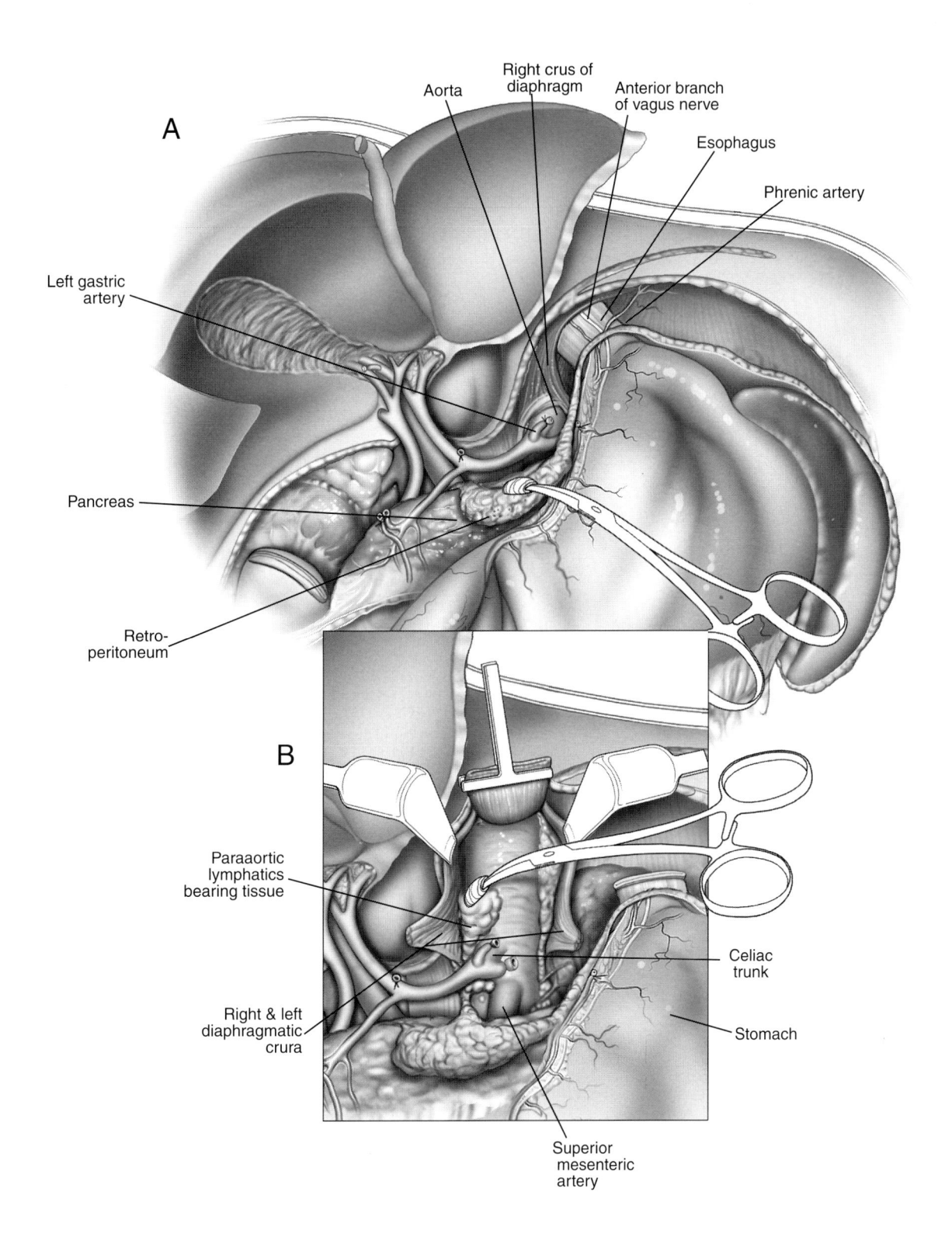

Figure 22-10 • **A,** The left gastric artery is divided and the esophagogastric junction is mobilized. All nodal tissue is mobilized inferiorly.

B, The esophagus is divided and the aorta is exposed between the diaphragmatic crura. Paraaortic lymph nodes are dissected.

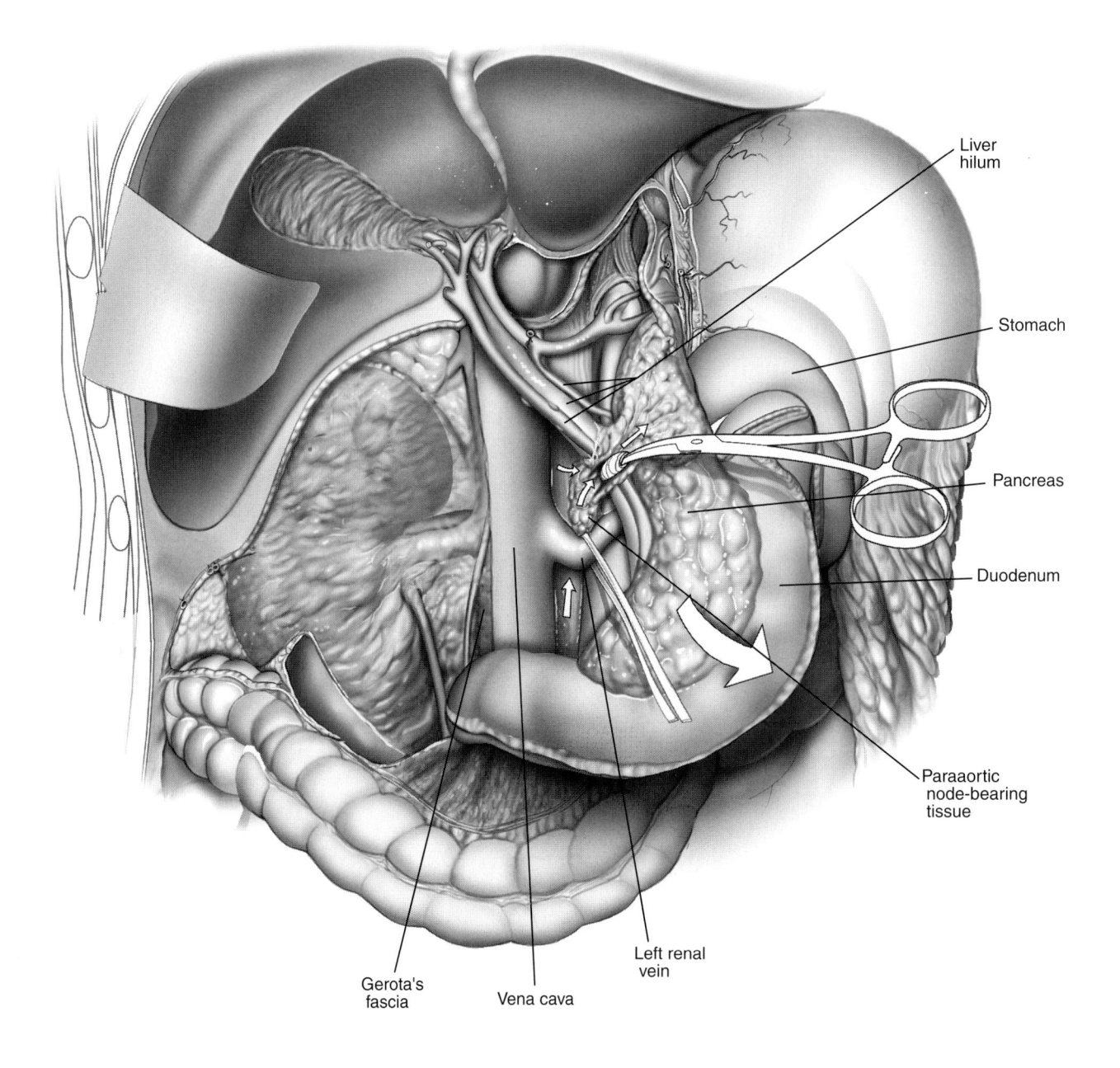

Figure 22-11 • All paraaortic nodes are dissected to the level of the renal arteries.

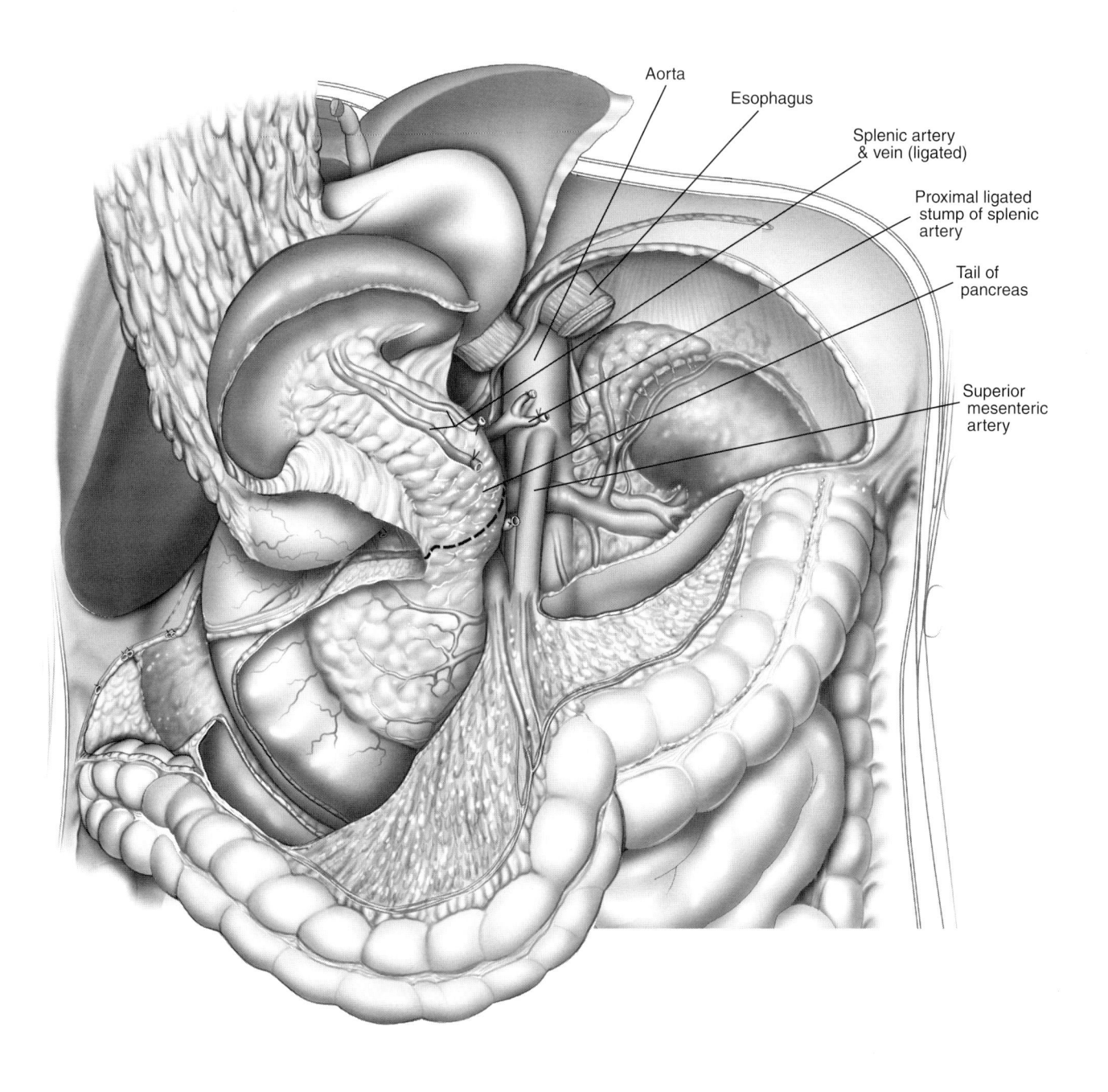

Clinical Case: Extended Gastrectomy with Radical Lymphadenectomy • 179

Figure 22–12 • The splenic artery and vein are divided, and the line of resection on the body of the pancreas is defined.

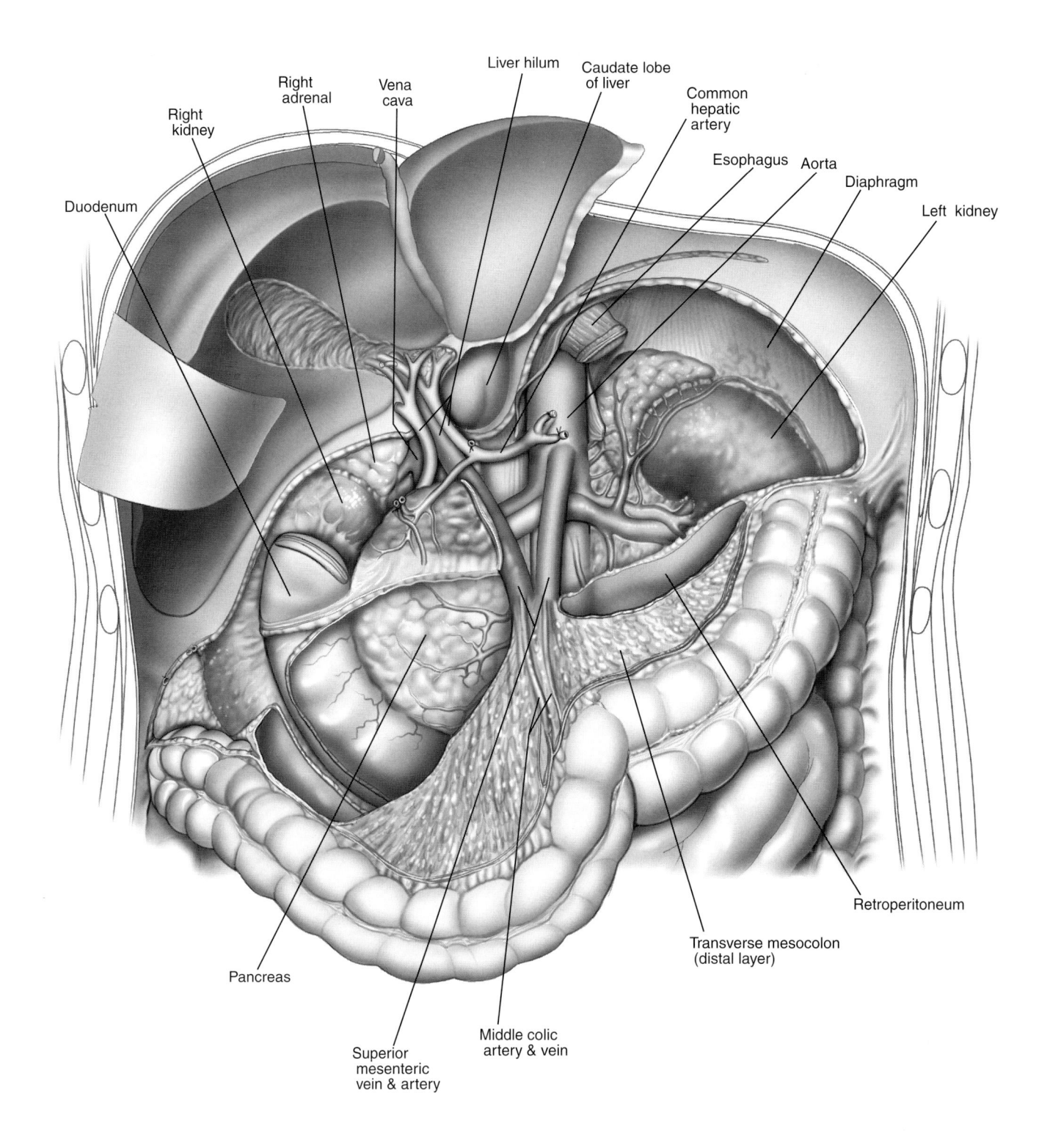

Figure 22–13 • The completed resection is depicted.

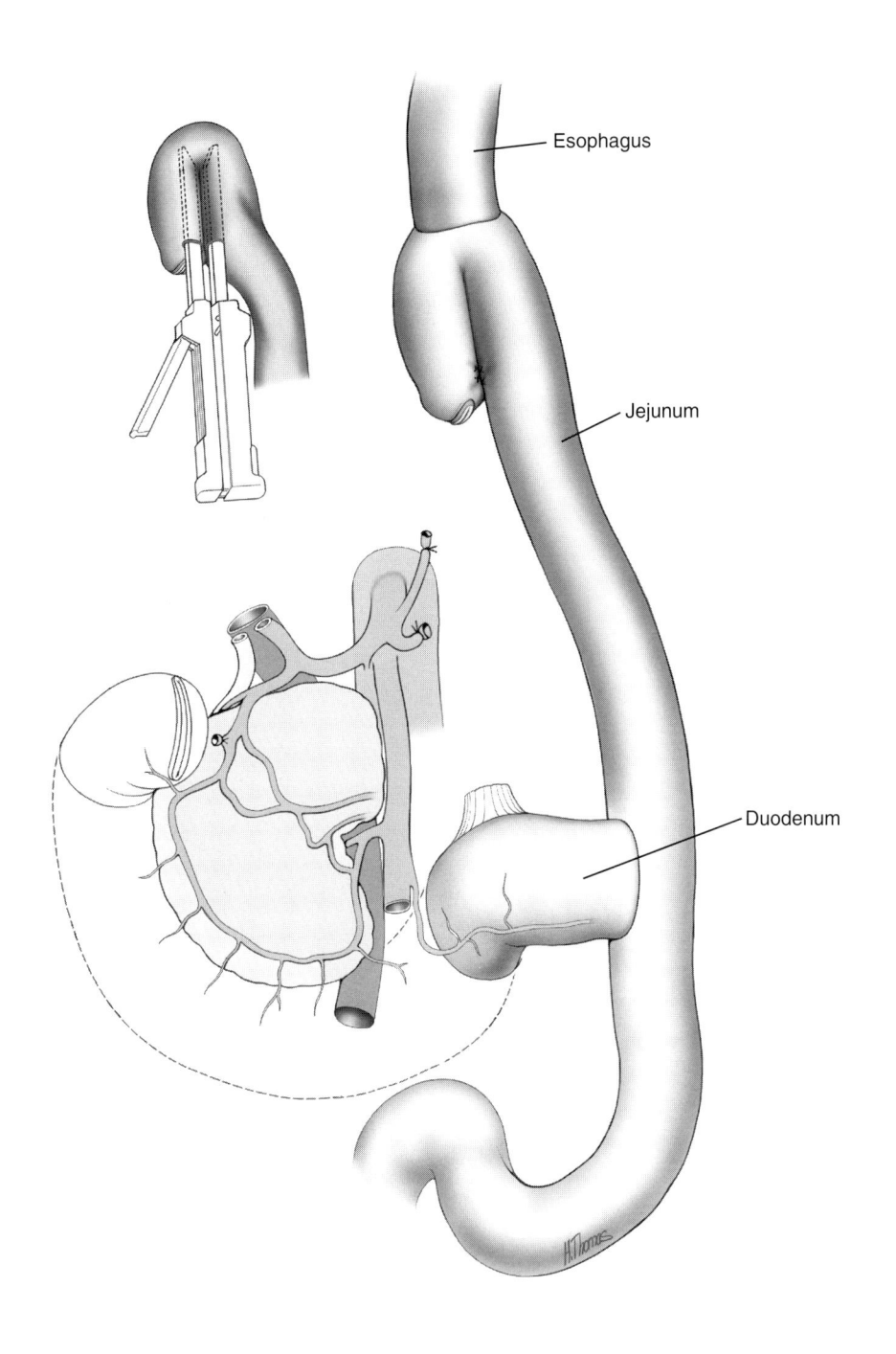

Clinical Case: Extended Gastrectomy with Radical Lymphadenectomy • 181

Figure 22–14 • A Roux-en-Y anastomosis is created.

Chapter 23
Right Hepatic Lobectomy

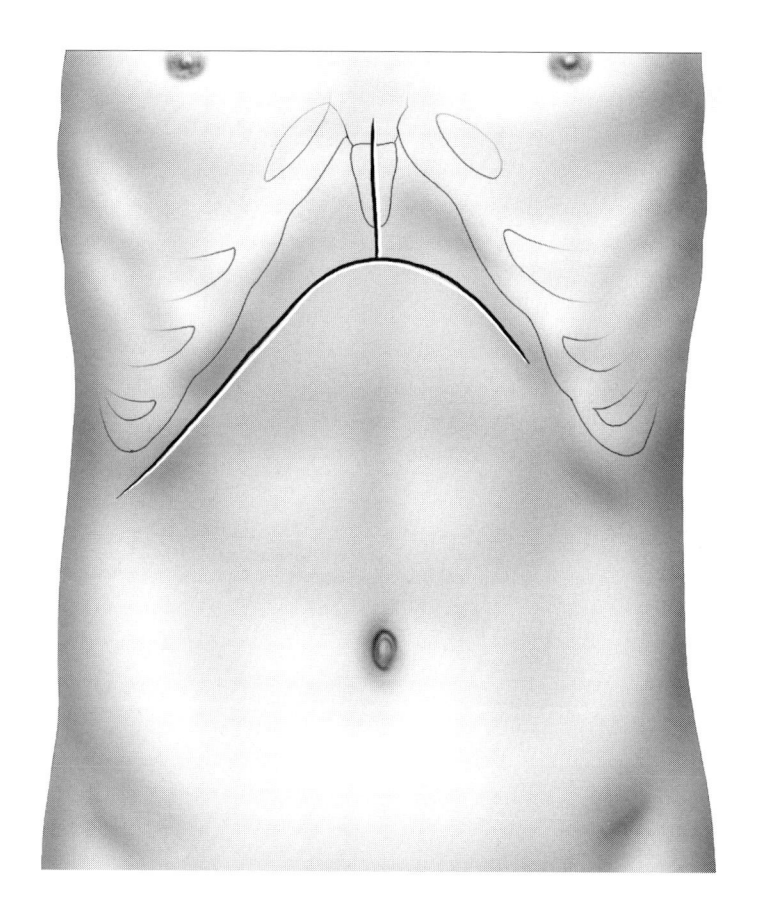

Figure 23–1 • A transverse upper abdominal incision is preferred, with the potential for a vertical extension.

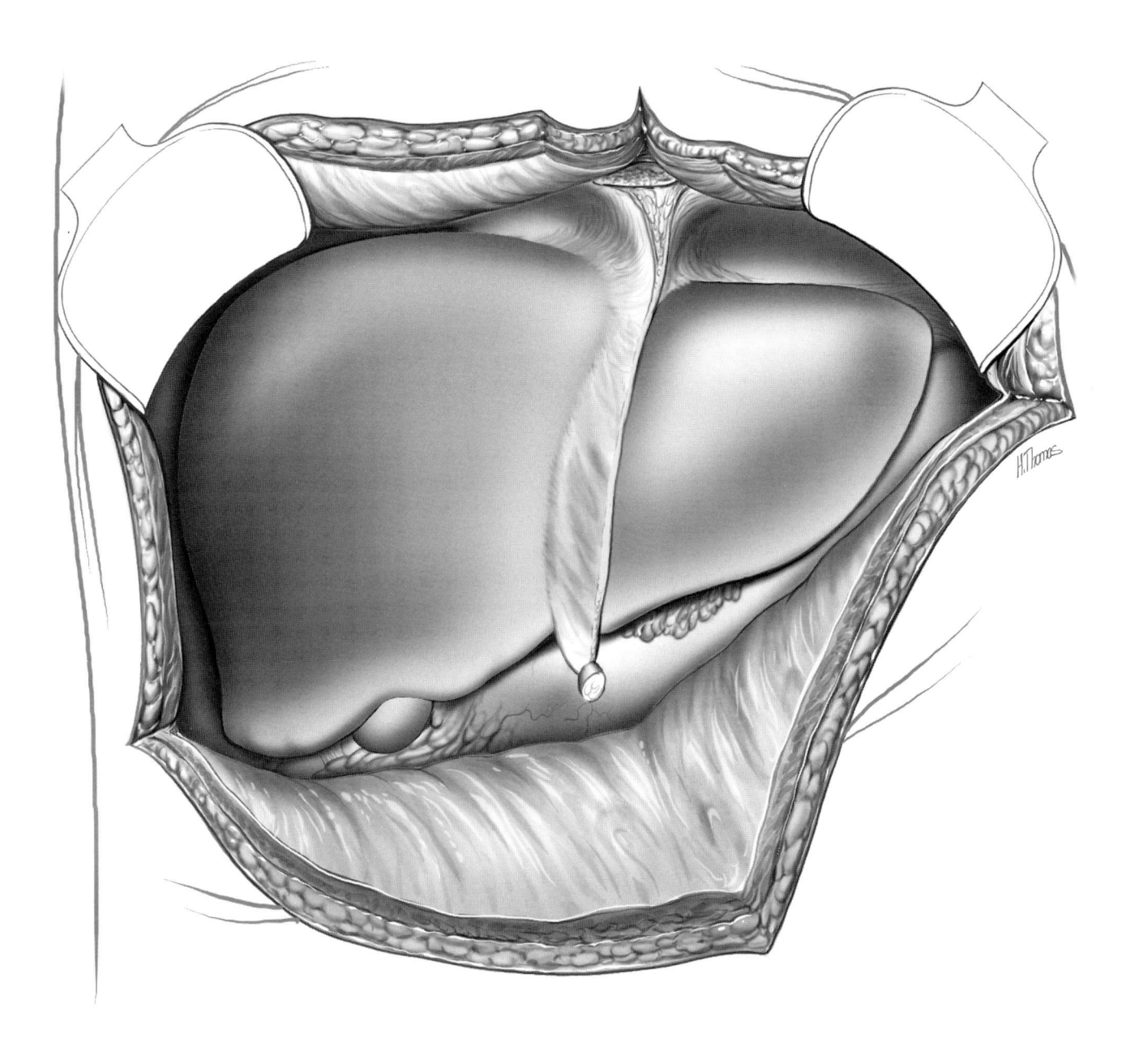

Figure 23–2 • Following completion of the abdominal incision, the falciform ligament is divided.

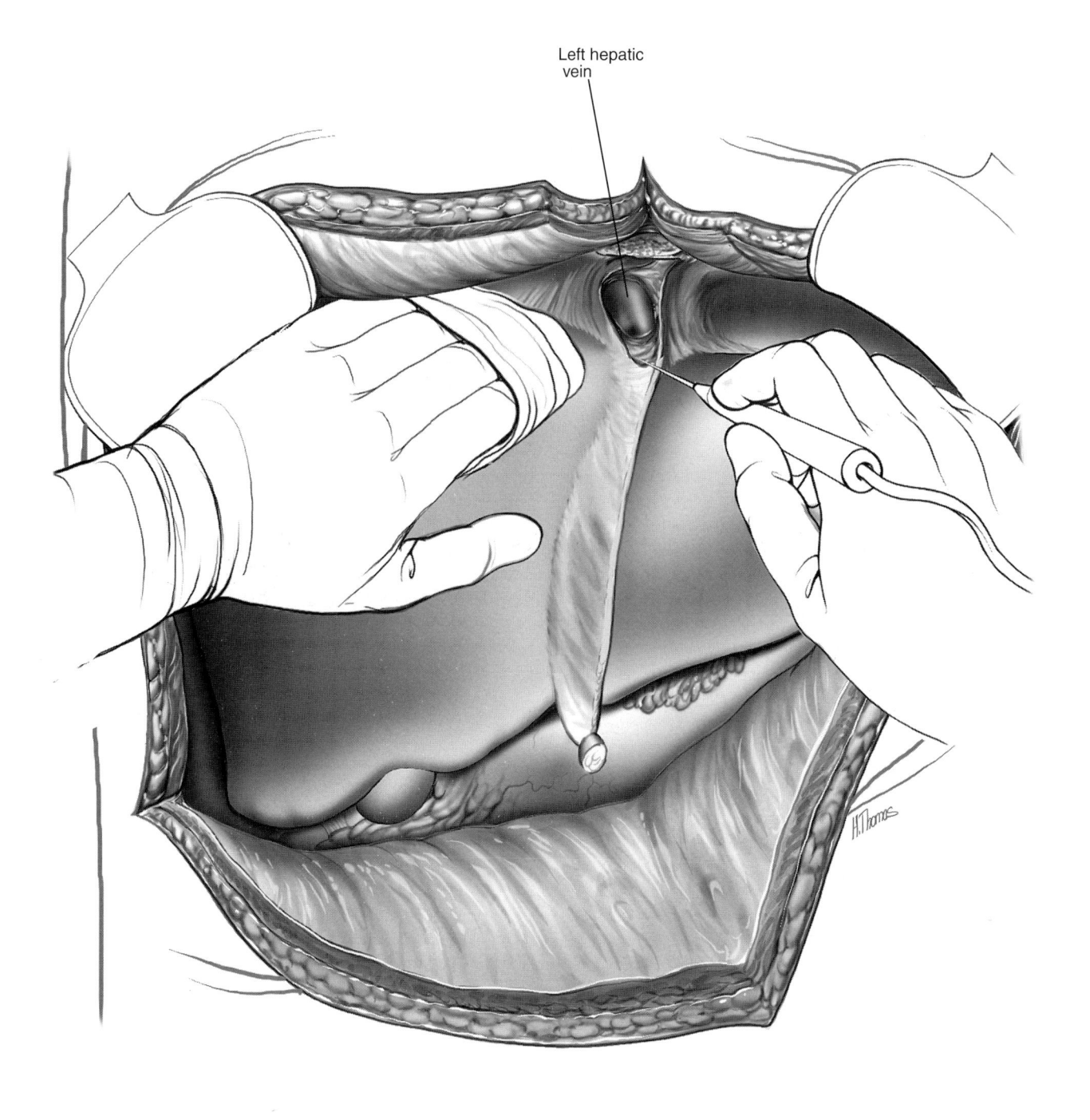

Figure 23–3 • Using a cautery, the apex of the falciform ligament is incised and the hepatic veins are identified.

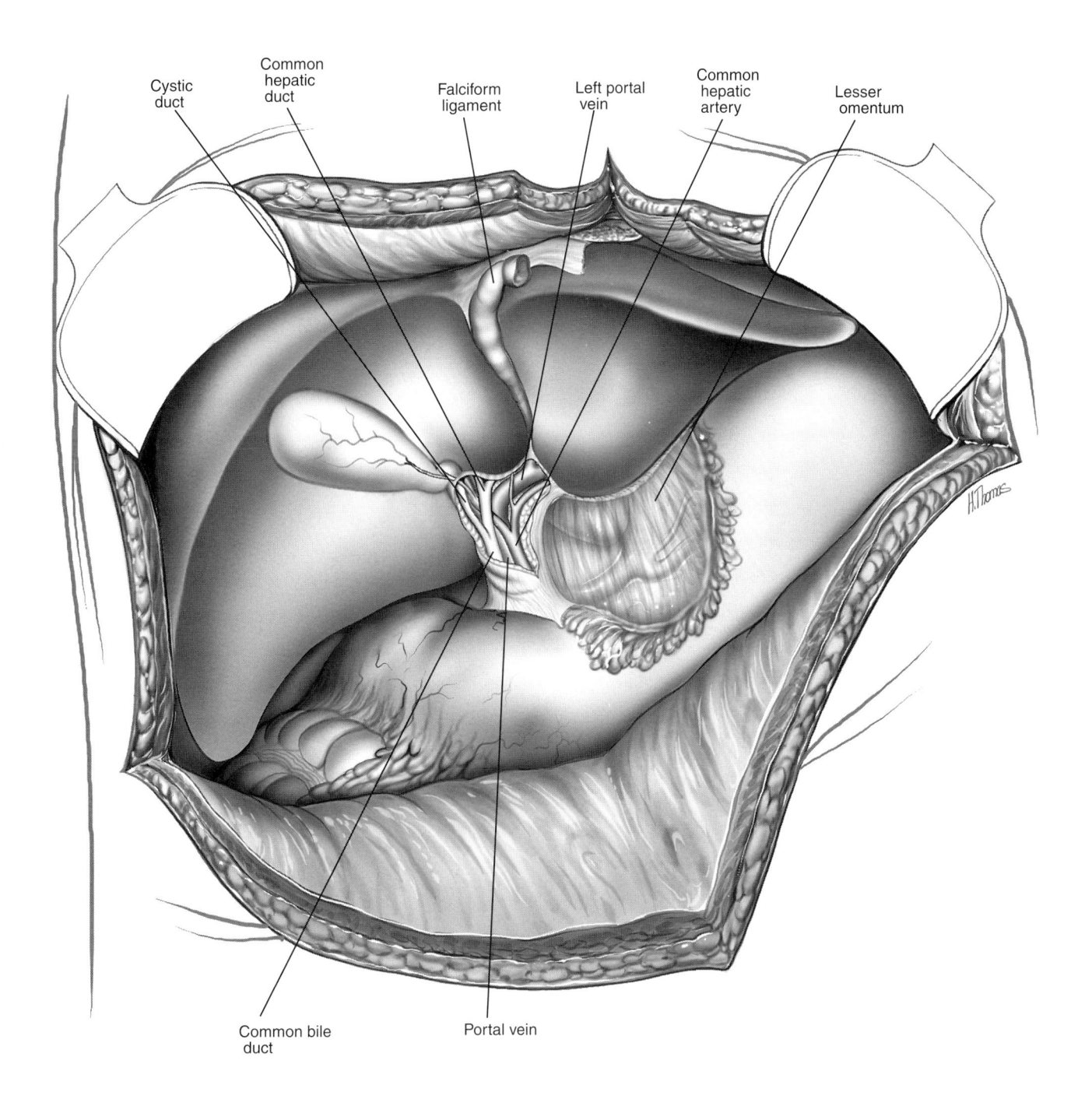

Figure 23–4 • The porta hepatis is exposed and the major structures are identified.

186 • Part III UPPER ABDOMEN

Gallbladder   Cystic artery   Cystic duct   Right hepatic artery

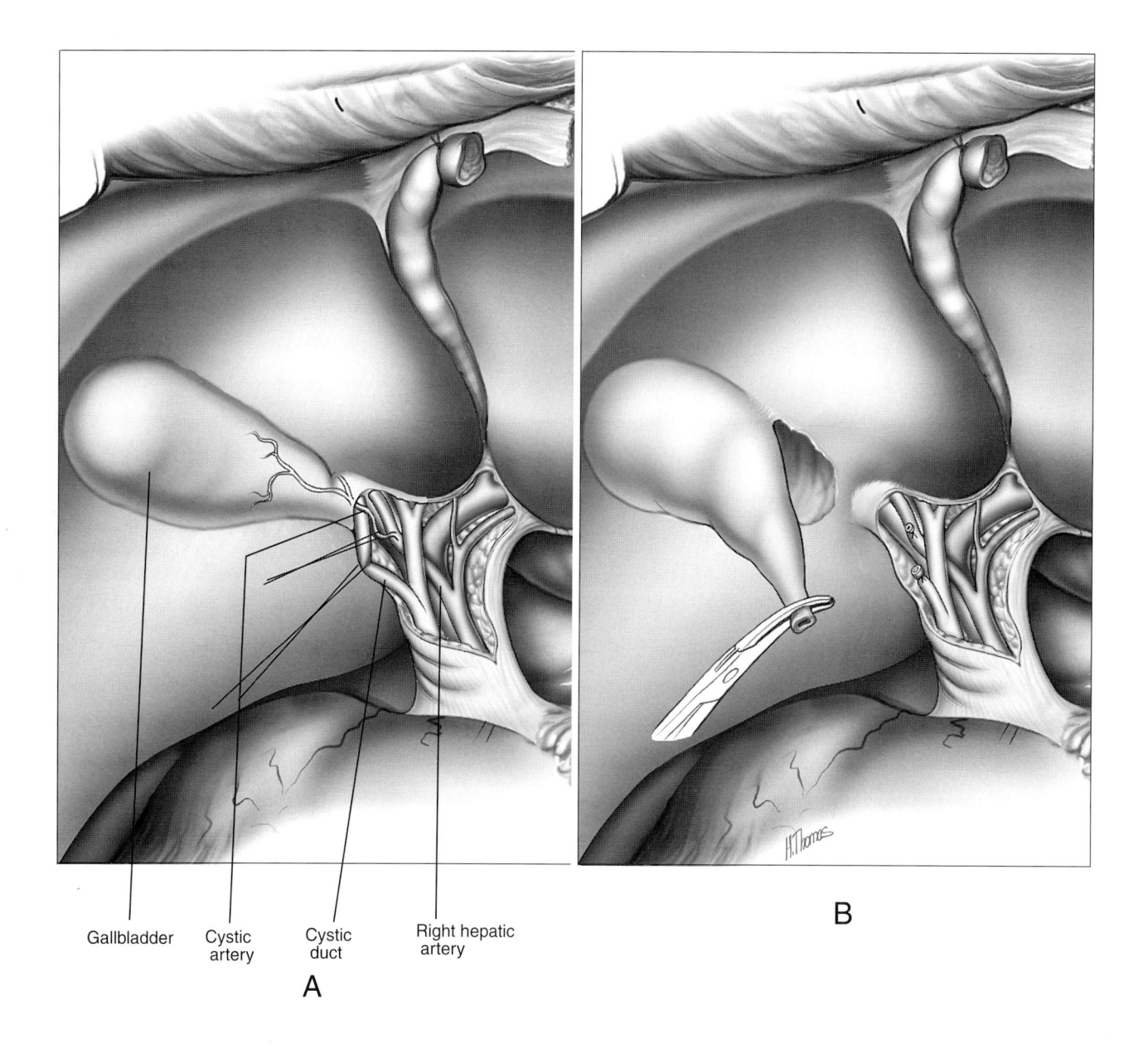

A

B

Figure 23–5 • **A,** The cystic duct and artery are divided.
B, The gallbladder is removed.

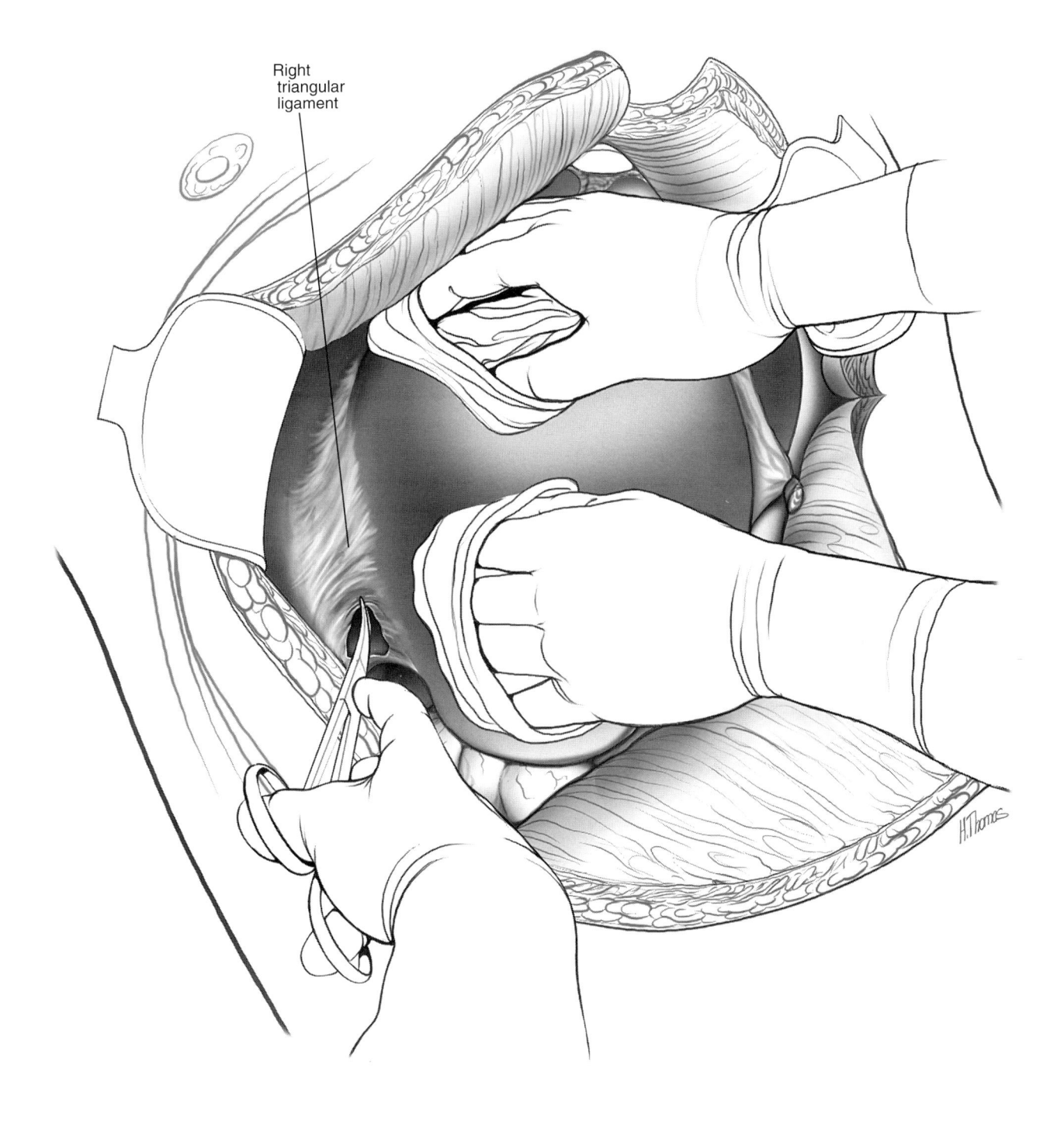

Figure 23–6 • The right triangular ligament is incised.

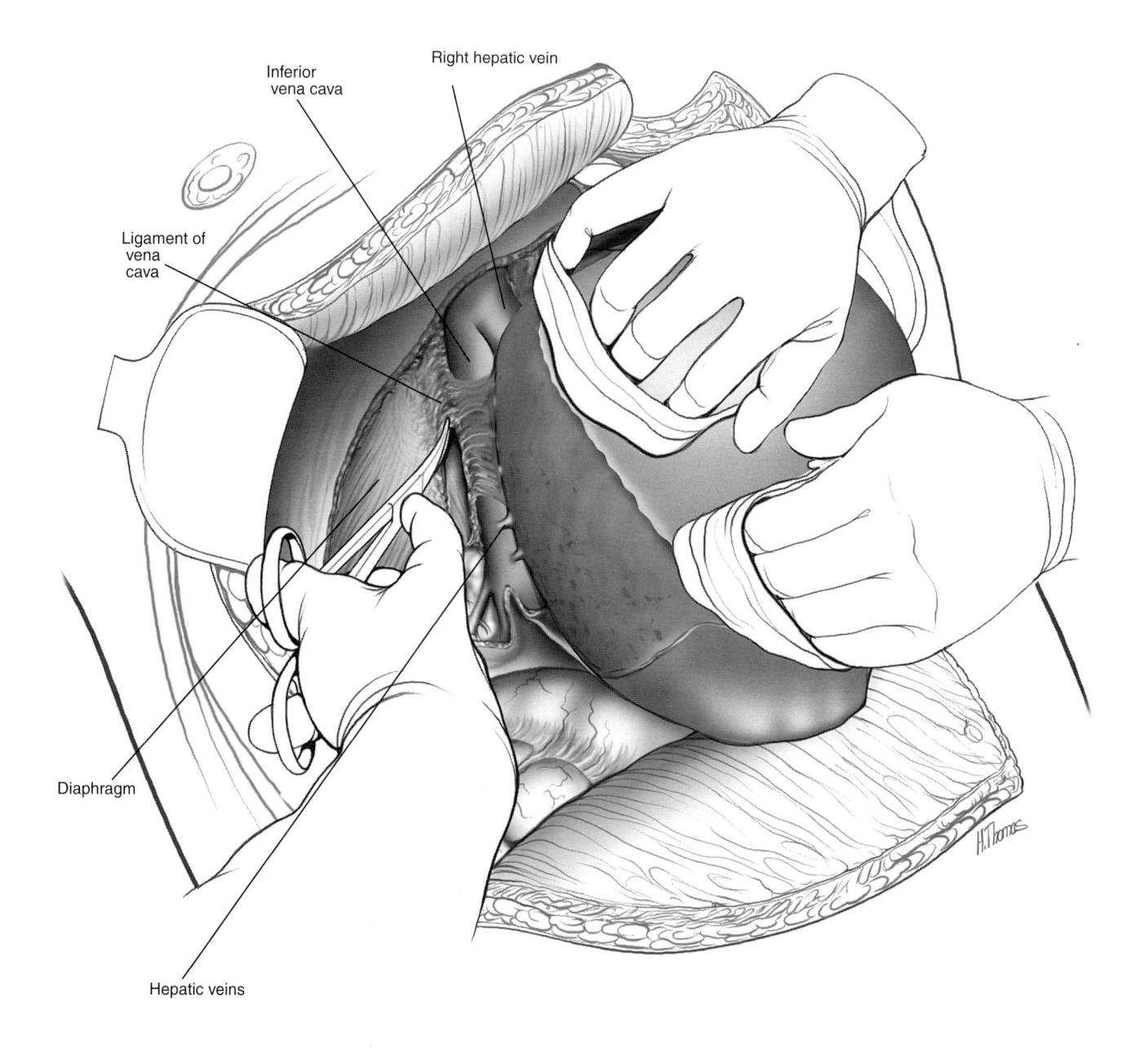

Figure 23–7 • With retraction of the right lobe of the liver, the vena cava is exposed.

Right Hepatic Lobectomy • 189

Right hepatic vein

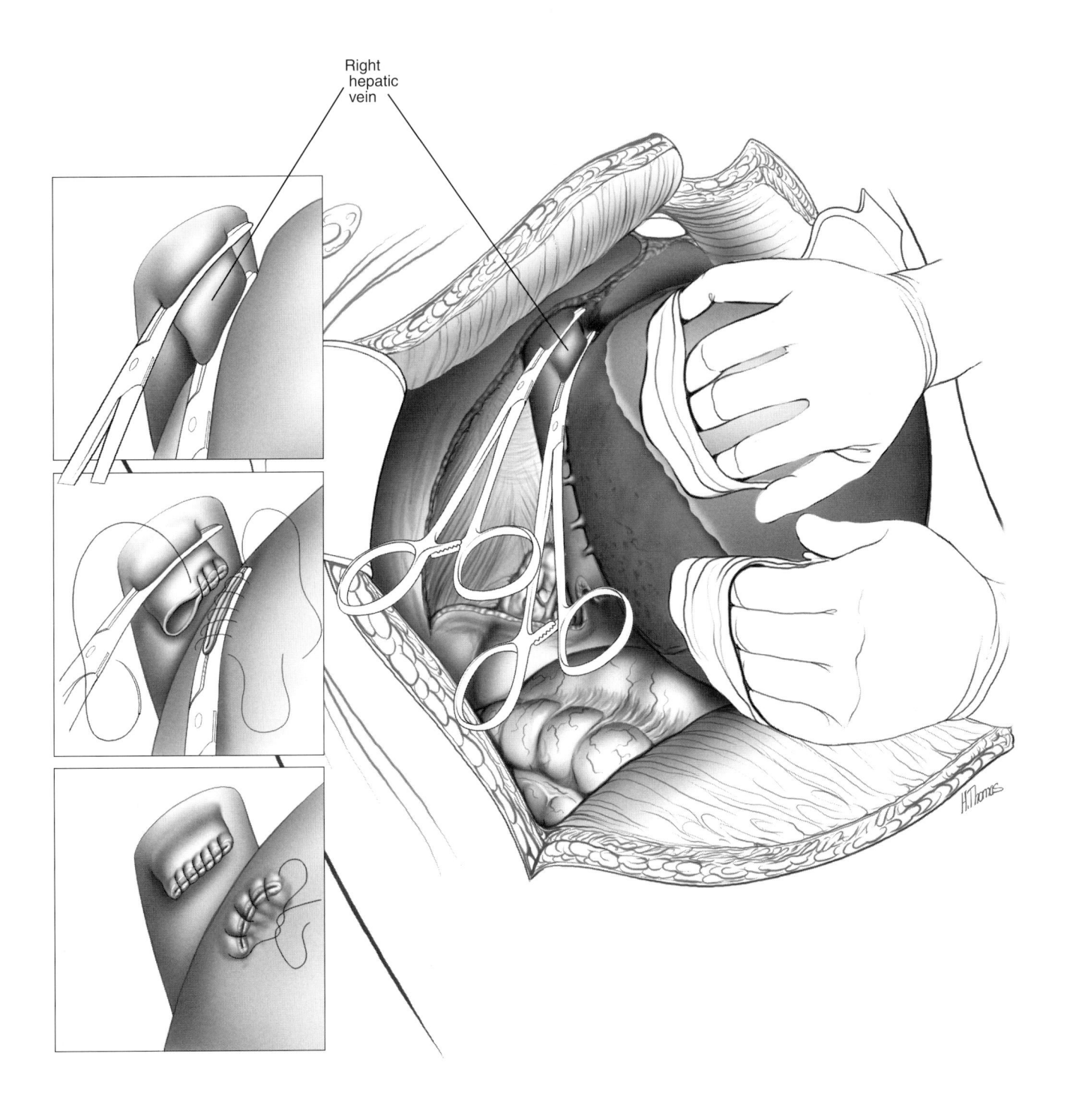

Figure 23–8 • The right hepatic vein is ligated and divided.

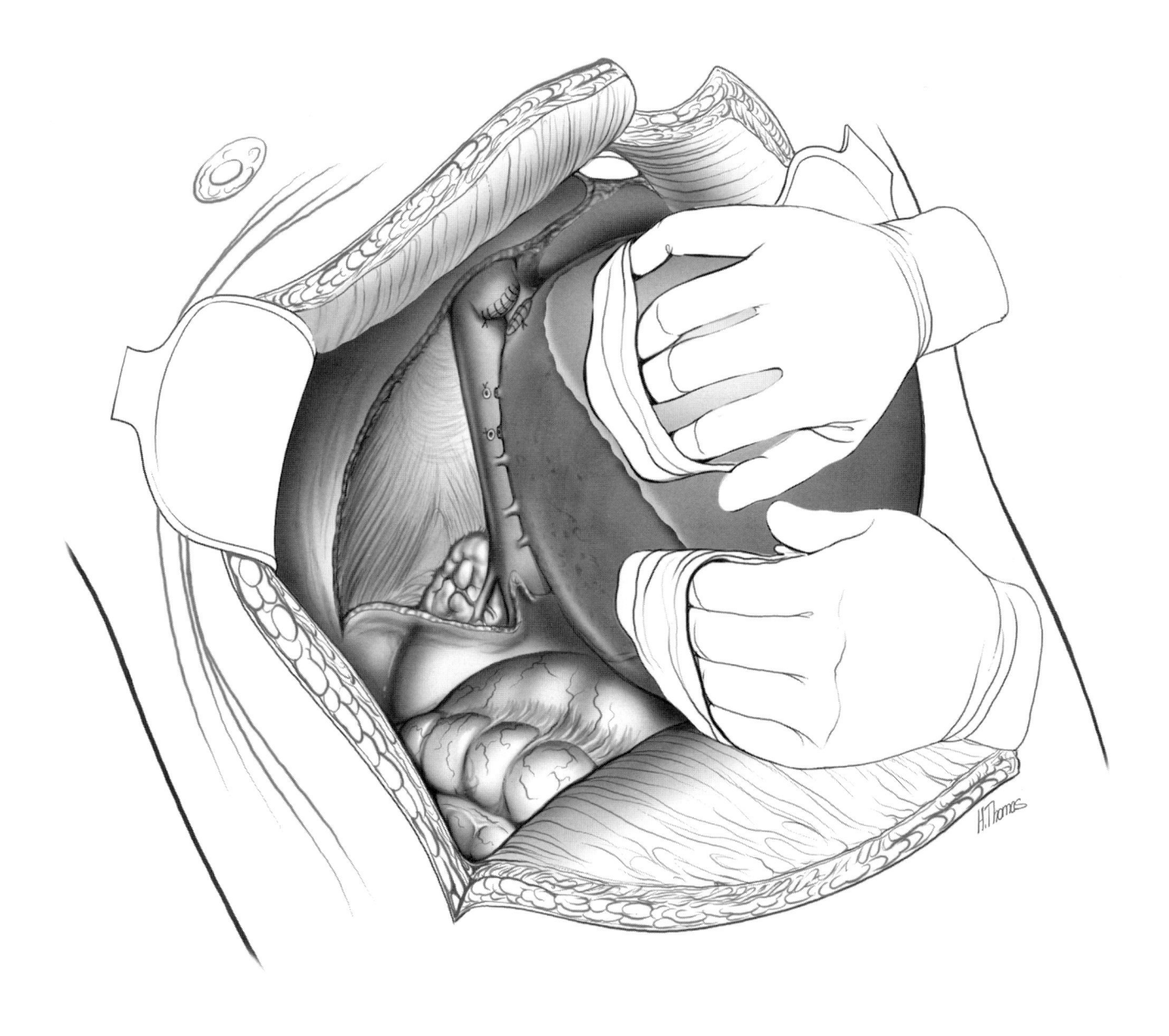

Figure 23-9 • Multiple branches off the vena cava are individually divided.

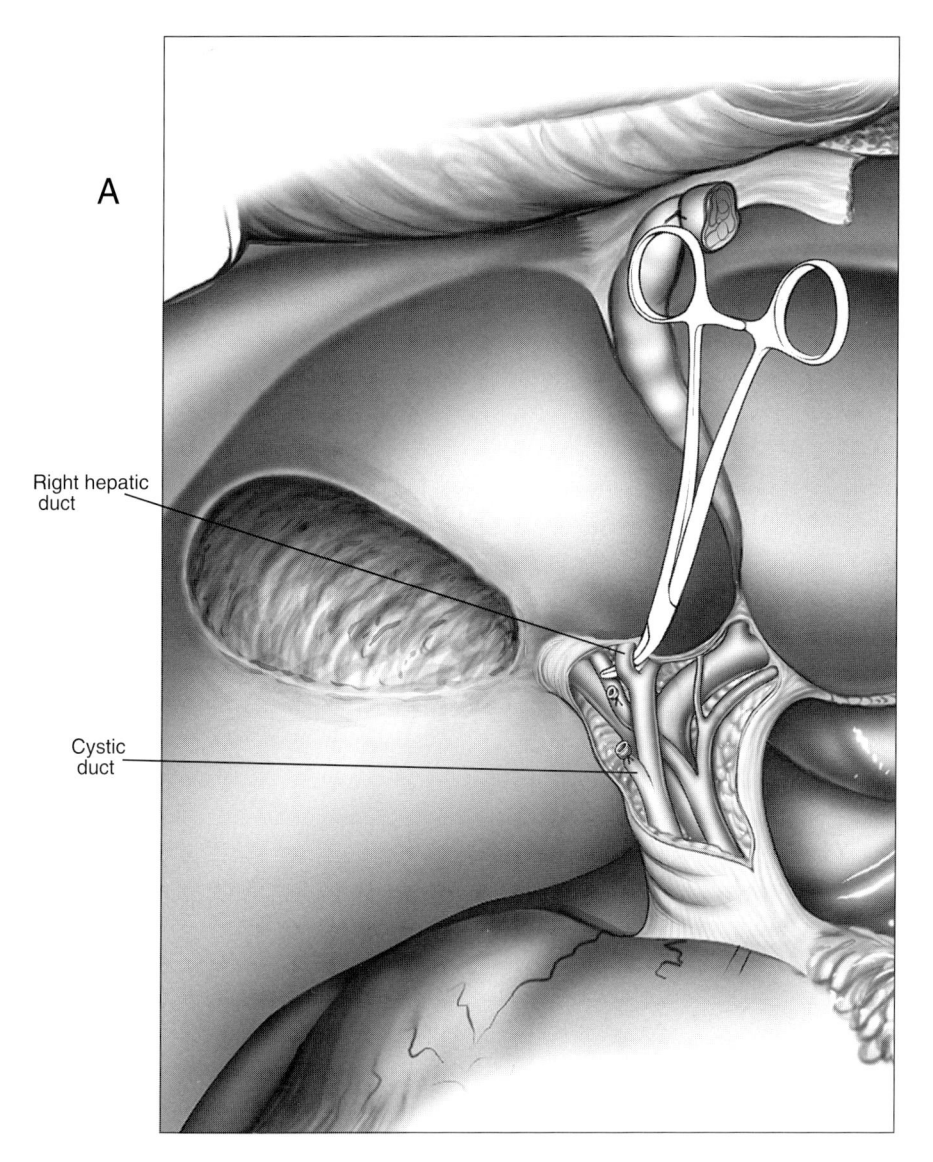

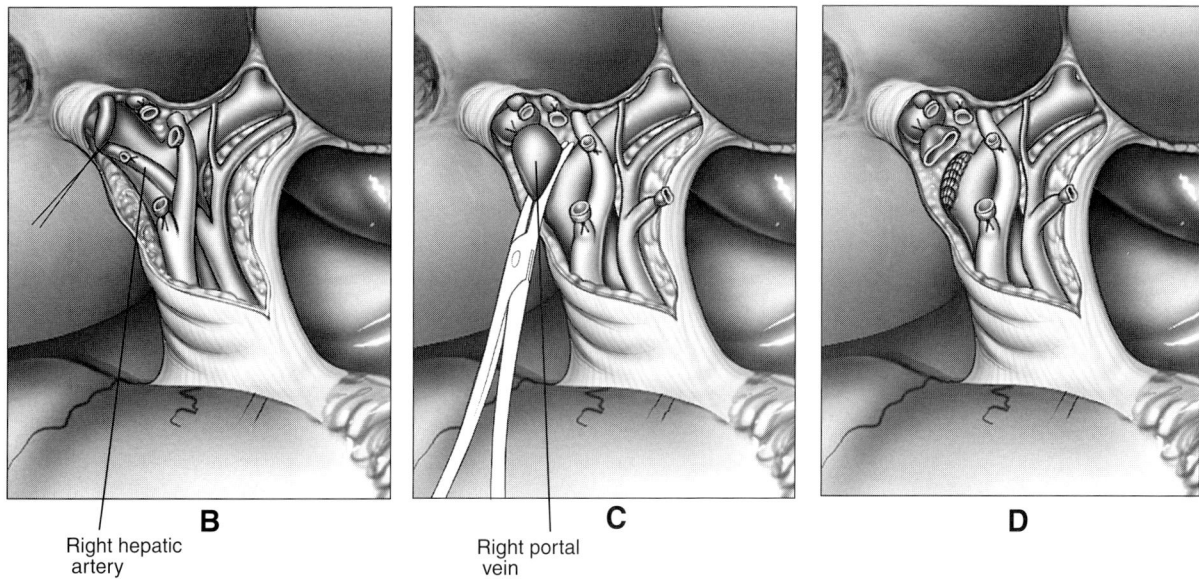

Figure 23–10 • **A,** Identification of the right hepatic duct.
B, Division of the right hepatic duct.
C, Identification and division of the right portal vein and right hepatic artery.
D, Completed division of the structures in the porta hepatis.

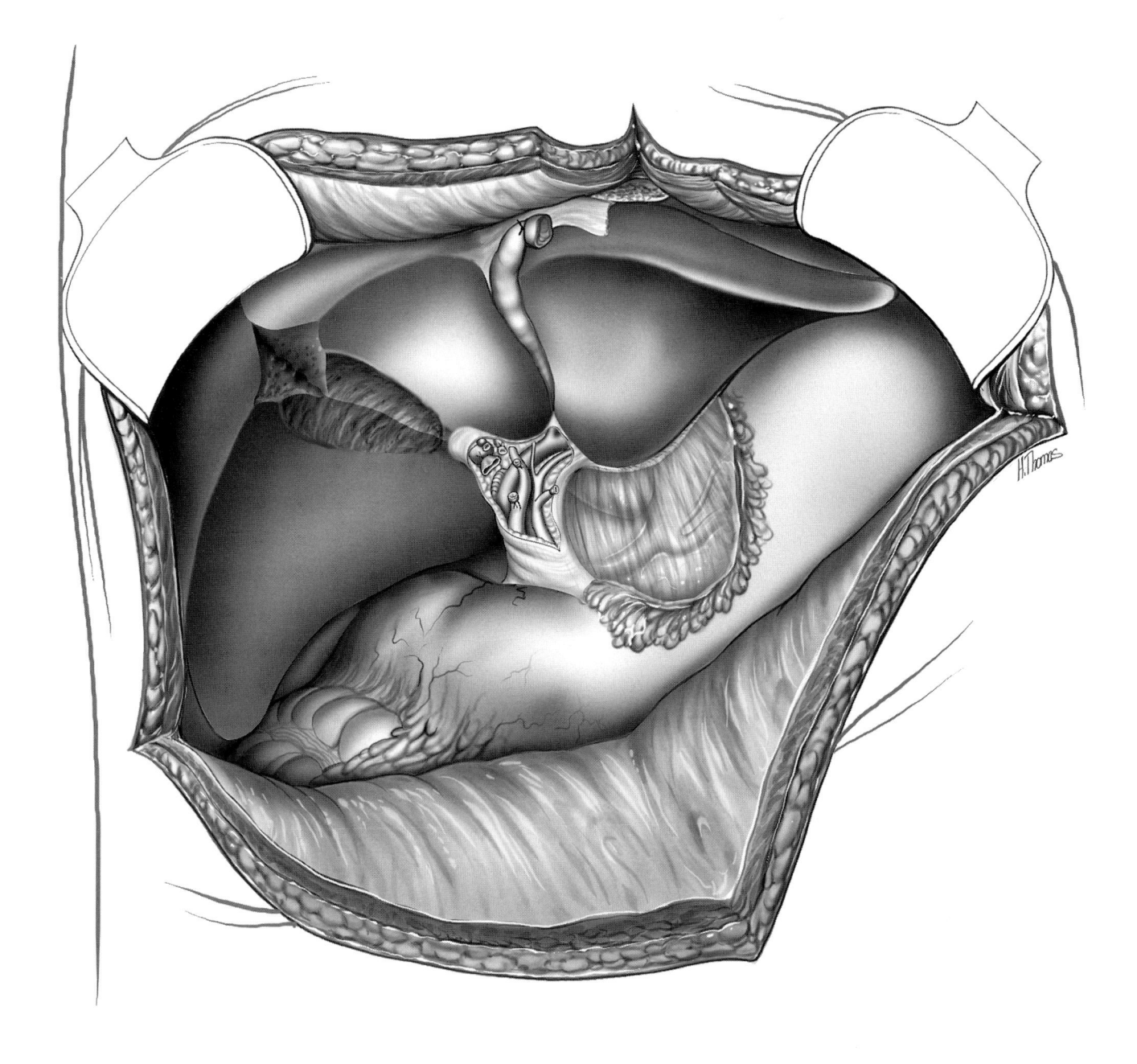

Figure 23–11 • Completed division of the branches to the right lobe of the liver, with demarcation of the devascularized segments.

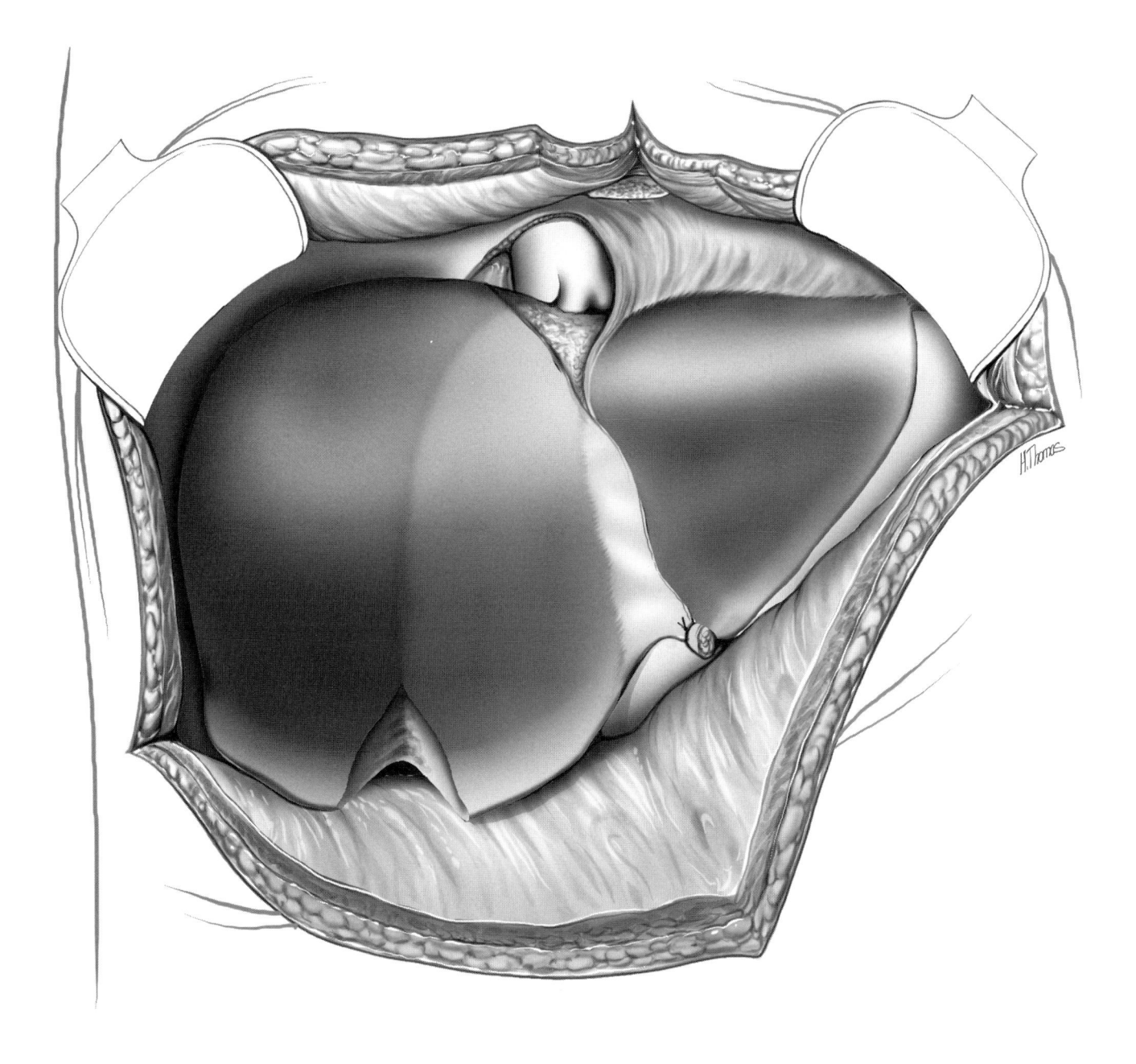

Figure 23-12 • Division of the hepatic parenchyma along the line of demarcation, using cautery, finger fracture technique, or Cavitron ultrasonic aspirator (CUSA).

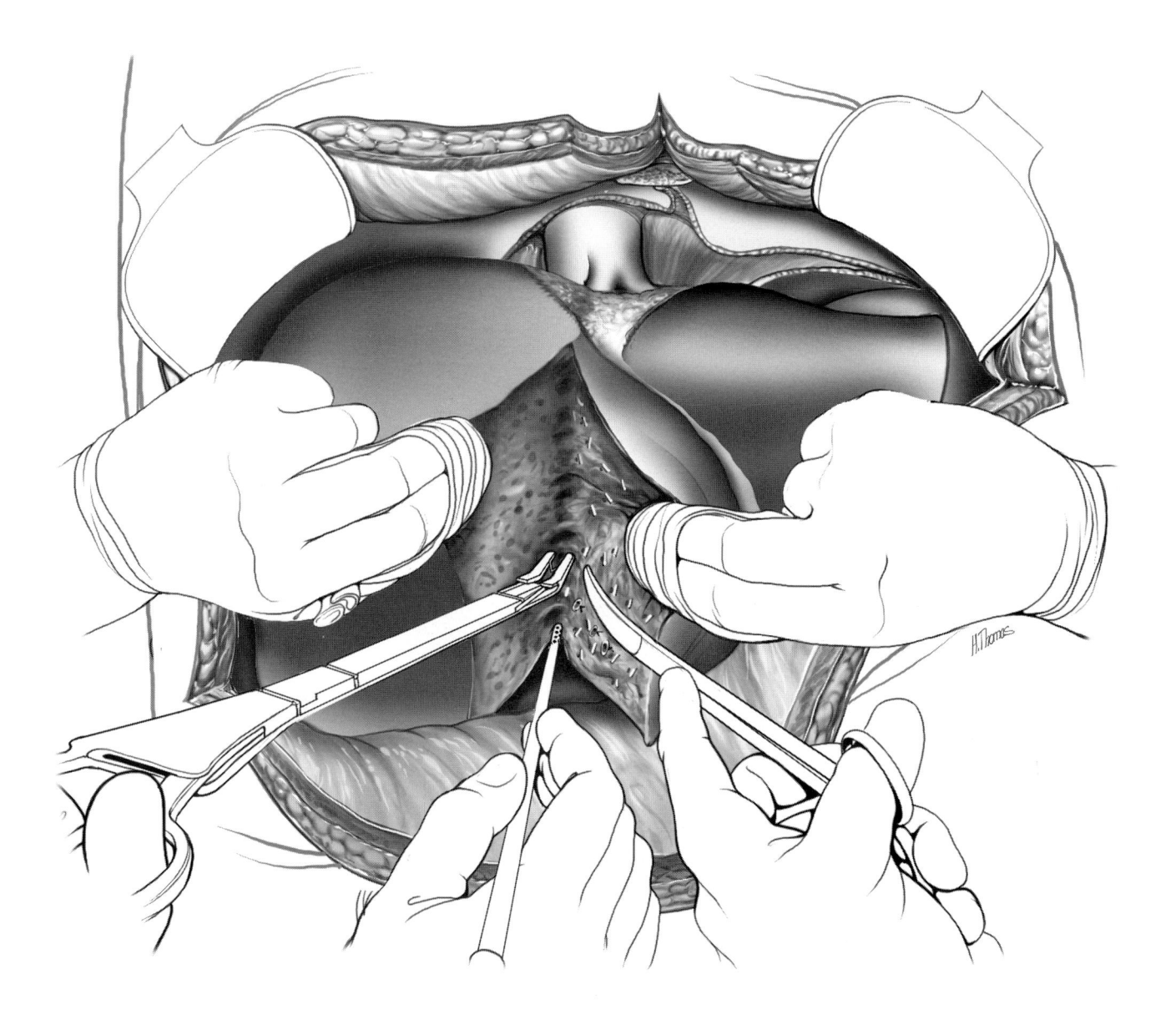

Figure 23–13 • Completing the division of the hepatic parenchyma, with division of the remaining vascular channels.

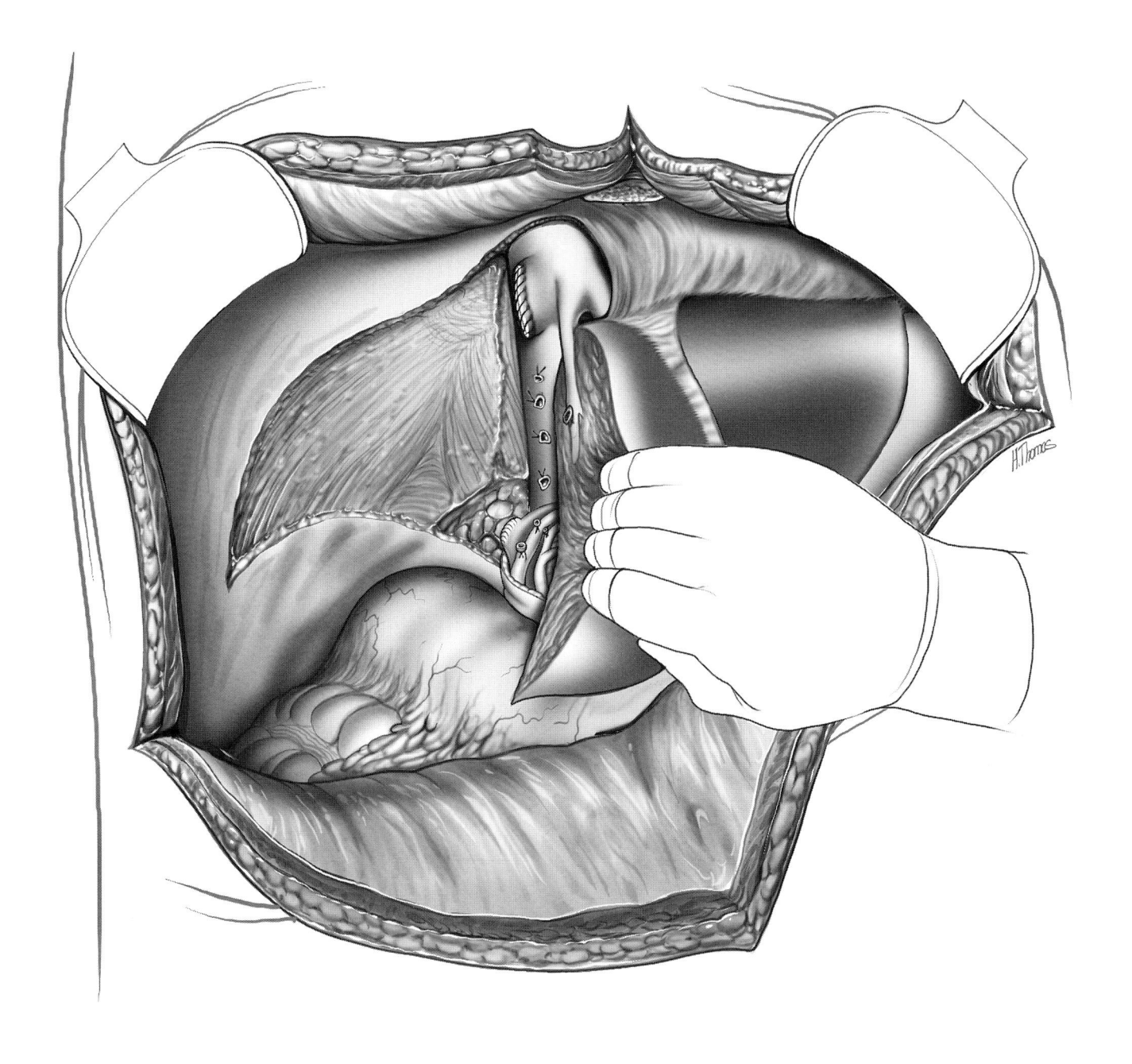

Figure 23–14 • Completed right hepatic lobectomy.

Chapter 24
Left Hepatic Lobectomy

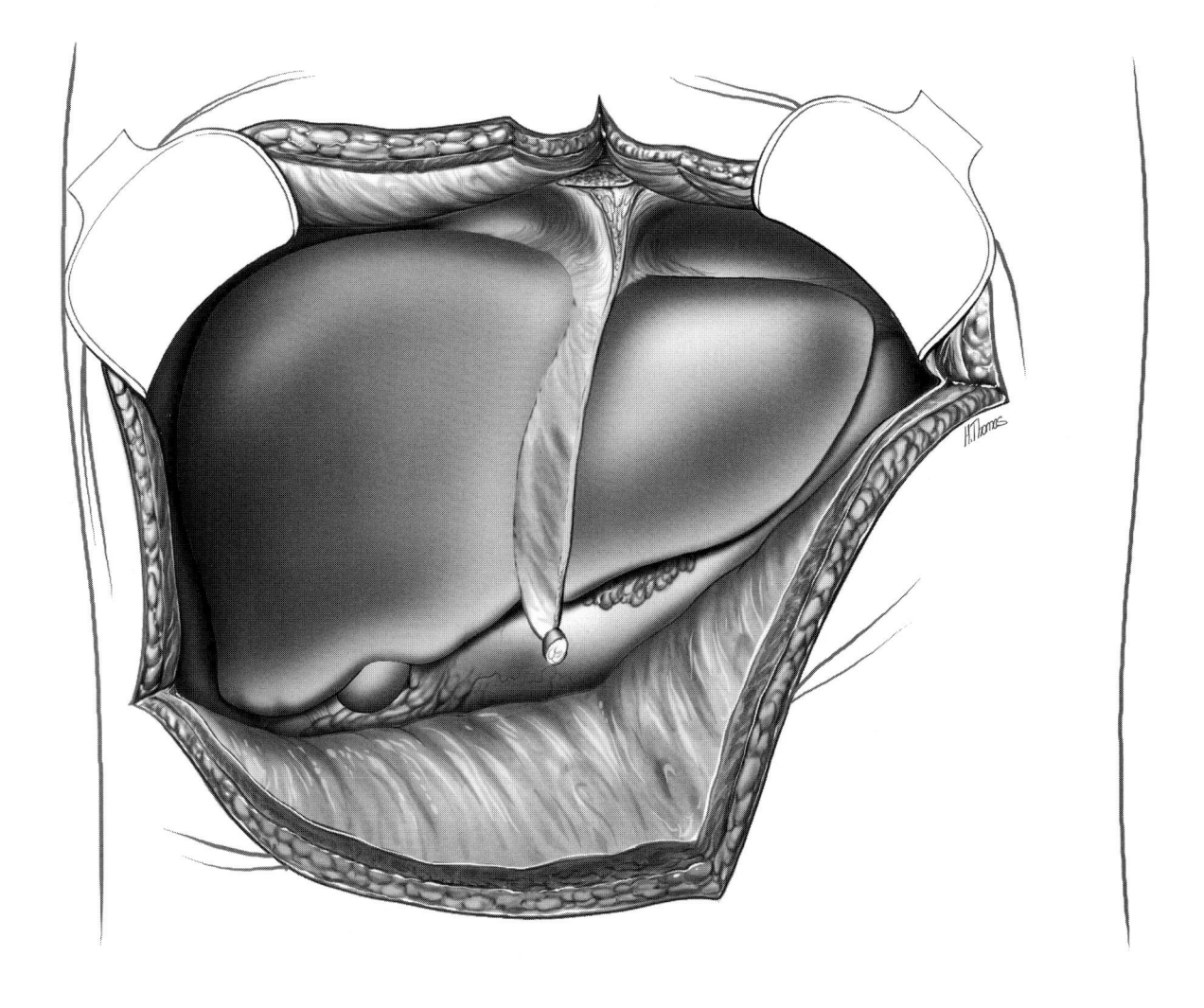

Figure 24–1 • Following the abdominal incision, the falciform ligament is divided.

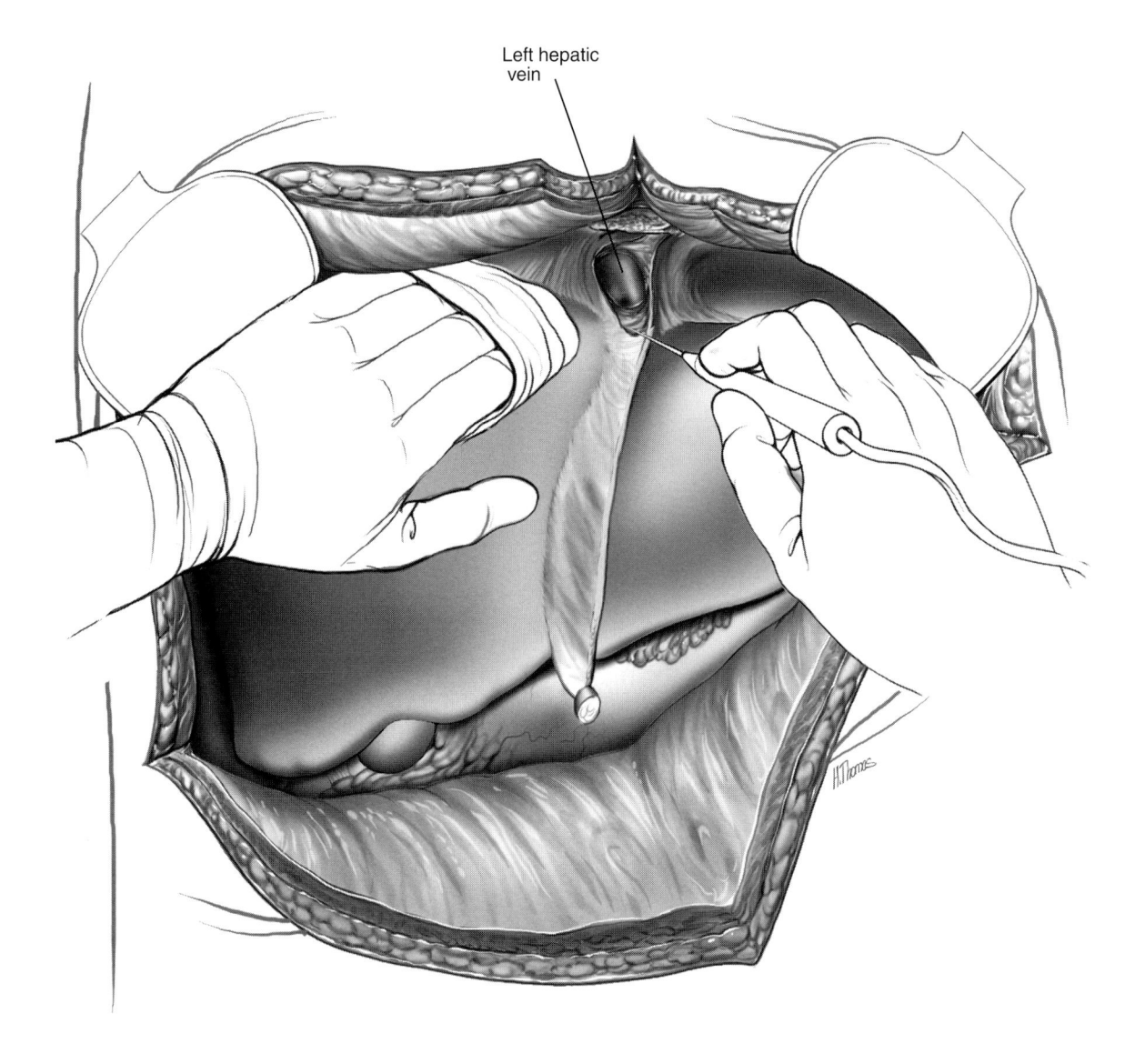

Figure 24–2 • At the base of the falciform ligament, the hepatic veins are exposed.

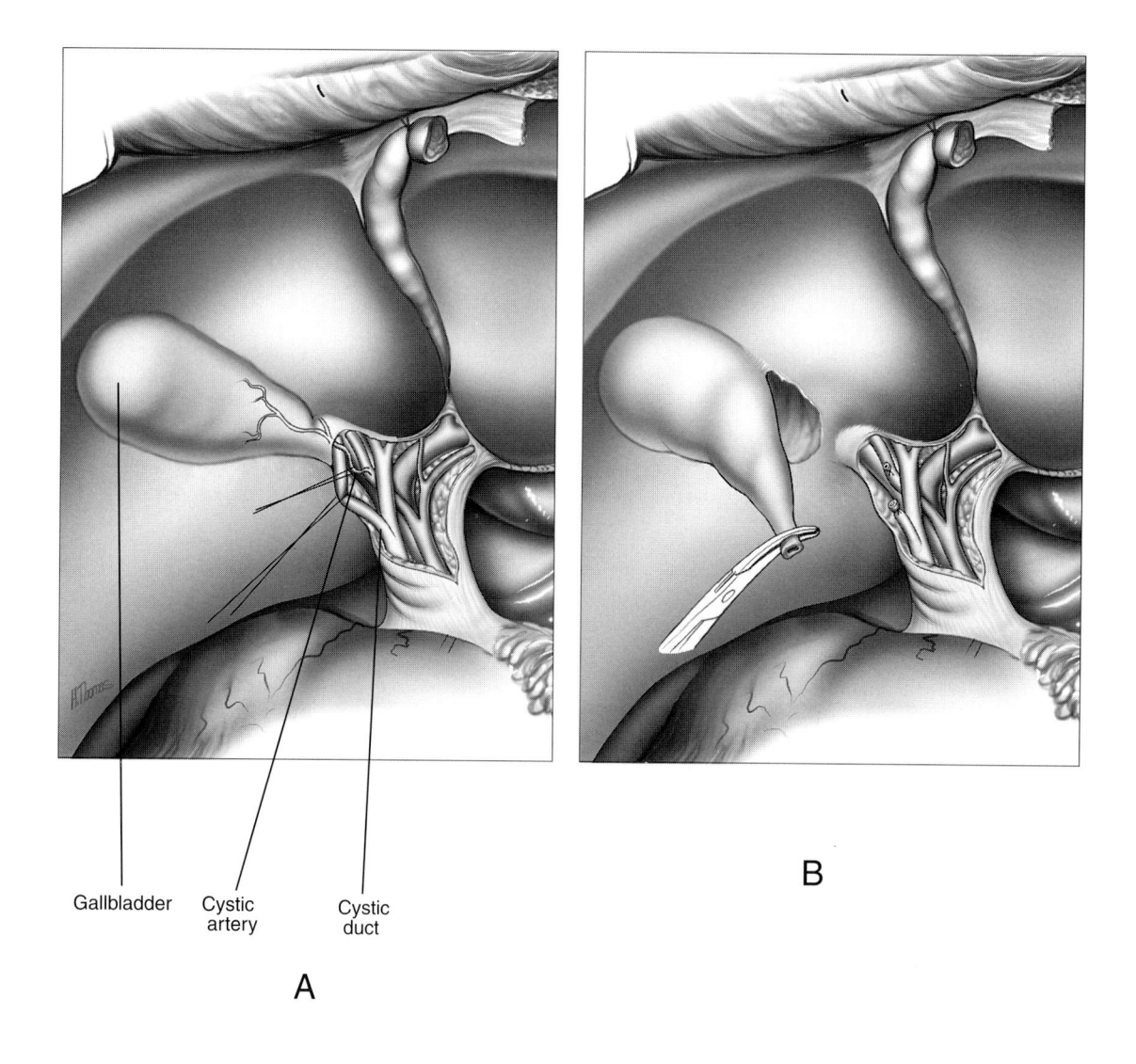

Figure 24–3 • **A,** The cystic artery and duct are isolated and divided.
B, The gallbladder is removed.

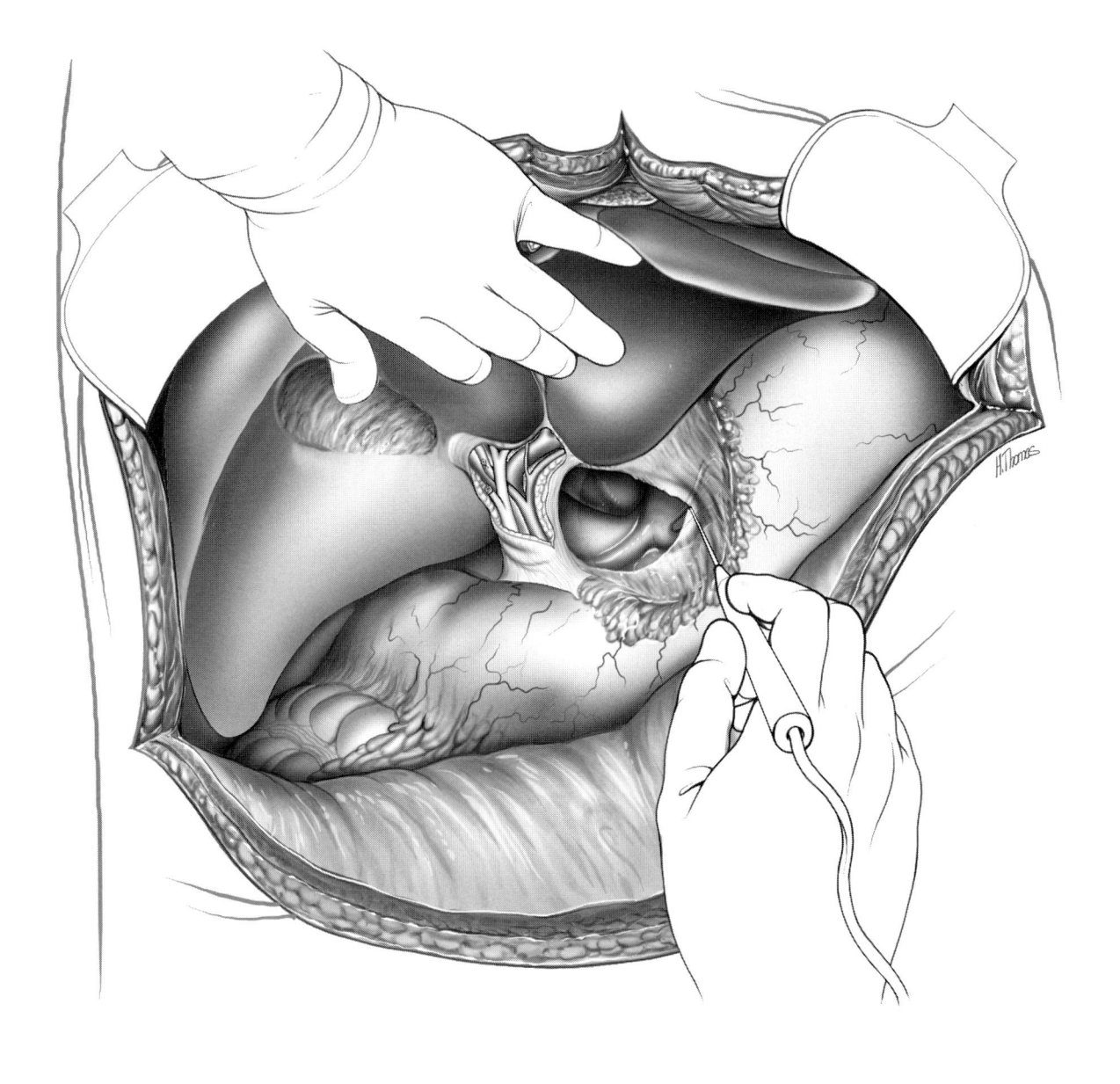

Figure 24–4 • The gastrohepatic ligament is divided, and the celiac axis is exposed.

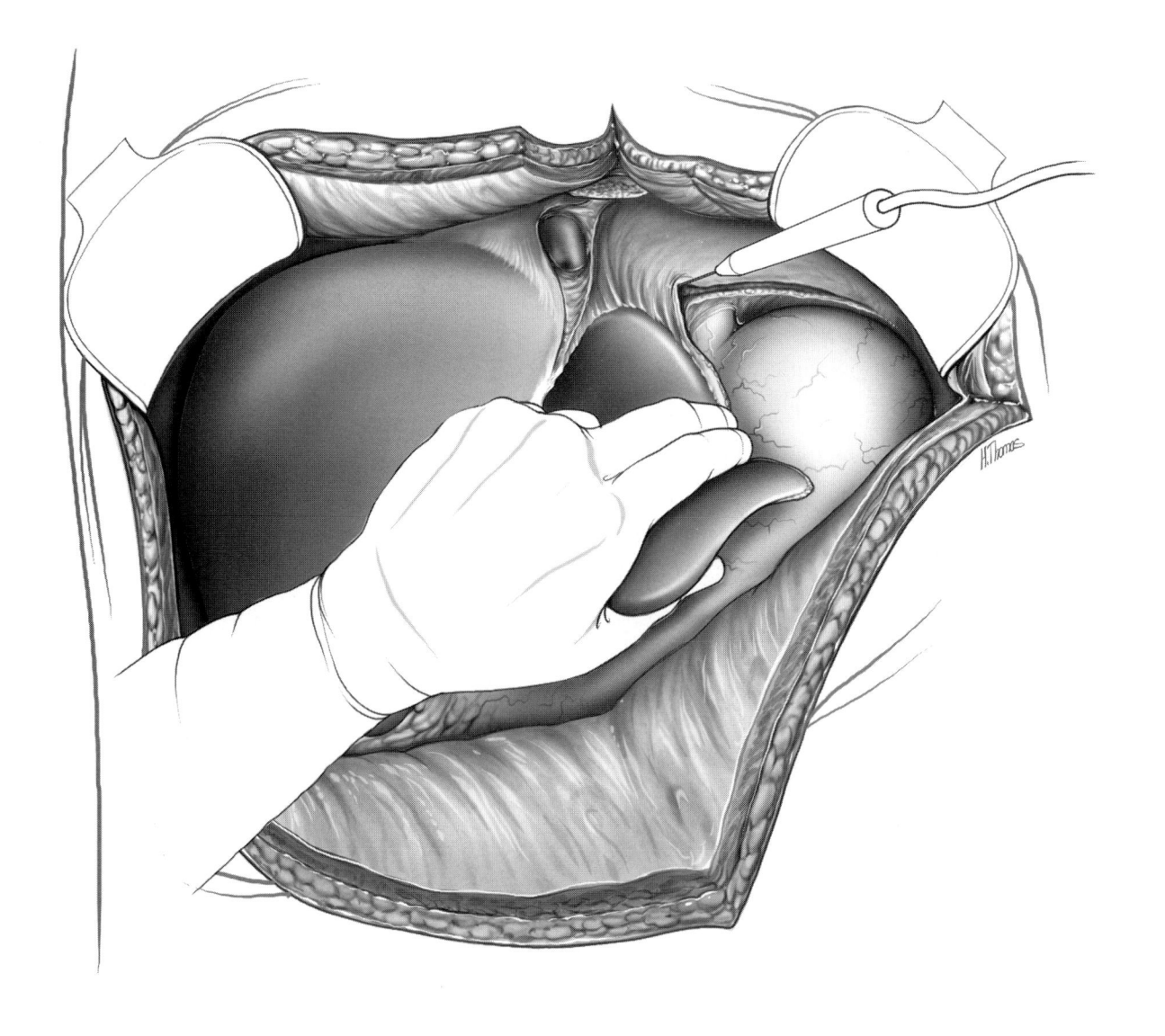

Figure 24–5 • The left triangular ligament is divided completely.

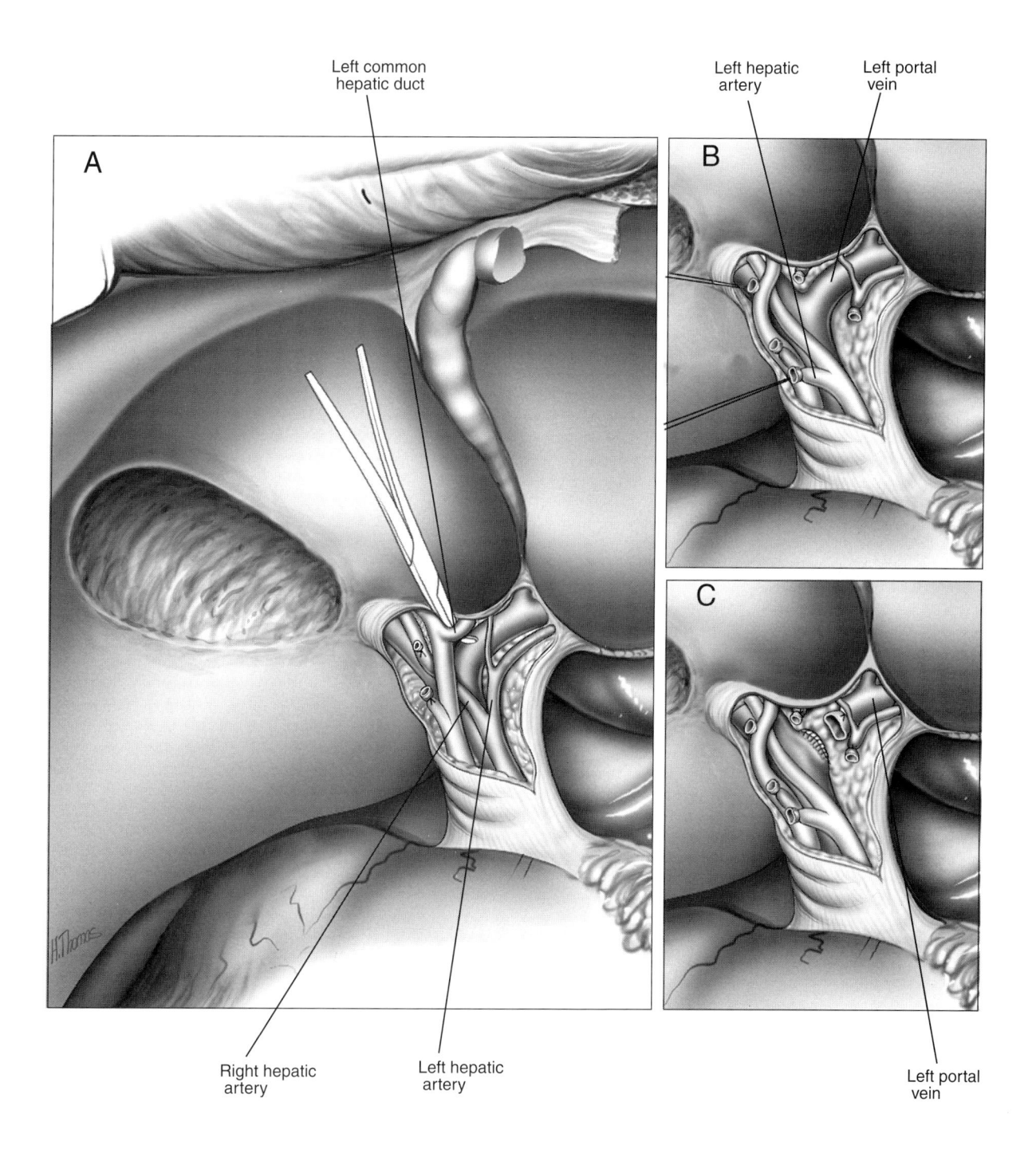

Figure 24–6 • **A,** The left hepatic duct is identified and divided.
B, The left hepatic artery is divided and the portal vein is exposed.
C, The left portal vein is divided.

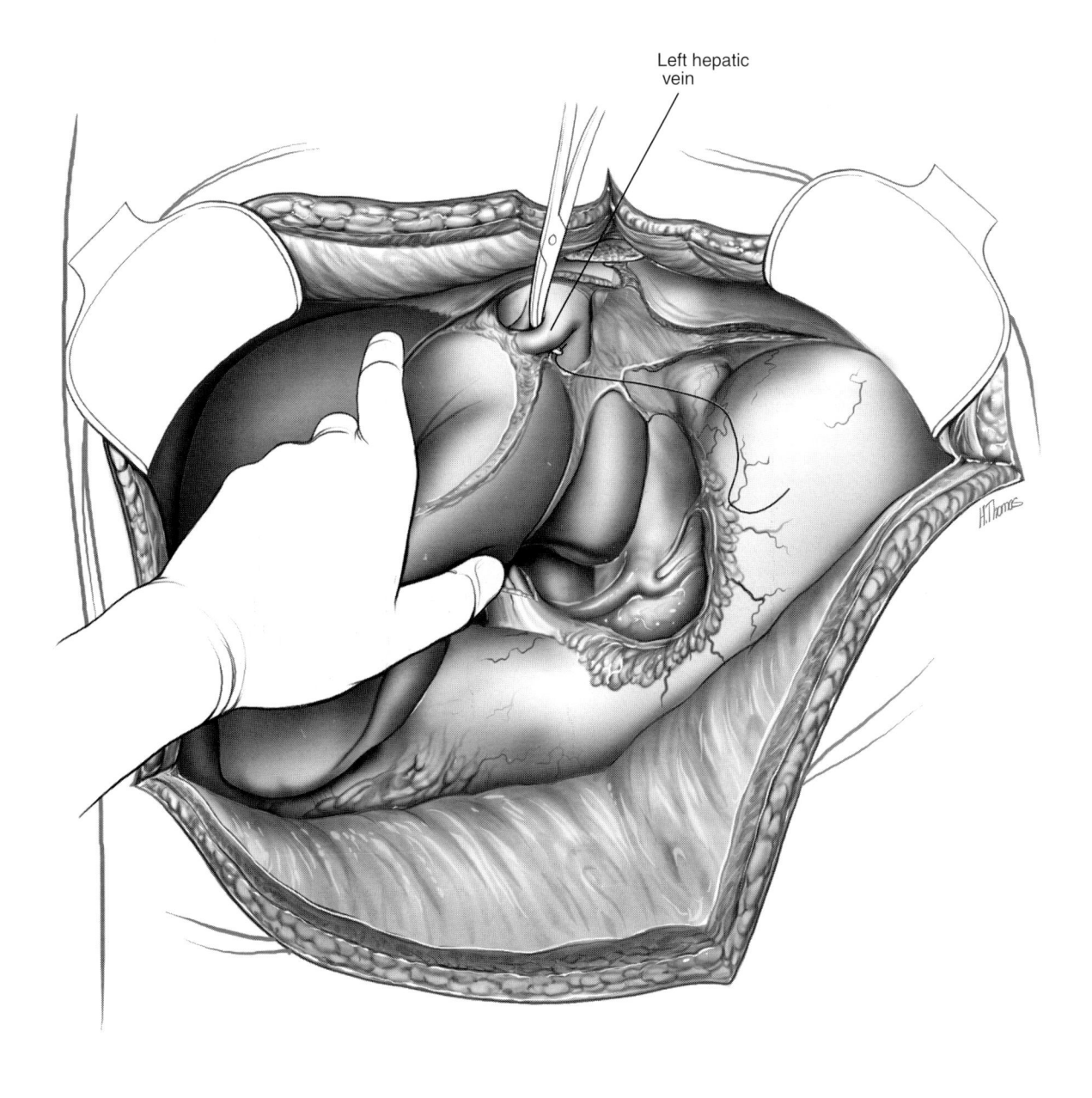

Figure 24–7 • The left hepatic vein is divided after completely mobilizing the left lobe.

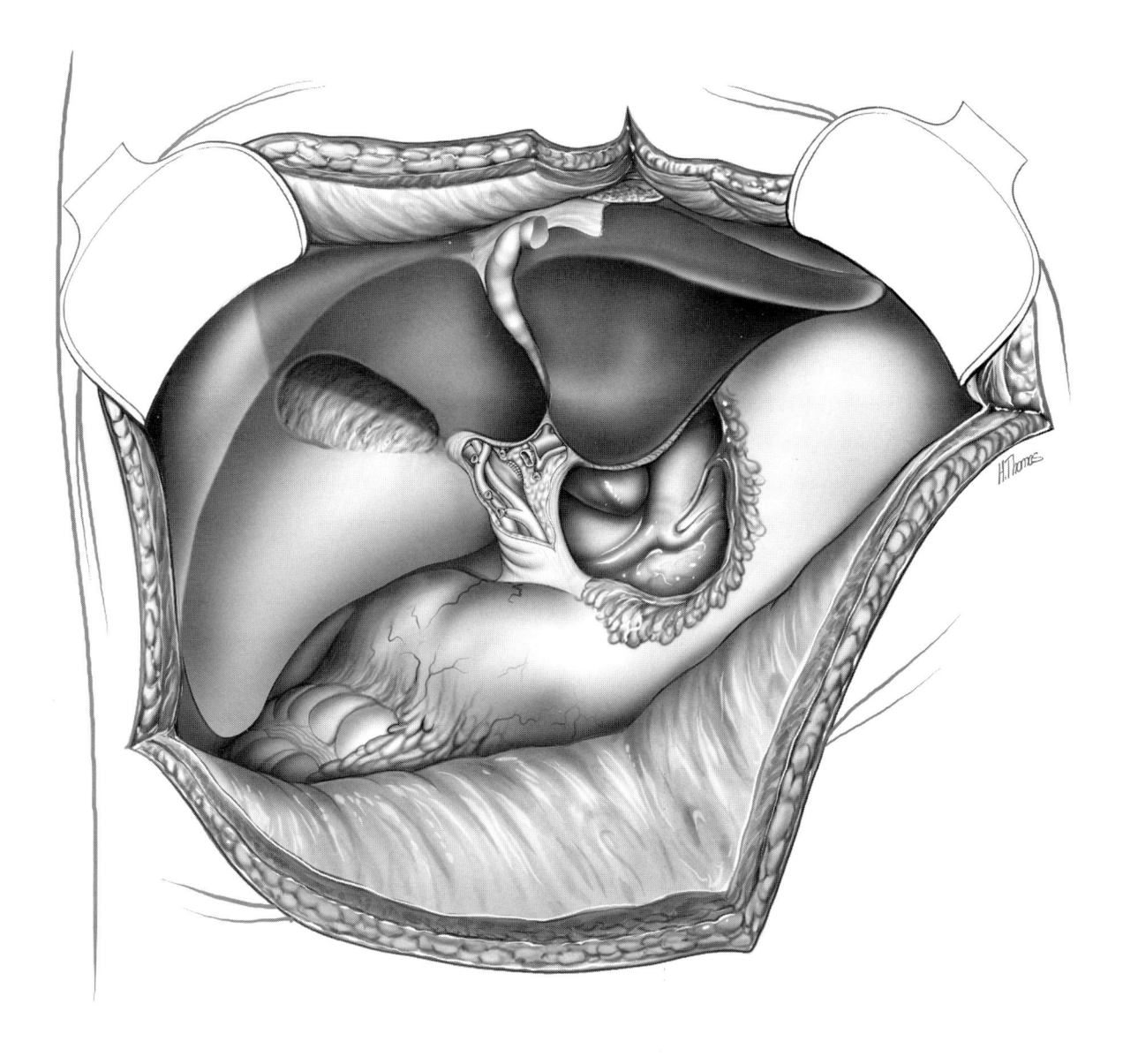

Figure 24–8 • The left lobe is completely devascularized and begins to demarcate.

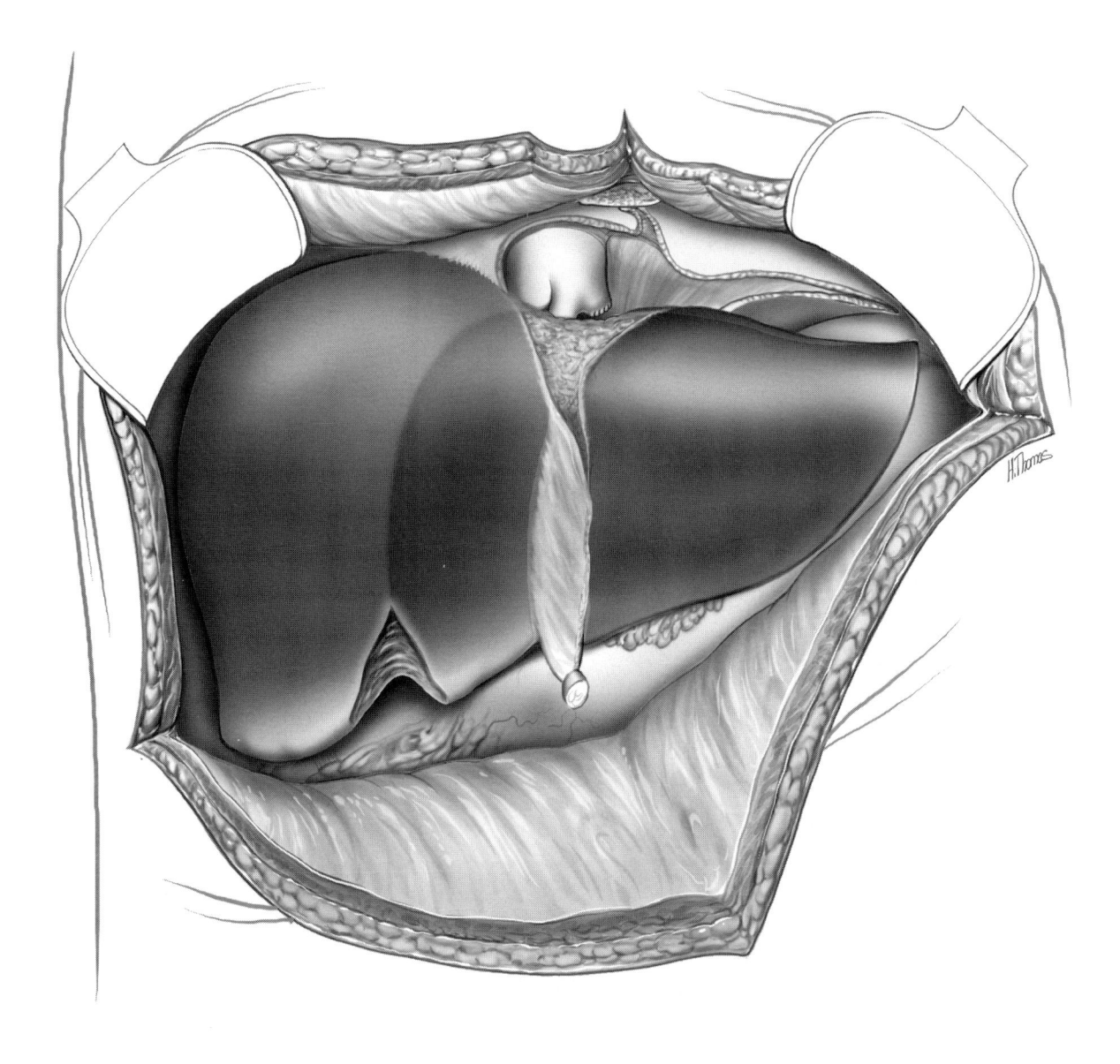

Figure 24–9 • Division of the hepatic parenchyma along the line of demarcation is begun, using the cautery, finger fracture, or Cavitron ultrasonic aspirator (CUSA).

Left Hepatic Lobectomy • 205

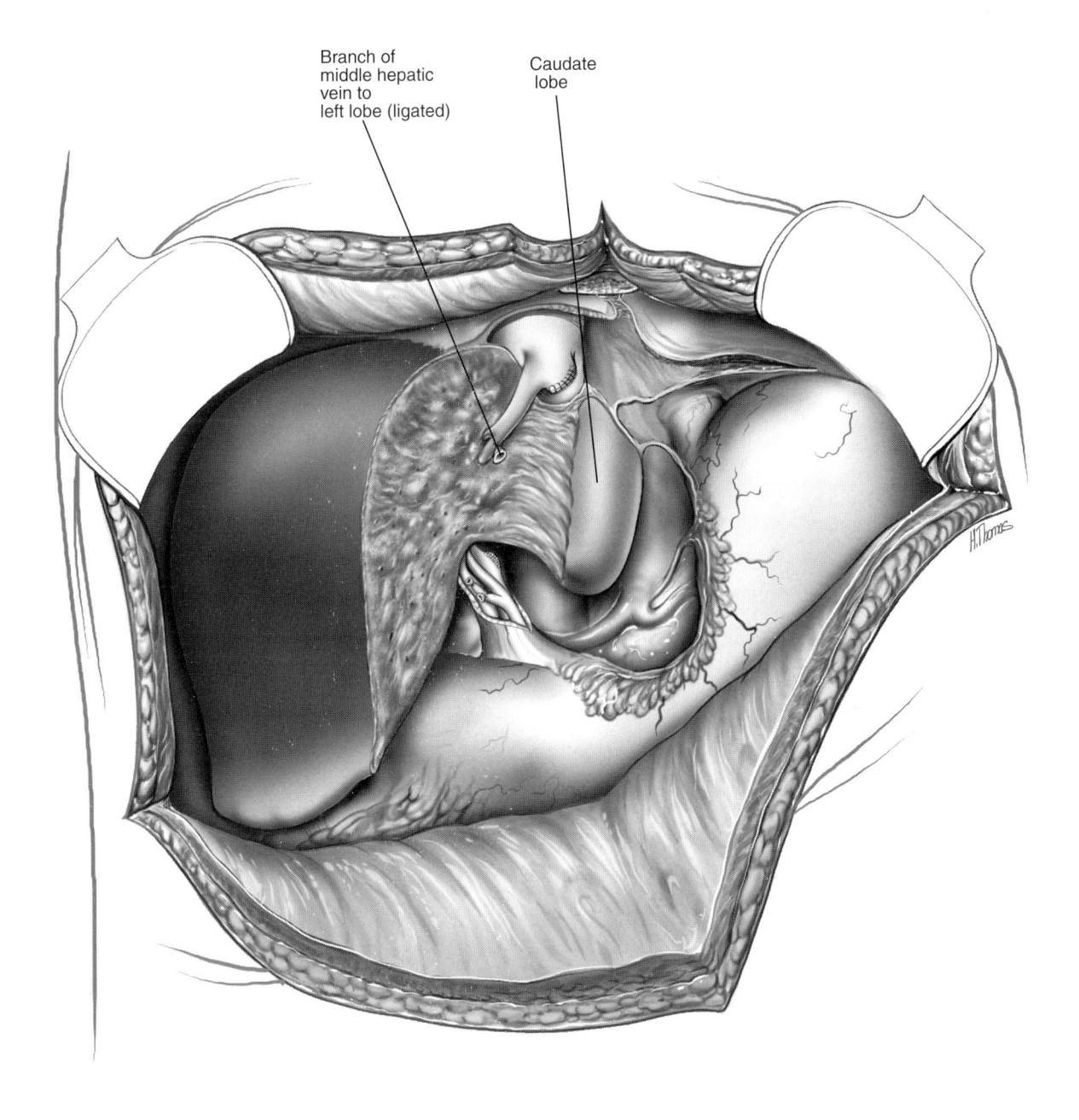

Figure 24–10 • The left lobe is removed, often leaving the caudate lobe. A large branch off the middle hepatic vein to the left lobe is common and is divided.

Chapter 25
Trisegmentectomy

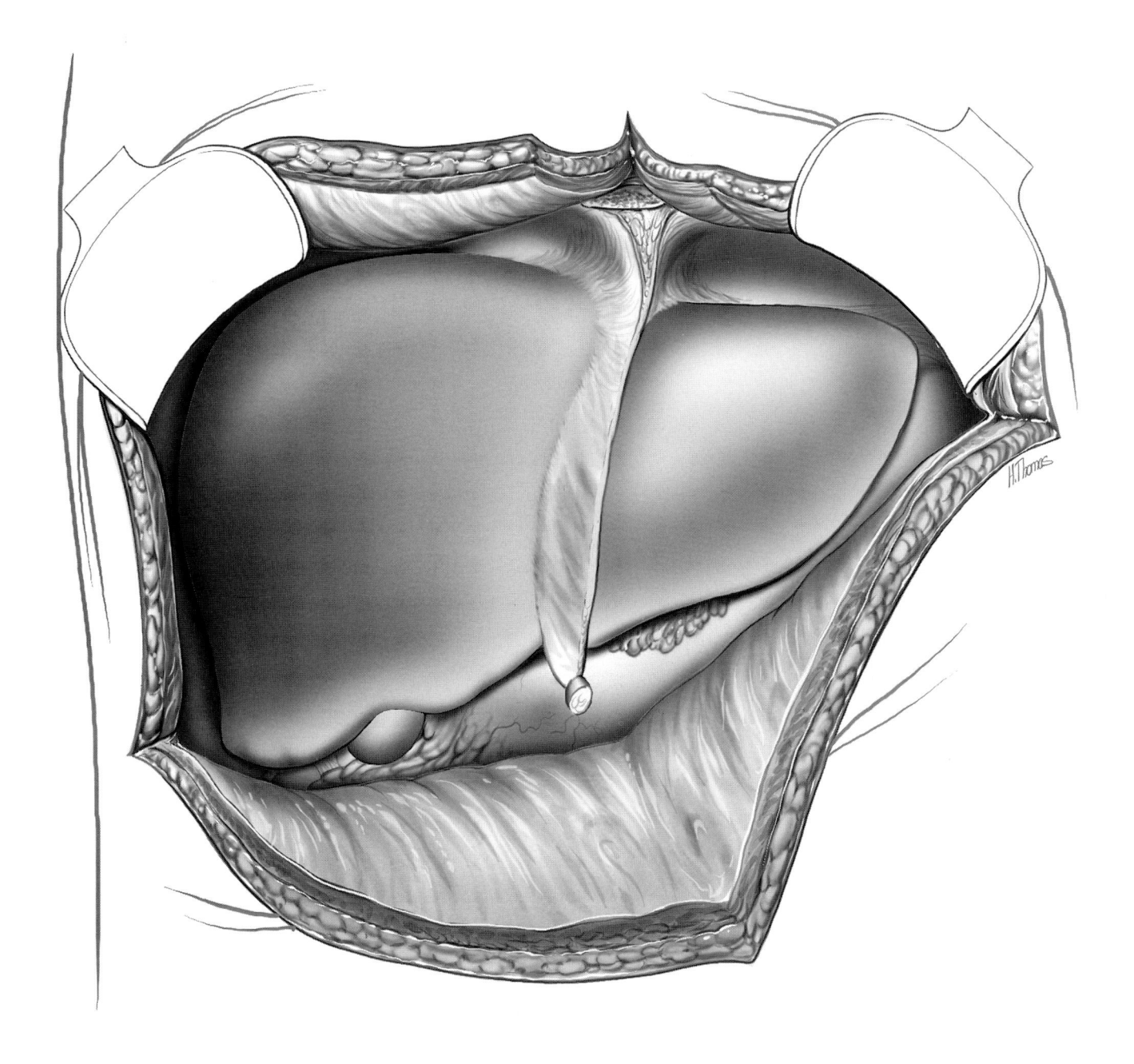

Figure 25–1 • Following a transverse abdominal incision, the falciform ligament is divided.

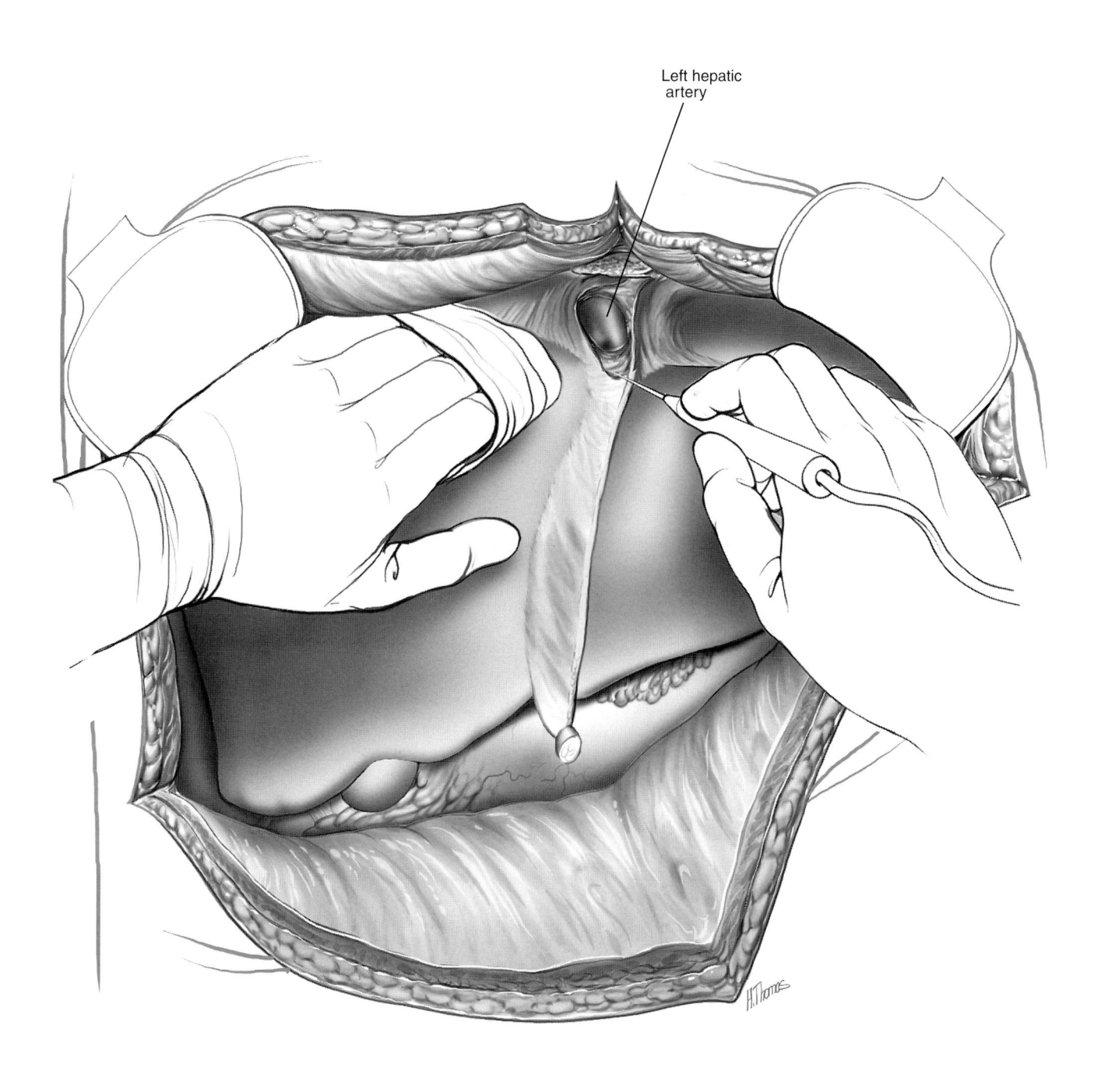

Figure 25–2 • The hepatic veins are exposed at the base of the falciform ligament.

208 • Part III UPPER ABDOMEN

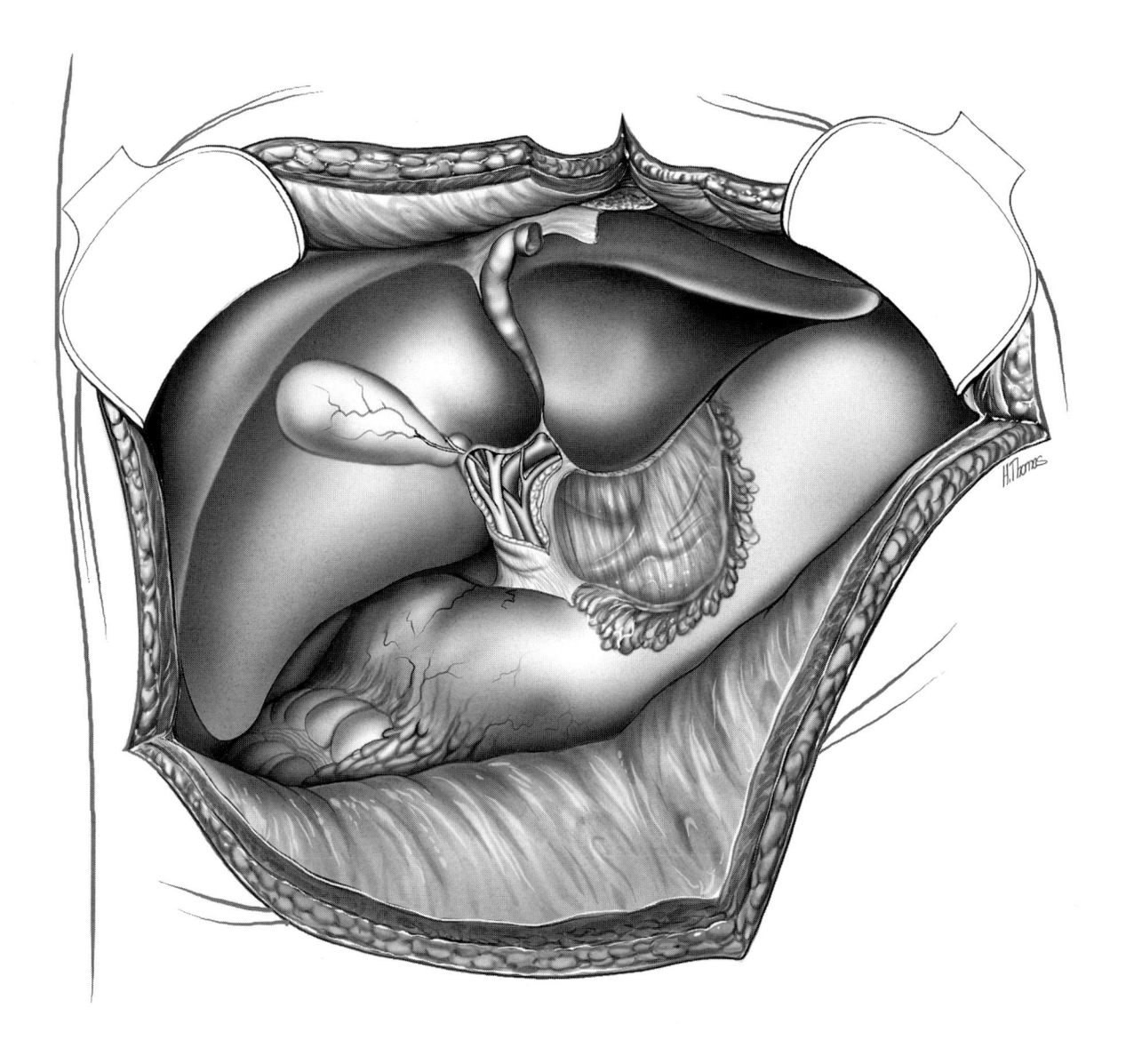

Figure 25–3 • The major structures in the porta hepatis are identified.

Trisegmentectomy • 209

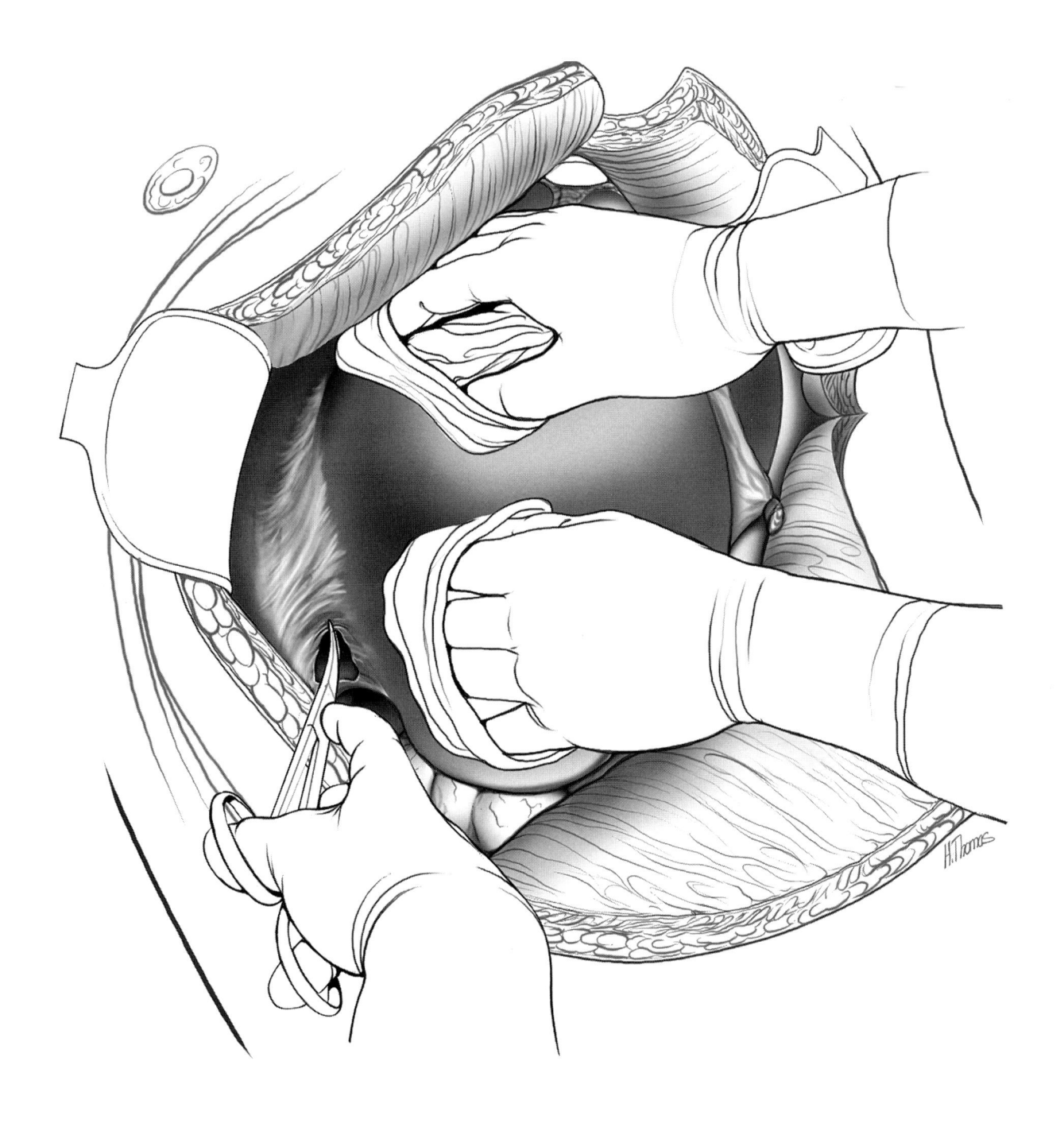

Figure 25–4 • The right triangular ligament is incised in order to mobilize the right lobe of the liver.

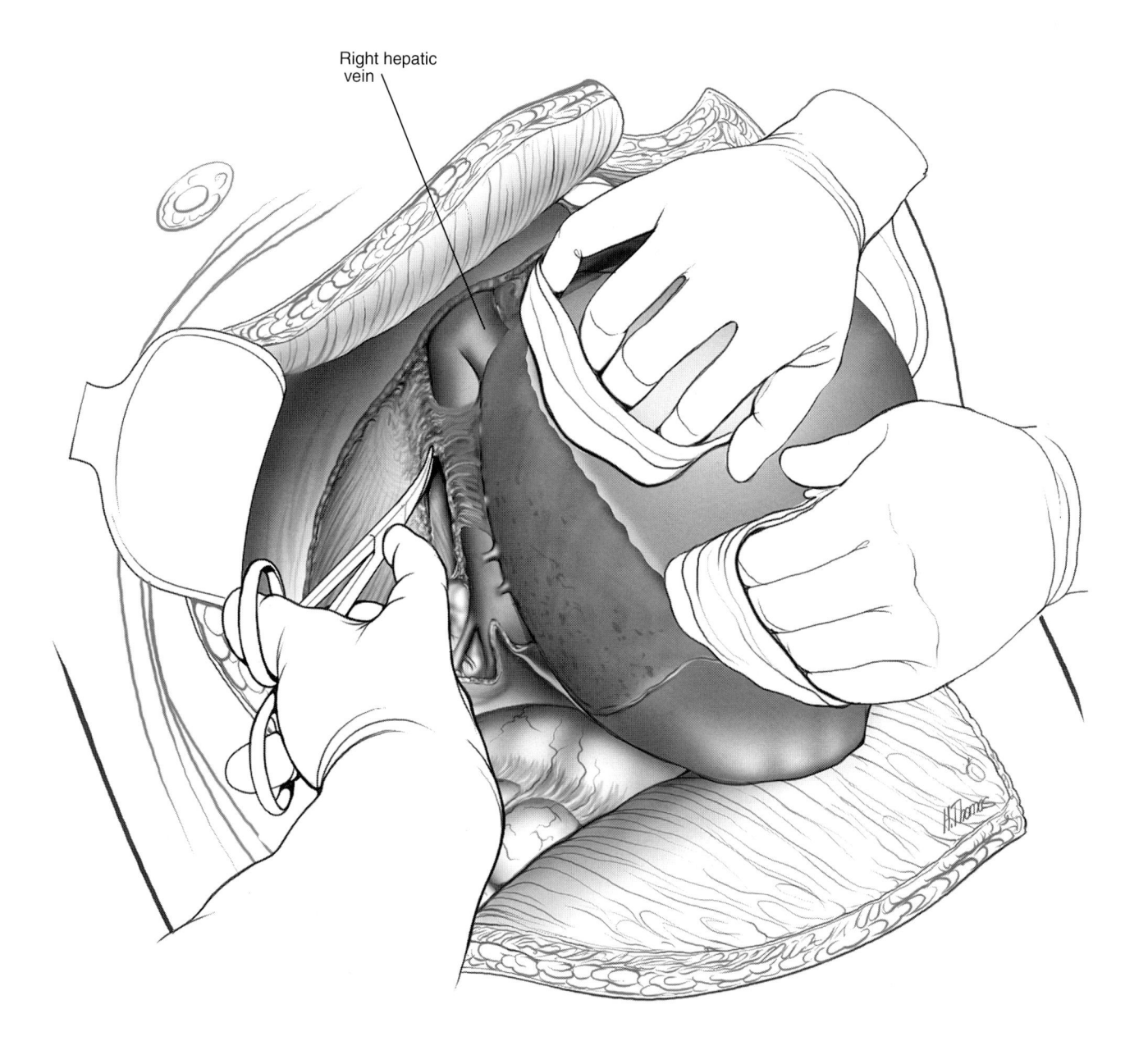

Figure 25–5 • The vena cava is exposed by retracting the right lobe of the liver and incising the investing fascia.

Trisegmentectomy • 211

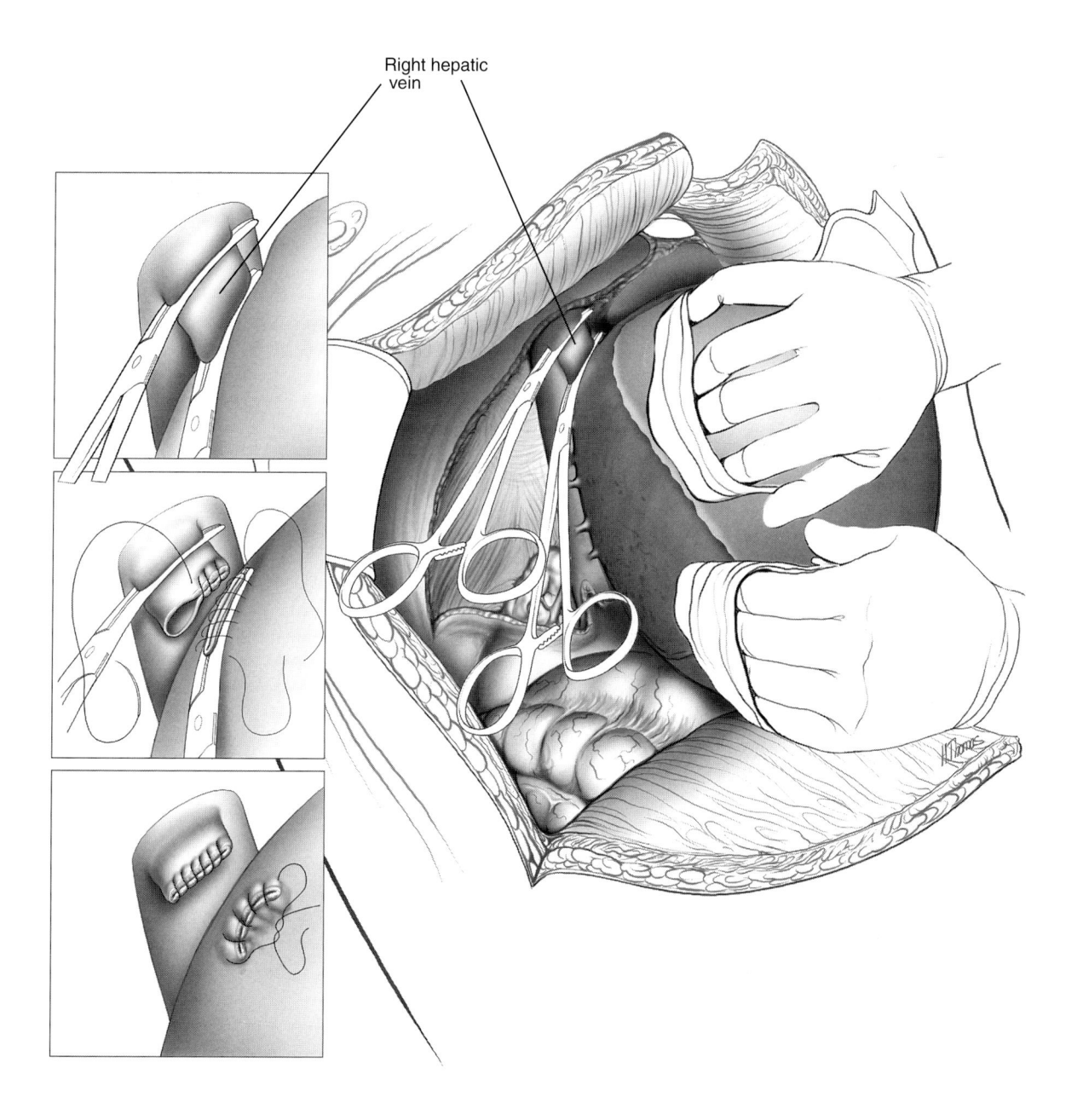

Figure 25–6 • The right hepatic vein is identified, ligated, and divided.

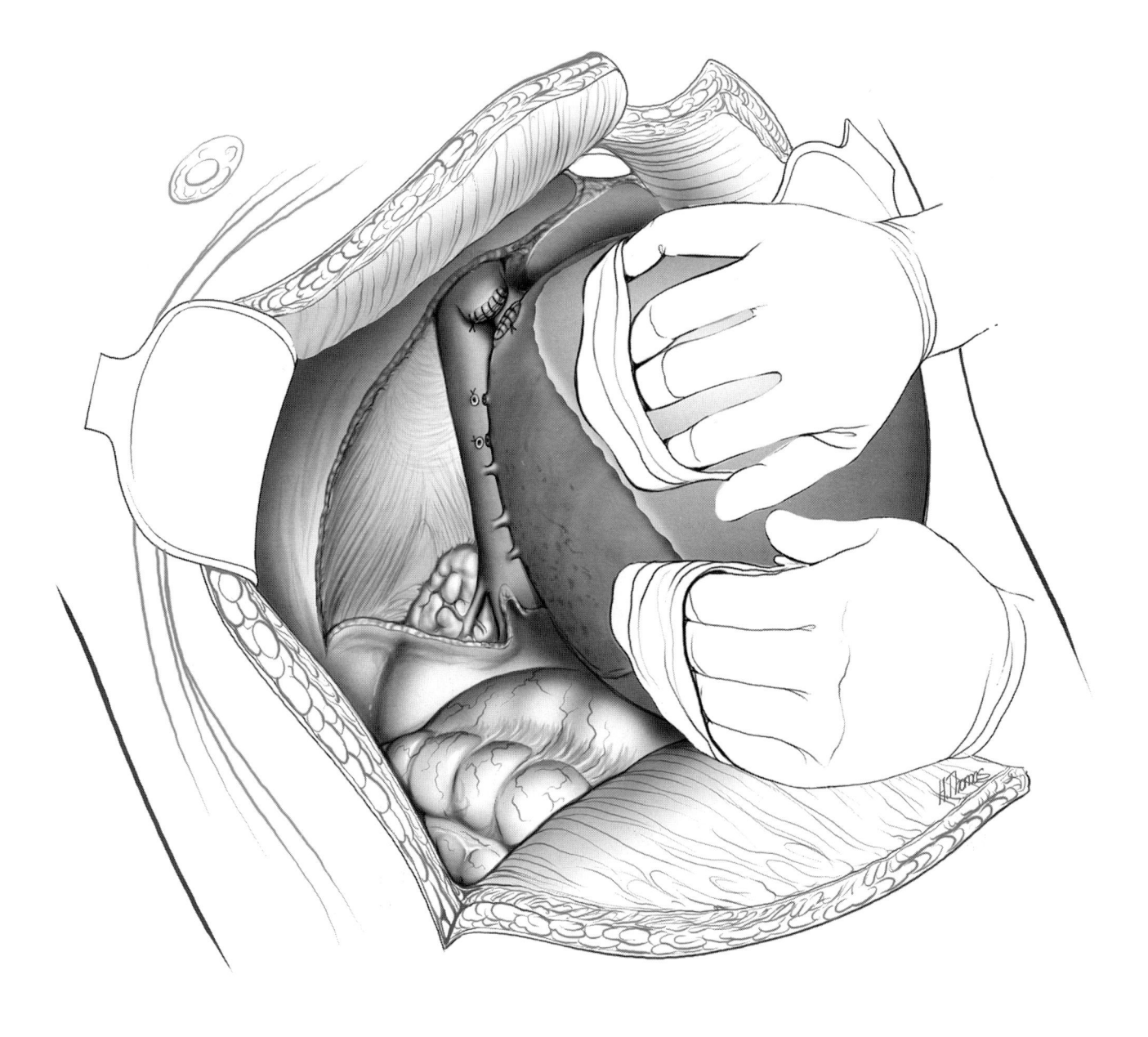

Figure 25–7 • Additional branches off the vena cava to the right lobe of the liver are individually ligated and divided.

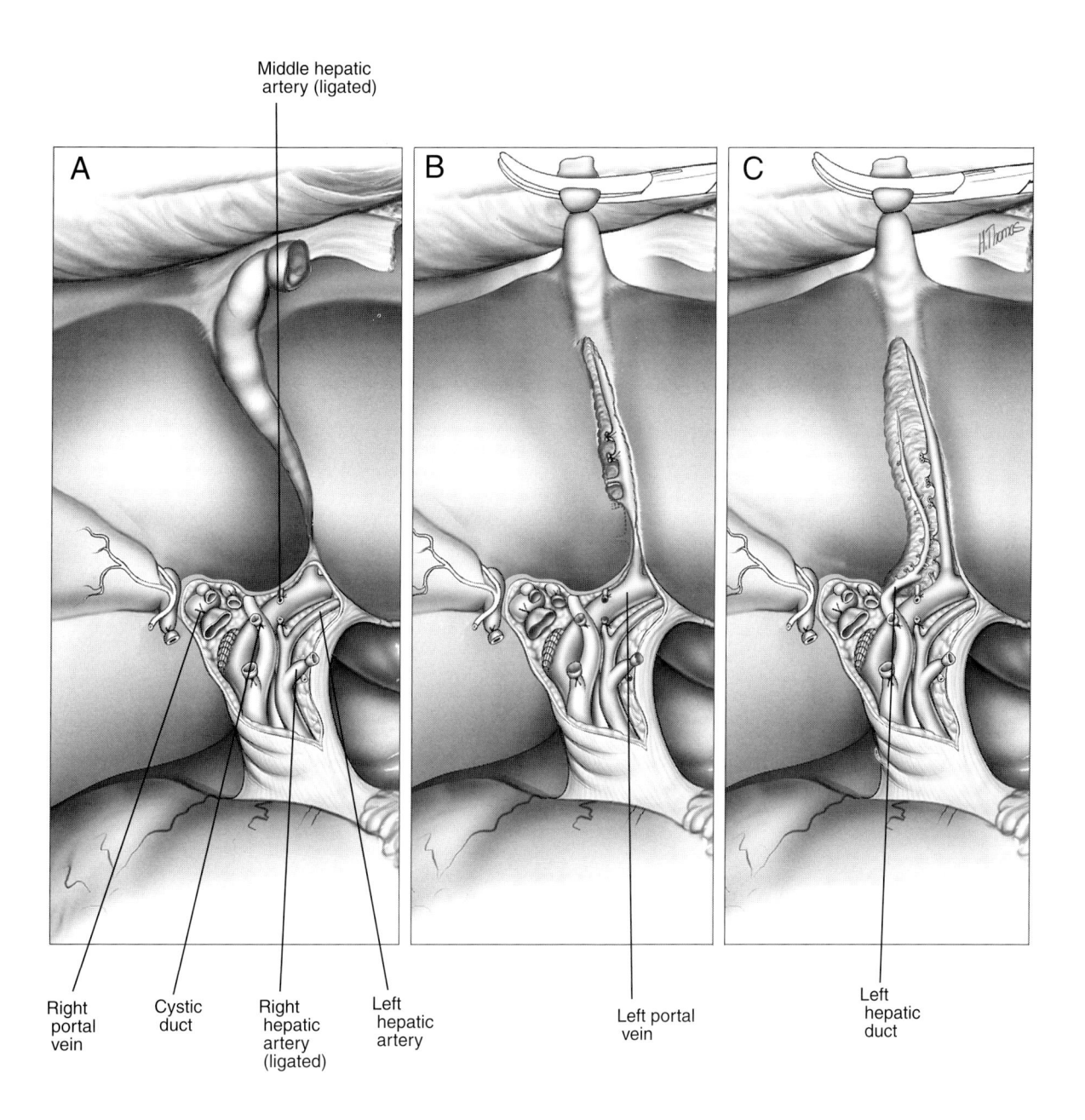

Figure 25–8 • **A,** Division of all the major structures in the porta hepatis is performed.
B, An incision into the hepatic parenchyma along the falciform ligament is made, and multiple branches off the hepatic duct and portal vein are ligated.
C, The dissection is completed, preserving the branches off the portal vein and left hepatic duct to the lateral liver segments.

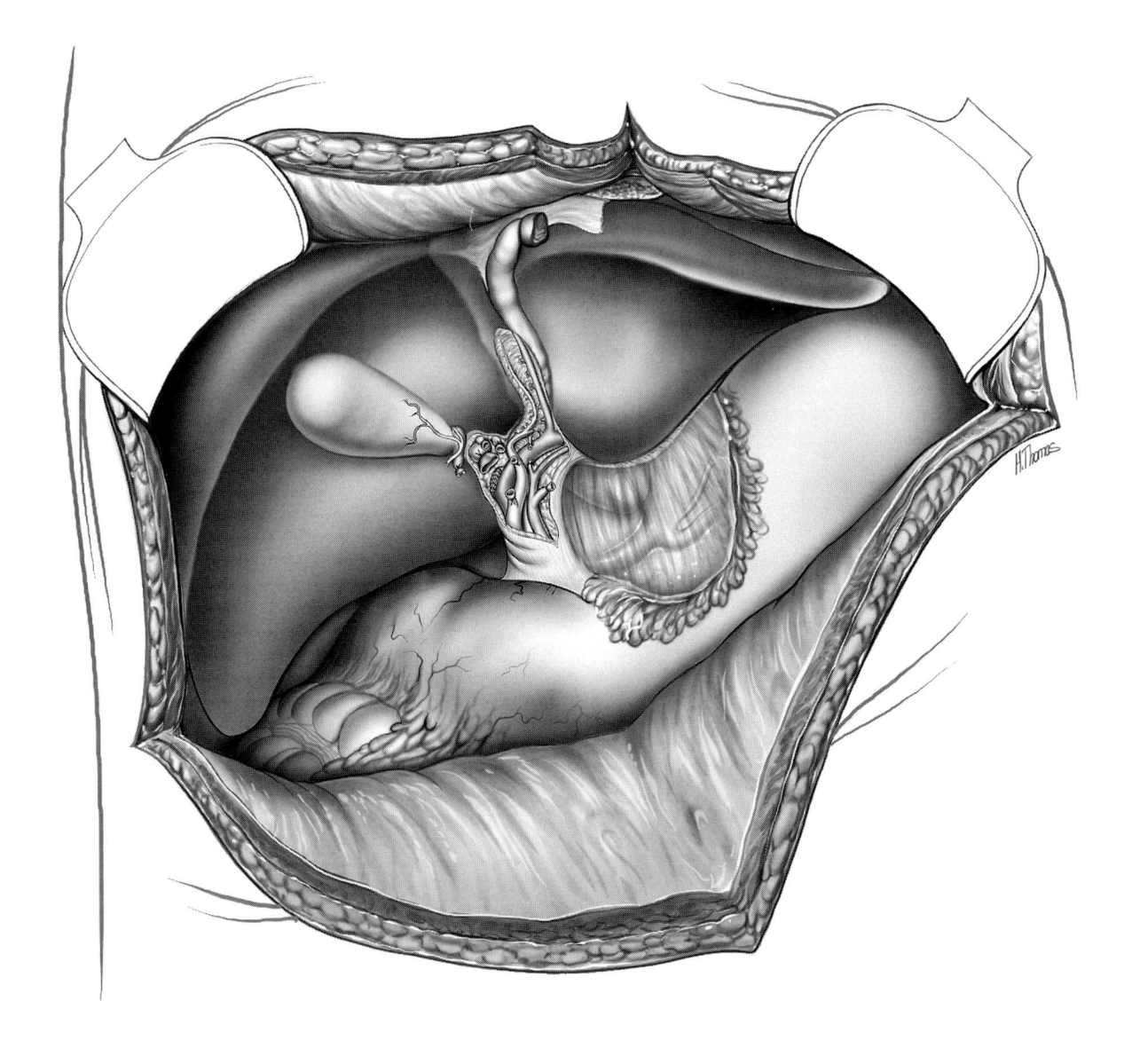

Figure 25–9 • The hepatic parenchyma demarcates just to the right of the falciform ligament.

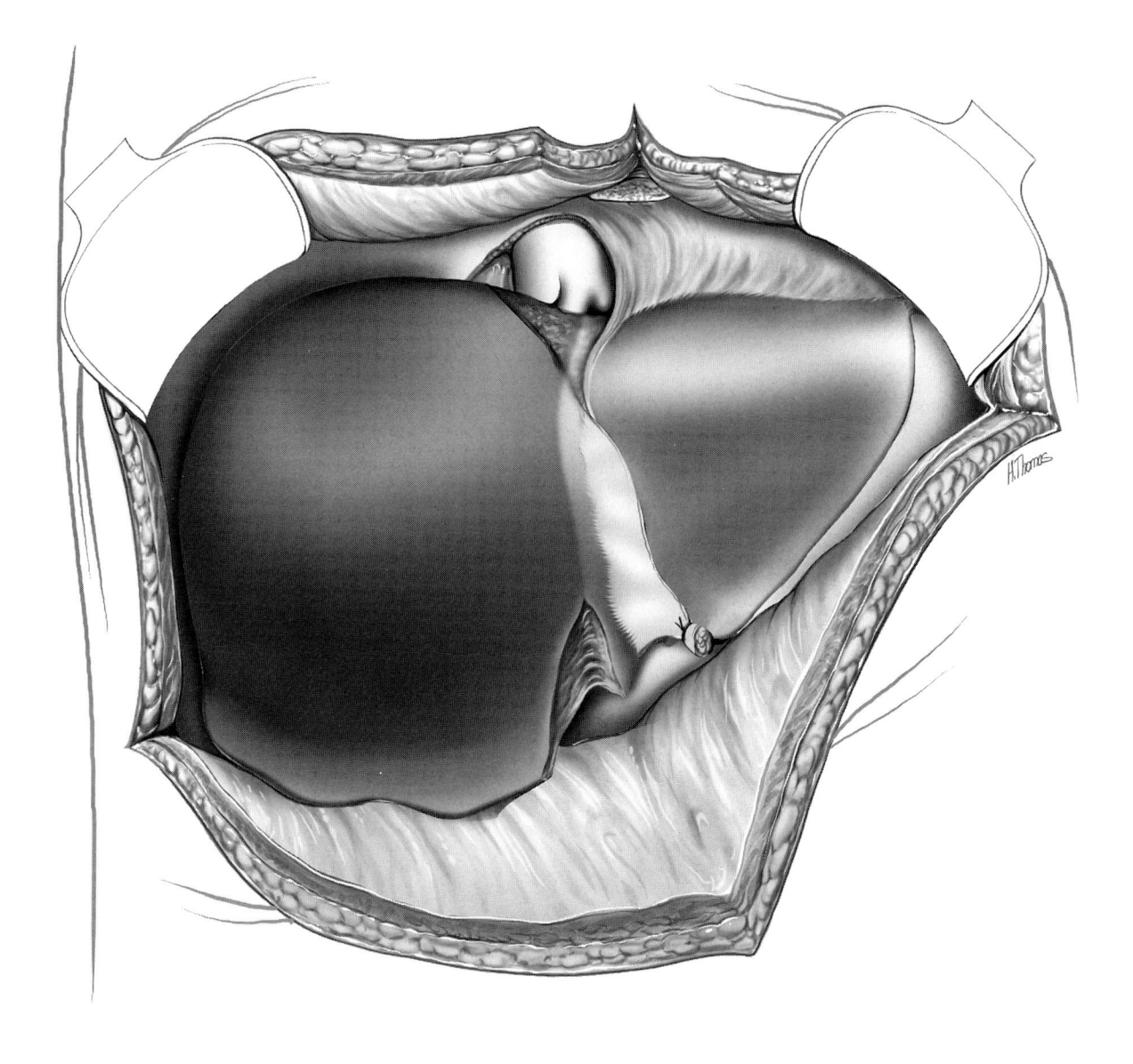

Figure 25–10 • The hepatic parenchyma is divided along the falciform ligament anteriorly.

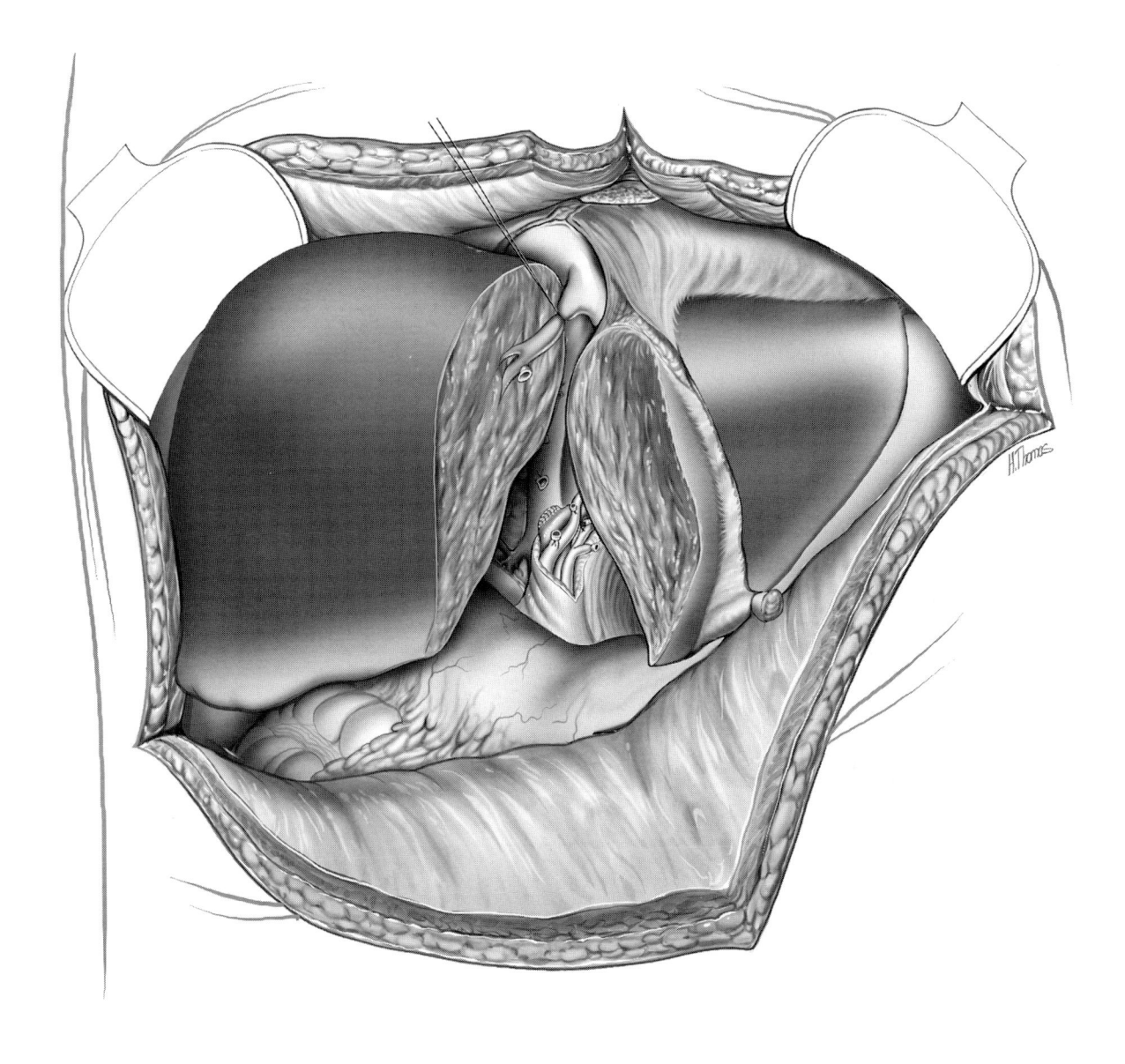

Figure 25–11 • The middle hepatic vein is identified and divided.

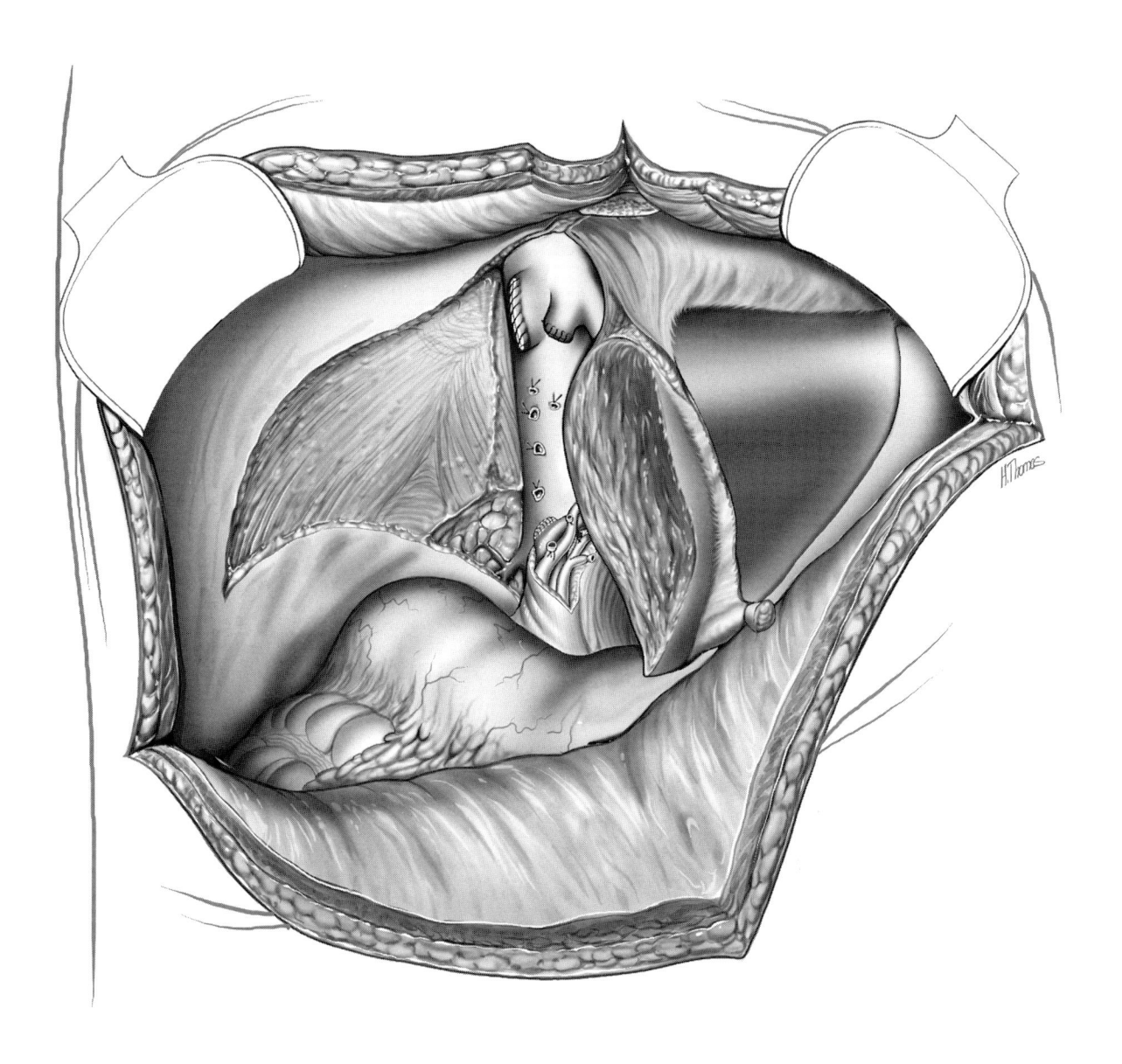

Figure 25–12 • The completed hepatic resection is depicted.

Chapter 26
Clinical Case: Hepatic Lobectomy: Vascular Isolation Technique

Charles Miller • Myron Schwartz

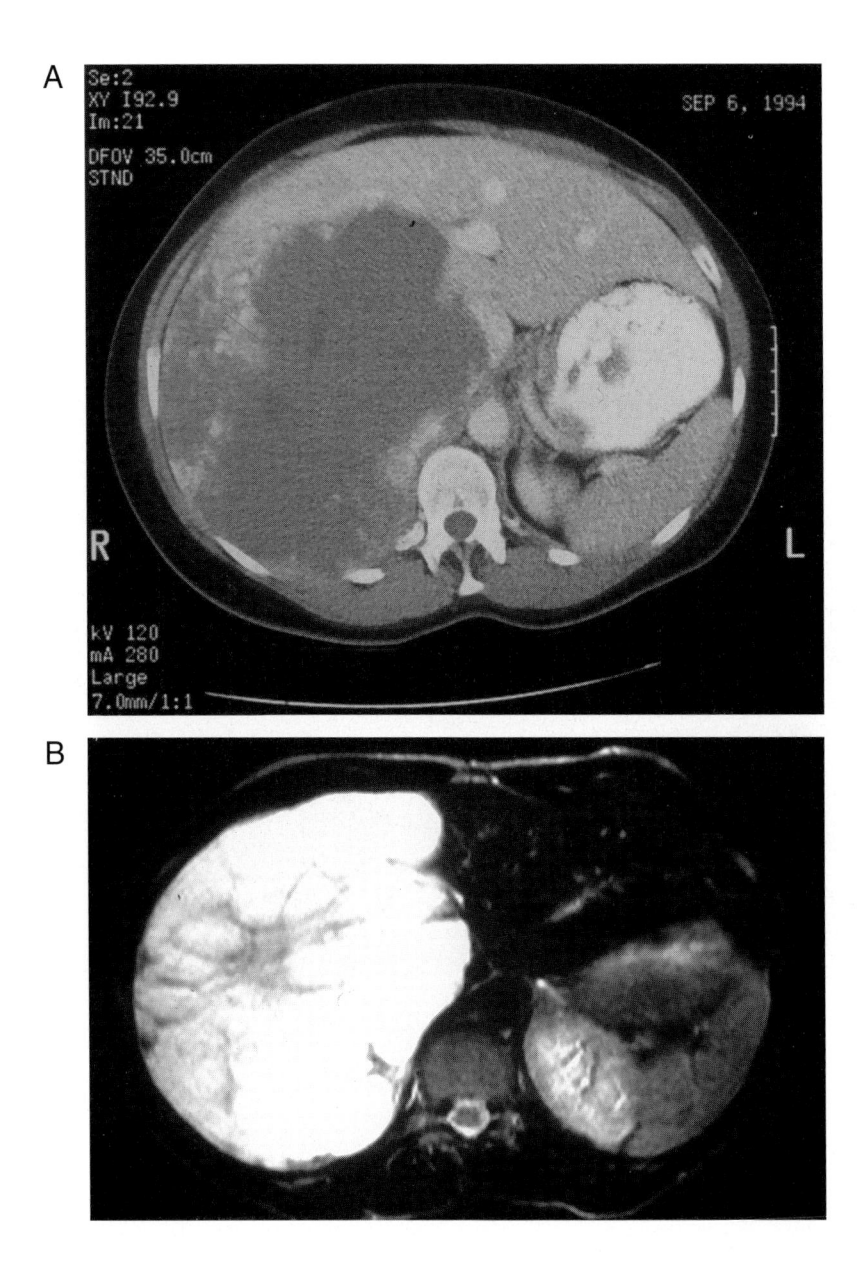

Figure 26–1 • A 36-year-old man presented with a large vascular lesion occupying the entire right lobe of the liver involving the vena cava. Over time he became progressively more symptomatic as the tumor continued to increase in size. The T1 MR image demonstrates the lesion (**A**). The T2 image shows that this is a vascular tumor (**B**). A vascular isolation technique was used for the hepatic lobectomy.

Clinical Case: Hepatic Lobectomy: Vascular Isolation Technique • 219

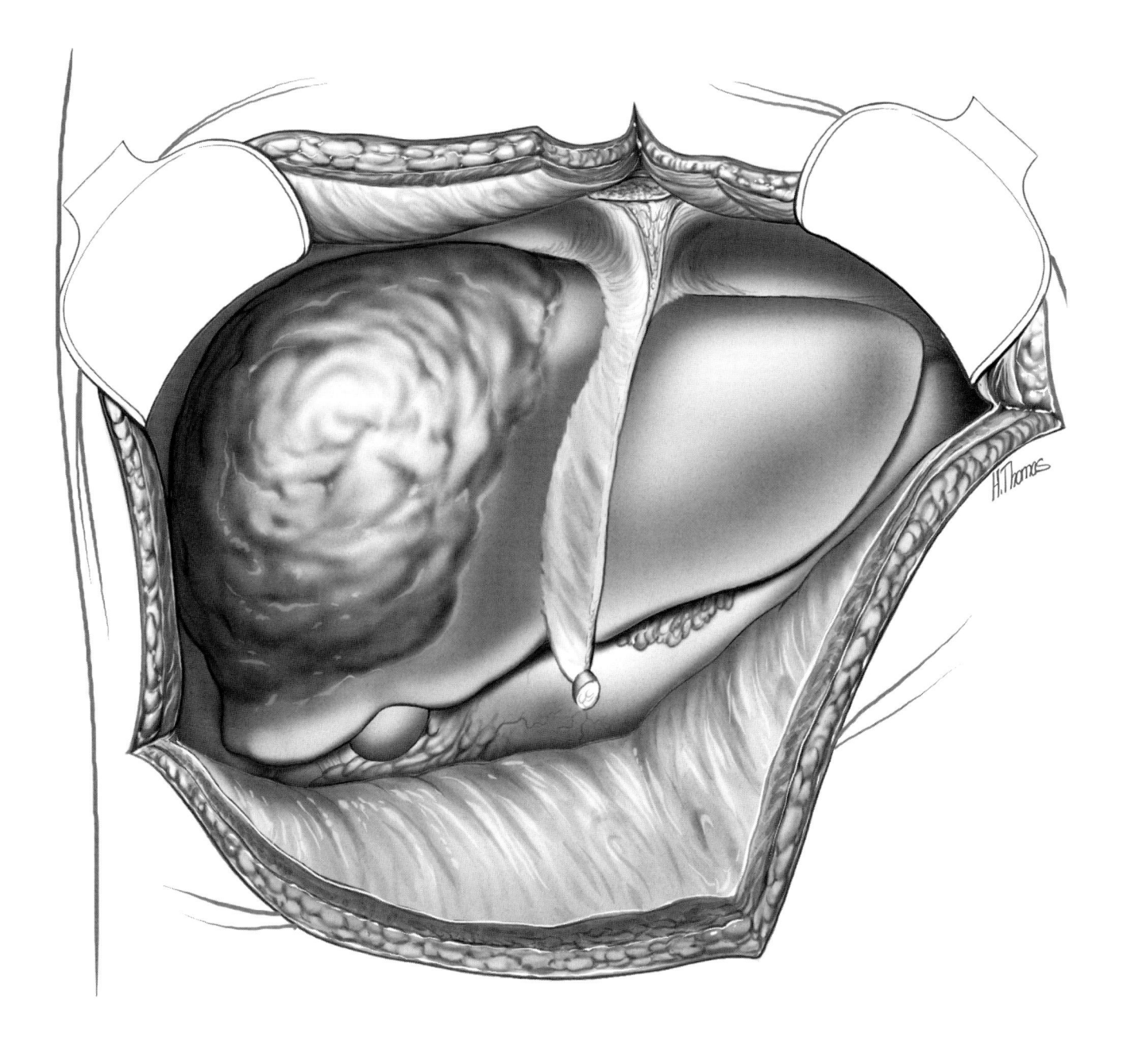

Figure 26–2 • Through a chevron incision, the falciform ligament is divided and the lesion is exposed.

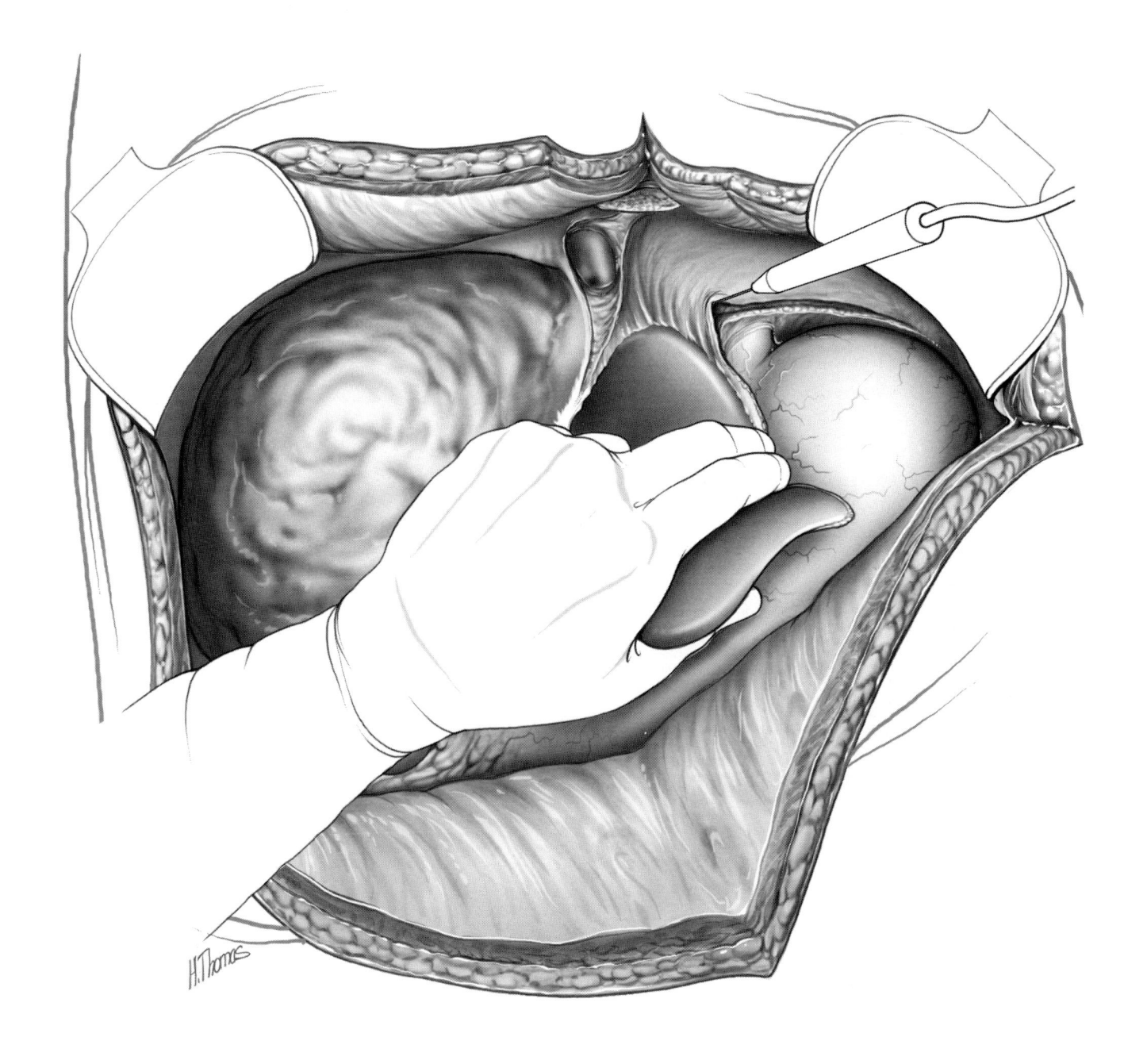

Figure 26–3 • The left triangular ligament is mobilized and the hepatic veins are identified.

Clinical Case: Hepatic Lobectomy: Vascular Isolation Technique • 221

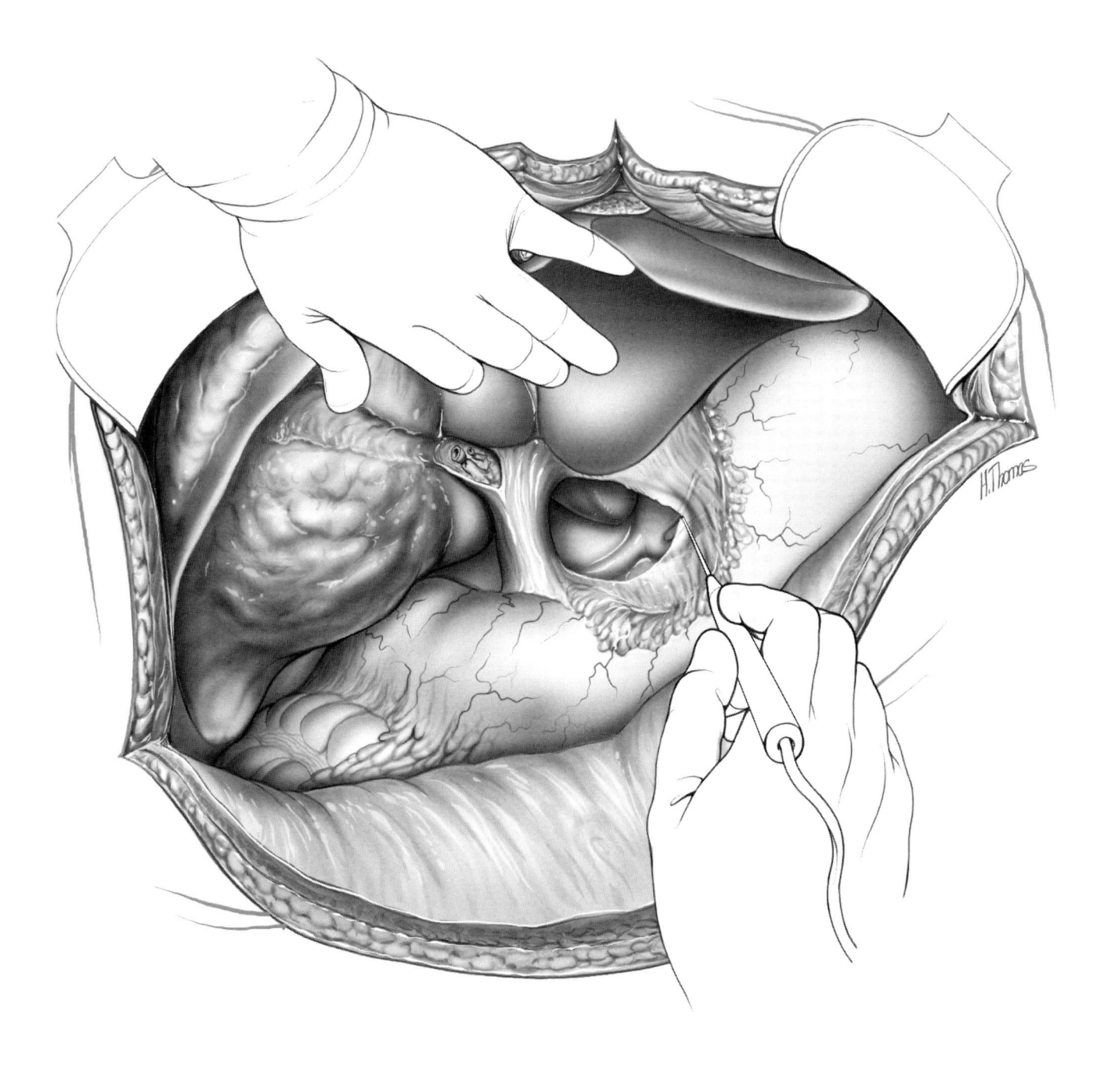

Figure 26–4 • A cholecystectomy is performed and the celiac axis is identified.

222 • Part III UPPER ABDOMEN

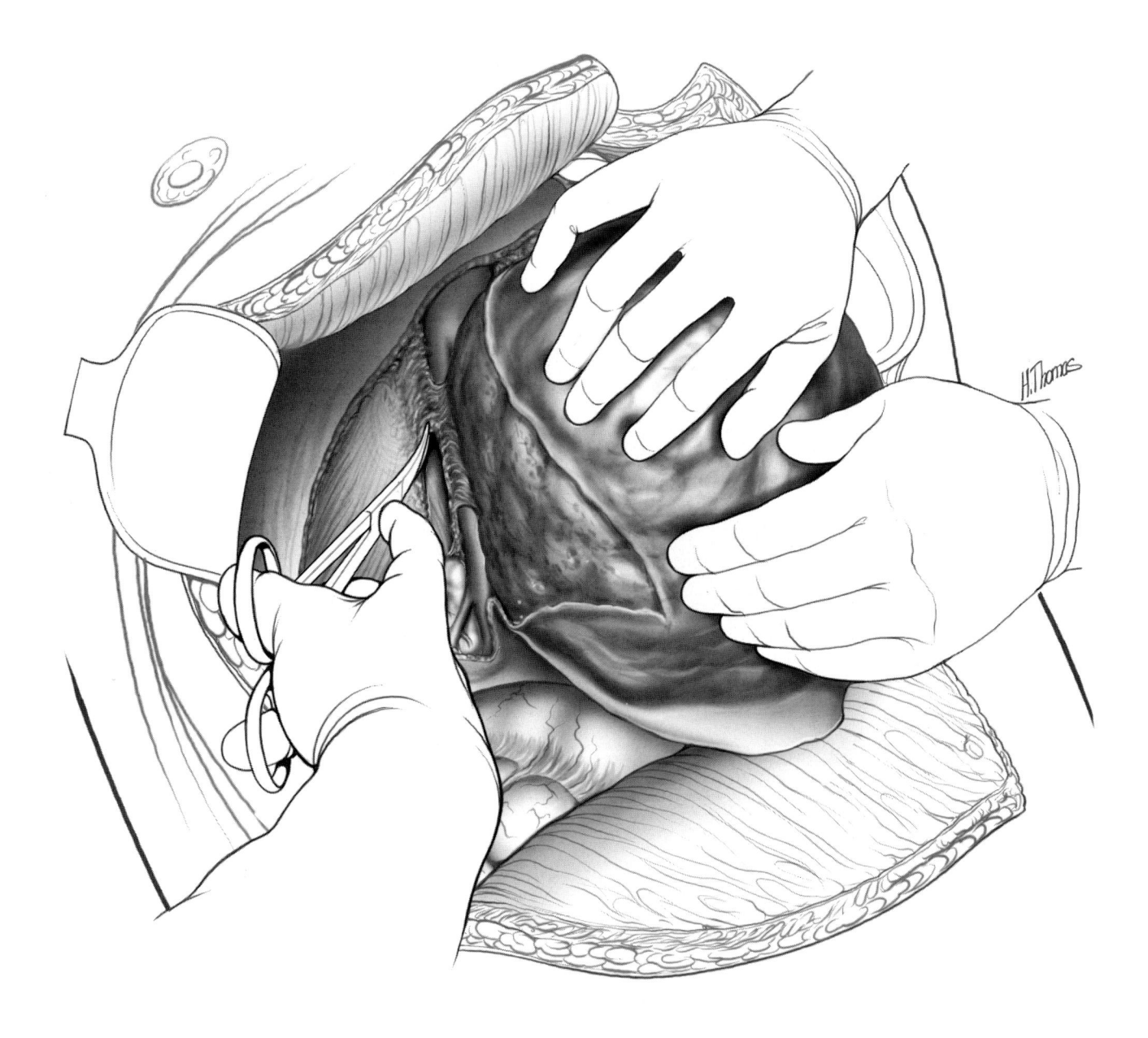

Figure 26–5 • The right lobe of the liver is fully mobilized, exposing the vena cava.

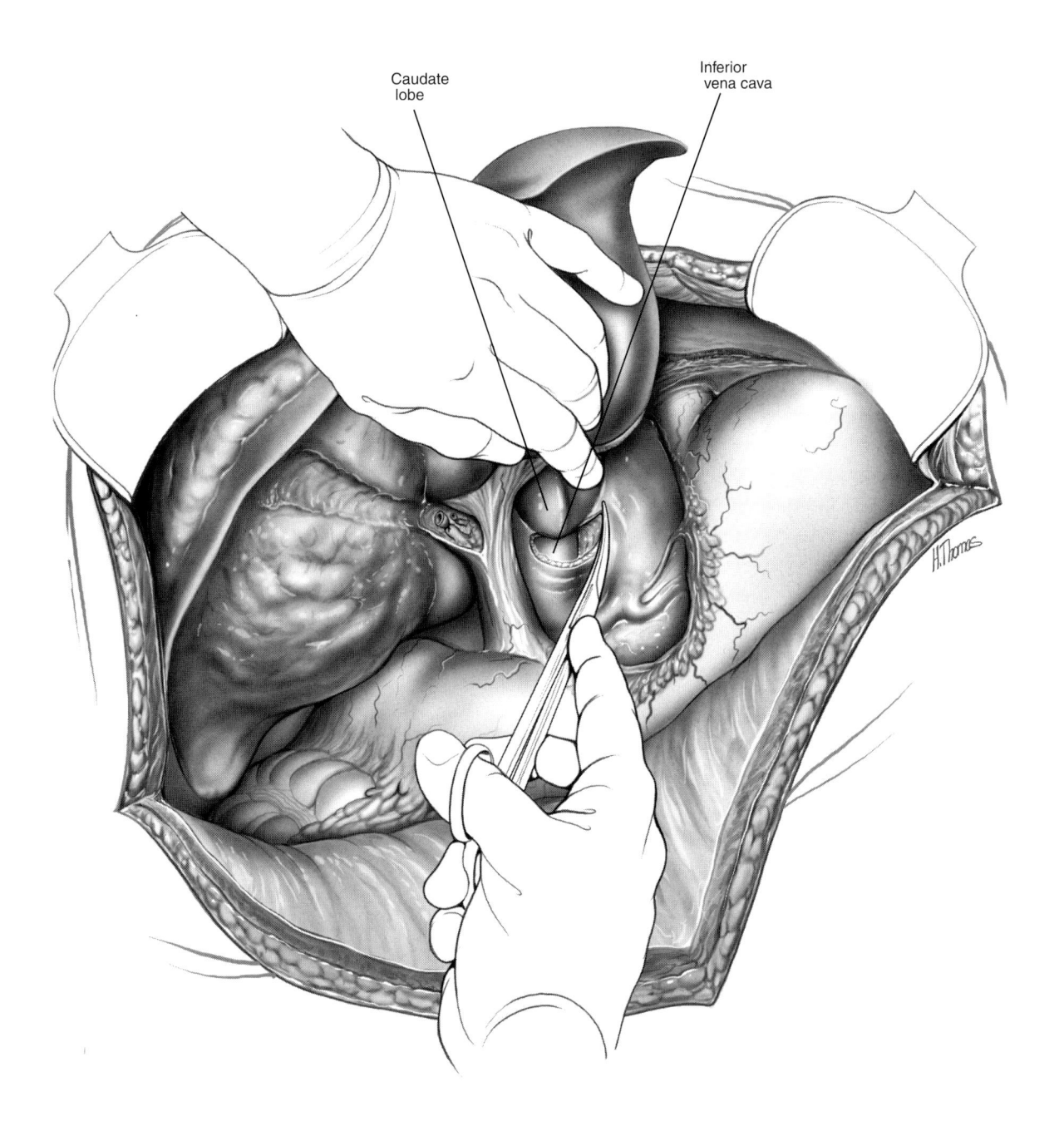

Figure 26–6 • The inferior vena cava is exposed below the caudate lobe.

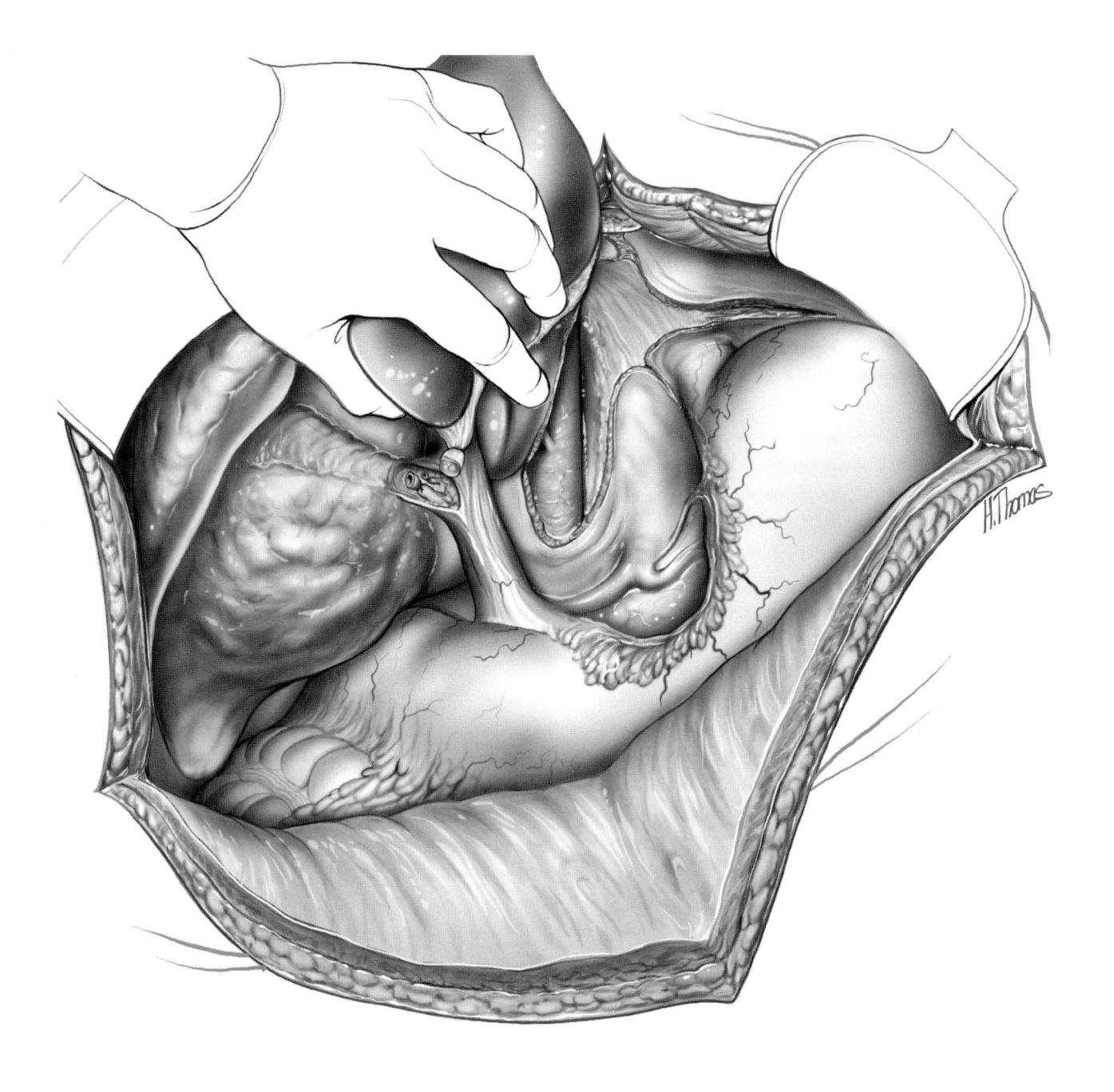

Figure 26–7 • The caudate lobe is mobilized off the vena cava, and several small branches are identified.

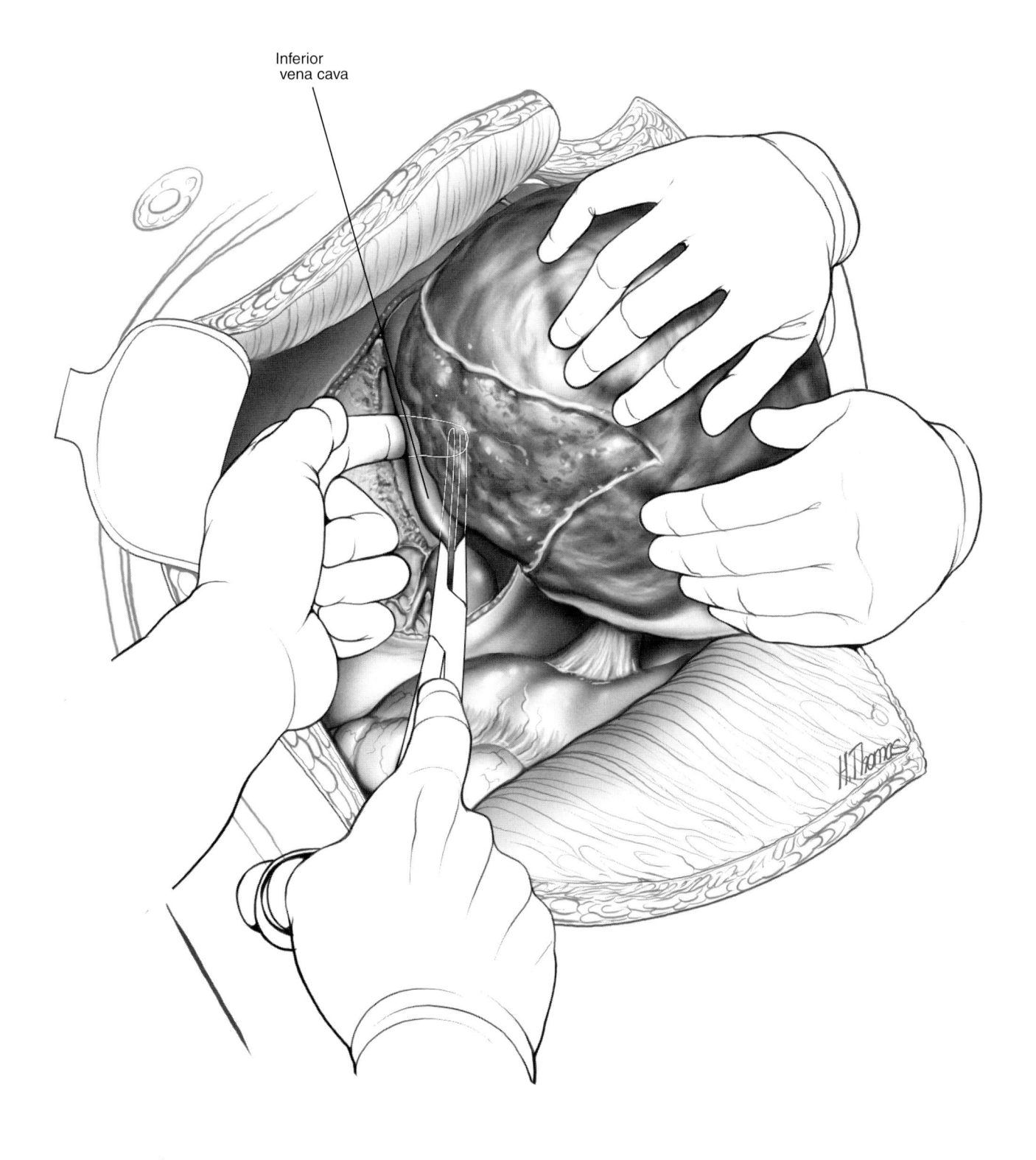

Figure 26–8 • A vascular clamp is placed across the inferior vena cava.

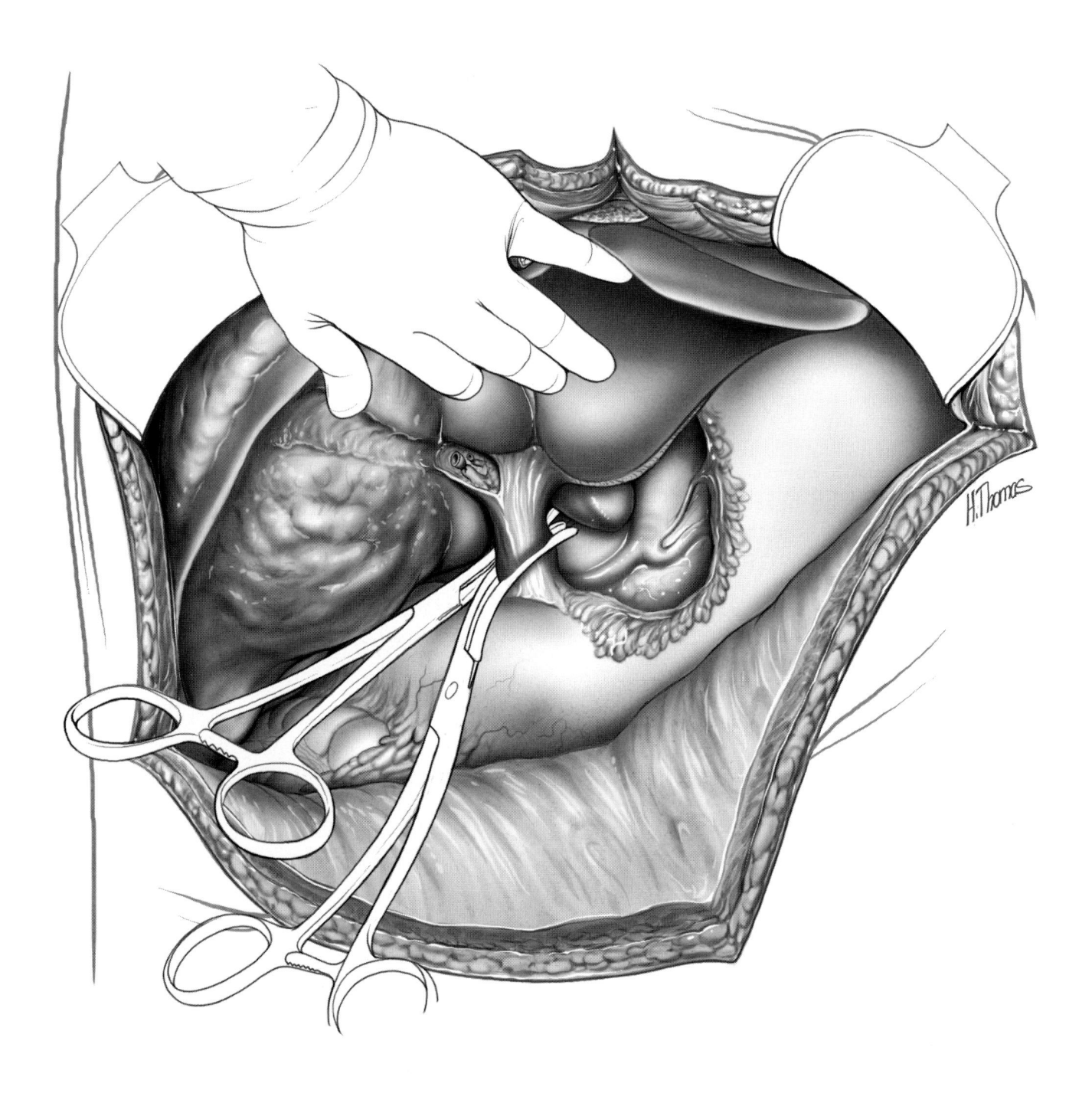

Figure 26-9 • A vascular clamp is placed across the porta hepatis. The right hepatic artery is divided, as is the right hepatic duct.

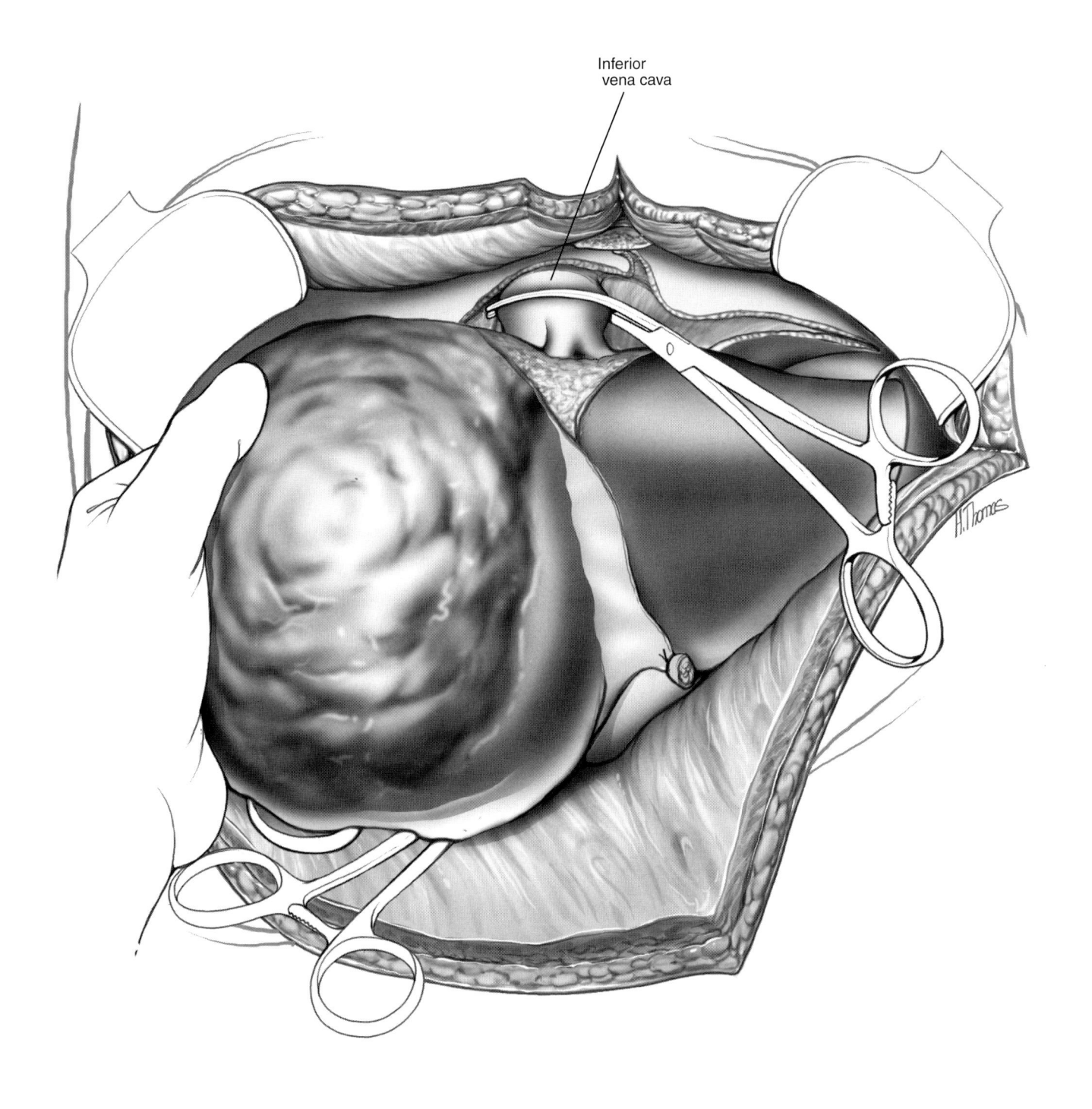

Clinical Case: Hepatic Lobectomy: Vascular Isolation Technique • 227

Figure 26–10 • A vascular clamp is placed across the inferior vena cava proximal to the hepatic veins.

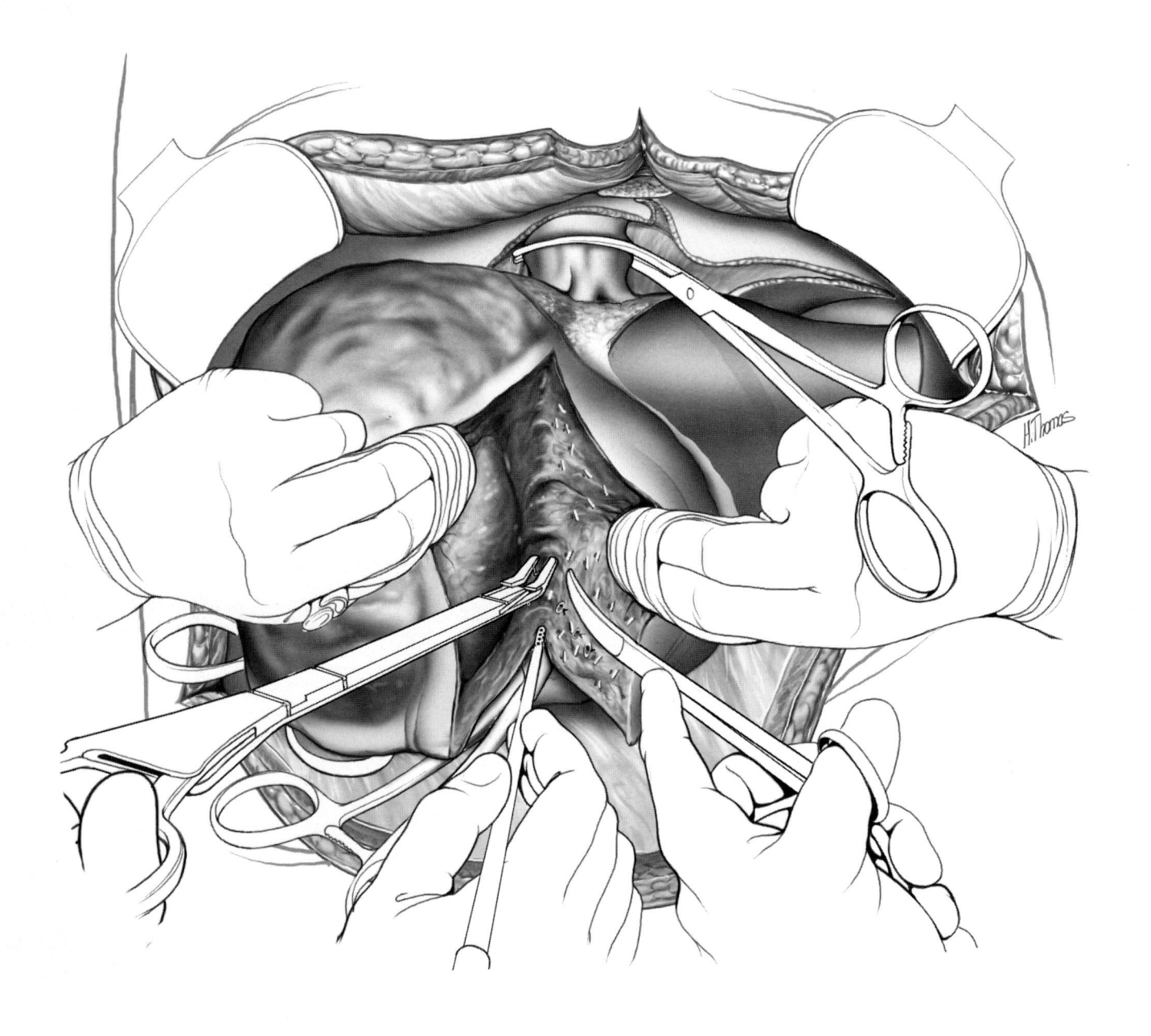

Figure 26–11 • The right lobe of the liver is divided.

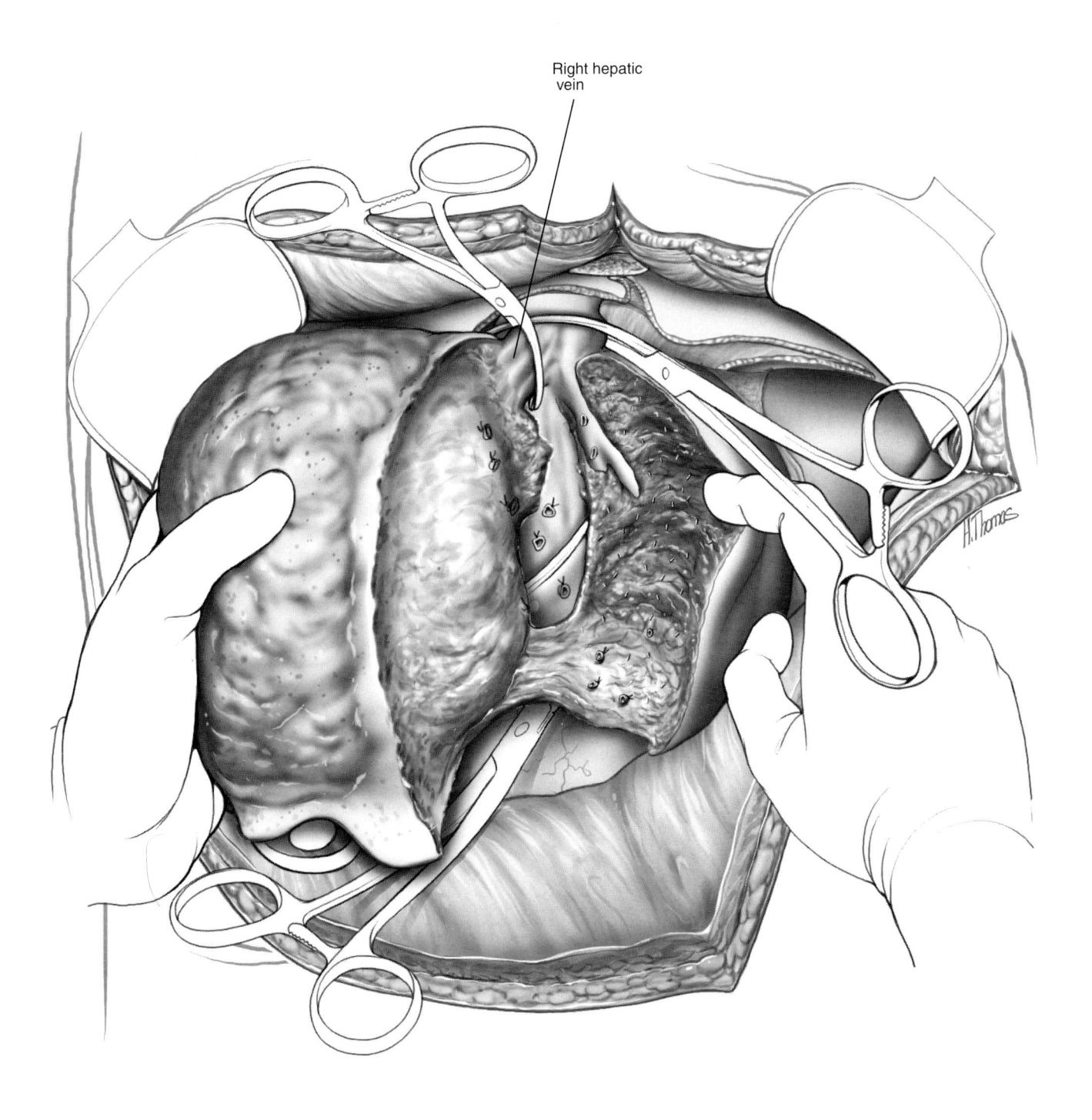

Figure 26–12 • Several branches off the middle hepatic vein are ligated and divided. A clamp is placed across the right hepatic vein, and the direct extension of the tumor into the vena cava is identified.

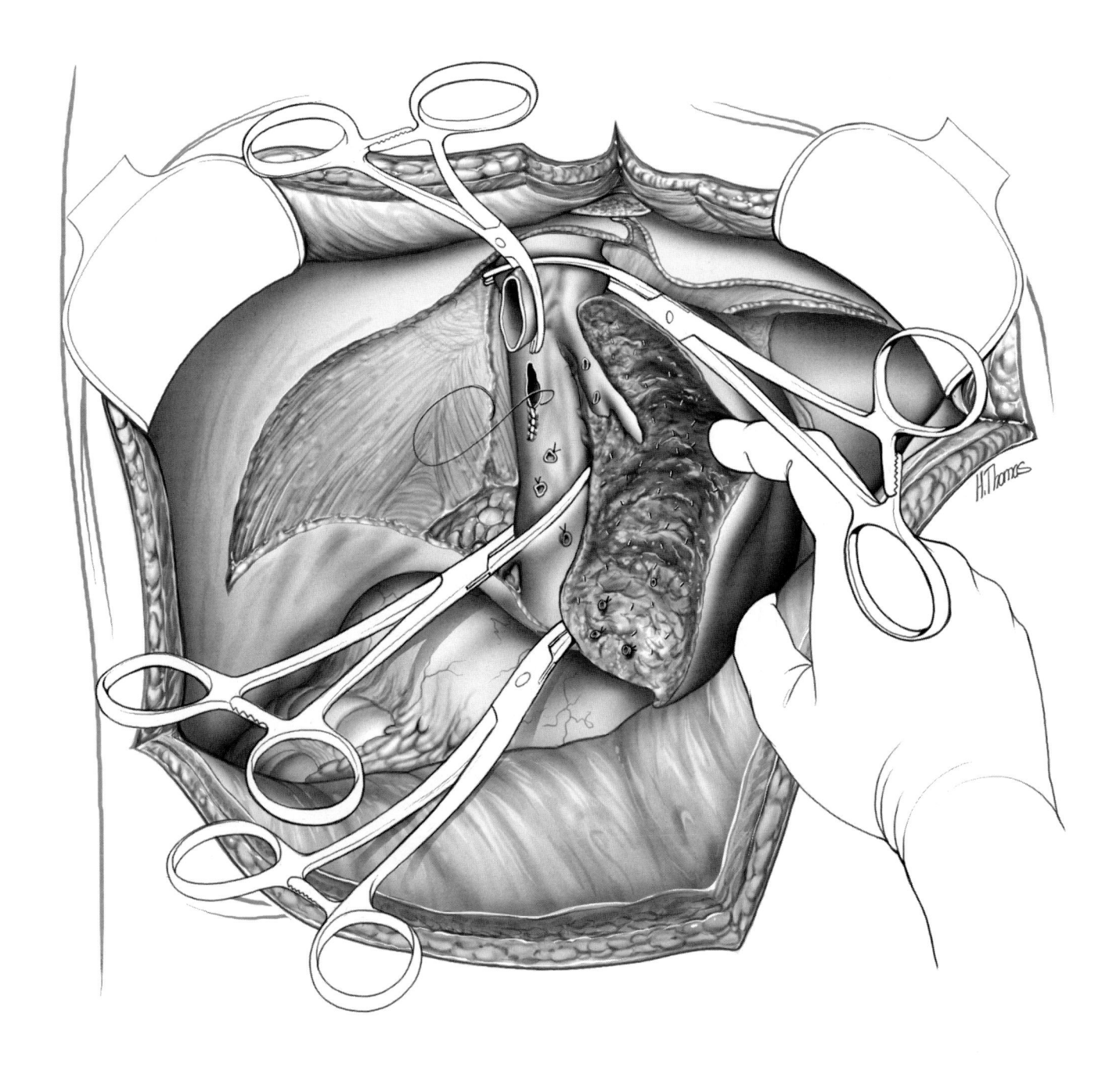

Figure 26-13 • The right hepatic vein is divided and the tumor is removed. The hole in the vena cava is repaired.

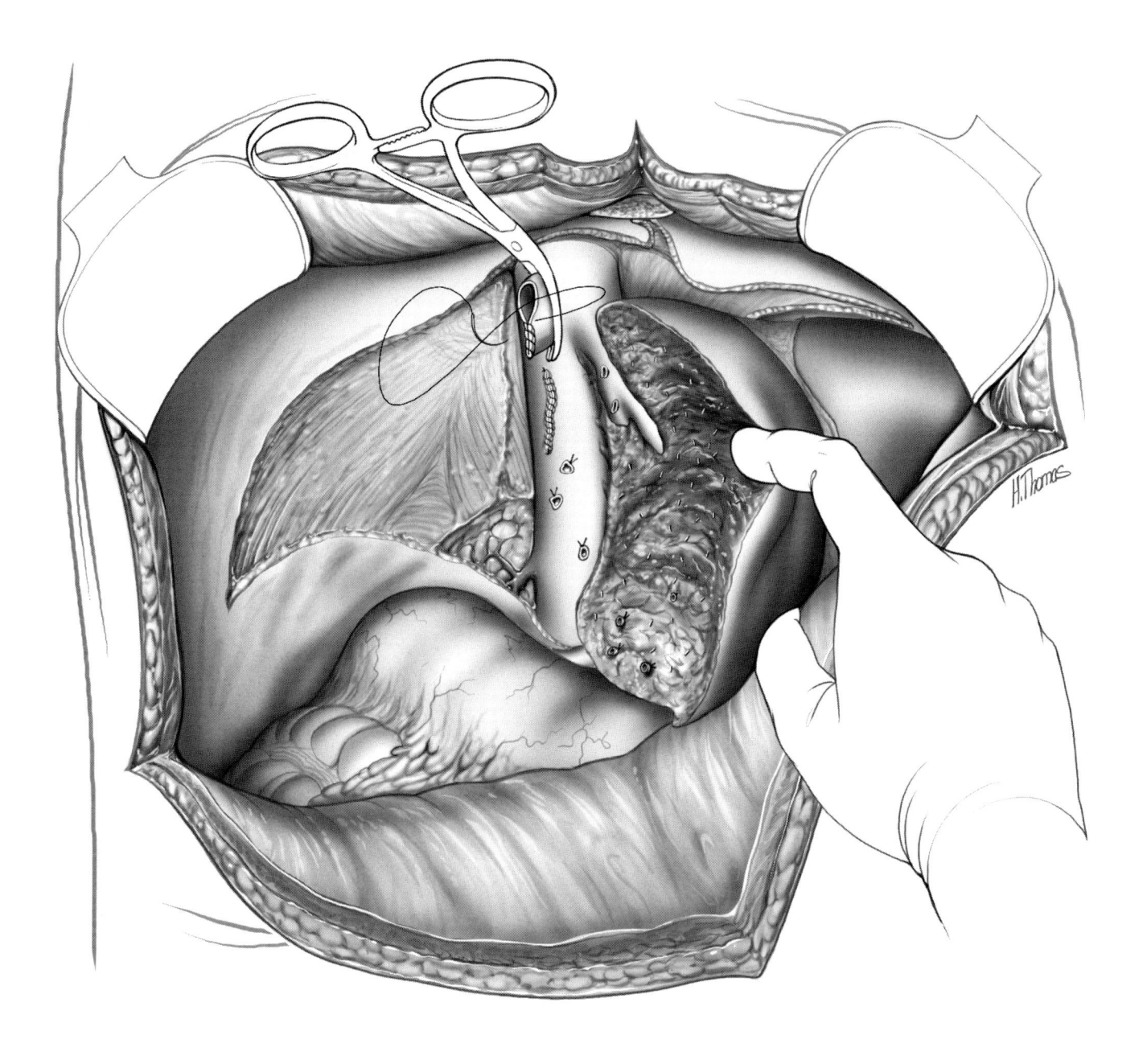

Figure 26–14 • All vascular clamps are removed, and the right hepatic vein is oversewn.

Chapter 27
Radical Cholecystectomy

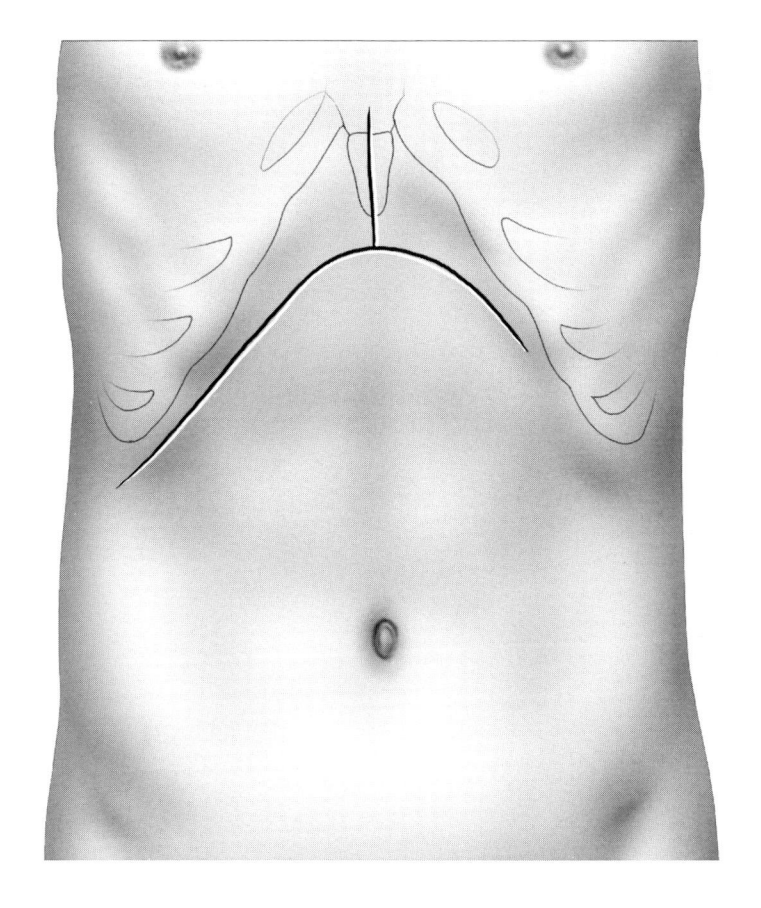

Figure 27–1 • A subcostal incision is performed.

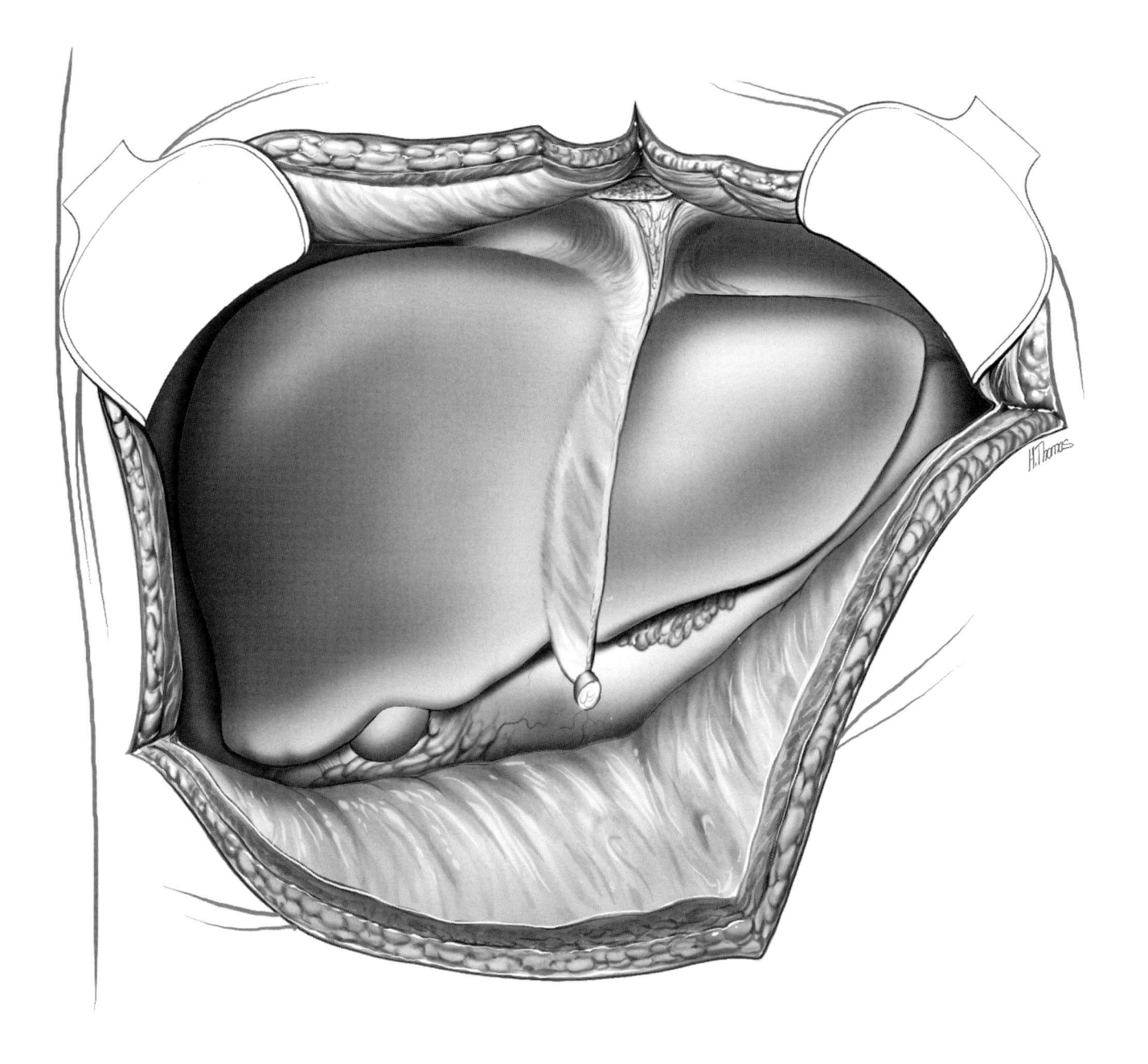

Figure 27-2 • Upon opening of the abdominal cavity, the falciform ligament is divided.

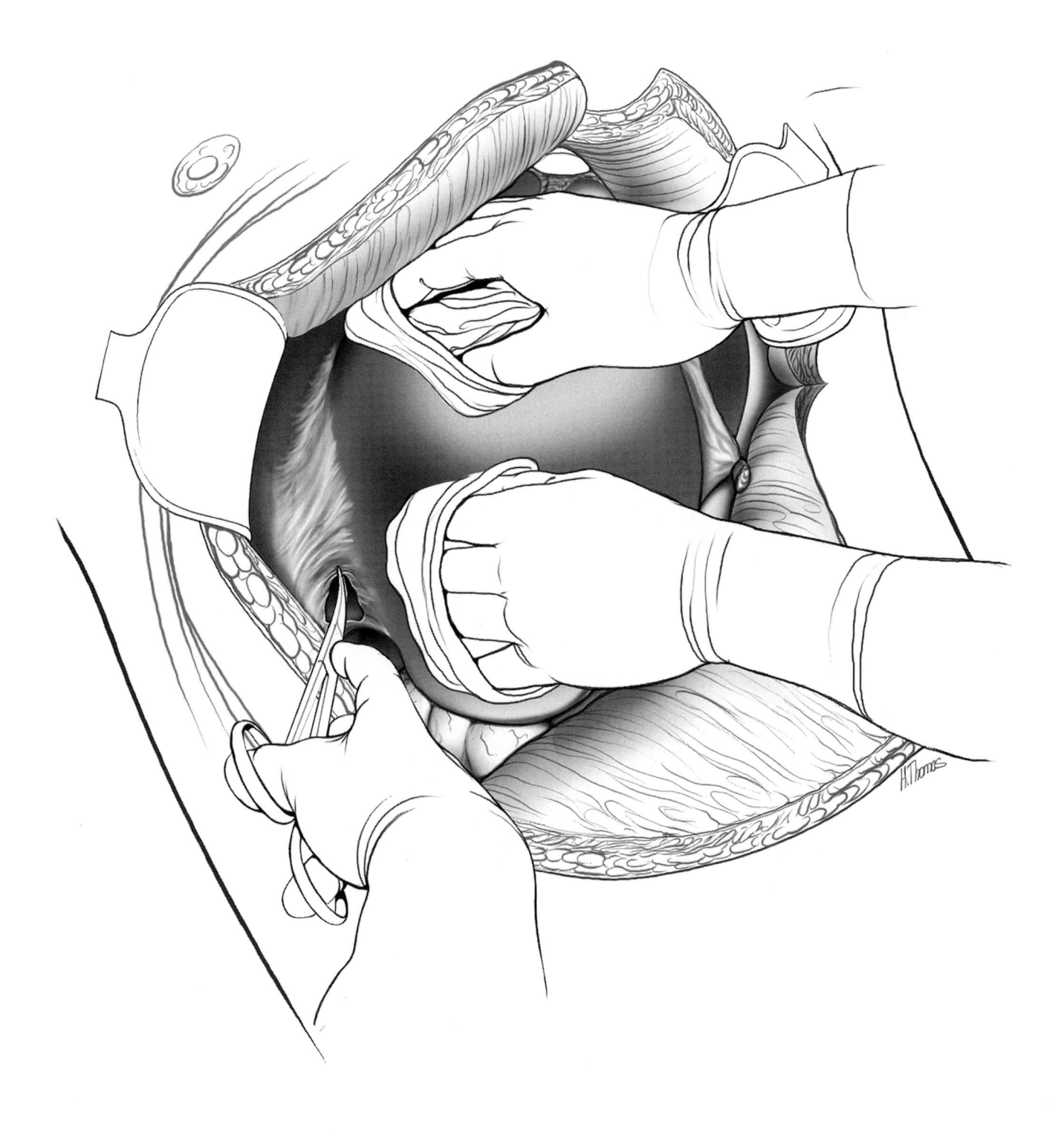

Figure 27–3 • The right triangular ligament is divided and the right hepatic lobe is mobilized.

Radical Cholecystectomy • 235

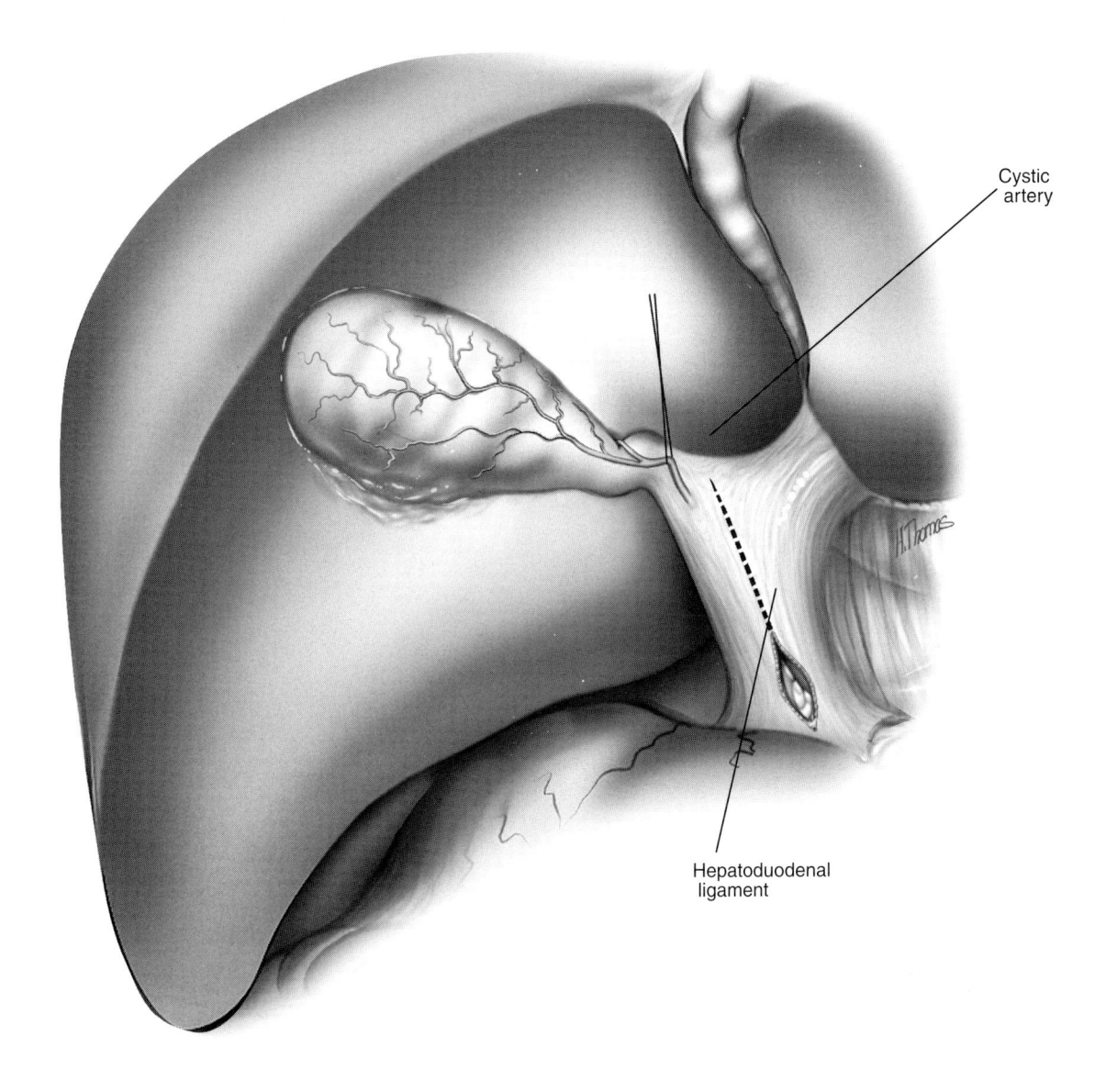

Figure 27–4 • The dissection of the porta hepatis is commenced.

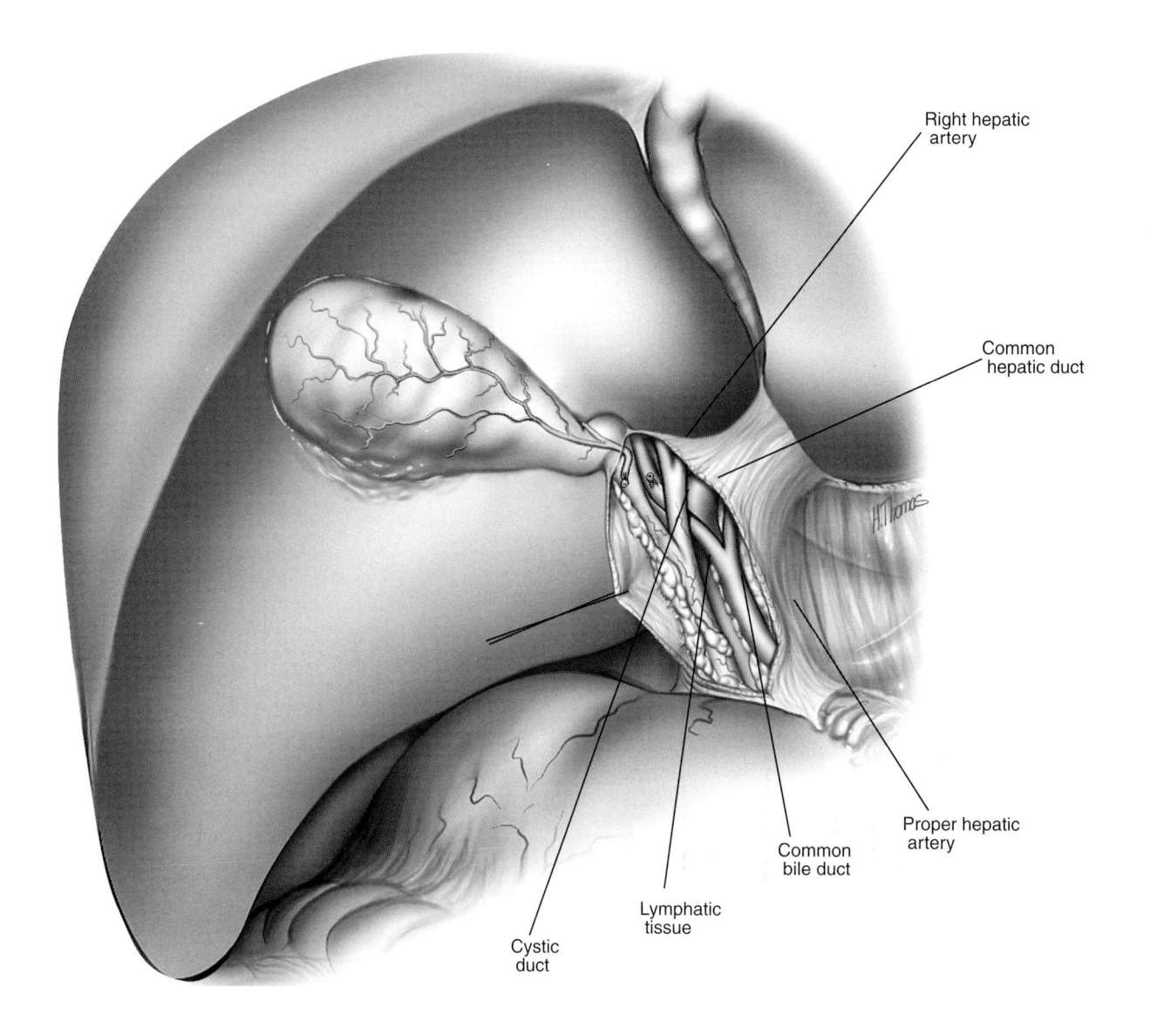

Figure 27–5 • All nodal tissue is dissected off the common hepatic artery and common bile duct, and the cystic artery is divided.

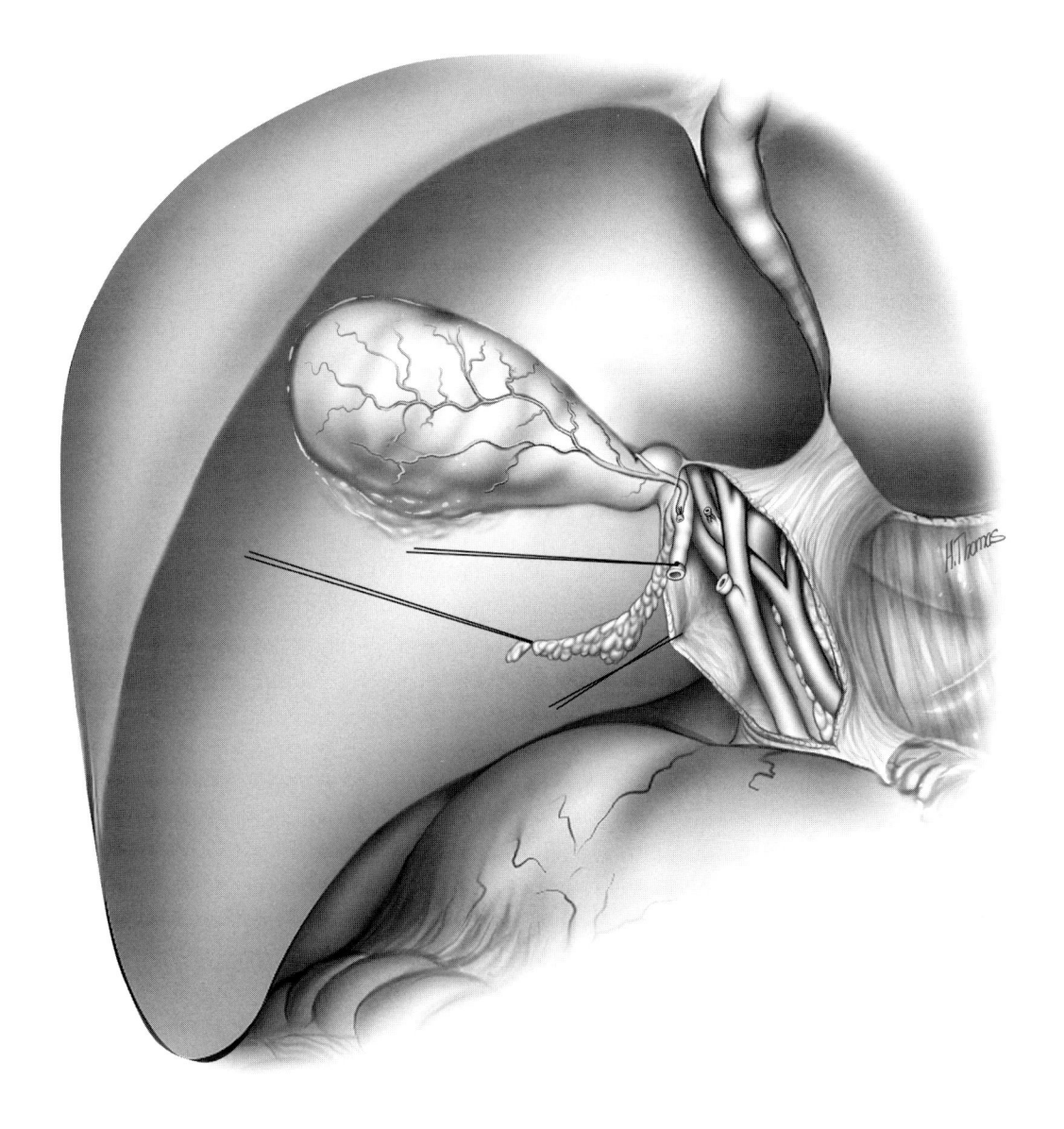

Figure 27–6 • The cystic duct is divided and the nodal dissection is completed.

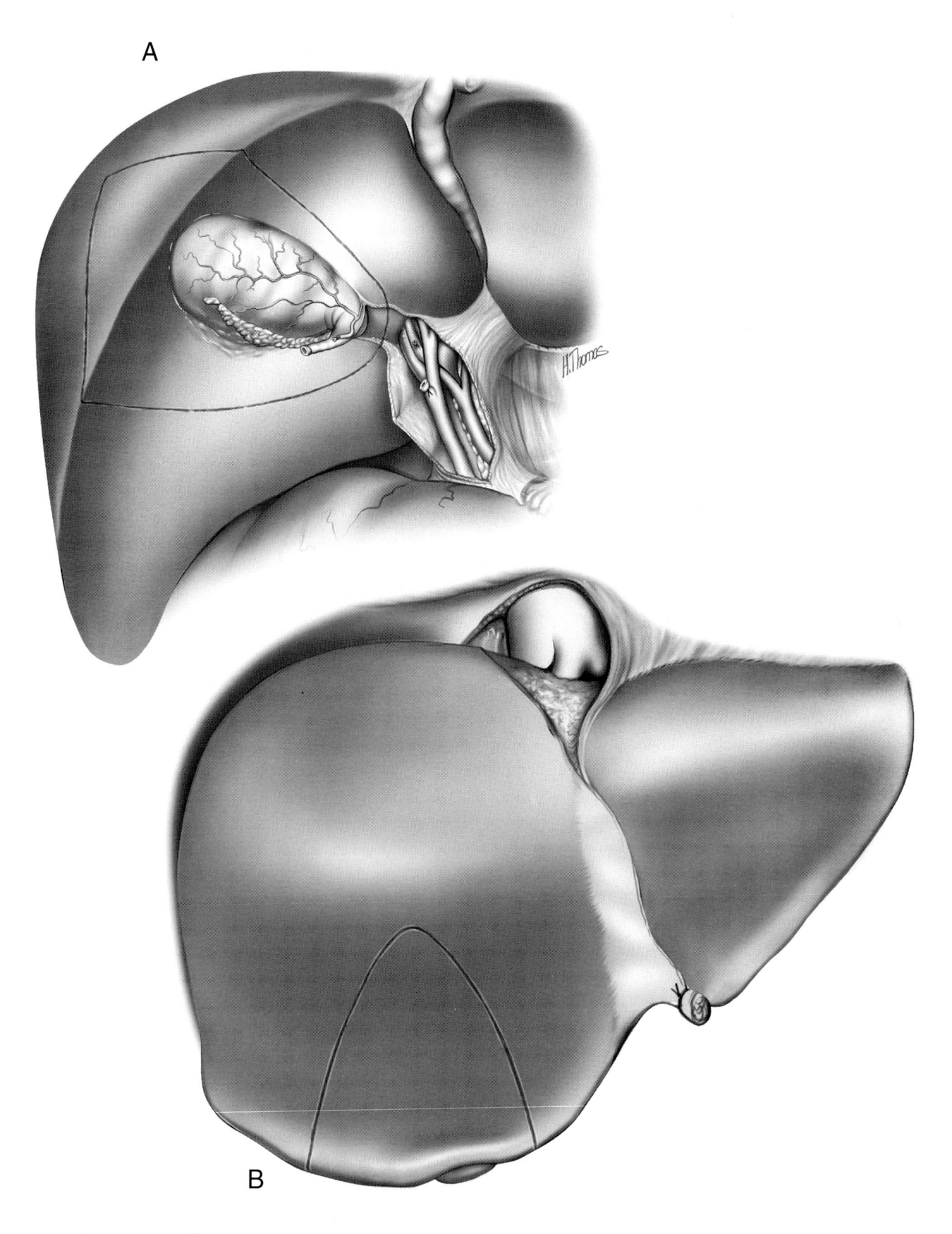

Figure 27–7 • The portion of the liver to be resected is defined. The capsule is scored with a cautery on the posterior (**A**) and anterior (**B**) aspects of the liver.

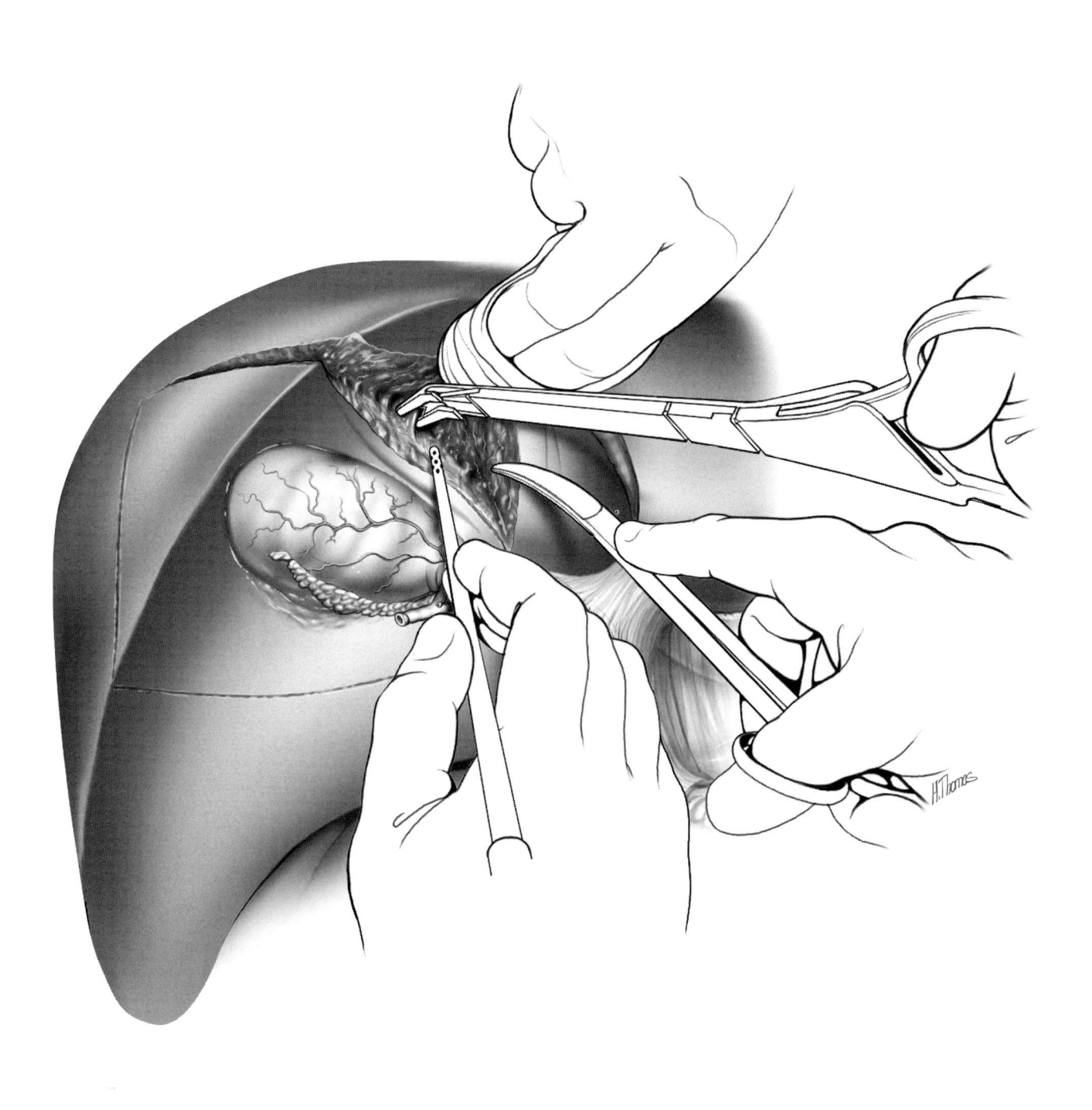

Figure 27–8 • Utilizing sharp dissection, cautery, and clips, the hepatic parenchyma is resected.

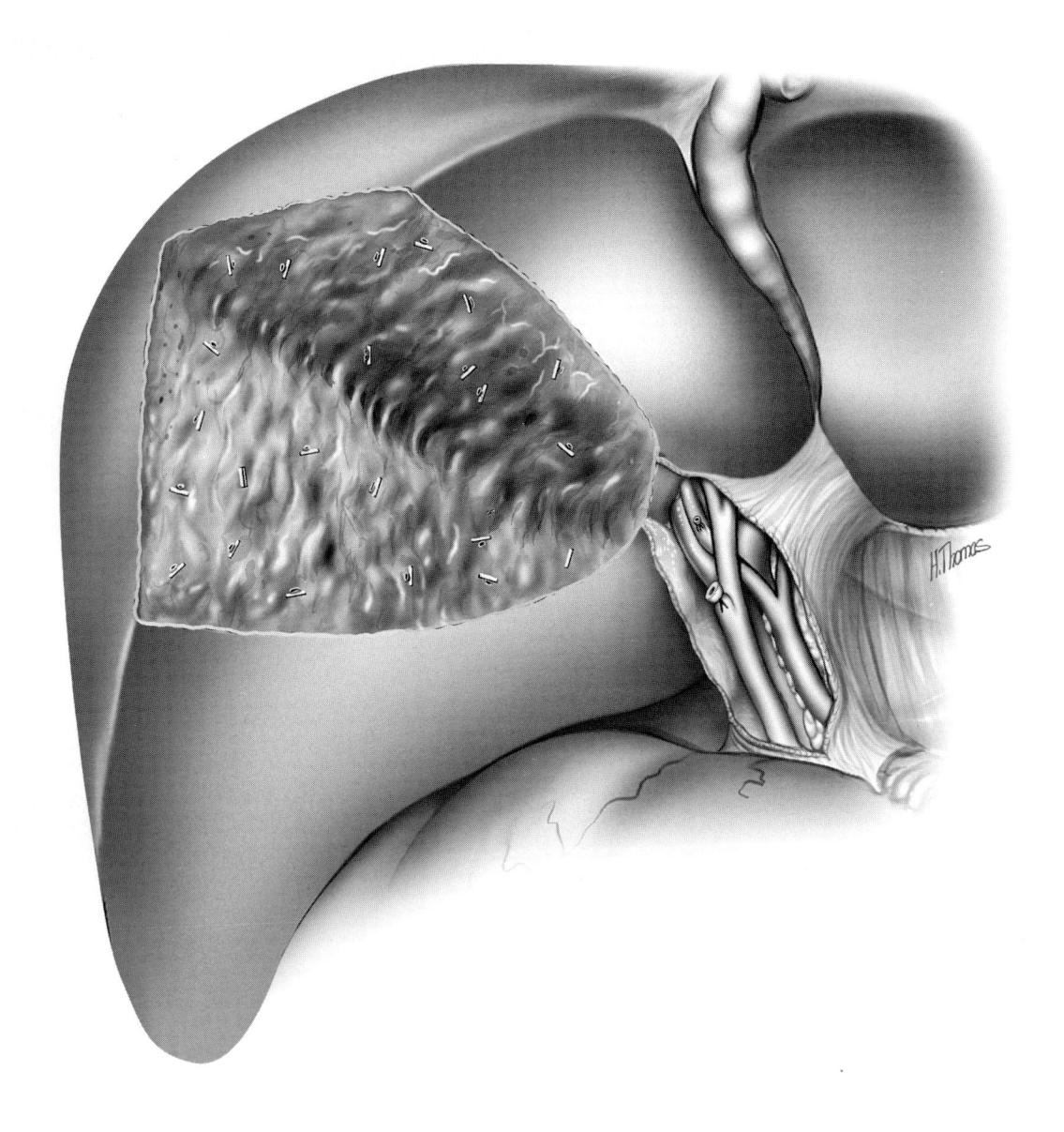

Figure 27-9 • The completed resection is depicted.

Chapter 28
Pancreatectomy (Whipple Procedure)

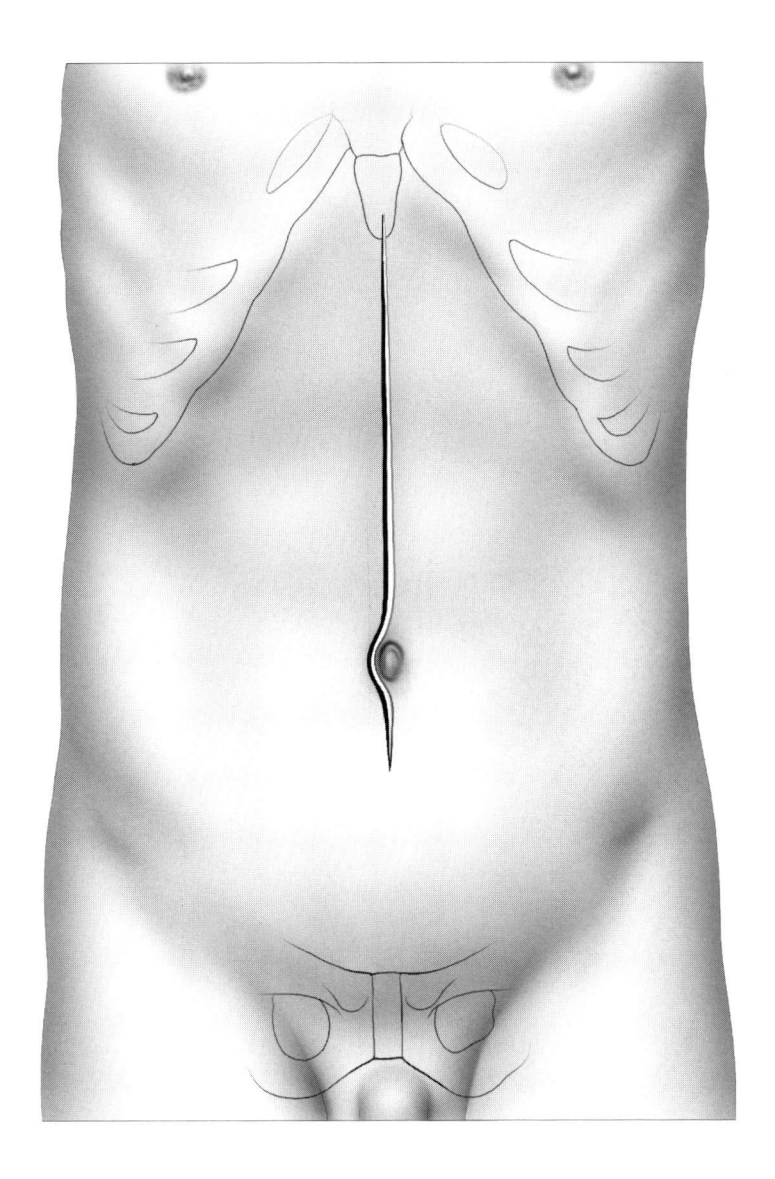

Figure 28–1 • A midline abdominal incision is the preferred incision for this procedure.

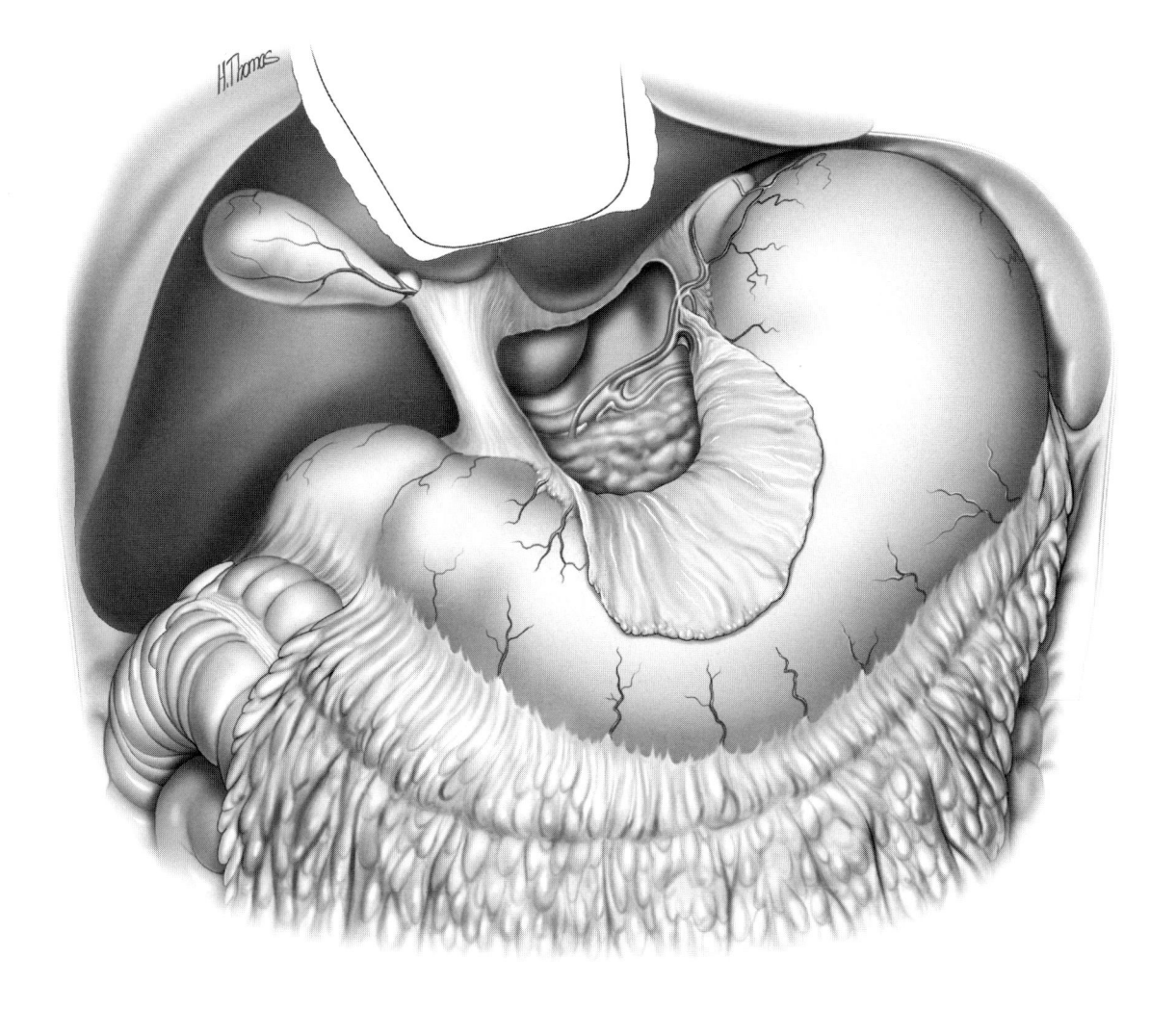

Figure 28–2 • The gastrohepatic ligament is incised to expose the celiac axis and the right and left gastric and pancreaticoduodenal arteries.

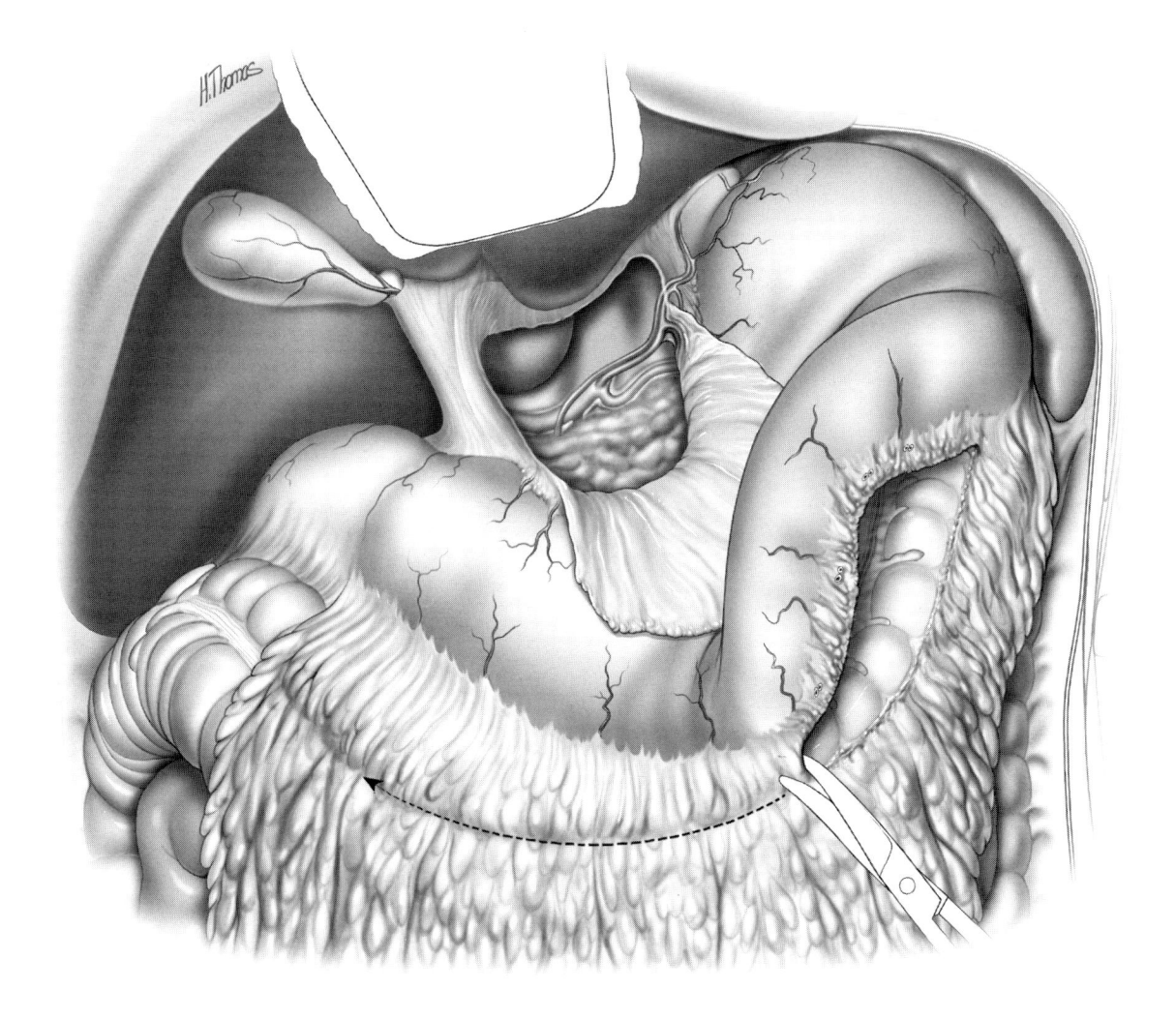

Figure 28-3 • The gastrocolic mesentery is incised in order to enter the lesser sac.

244 • Part III UPPER ABDOMEN

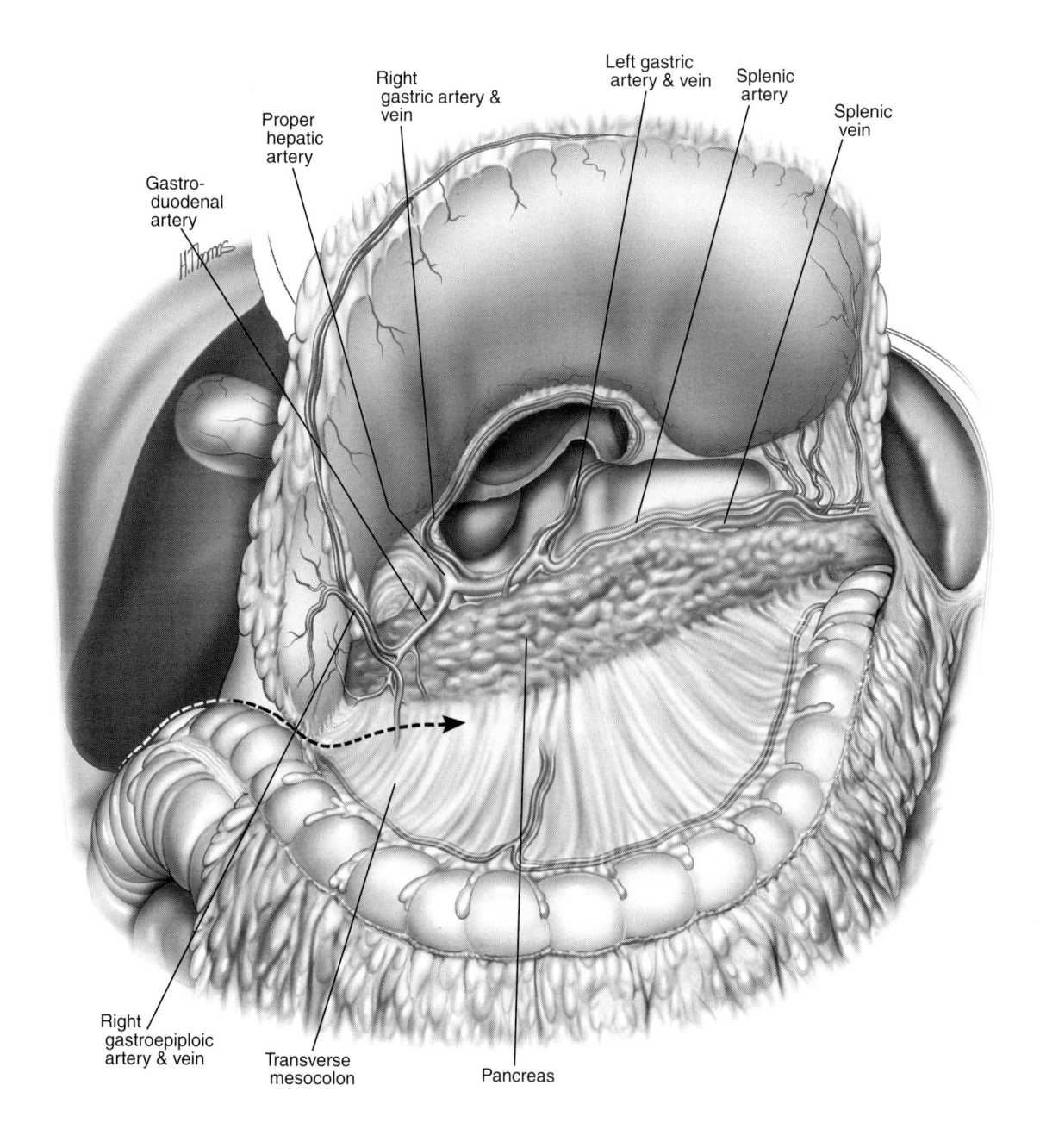

Figure 28–4 • An incision is made in the transverse mesocolon to expose the third and fourth portions of the duodenum.

Pancreatectomy (Whipple Procedure) • 245

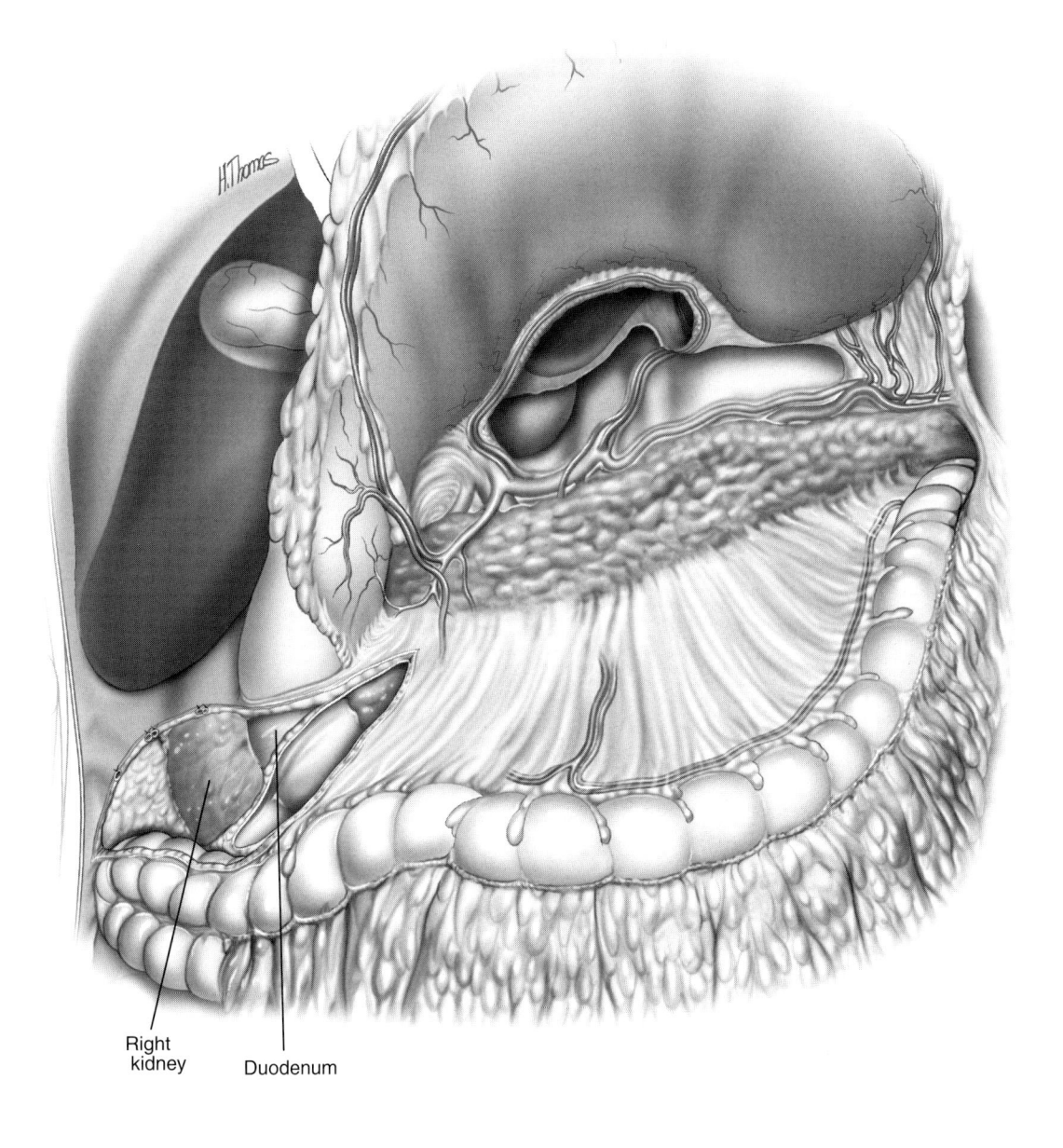

Right kidney
Duodenum

Figure 28–5 • The incision is carried medially toward the superior mesenteric vessels.

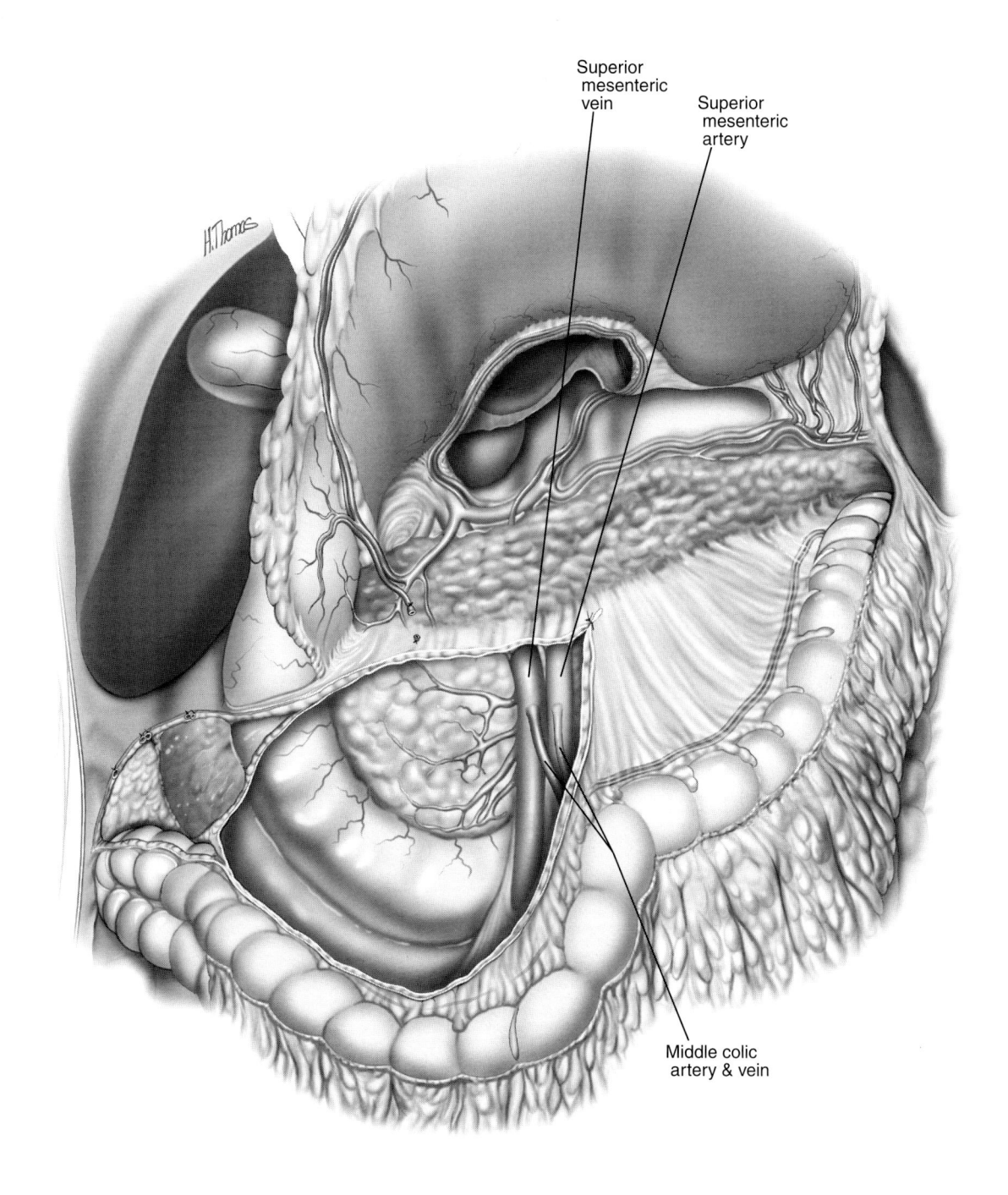

Figure 28–6 • By completing the mesenteric incision, the superior mesenteric artery and vein can be exposed and their course mobilized below the inferior border of the pancreas and above the fourth portion of the duodenum.

Pancreatectomy (Whipple Procedure) • 247

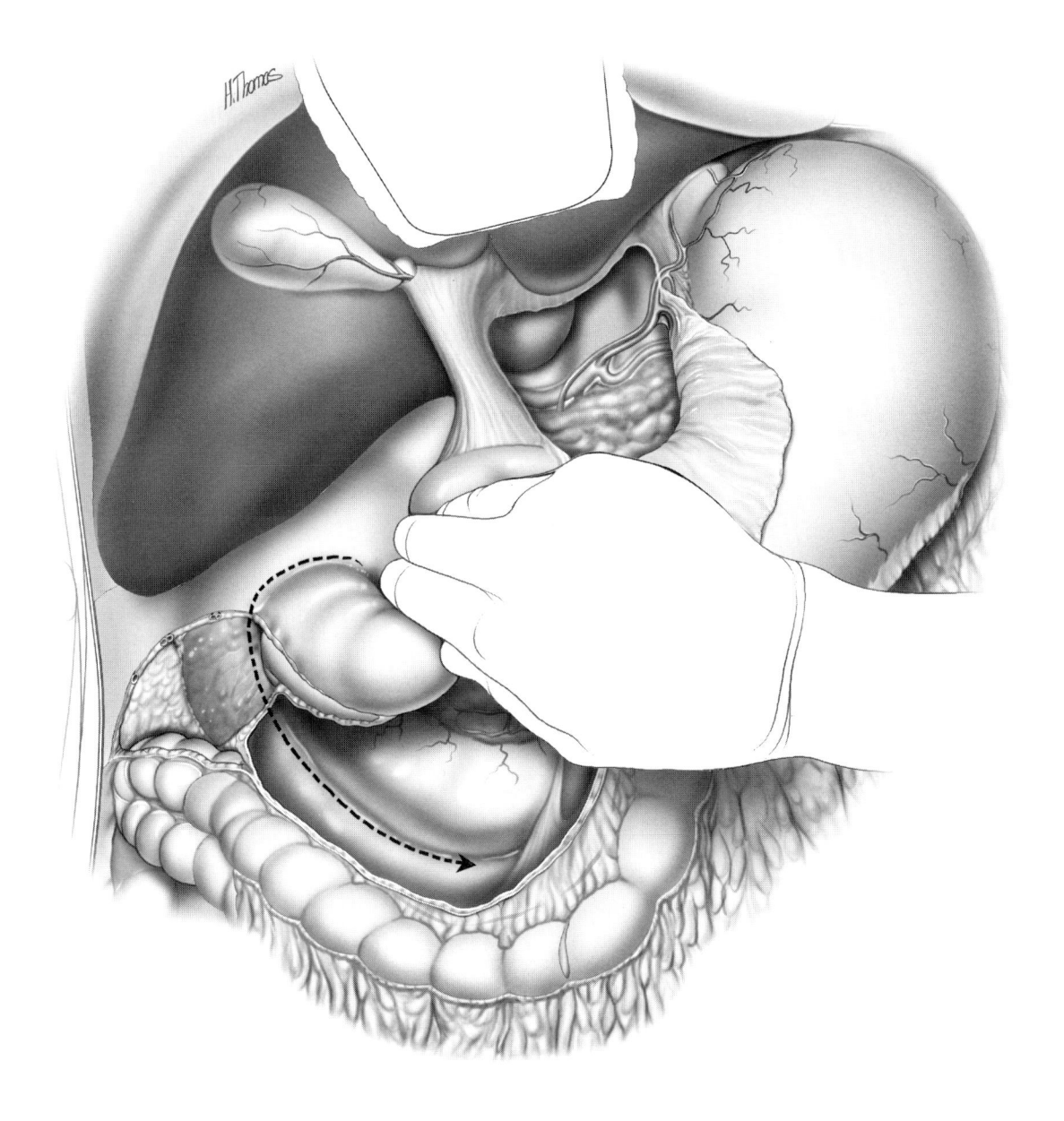

Figure 28-7 • The mesenteric attachments between the hepatic flexure and the liver are divided, and the duodenum is kocherized.

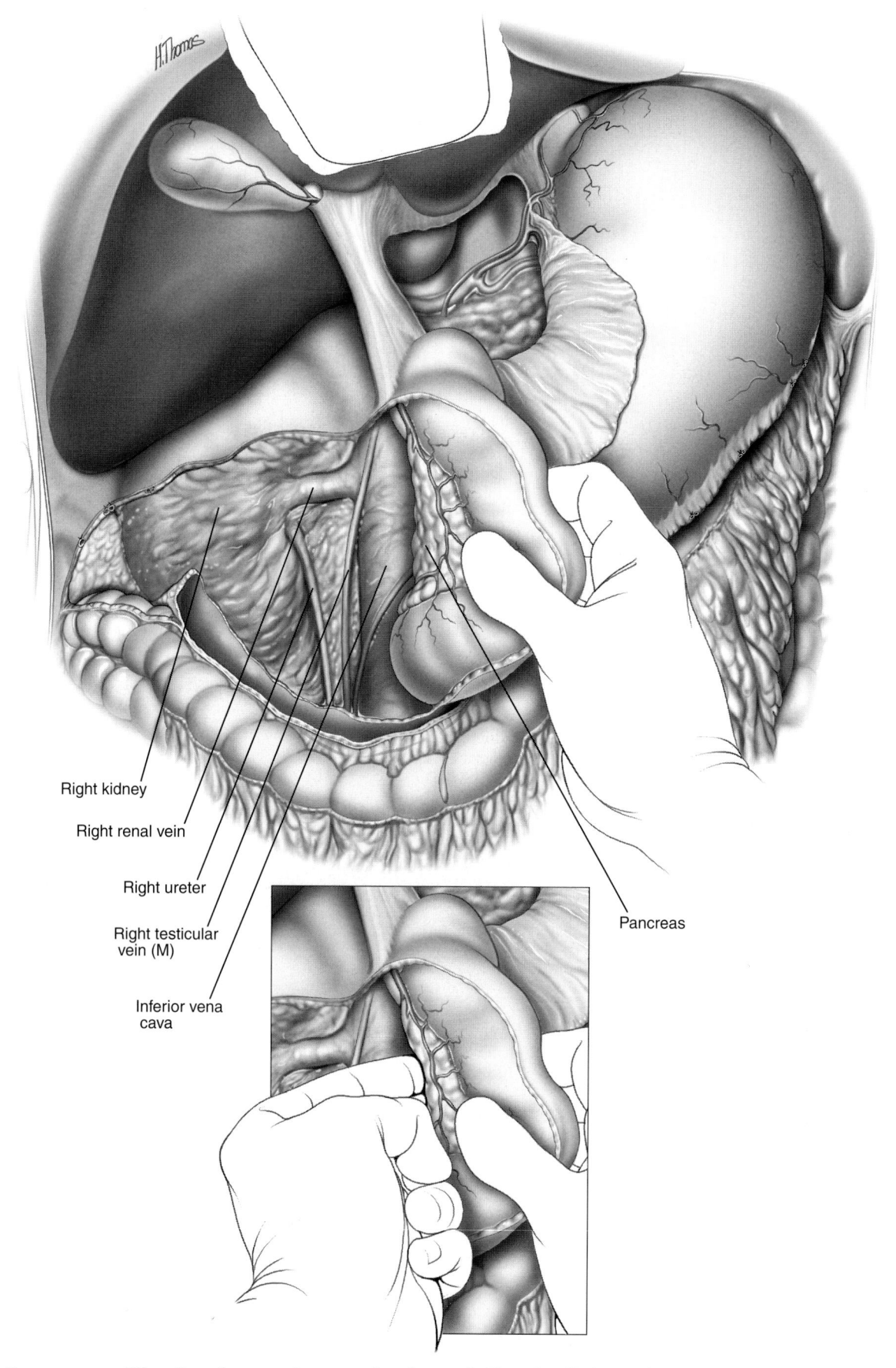

Figure 28–8 • The duodenum is completely mobilized off the inferior vena cava to assess the involvement of the portal vein.

Pancreatectomy (Whipple Procedure) • 249

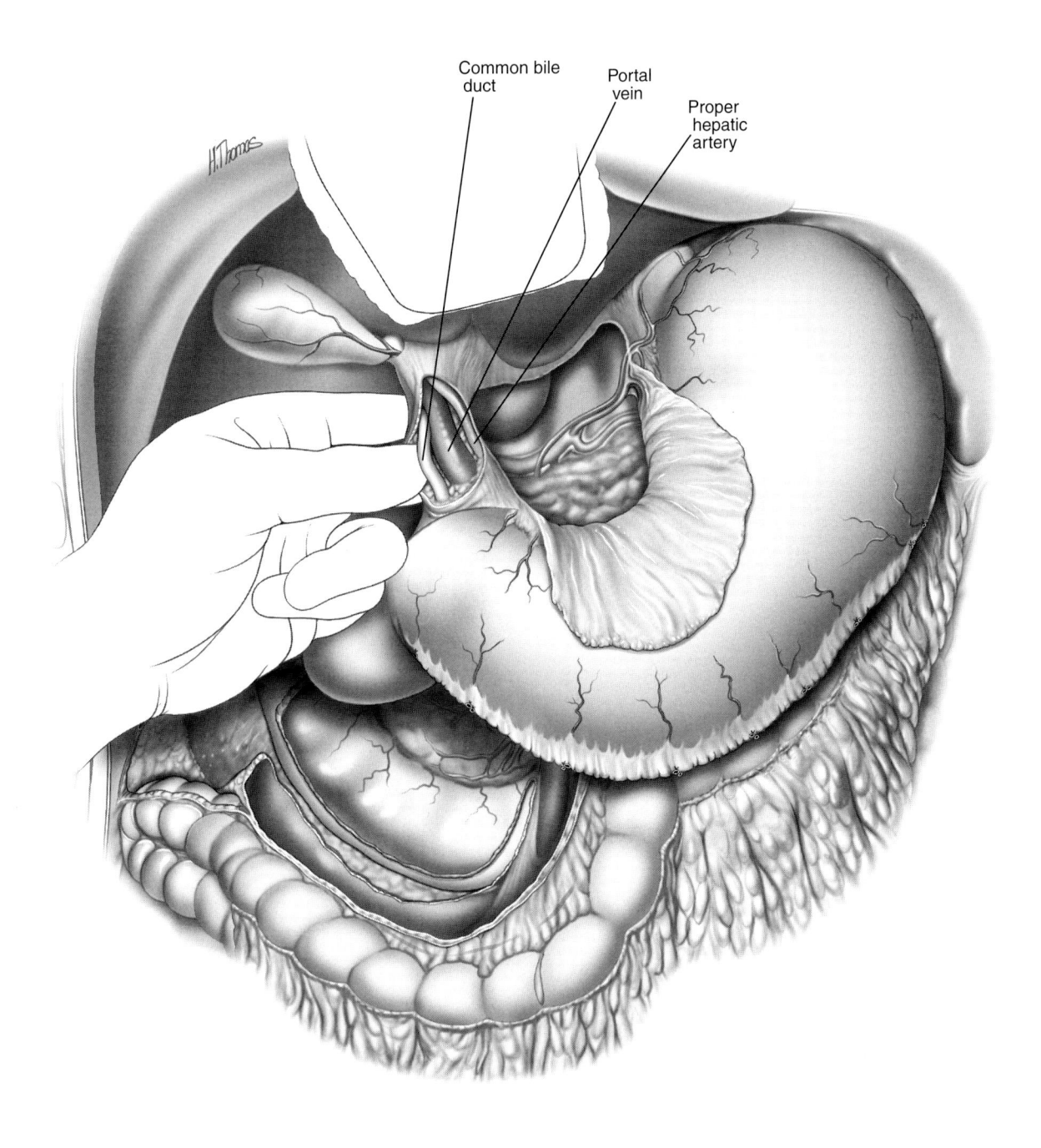

Figure 28-9 • The foramen of Winslow is assessed, and exposure of the portal vein, common bile duct, and hepatic artery is commenced. The structures of the portal triad are identified, and the mesentery along the lesser curvature is incised.

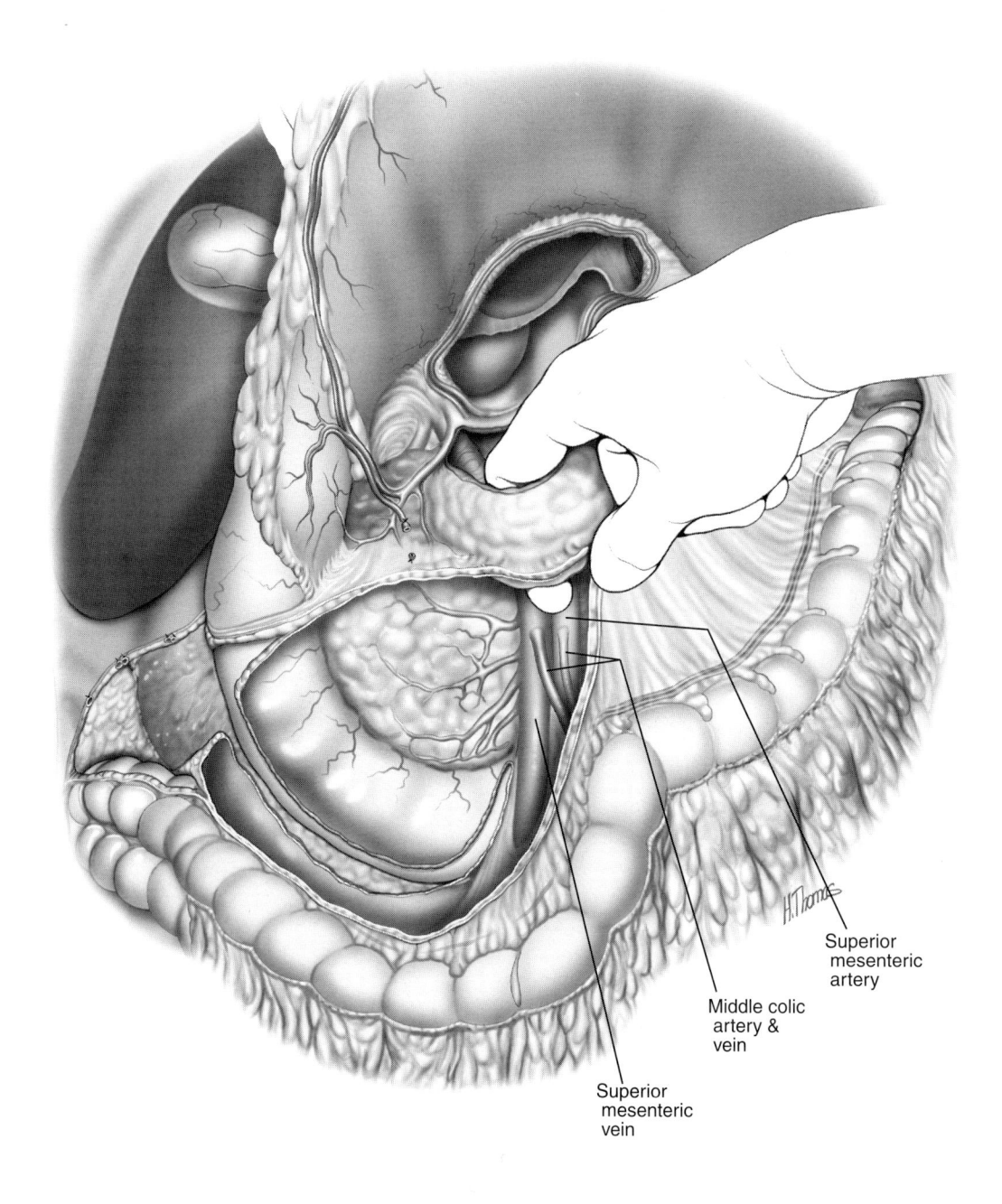

Figure 28–10 • The plane between the portal vein and the body of the pancreas is assessed.

Pancreatectomy (Whipple Procedure) • 251

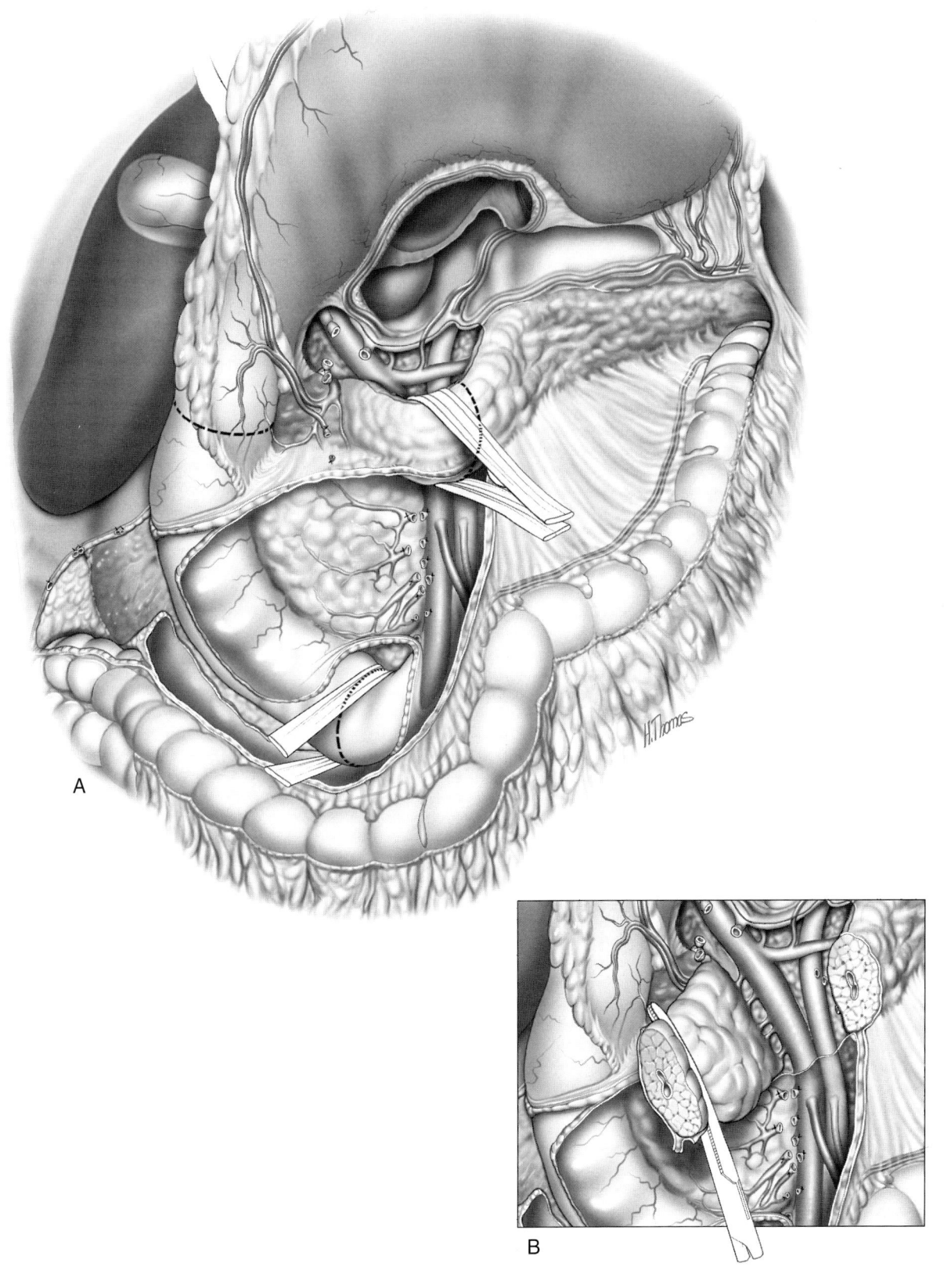

Figure 28–11 • **A,** Numerous branches to the uncinate process off the superior mesenteric vein are divided. The pancreaticoduodenal artery is divided, and the points of division of the duodenum are defined.
B, The body of the pancreas is divided.

252 • Part III UPPER ABDOMEN

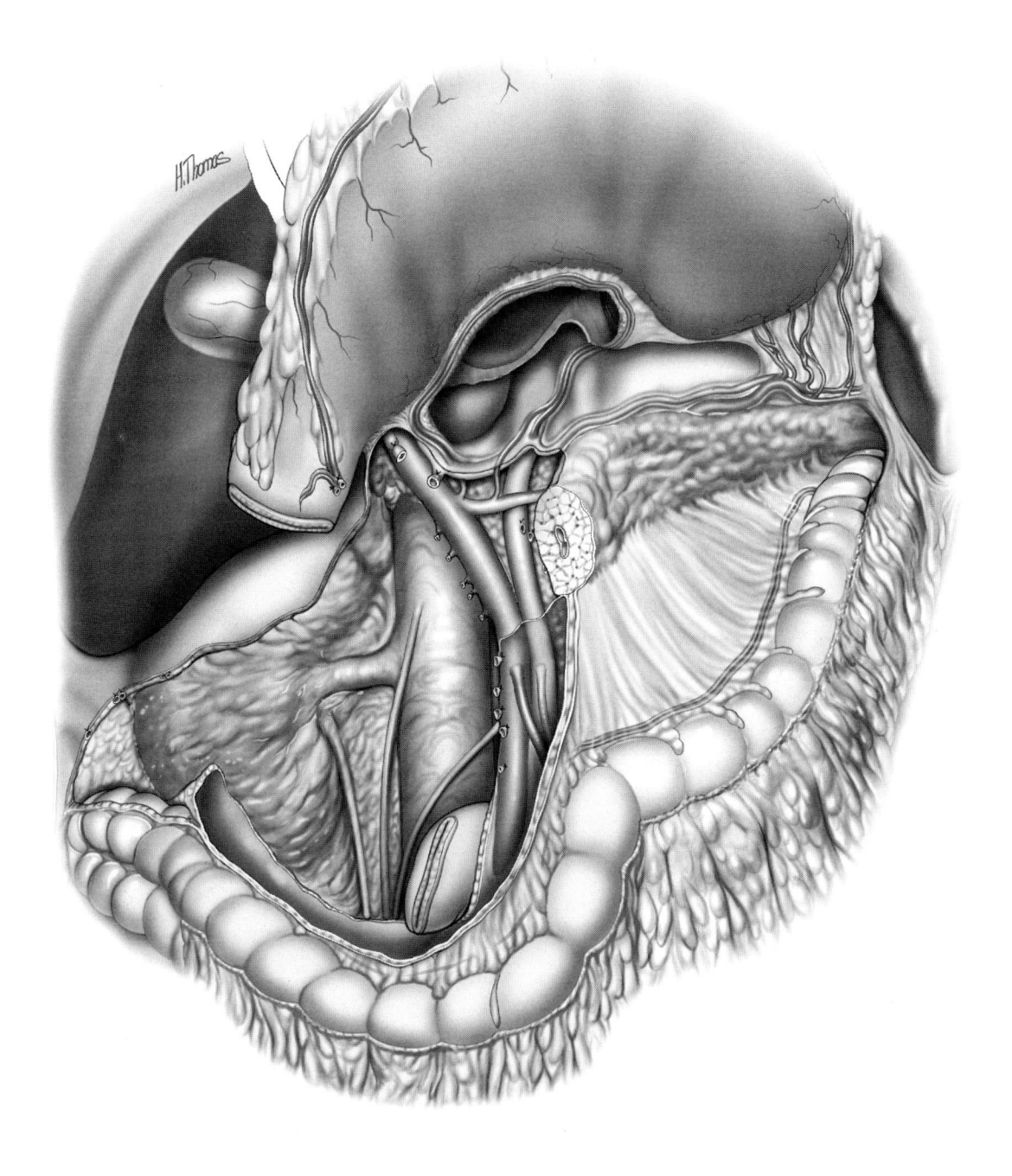

Figure 28-12 • The resected specimen with the resulting defect is illustrated. A pylorus-preserving procedure is depicted, but a distal gastric resection can be included easily.

Pancreatectomy (Whipple Procedure) • 253

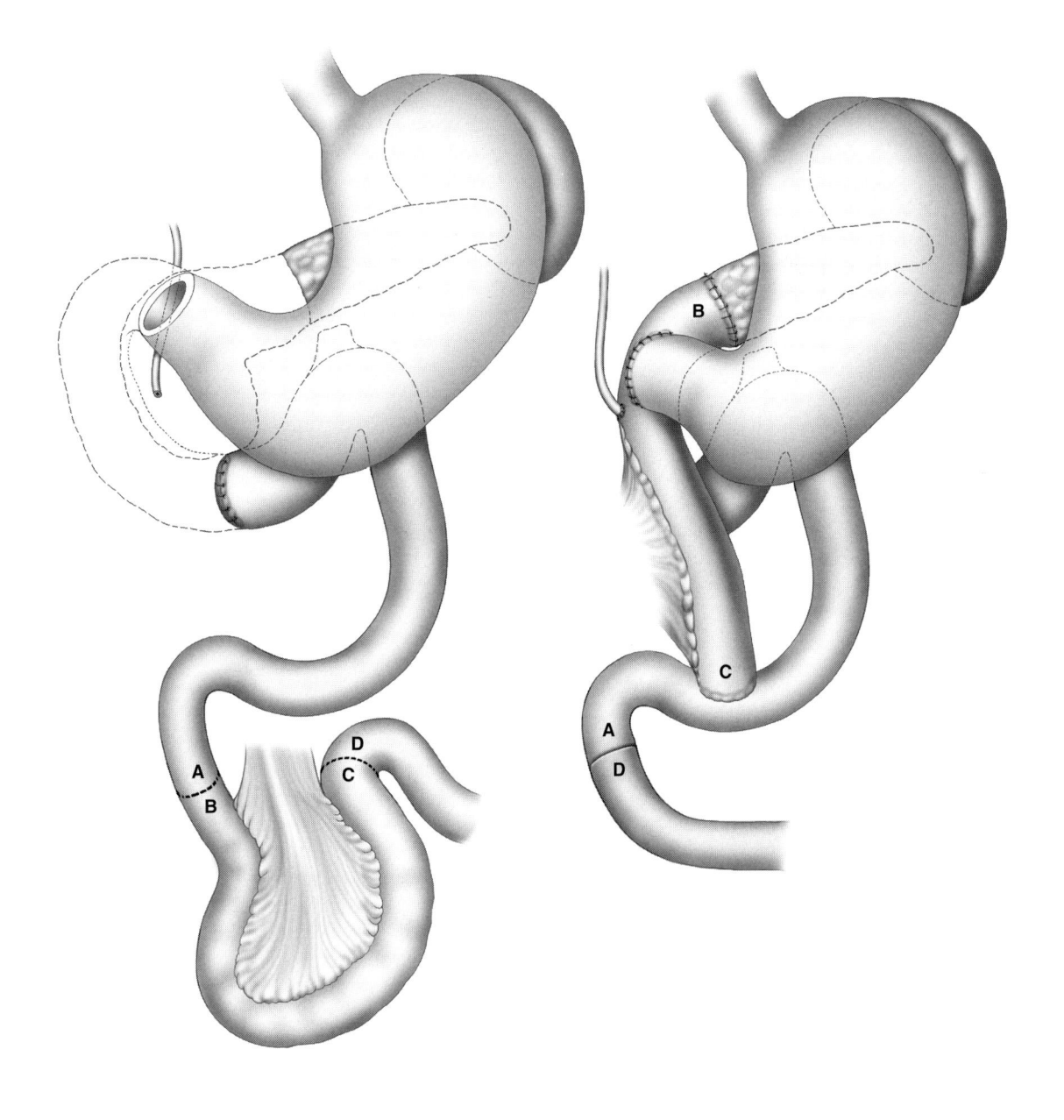

Figure 28-13 • A jejunal segment is utilized and a Roux-en-Y reconstruction is performed.

Chapter 29
Distal Pancreatectomy

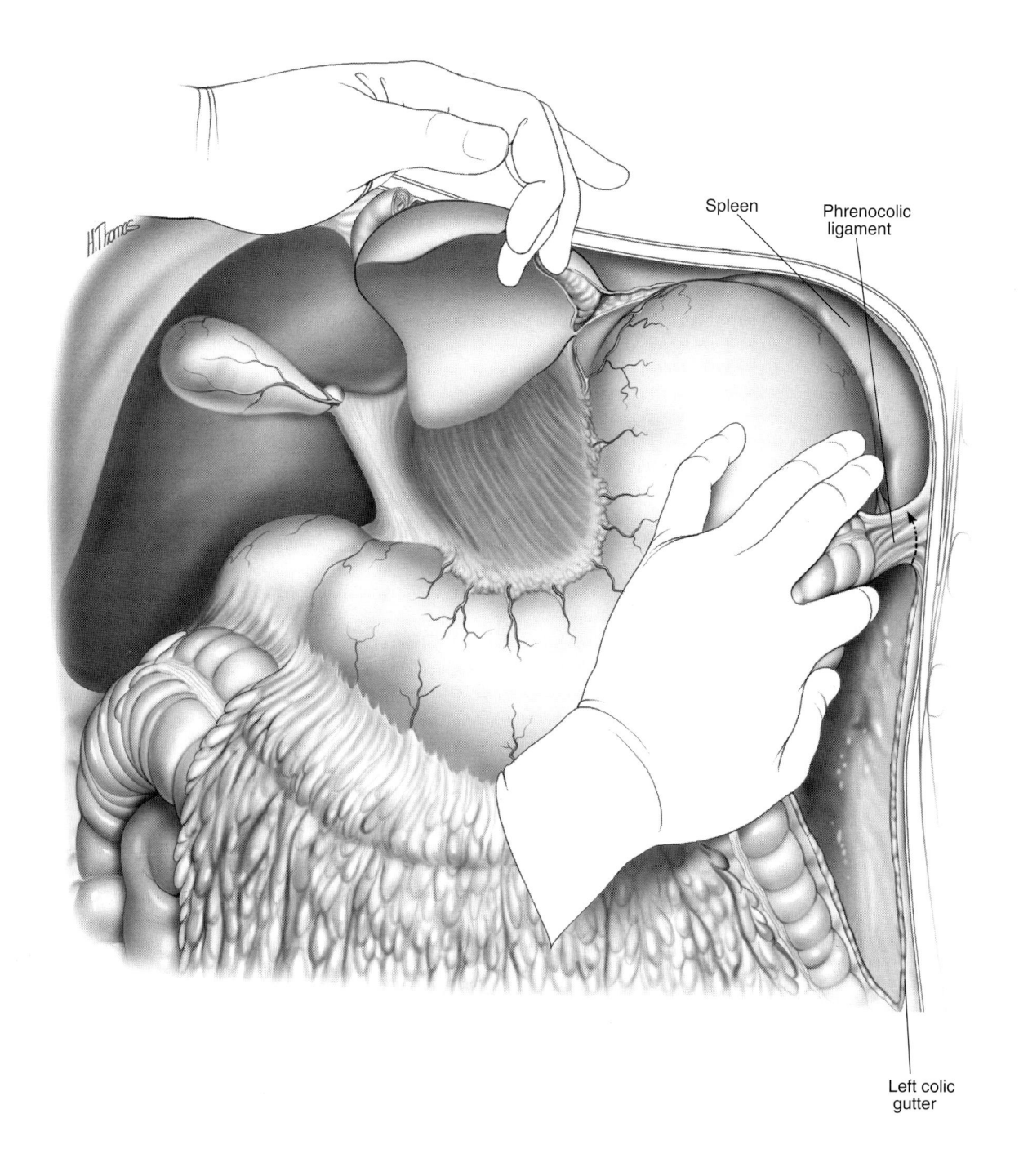

Figure 29–1 • Following a midline abdominal incision, the left colonic flexure is mobilized, the stomach and spleen are pulled medially, and the posterior splenic attachments are incised. The left triangular ligament is incised as well.

Distal Pancreatectomy • 255

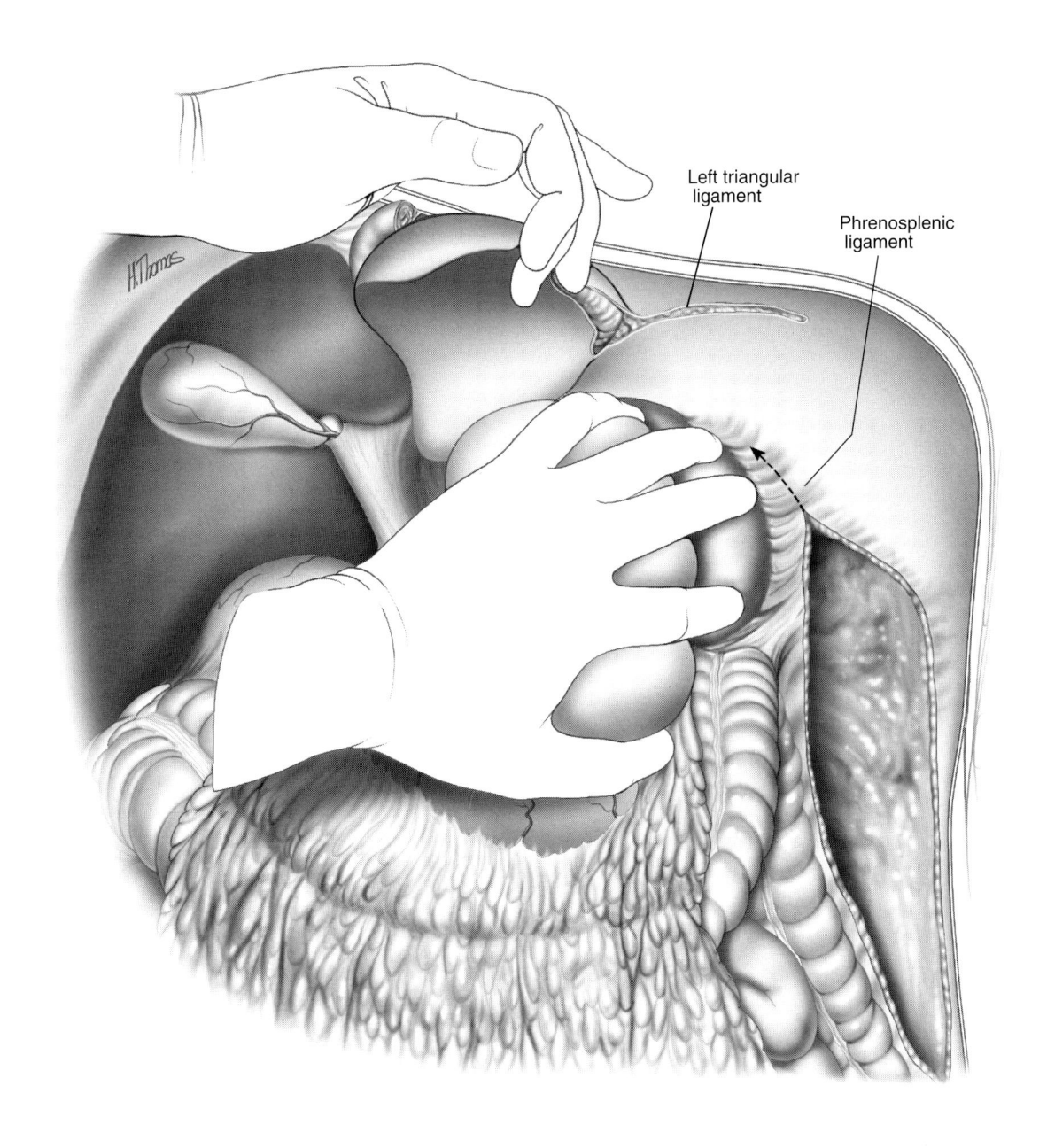

Figure 29–2 • The phrenosplenic ligament is divided in order to complete the mobilization of the spleen and tail of the pancreas.

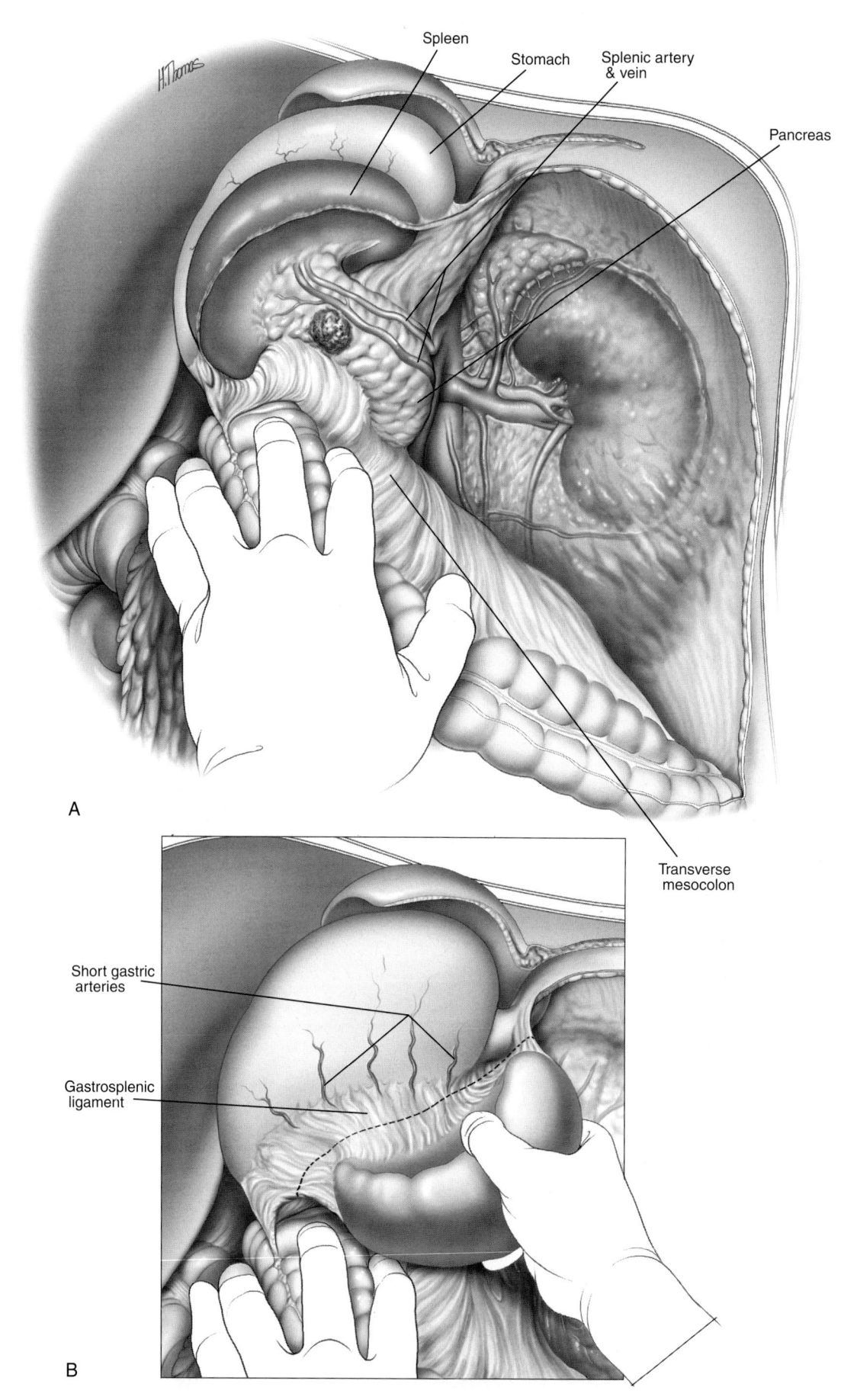

Figure 29–3 • **A**, The splenic attachments to the transverse colon are divided. **B**, The short gastrics are divided.

Distal Pancreatectomy • 257

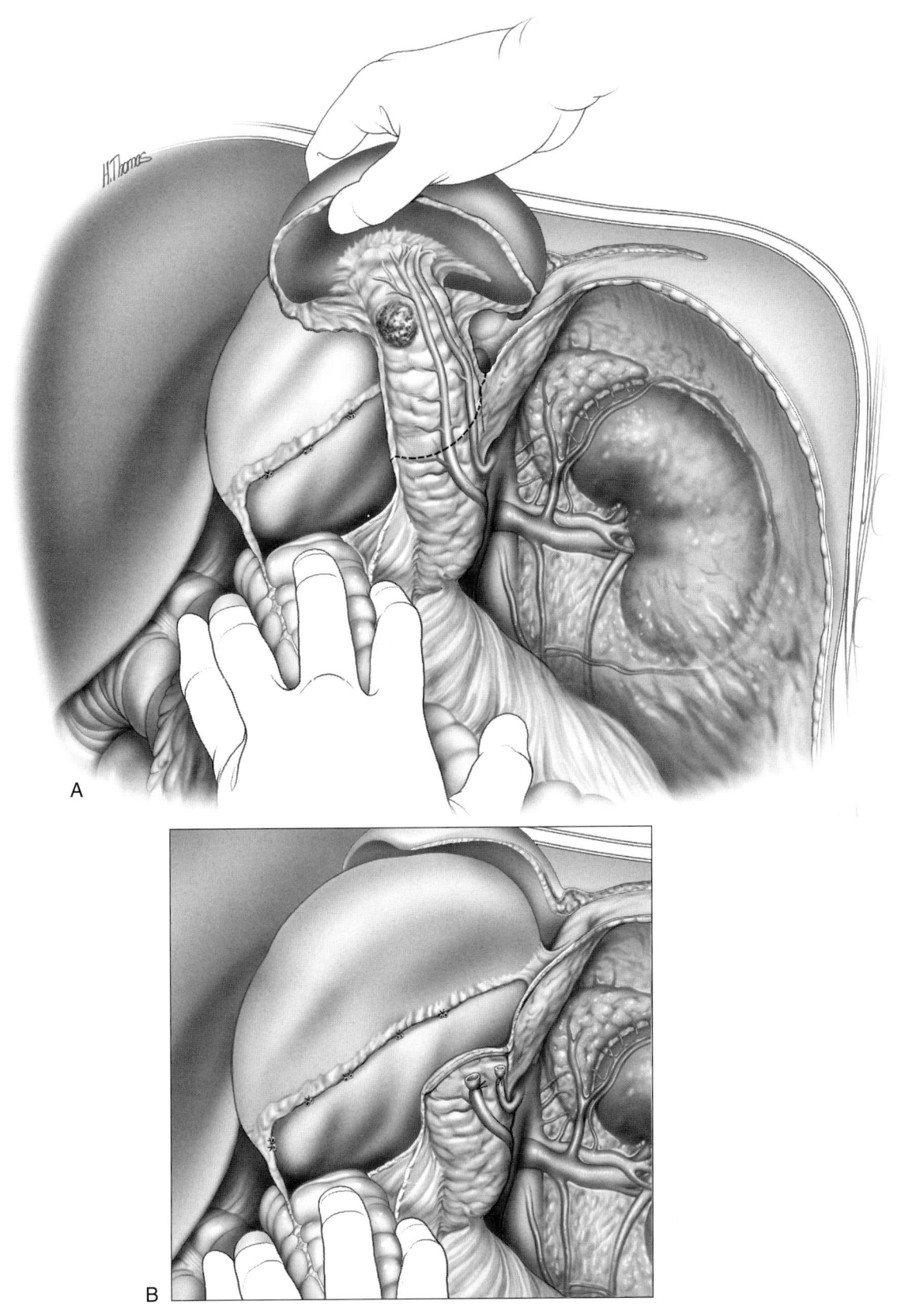

Figure 29–4 • **A,** The spleen and tail of the pancreas are elevated and reflected medially so that the splenic artery and vein can be identified.
 B, The pancreas is transected and the splenic artery and vein are ligated.

Chapter 30
Clinical Case: Regional Pancreatectomy for a Retroperitoneal Sarcoma

John Hoffman

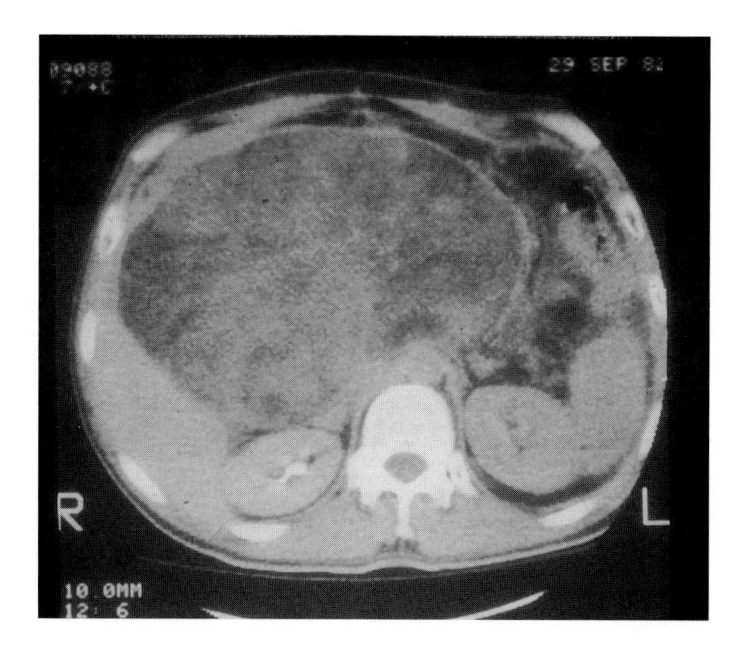

Figure 30–1 • A 56-year-old man presented for evaluation for resection of a large retroperitoneal sarcoma that was displacing the pancreas anteriorly and encasing the superior mesenteric artery. A resection of the tumor with a regional pancreatectomy was considered, but proximal control of the superior mesenteric artery had to be achieved by unconventional means.

Clinical Case: Regional Pancreatectomy for a Retroperitoneal Sarcoma • 259

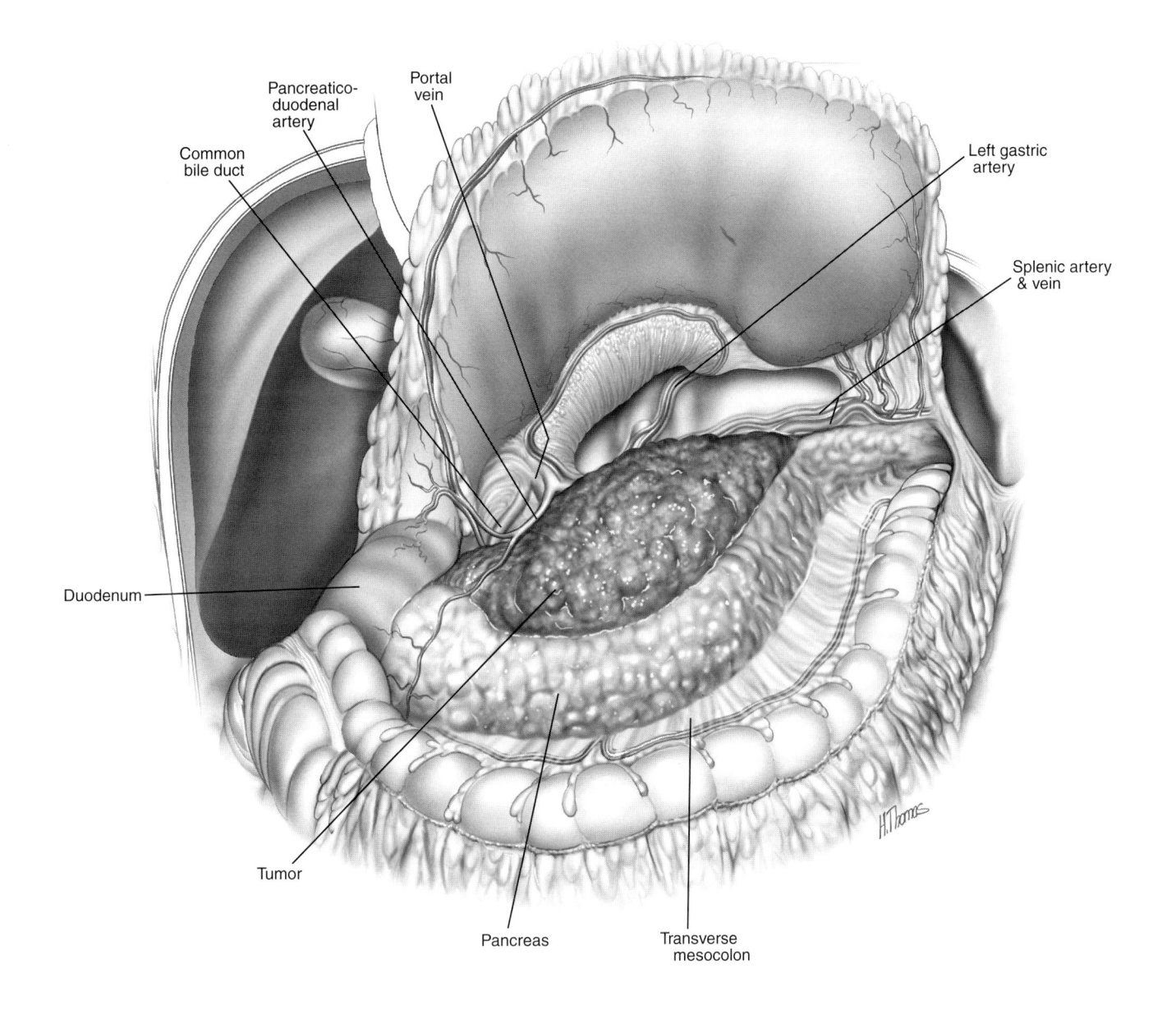

Figure 30–2 • Following a generous abdominal incision, the gastrocolic mesentery was divided and the stomach was elevated, exposing the tumor and the displaced pancreas.

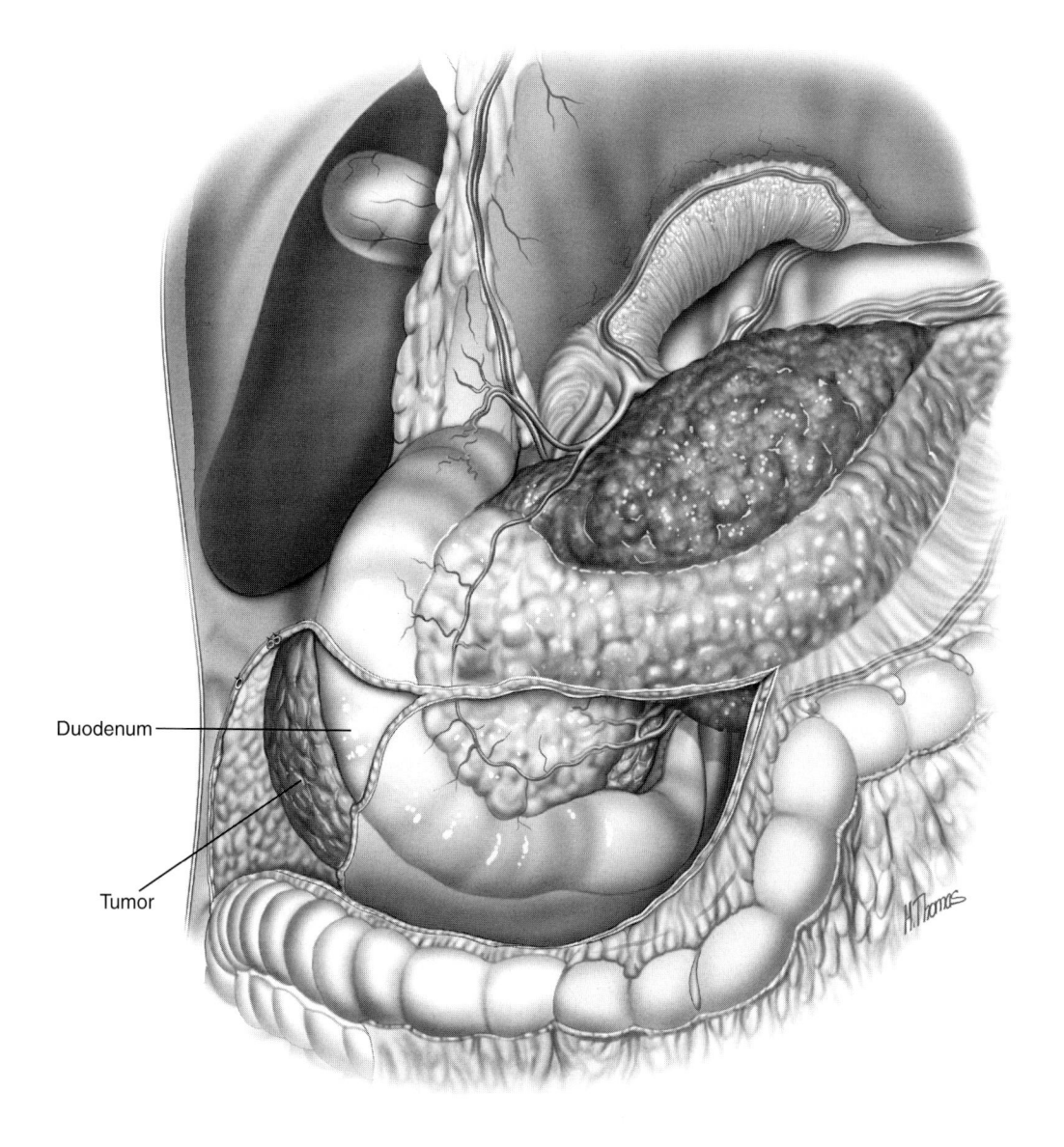

Figure 30–3 • The duodenum was kocherized and the mesentery of the colon was divided.

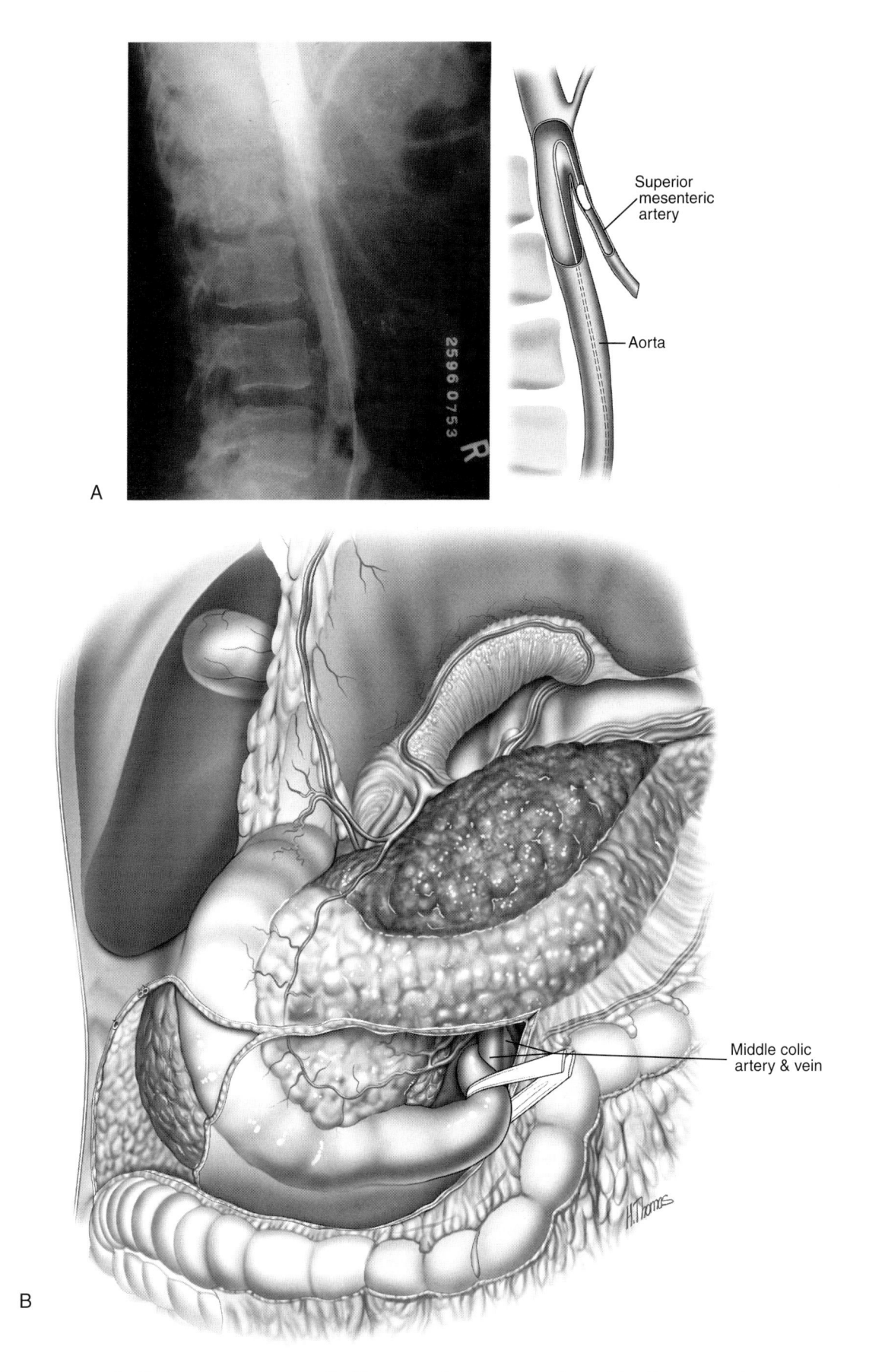

Figure 30–4 • **A,** Prior to surgery, a balloon catheter was placed in the superior mesenteric artery.

B, The fourth portion of the duodenum was mobilized, and the middle colic artery and vein were identified distal to the tumor mass.

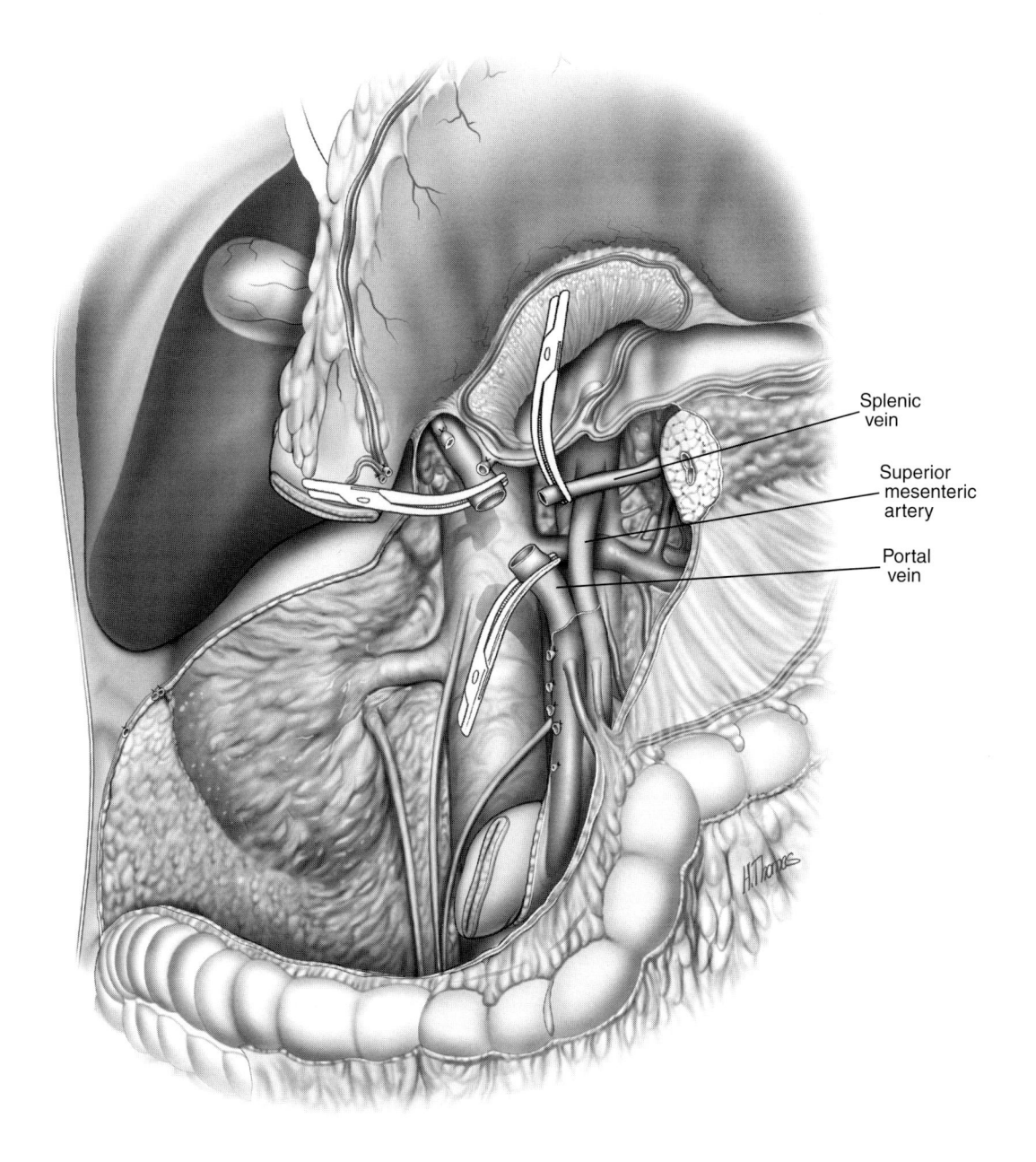

Figure 30–5 • The pancreatectomy was accomplished, with resection of a segment of the portal vein and preservation of the superior mesenteric artery.

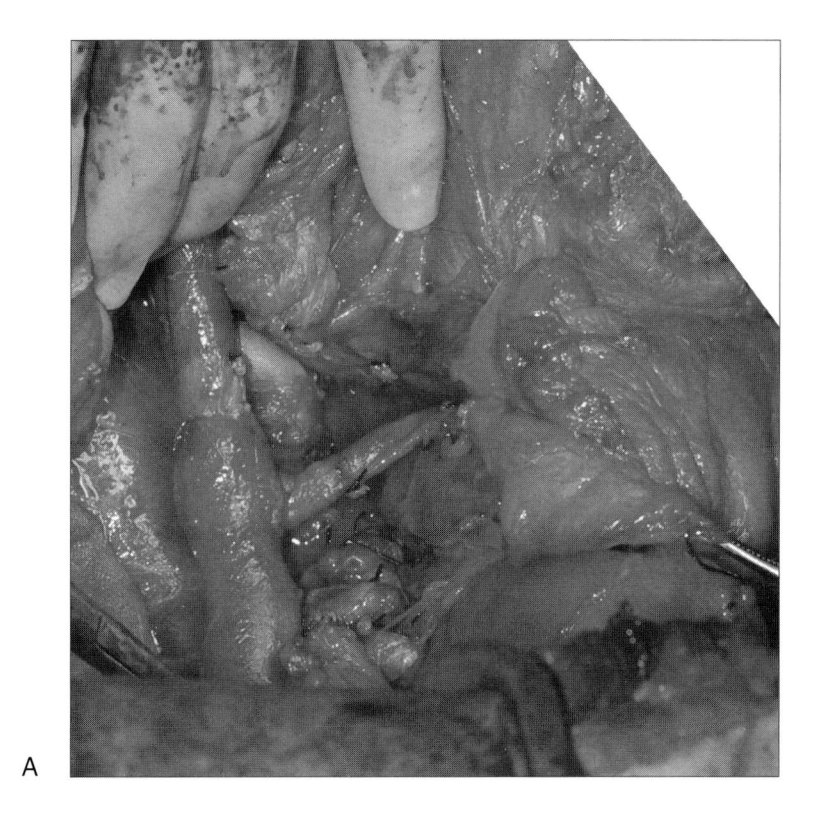

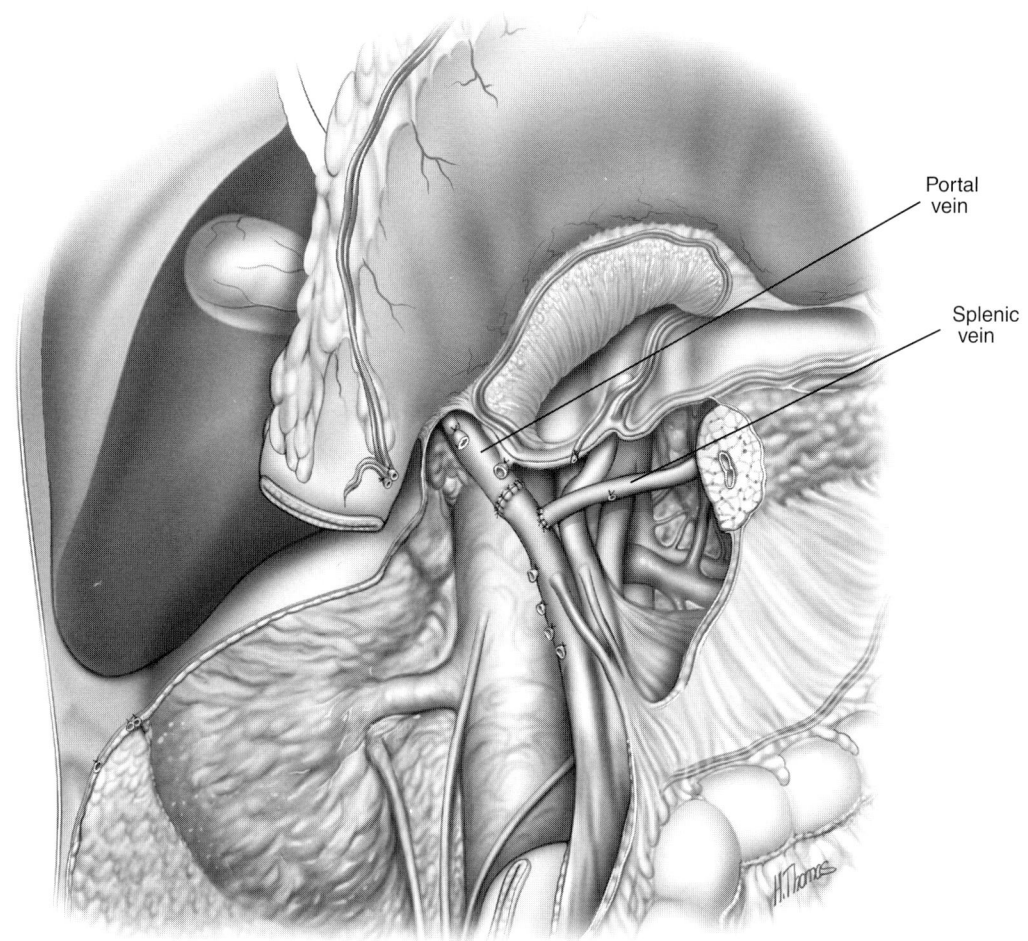

Figure 30–6 • **A,** The portal and splenic vein reanastomoses are depicted. **B,** A pylorus-preserving resection was performed, and the appropriate anastomoses were created.

Chapter 31
Right Adrenalectomy

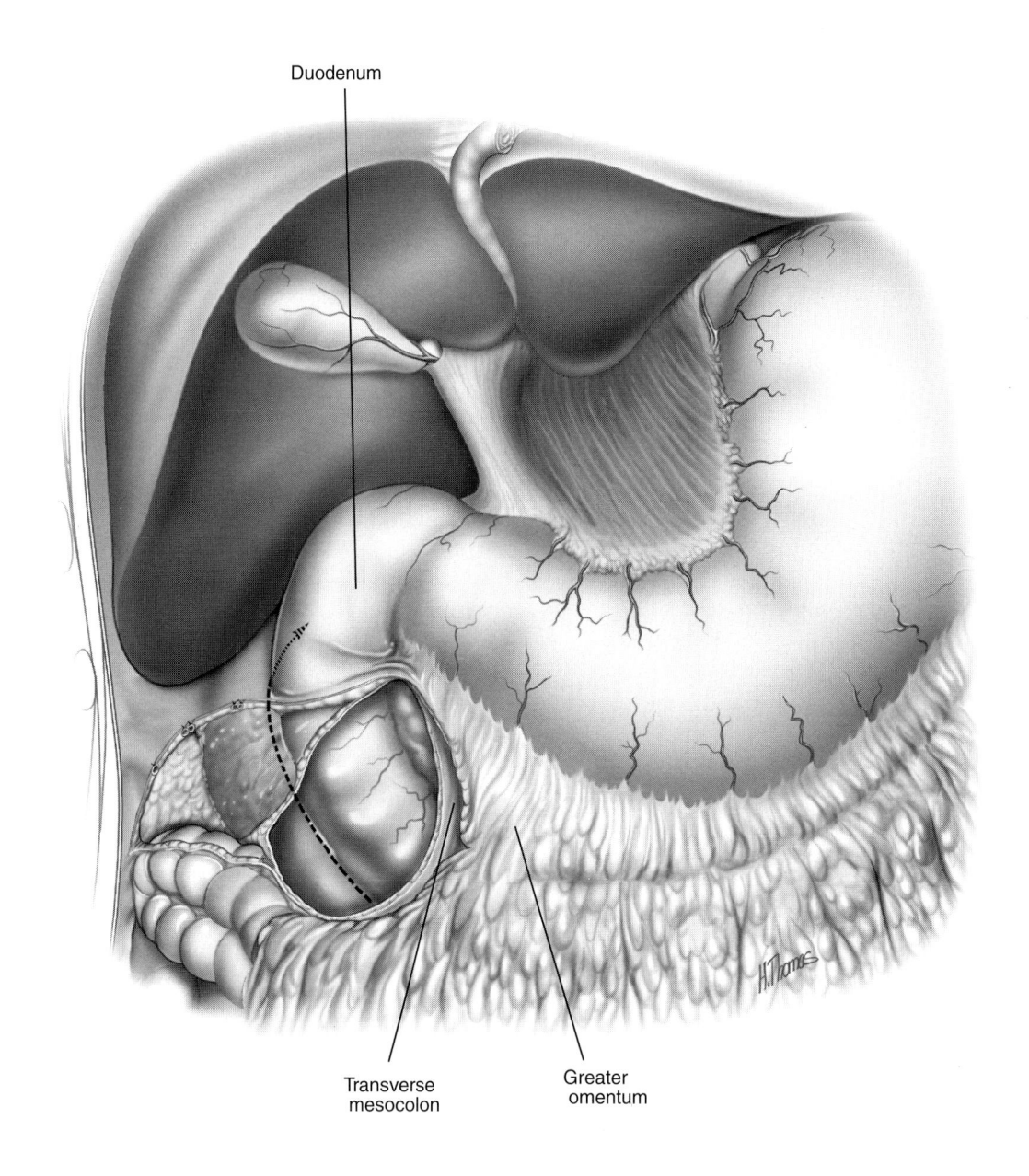

Figure 31–1 • Following an abdominal incision, the hepatic flexure is mobilized and the duodenum is kocherized.

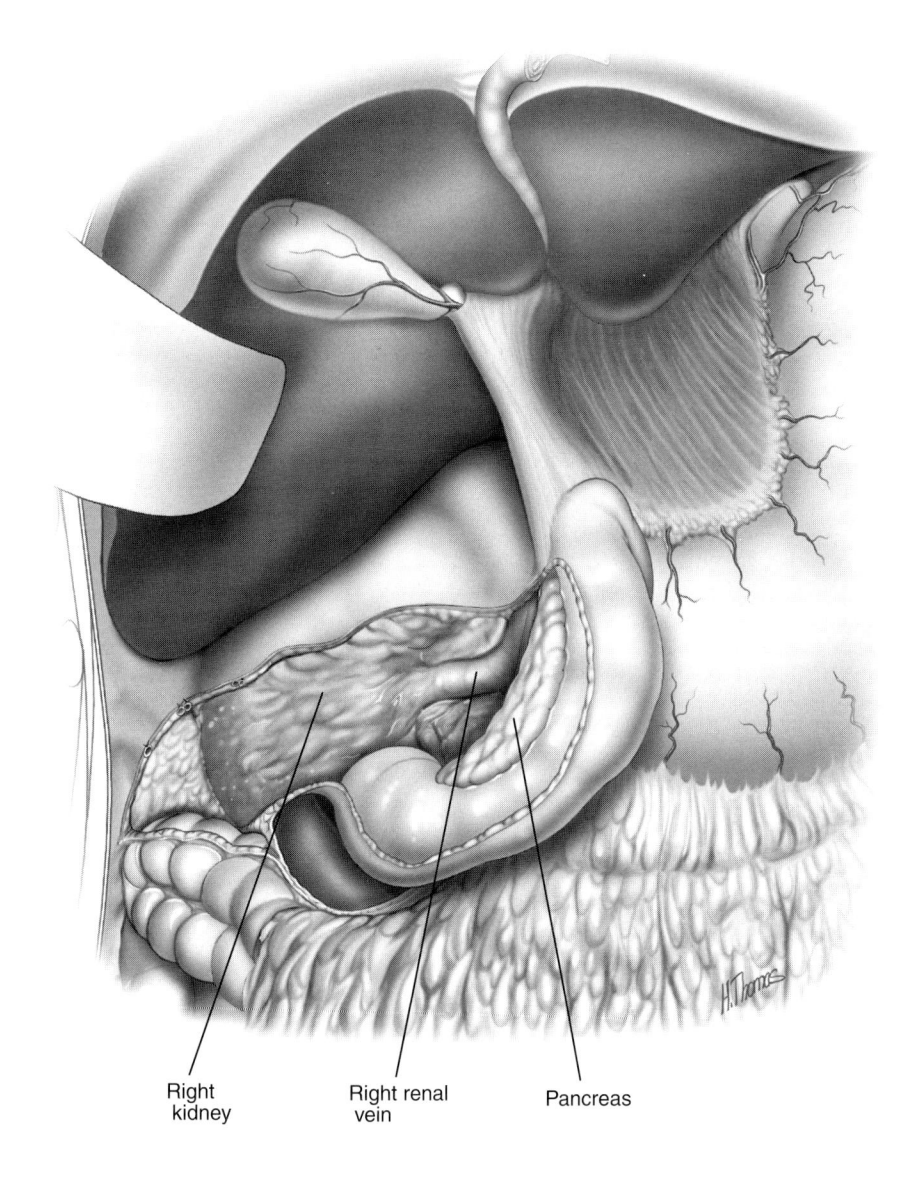

Figure 31–2 • The liver is retracted superiorly and the kidney is identified in Gerota's fascia. The inferior vena cava is identified medially.

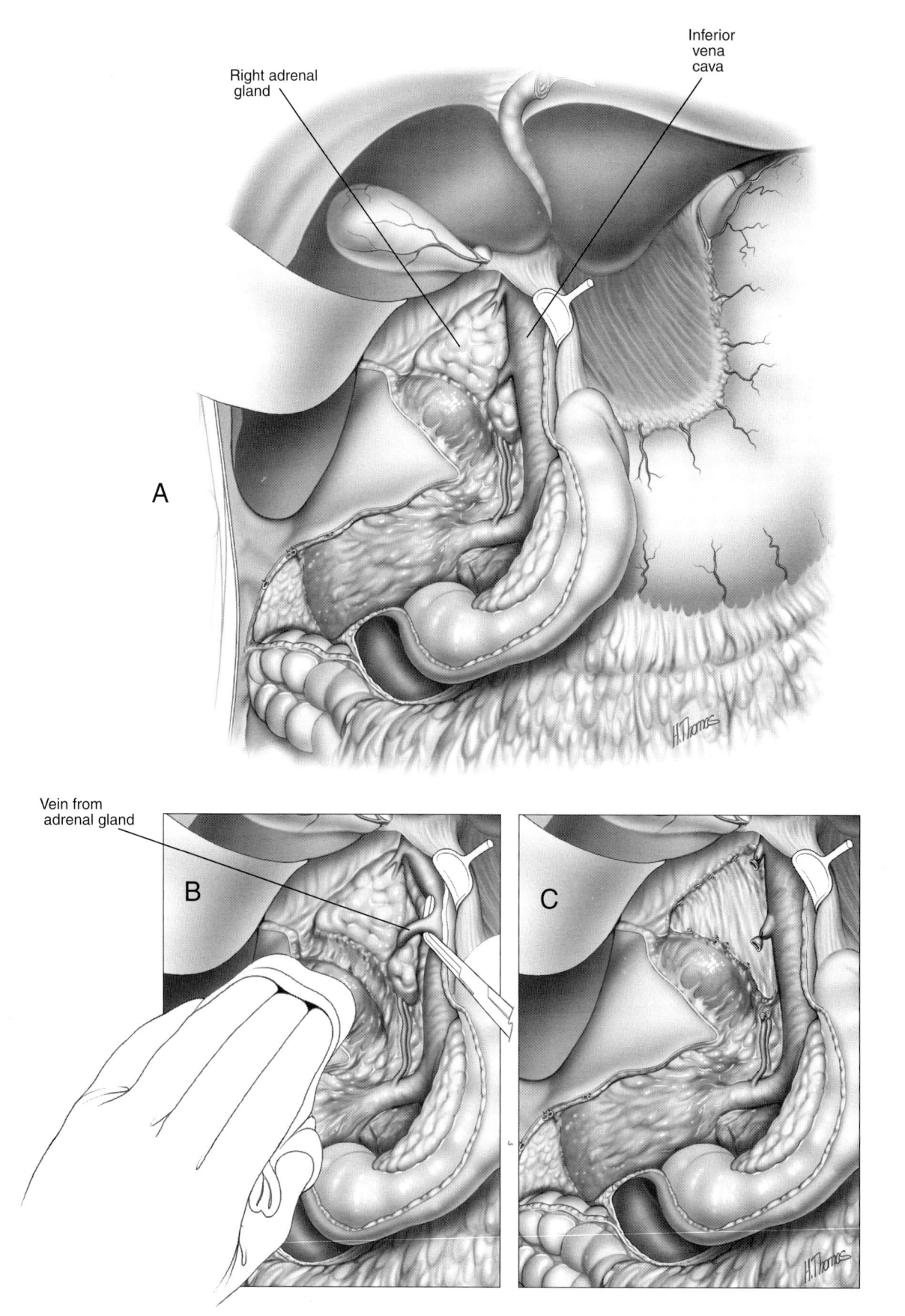

Figure 31–3 • **A,** The kidney is distracted inferiorly and the adrenal gland is visualized.
B, The adrenal vein is ligated.
C, Additional branches lateral to the vena cava off the renal vein and superior to the adrenal vein are ligated with clips and divided. The right adrenal gland is removed.

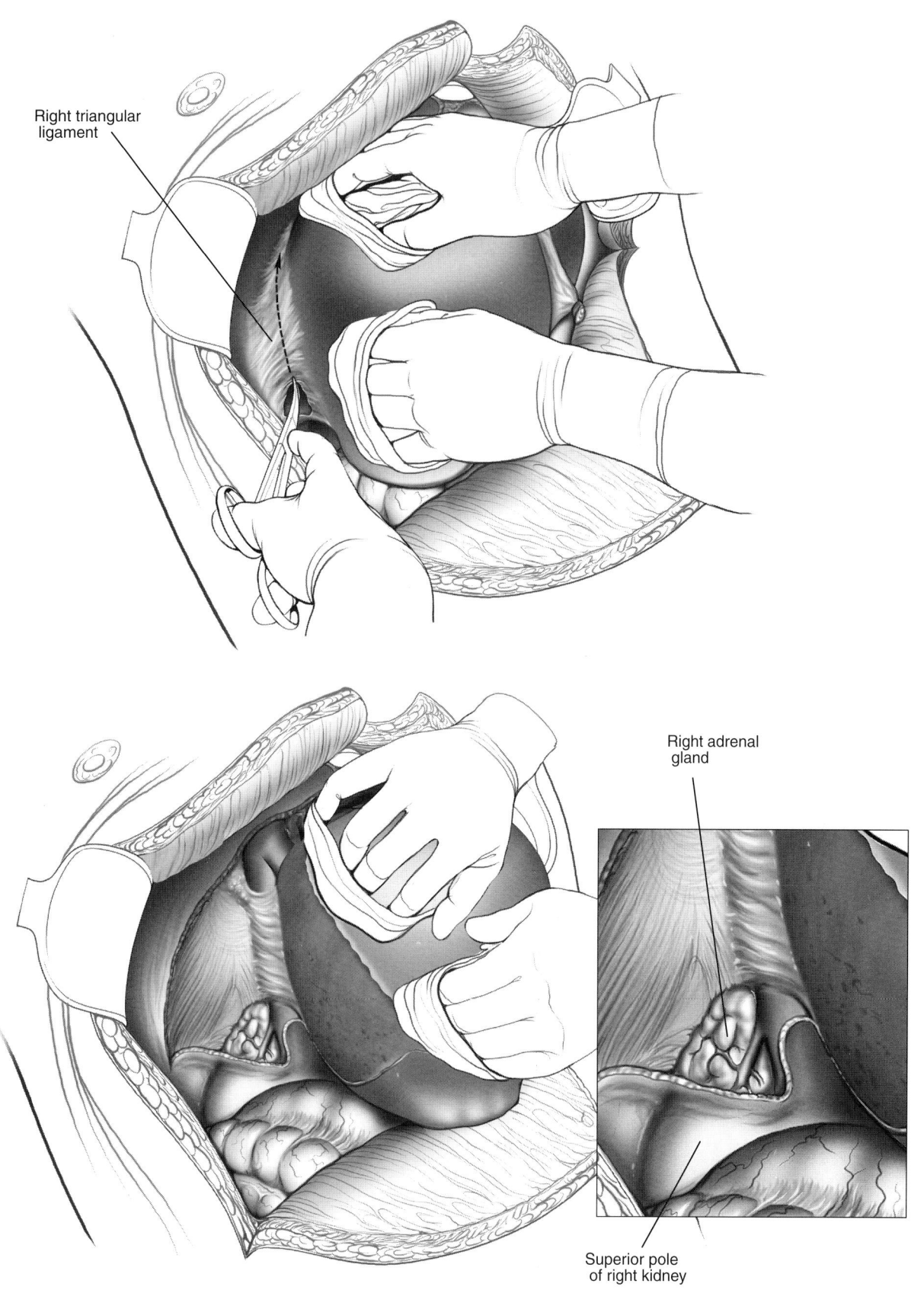

Figure 31–4 • An alternative exposure to the right adrenal gland involves complete mobilization of the right lobe of the liver. This is illustrated in greater detail in the description of a right hepatic lobectomy.

Chapter 32
Left Adrenalectomy

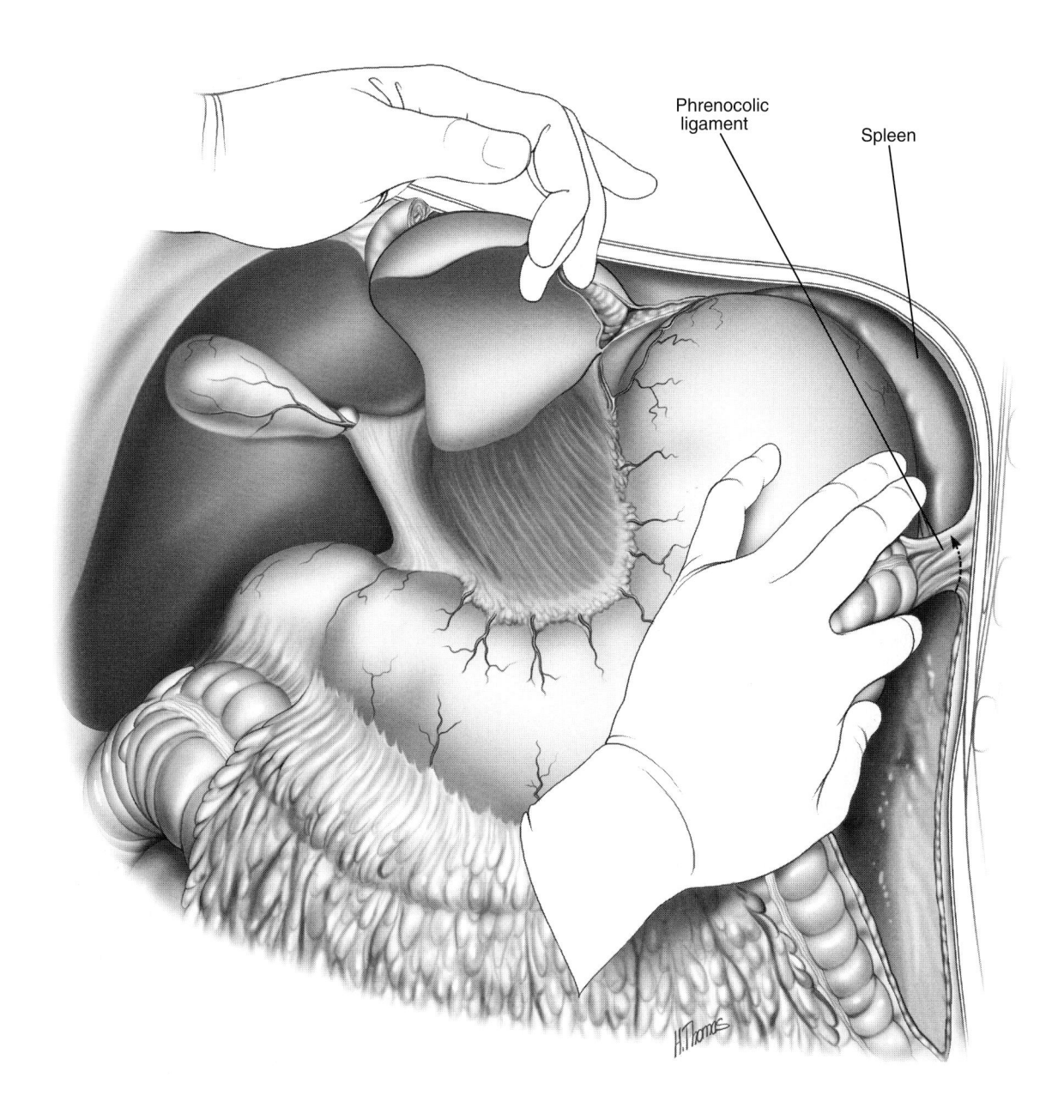

Figure 32–1 • Following a midline abdominal incision, the left colonic flexure is mobilized, the stomach and spleen are pulled medially, and the posterior splenic attachments are incised. The left triangular ligament is incised as well.

Left Adrenalectomy • 269

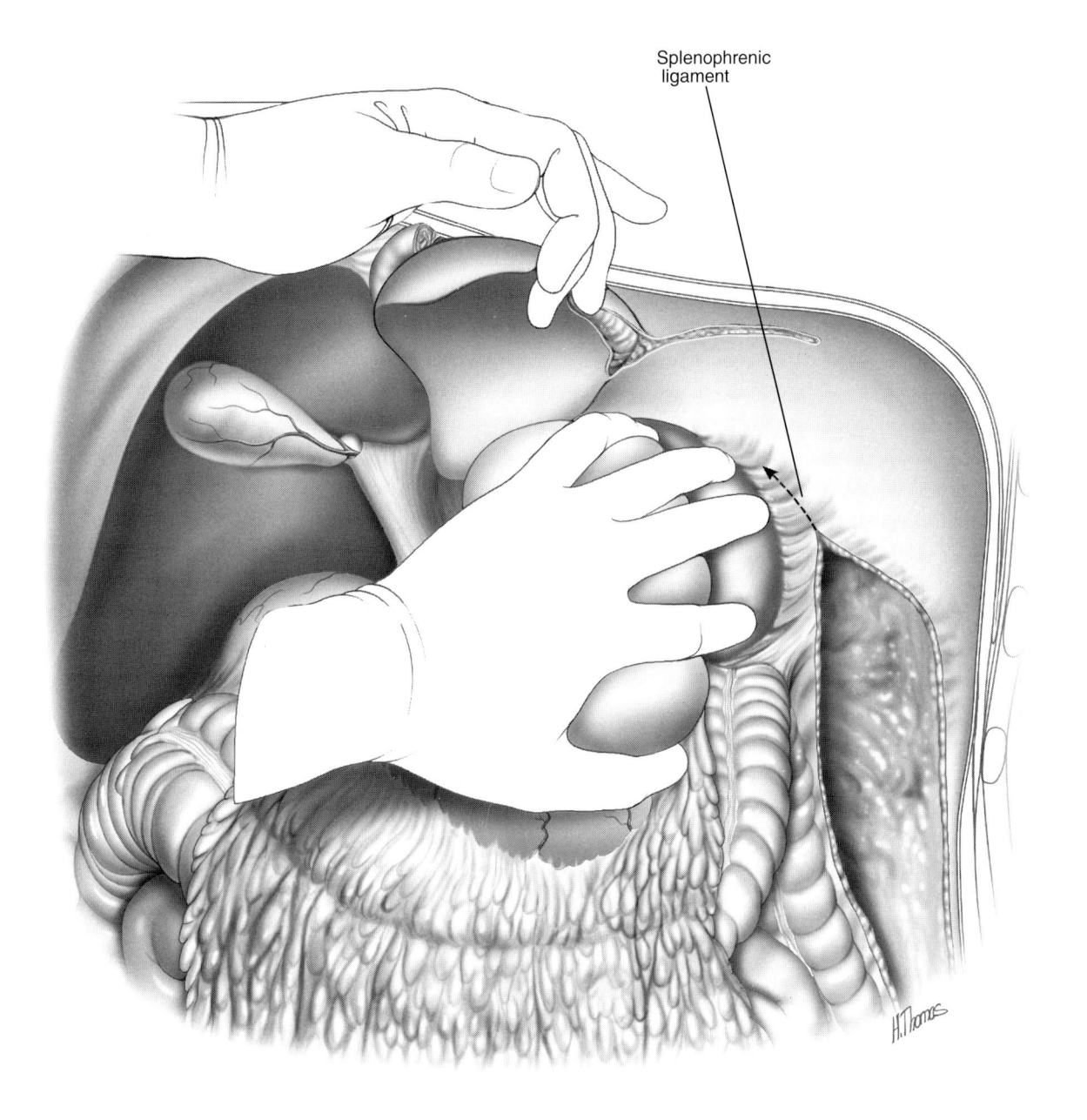

Figure 32–2 • The splenophrenic ligament is divided to expose the left kidney.

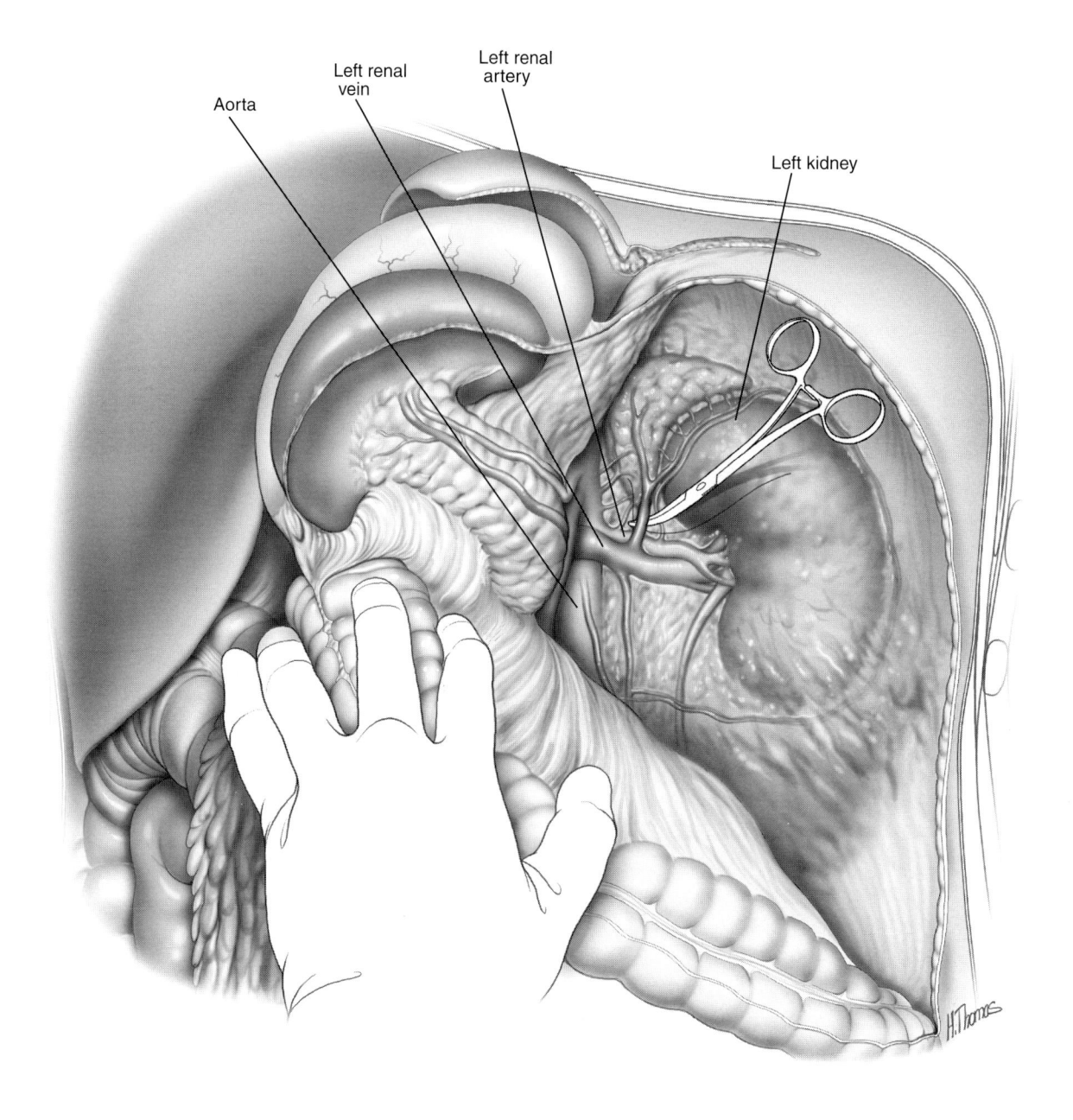

Figure 32–3 • Following complete mobilization of the spleen, pancreas, stomach, and colon, the renal vessels are identified. The adrenal vein is exposed at its point of entry into the renal vein.

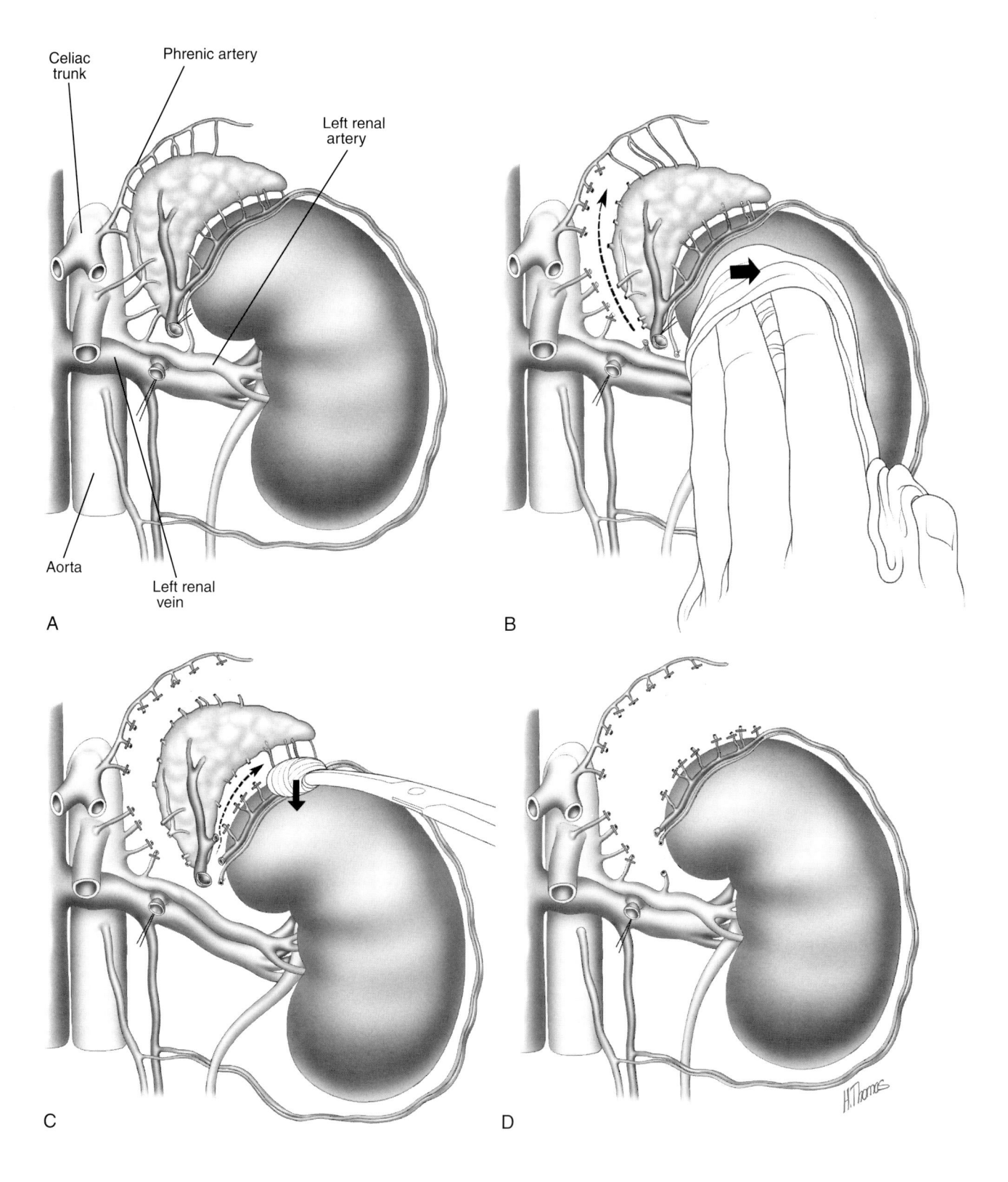

Figure 32–4 • **A,** The adrenal vein is ligated and divided.
B, All medial attachments are clipped and divided.
C, Small vessels off the phrenic artery are divided, and the adrenal gland is separated off the superior pole of the kidney.
D, The adrenalectomy is completed.

Part IV

LOWER ABDOMEN

Chapter 33
Surgical Anatomy of the Abdomen

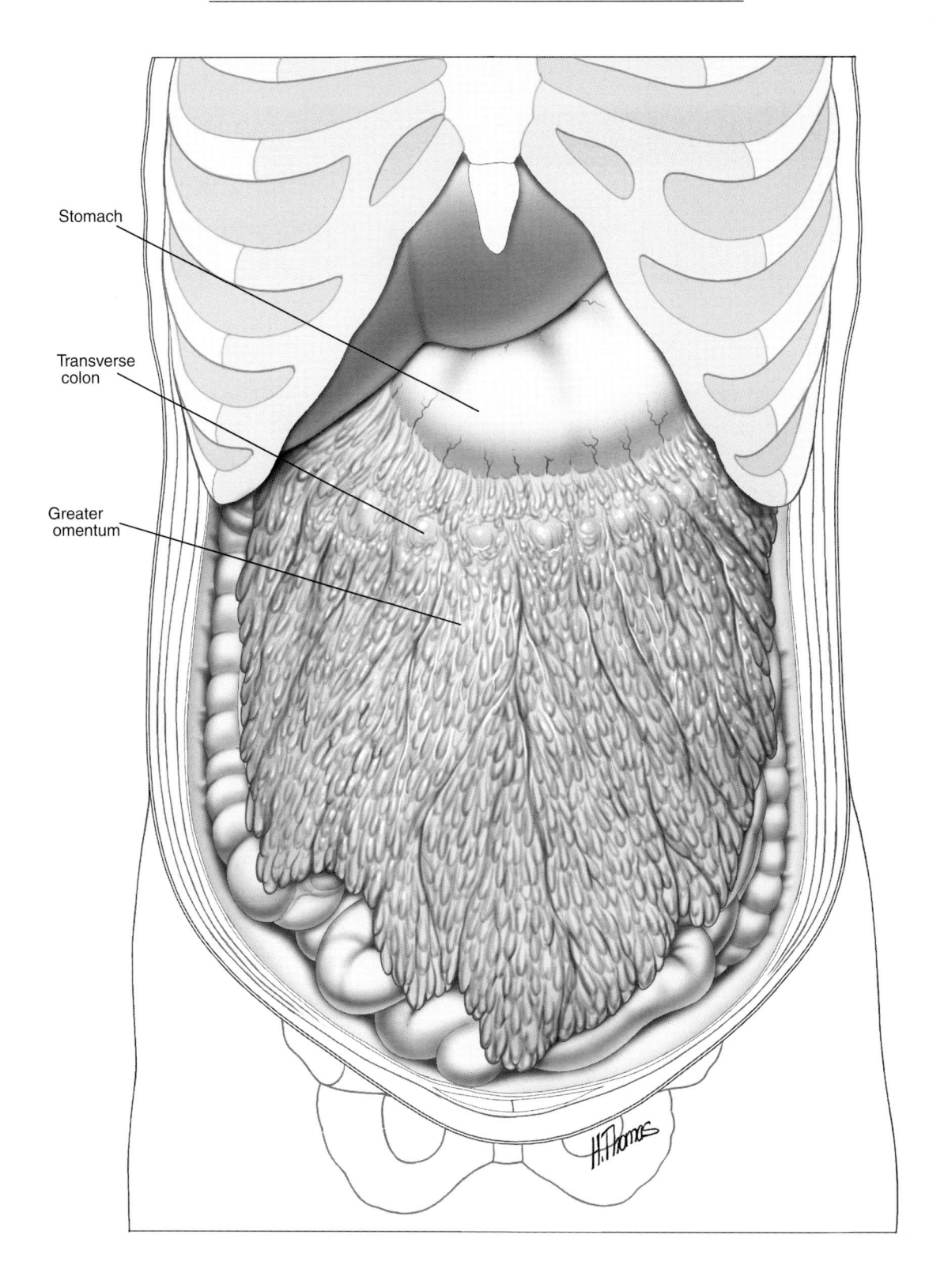

Figure 33–1 • This view of the open abdomen shows the greater omentum attached to the transverse colon and the greater curvature of the stomach.

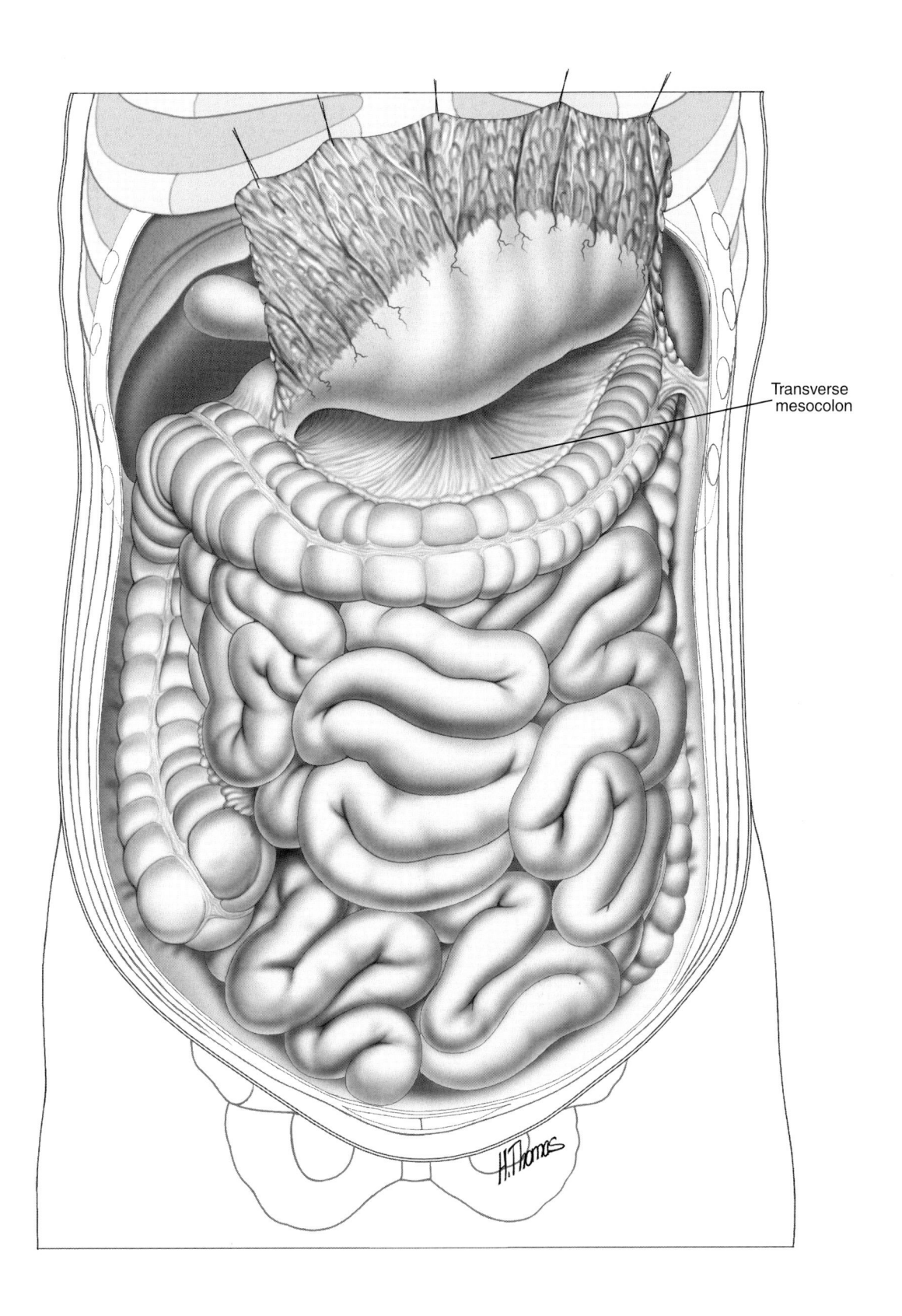

Figure 33–2 • With the greater omentum elevated, the lesser sac is opened and the abdominal viscera are seen.

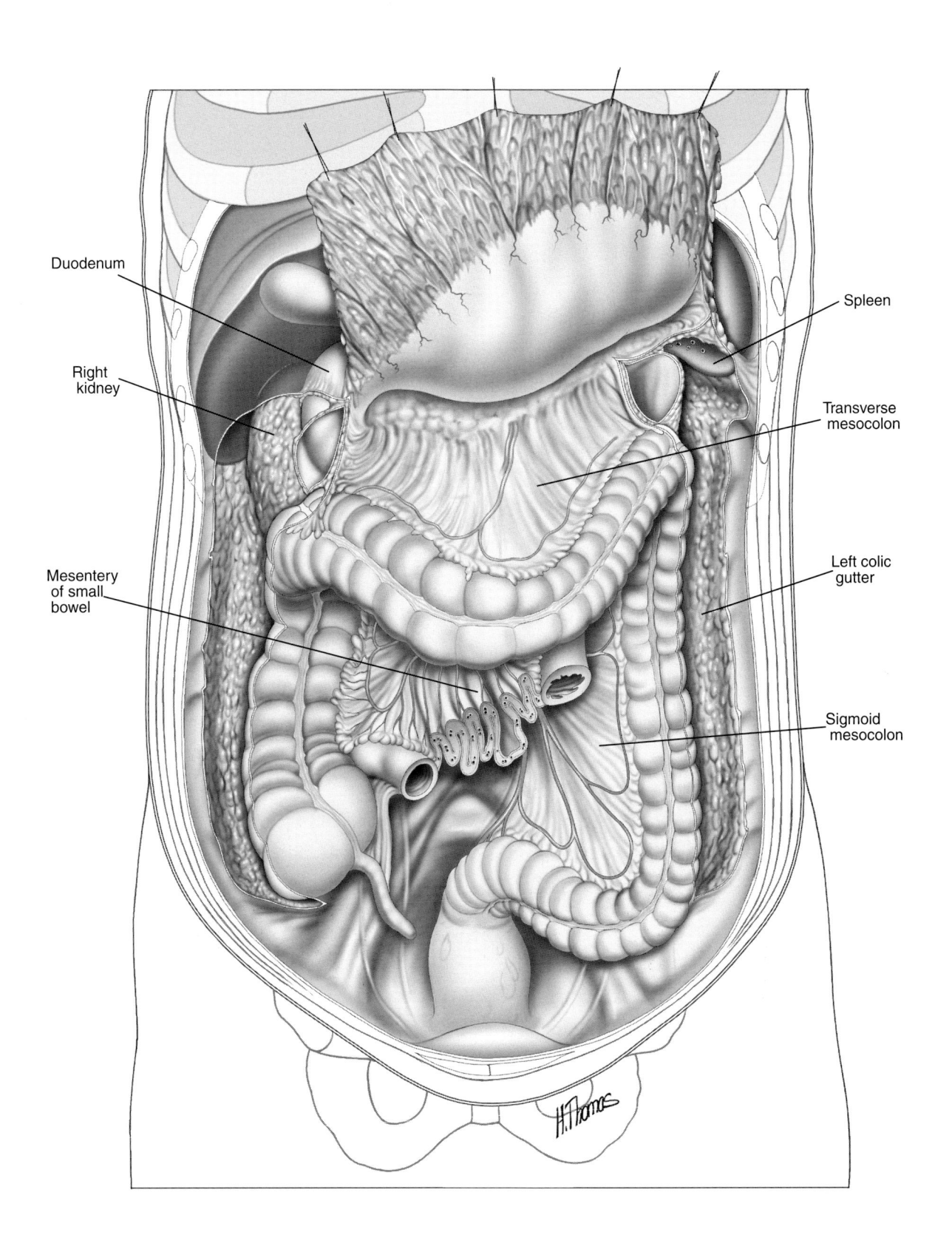

Figure 33–3 • The mesenteric attachments of the colon are demonstrated in this view.

Surgical Anatomy of the Abdomen • 277

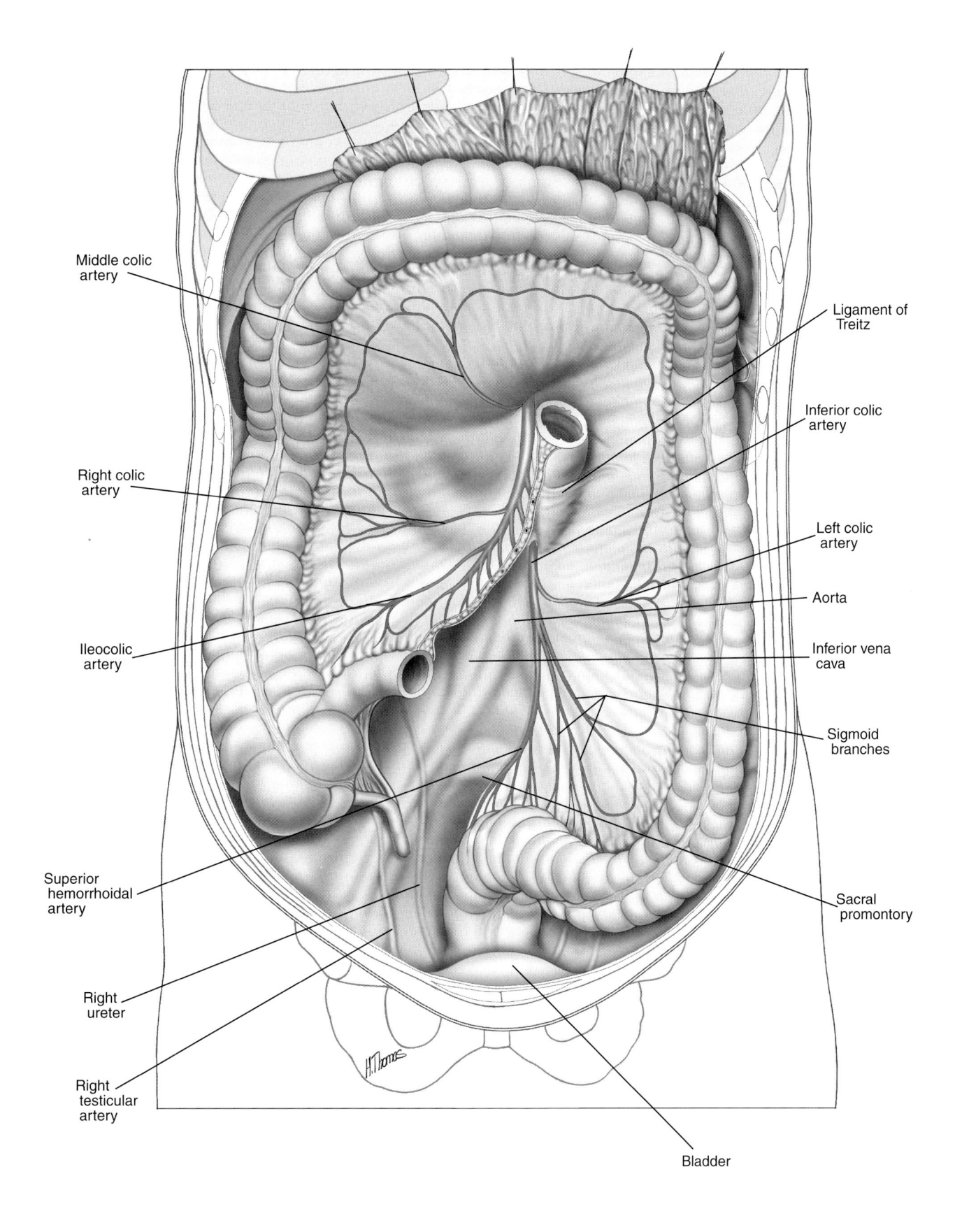

Figure 33–4 • The vascular anatomy to the large and small bowel is depicted.

278 • Part IV   LOWER ABDOMEN

A Right hemi-colectomy

B Transverse colectomy

C Left hemi-colectomy

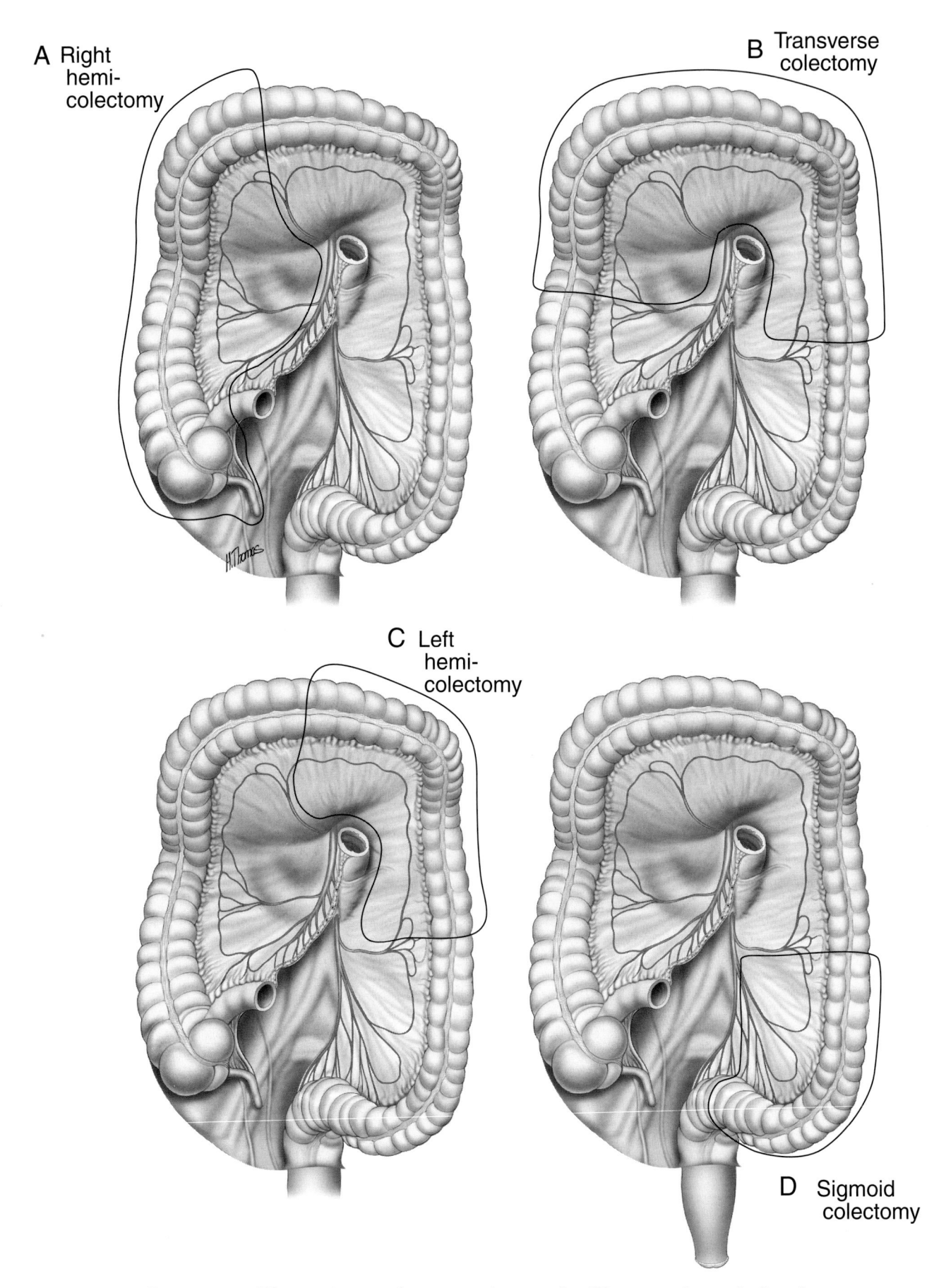

D Sigmoid colectomy

Figure 33–5 • The various colon resections to be illustrated are defined.

Chapter 34
Right Hemicolectomy

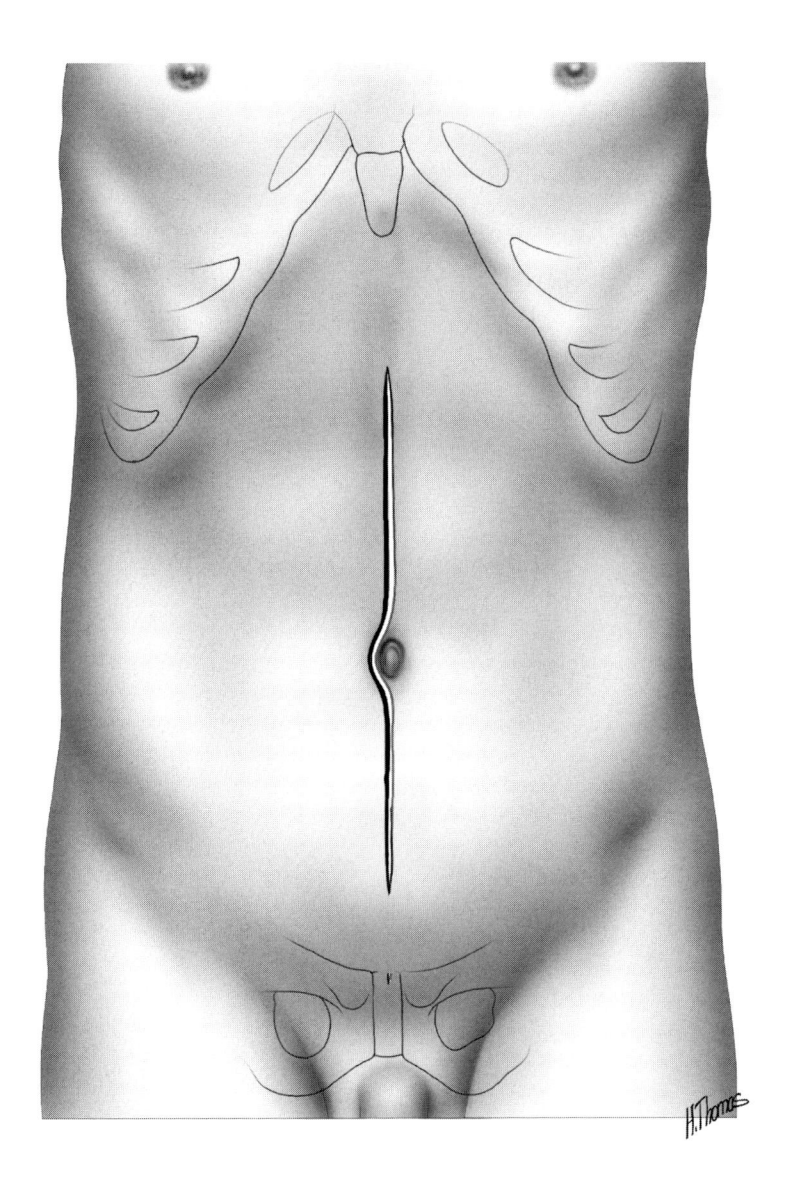

Figure 34–1 • A midline abdominal incision is employed, although a transverse incision can be utilized.

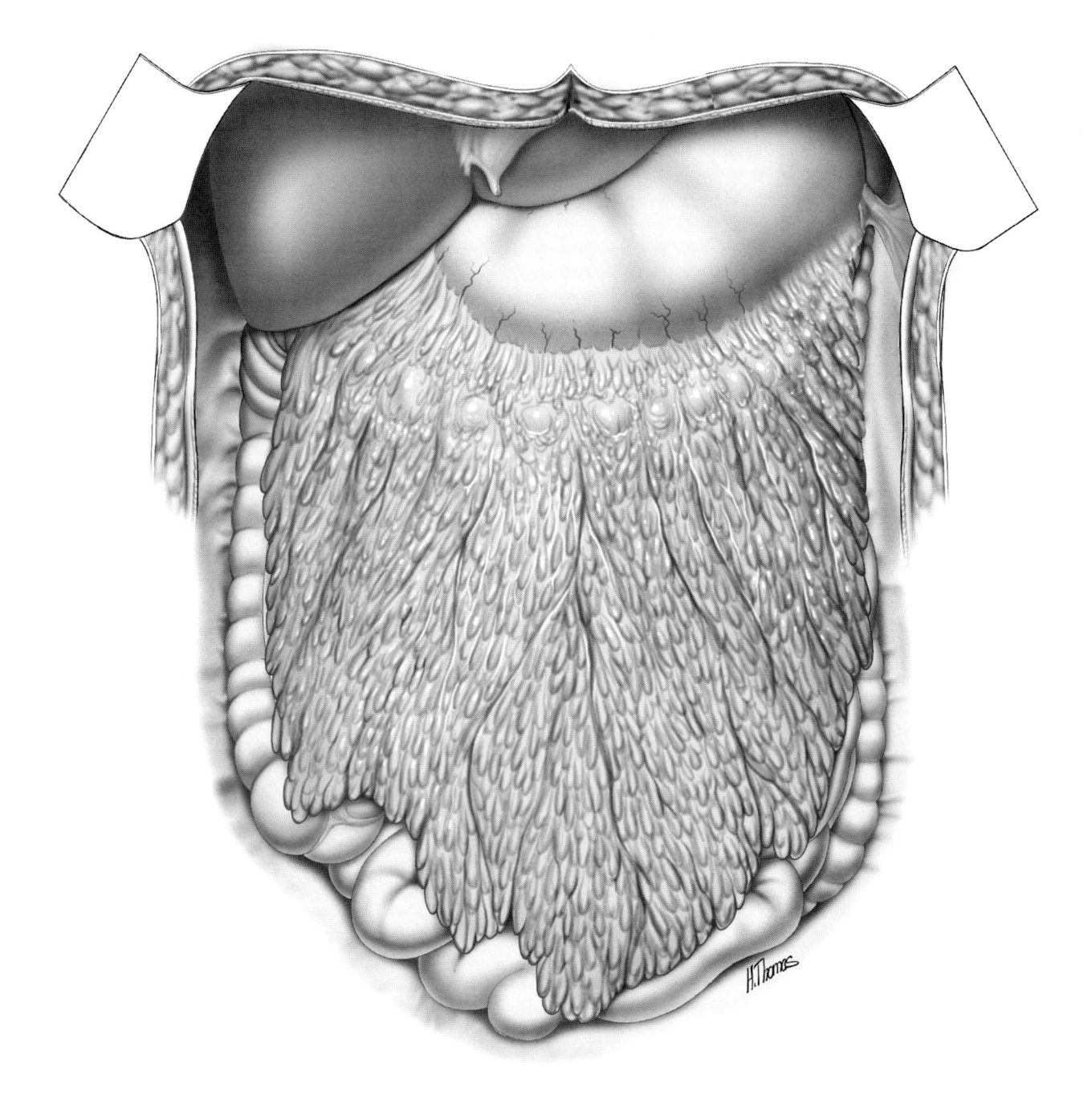

Figure 34–2 • Following the appropriate abdominal incision, the abdomen is explored and the liver is inspected.

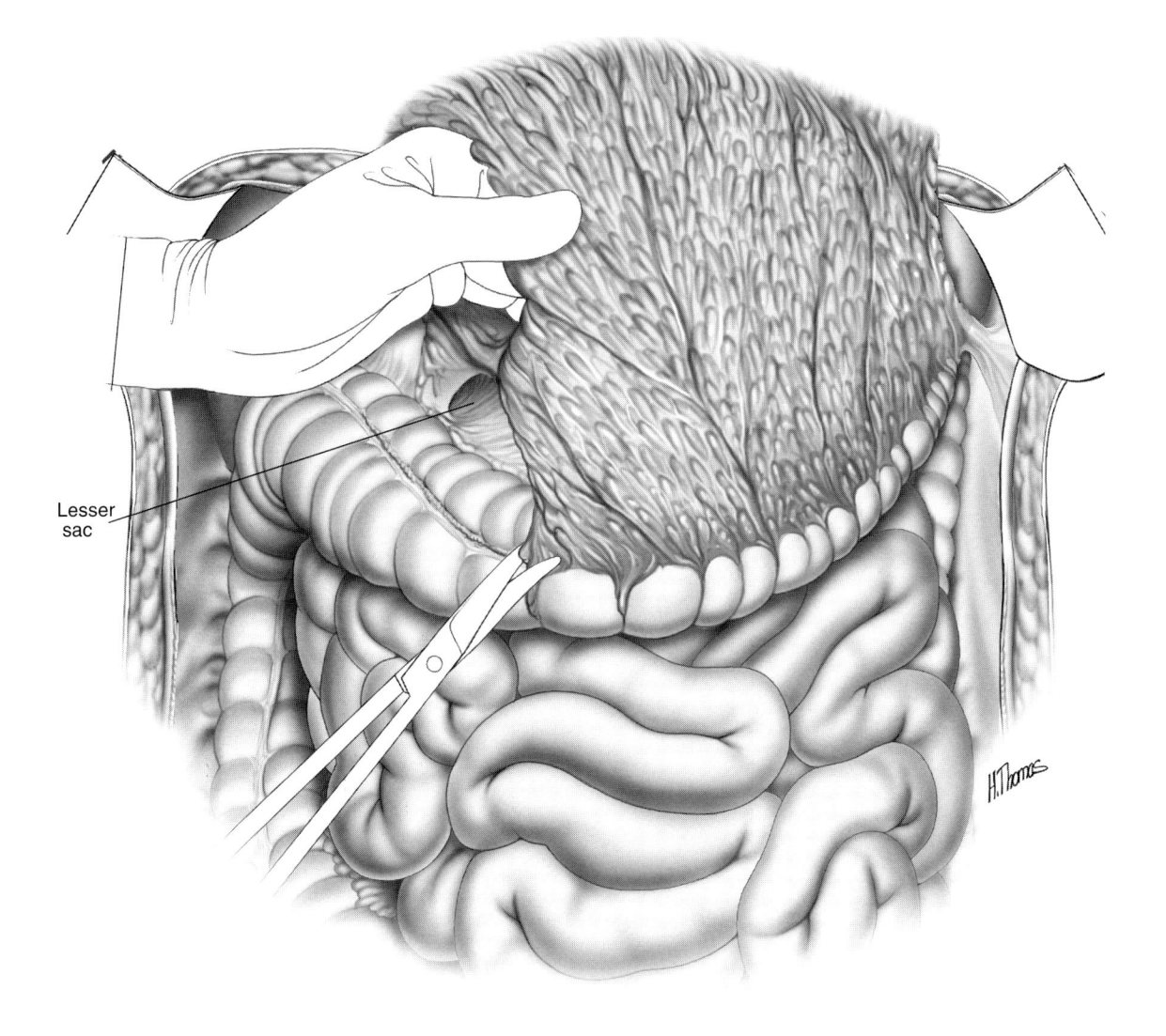

Figure 34–3 • The greater omentum is elevated superiorly and mobilized off the transverse colon by incising along an avascular plane.

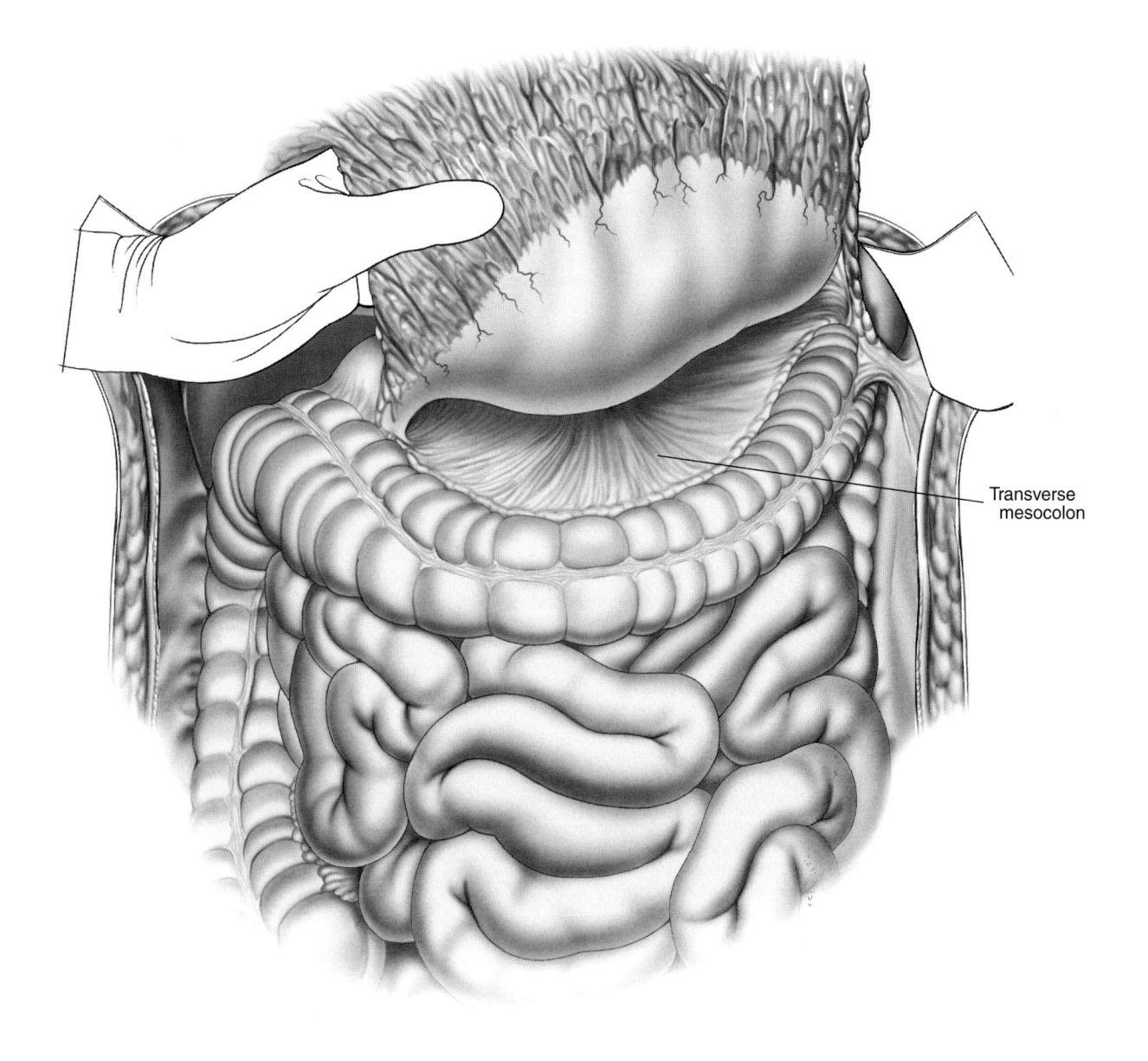

Figure 34-4 • Mobilization of the greater omentum proceeds from the hepatic flexure to the splenic flexure and opens the lesser sac with identification of the middle colic vessels.

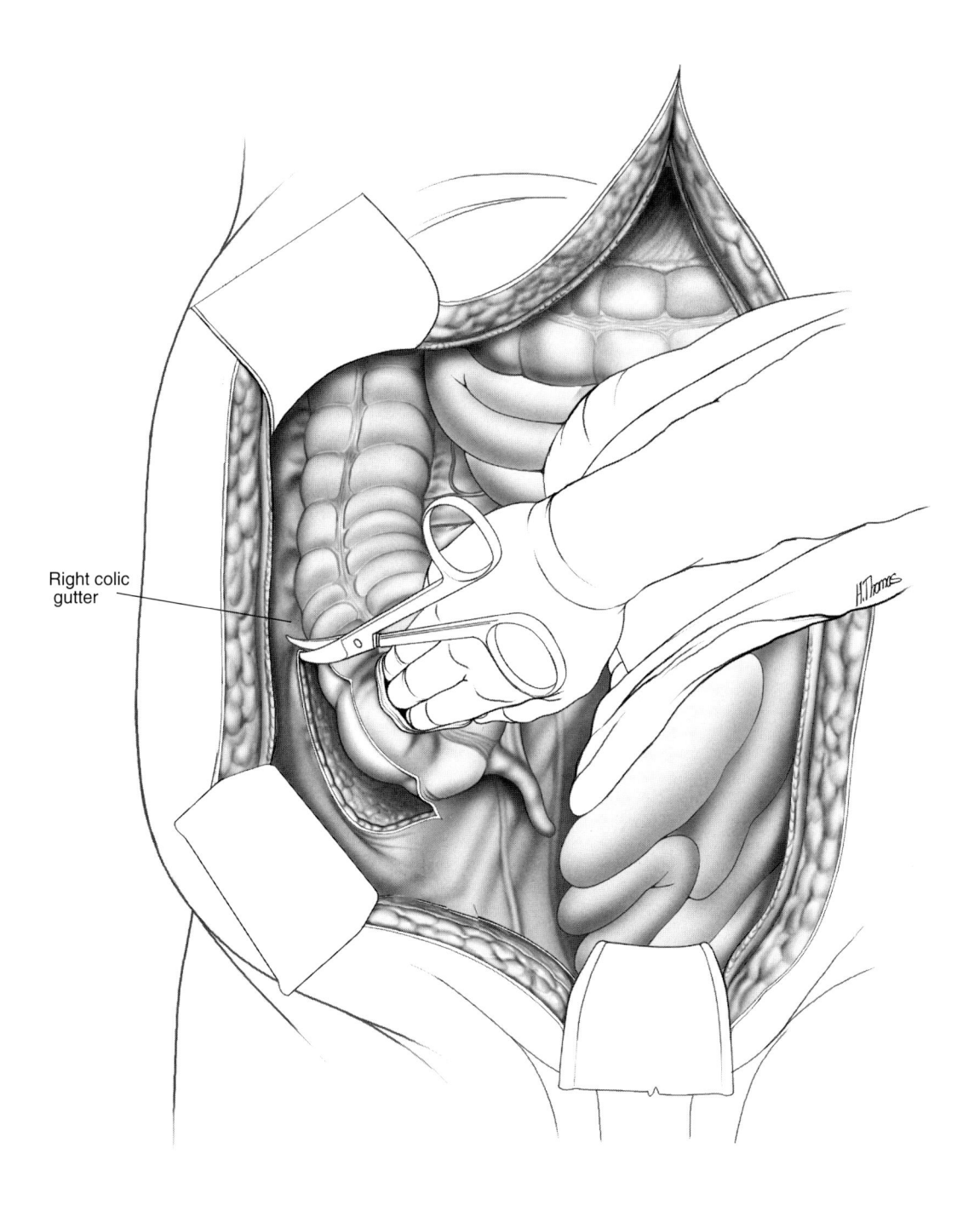

Figure 34–5 • The right colon is mobilized along the white line of Toldt to the hepatic flexure.

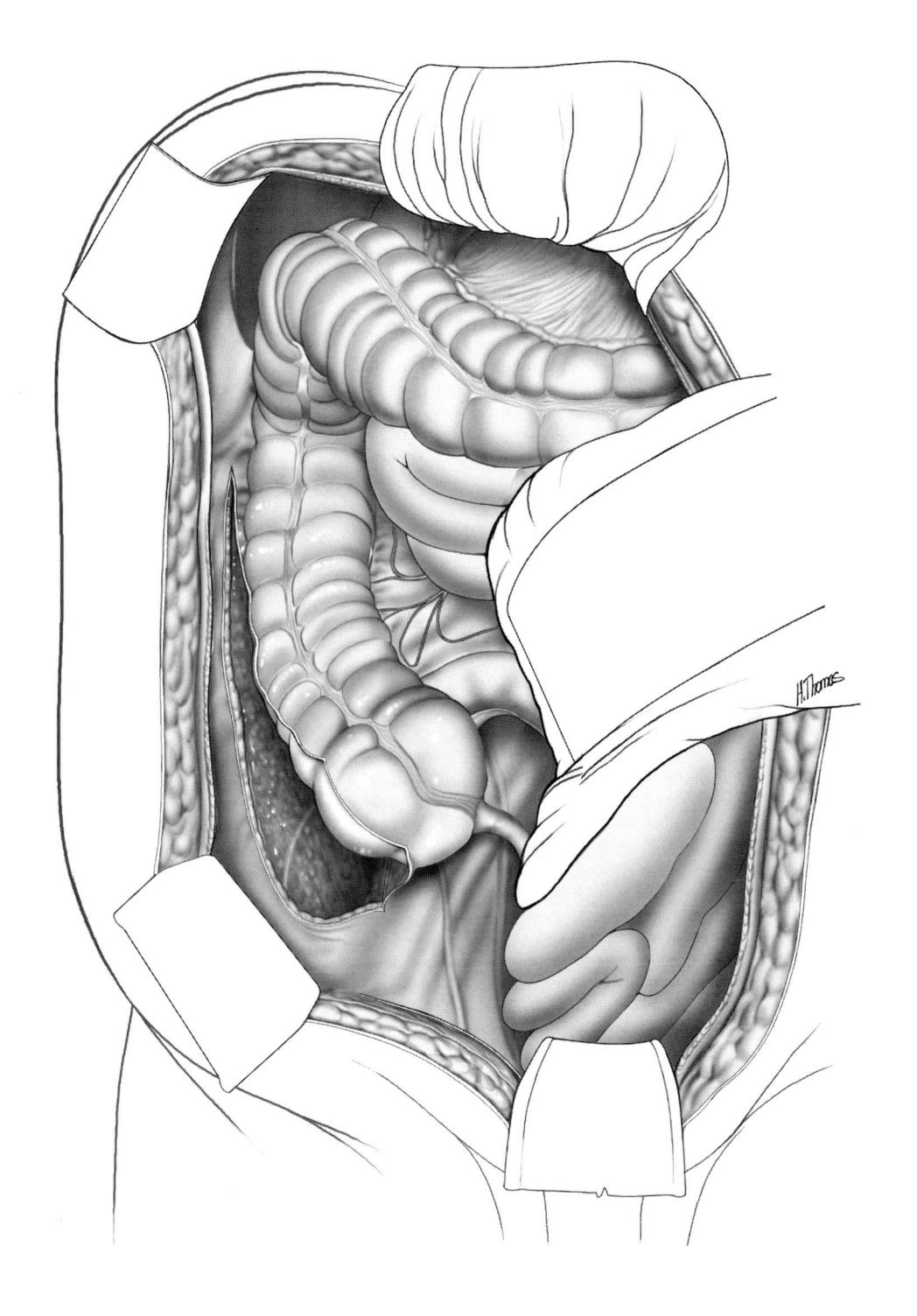

Figure 34–6 • Mobilization to the hepatic flexure is completed.

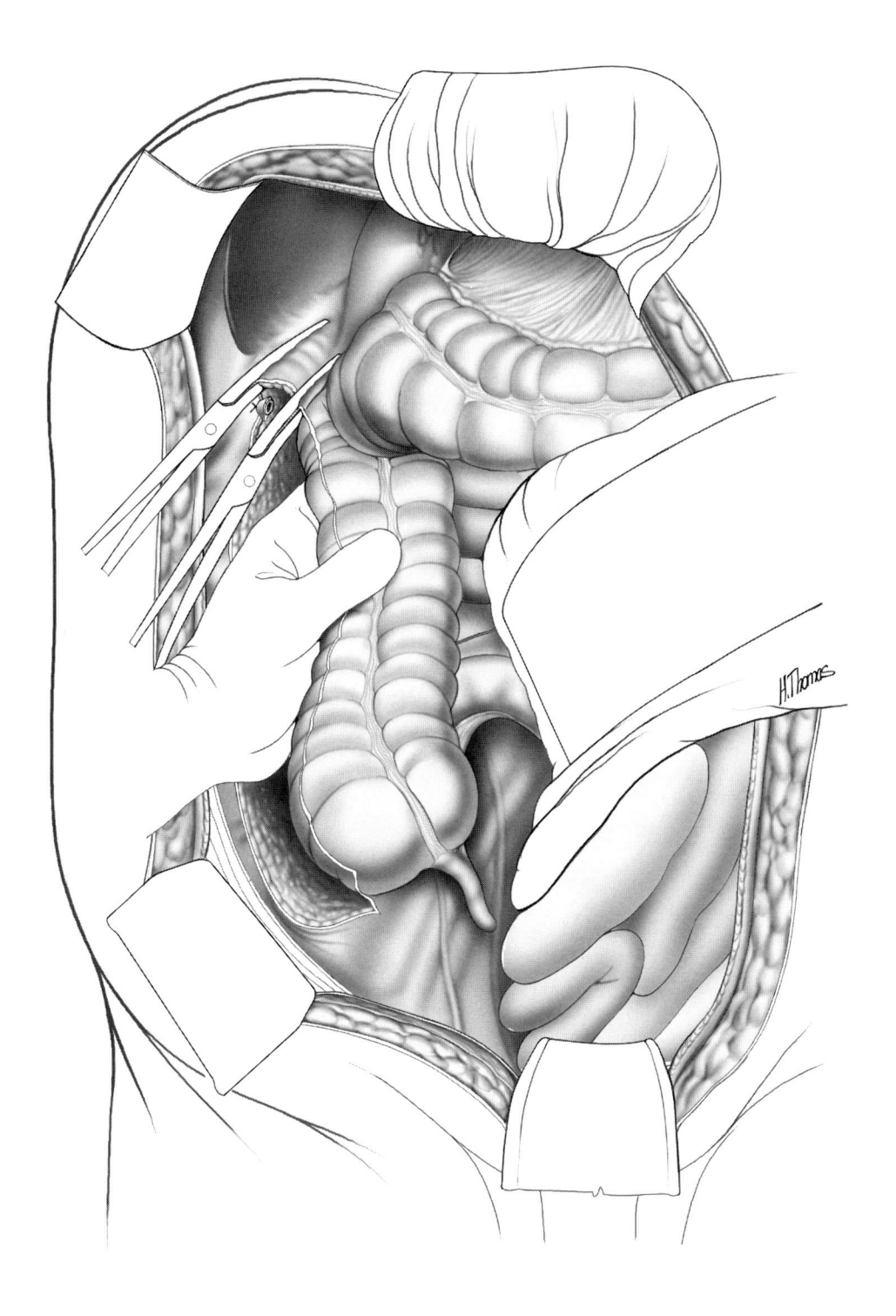

Figure 34-7 • The mesenteric attachments at the hepatic flexure are divided between clamps.

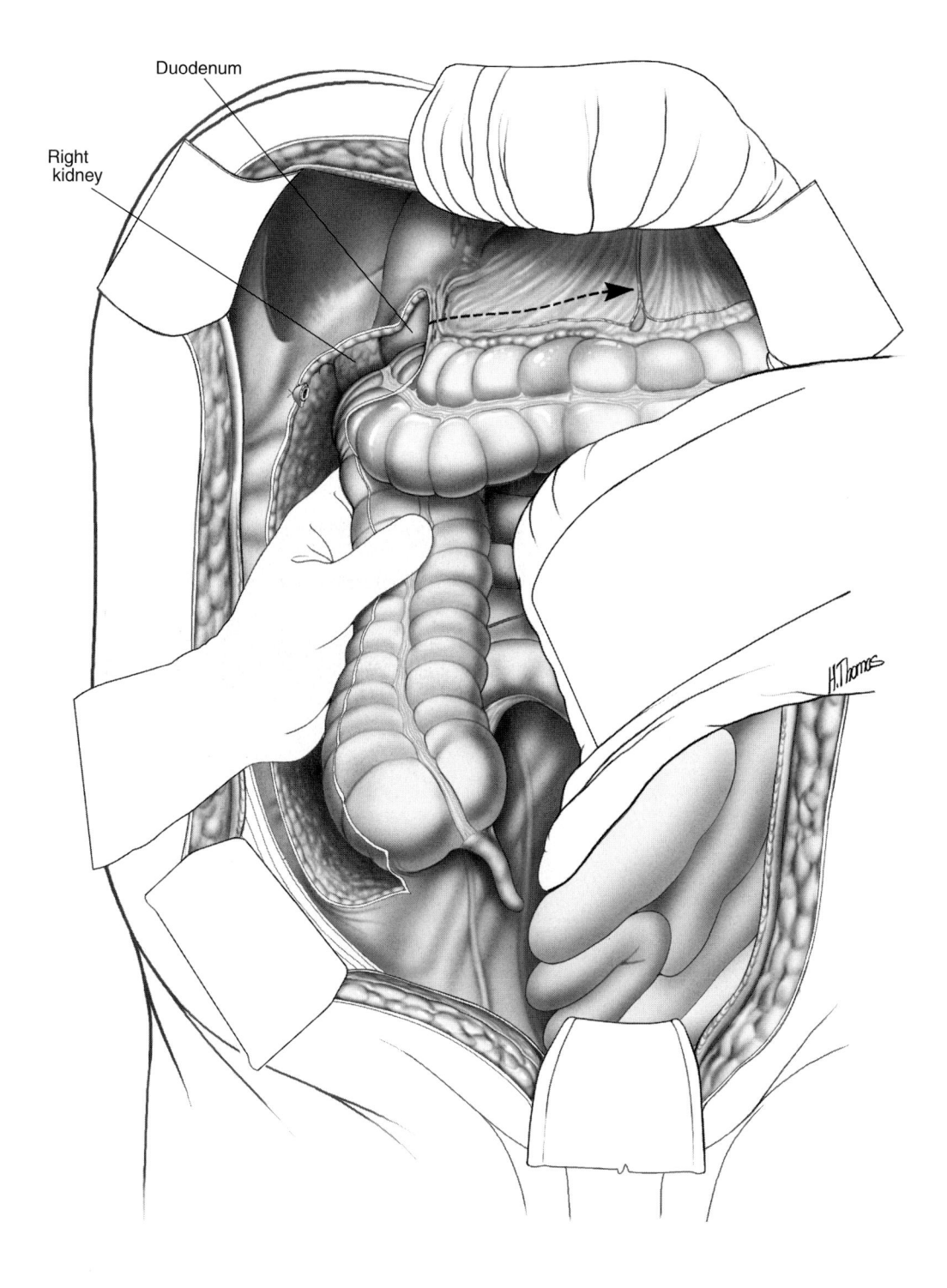

Figure 34–8 • Gerota's fascia and the duodenum are identified, and the line of resection on the transverse mesocolon is defined.

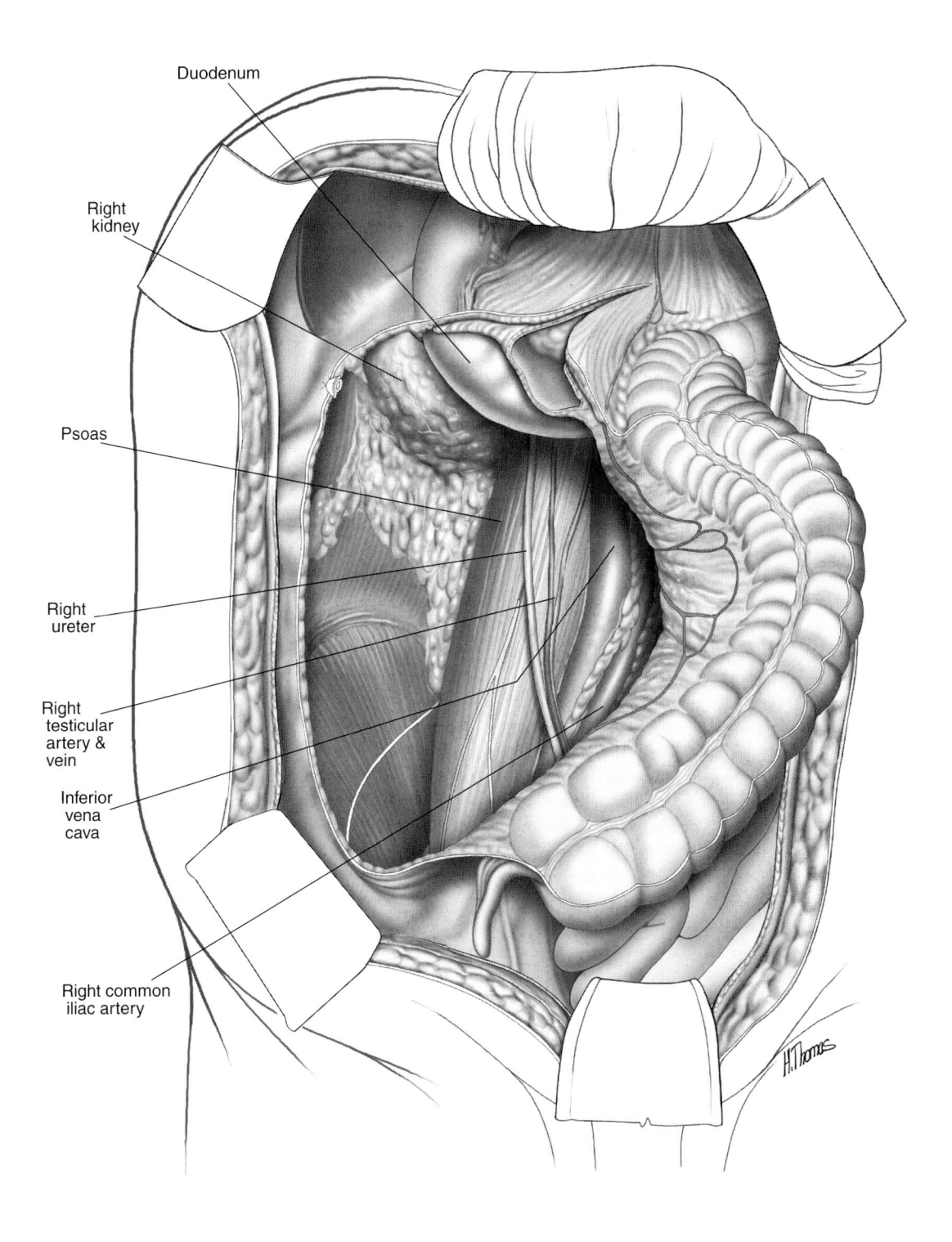

Figure 34–9 • The mobilization of the right colon is completed.

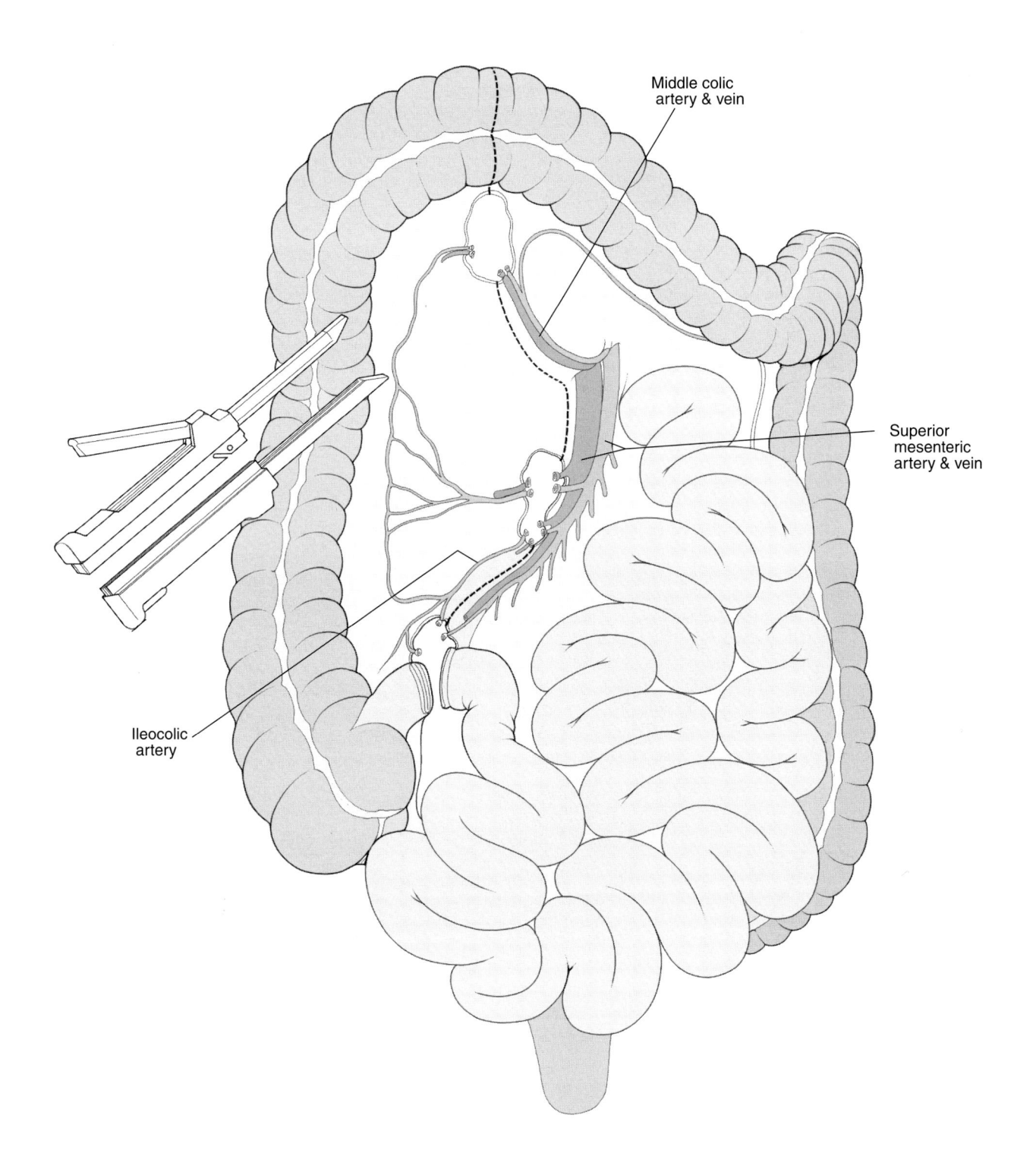

Figure 34–10 • The right branches of the middle colic, right colic, and ileocolic vessels are divided. The mesentery is completely divided, as indicated, and the bowel is divided using a stapler.

Right Hemicolectomy • 289

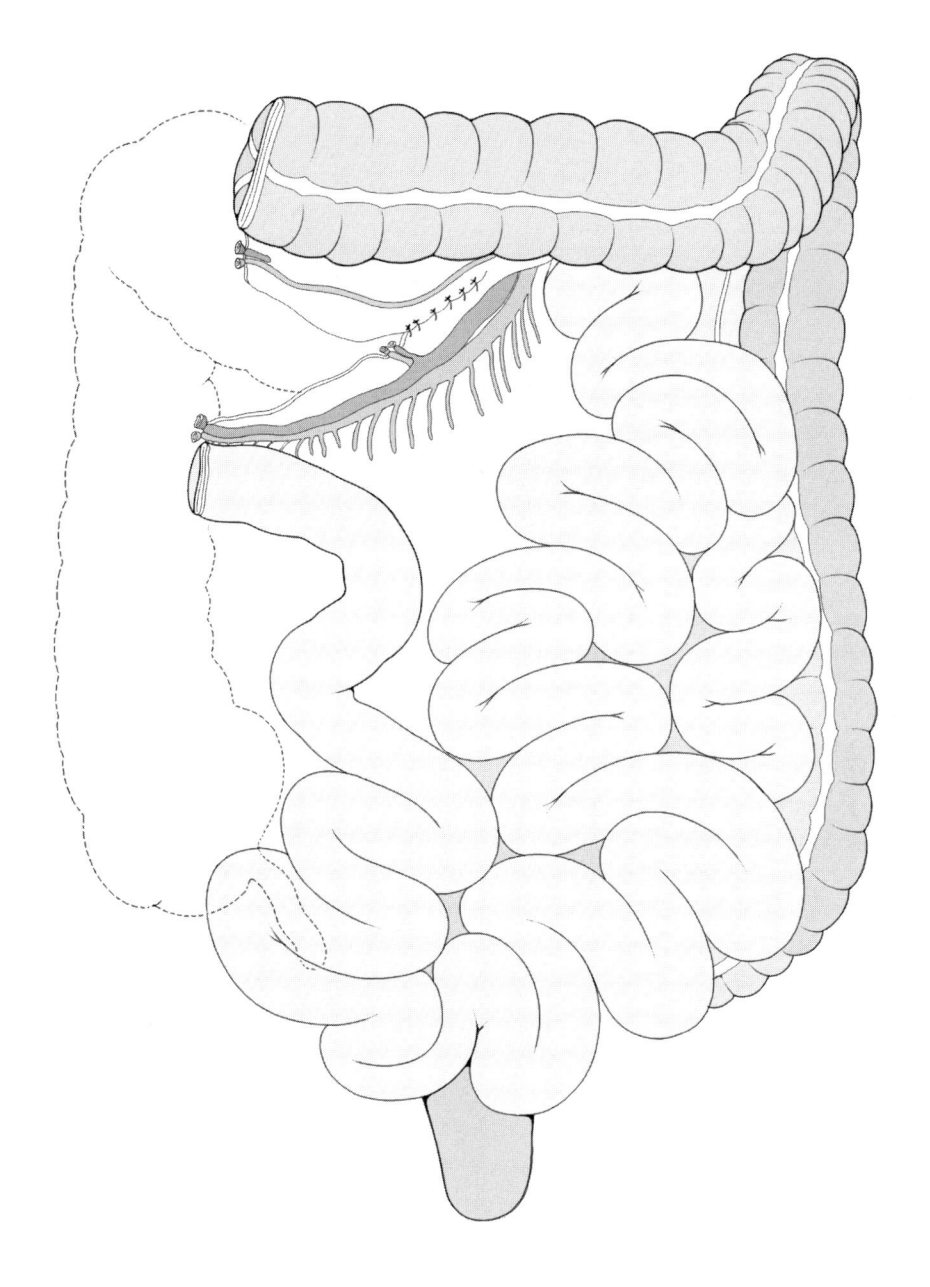

Figure 34–11 • The divided mesentery is reapproximated.

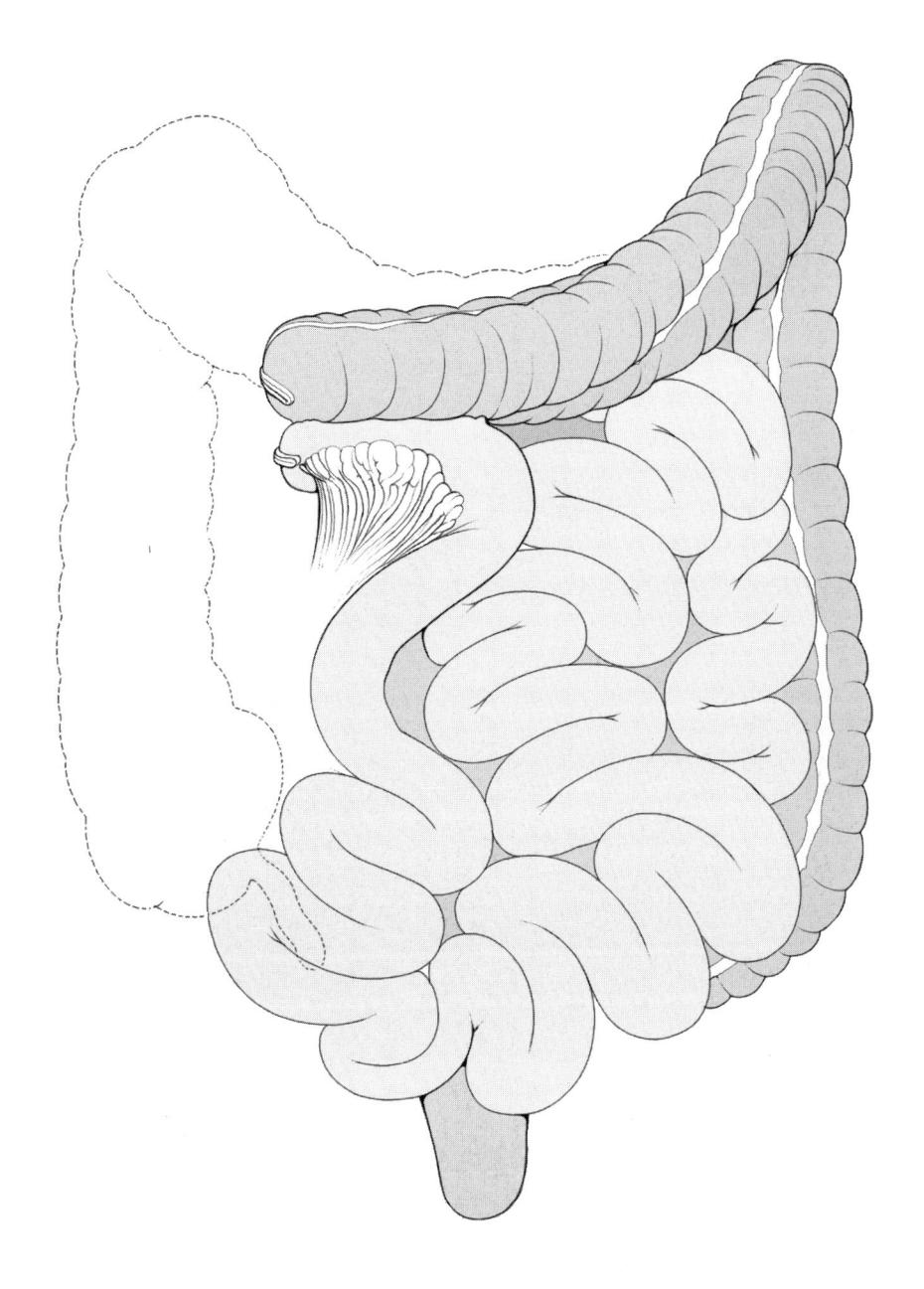

Figure 34–12 • The small bowel is aligned with the transverse colon in preparation for an anastomosis.

Right Hemicolectomy • 291

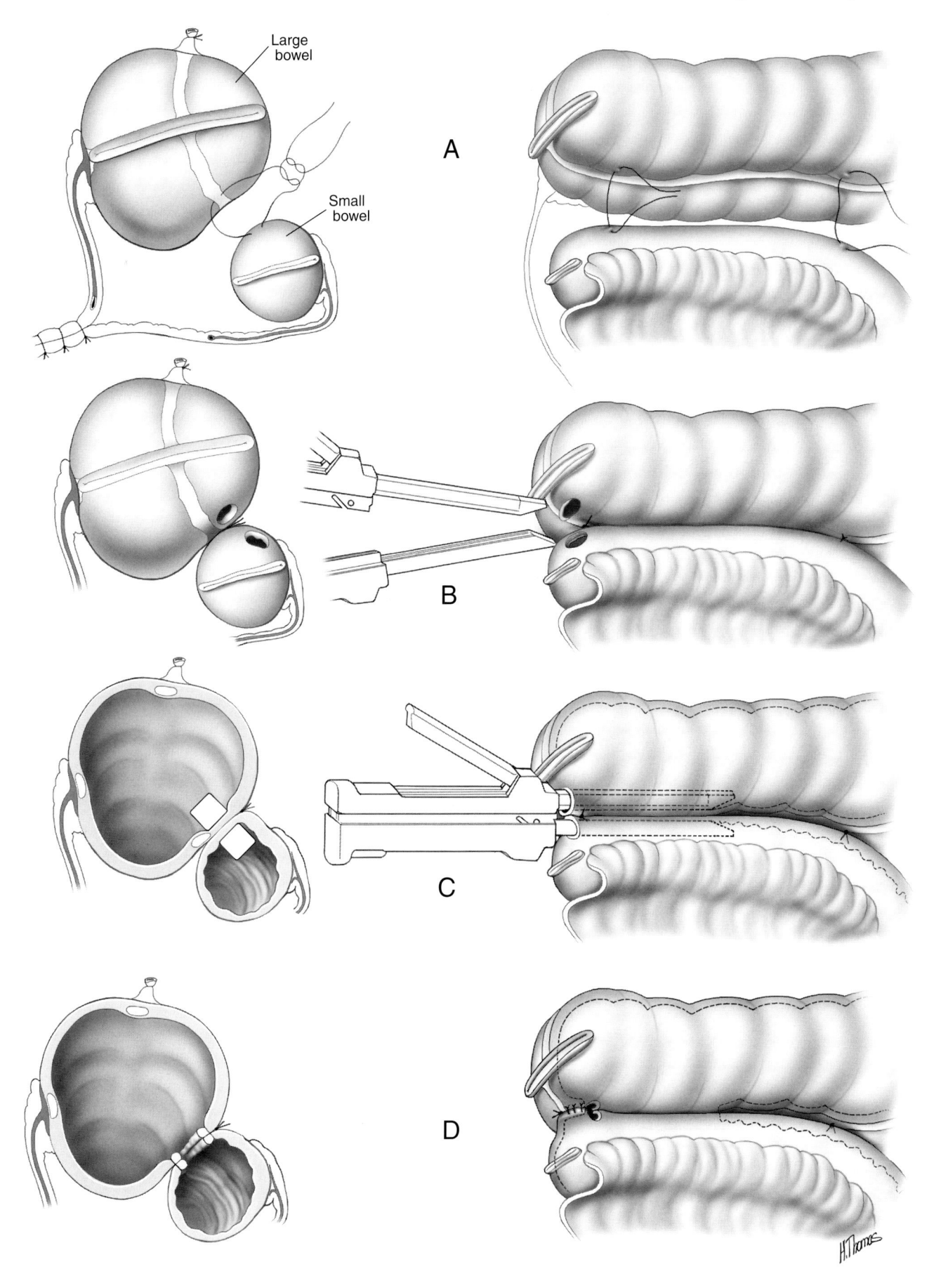

Figure 34–13 • A stapled anastomosis is illustrated.

Chapter 35
Left Hemicolectomy

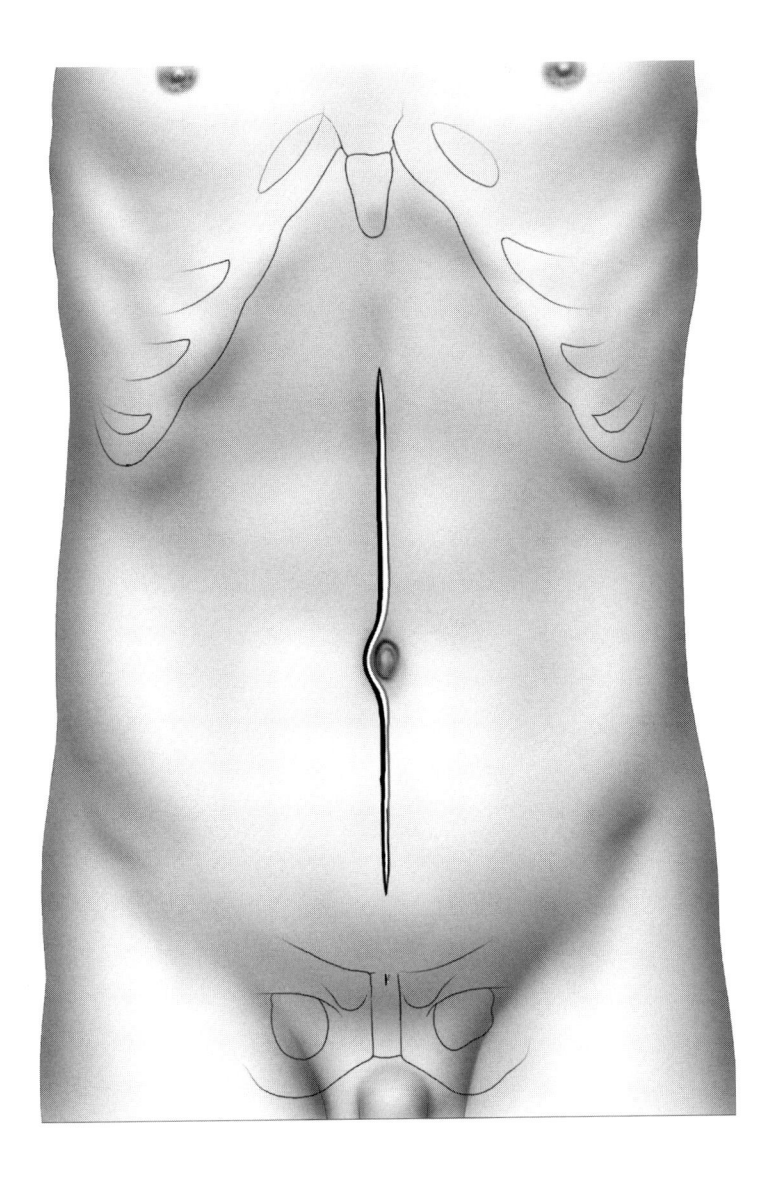

Figure 35–1 • The abdominal incision is completed, and the small bowel is packed out of the way.

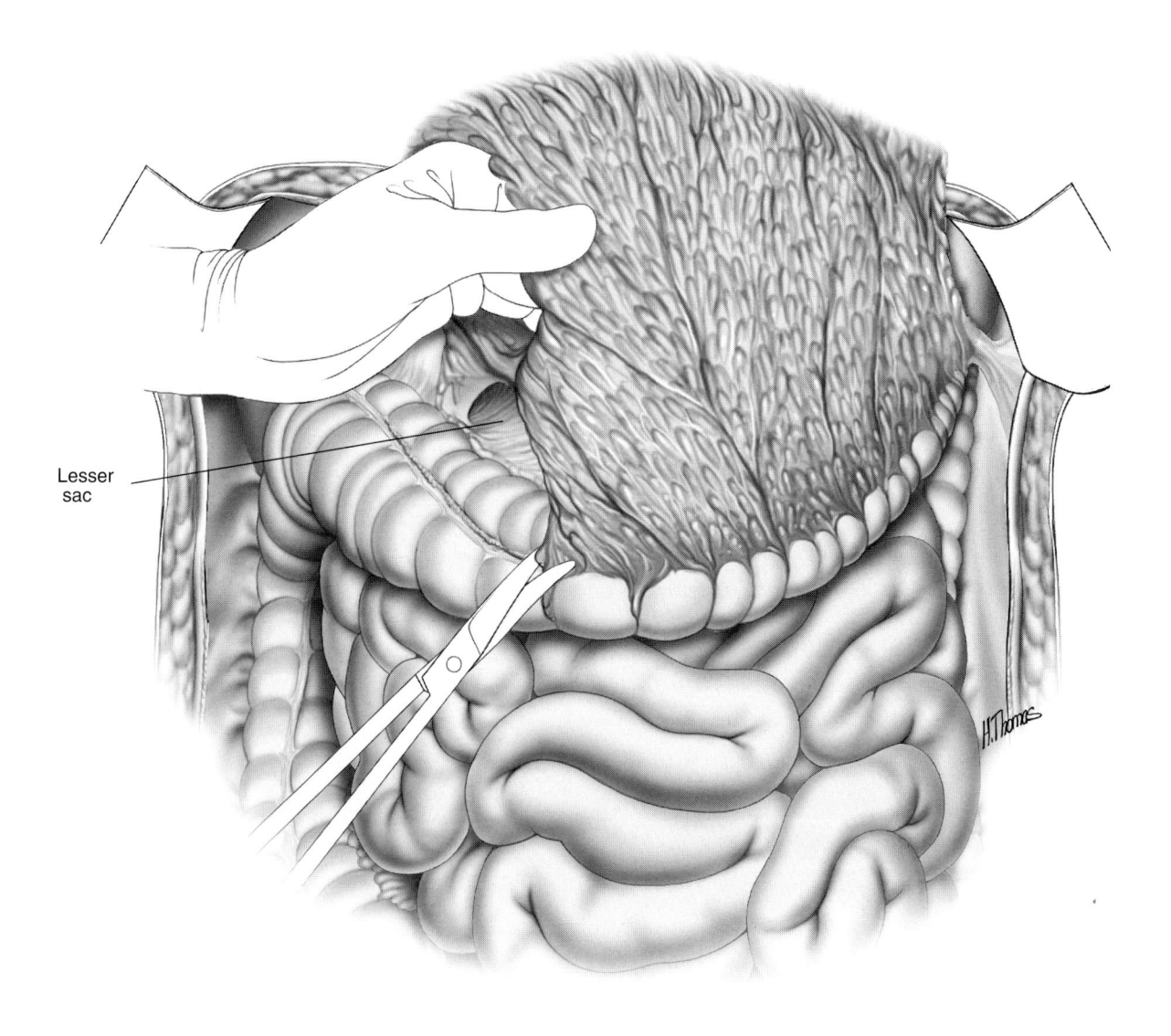

Figure 35-2 • The greater omentum is elevated off the transverse colon along the avascular plane.

Left Hemicolectomy • 295

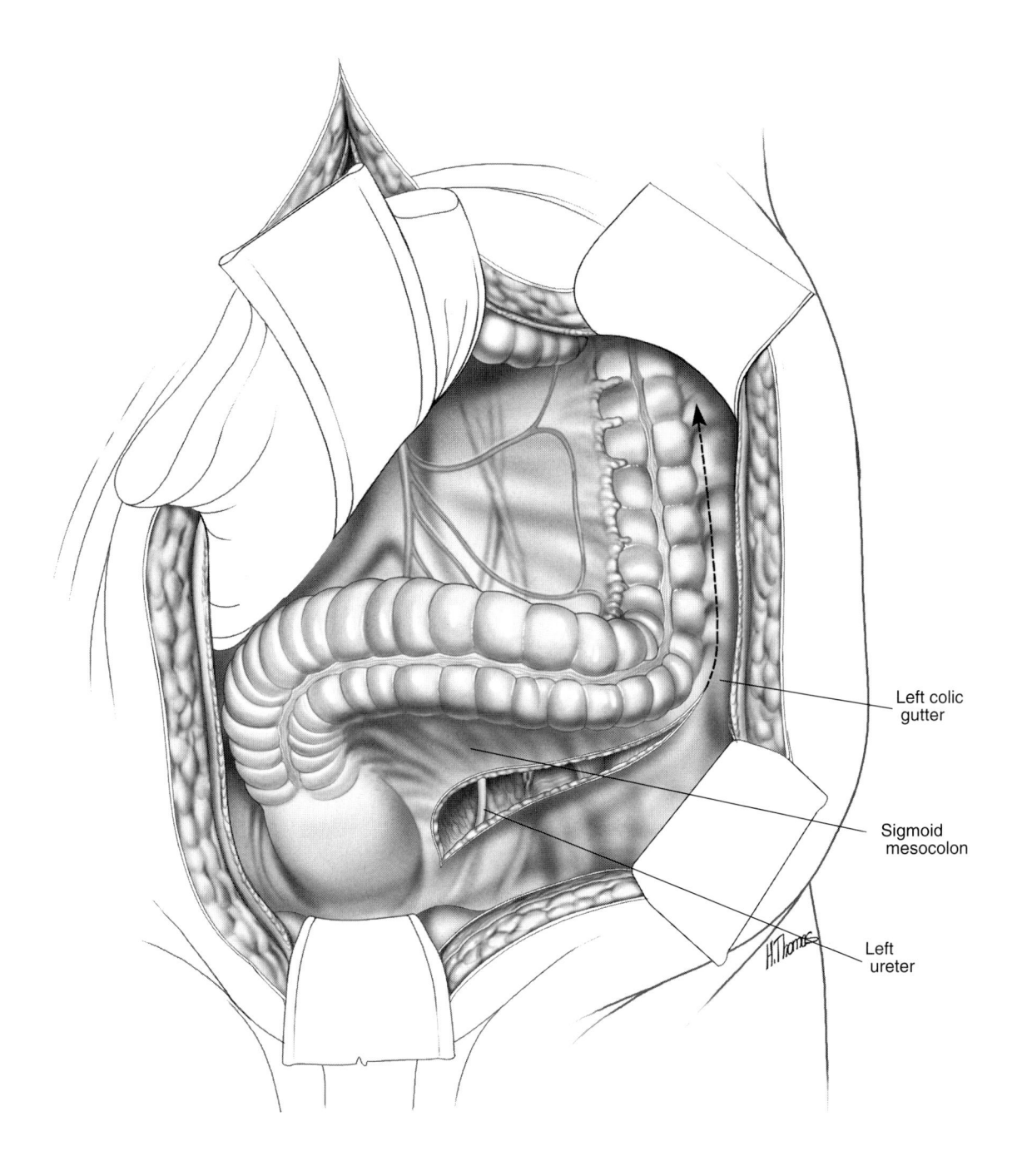

Figure 35–3 • An incision is made along the left colic gutter to the splenic flexure along the white line of Toldt.

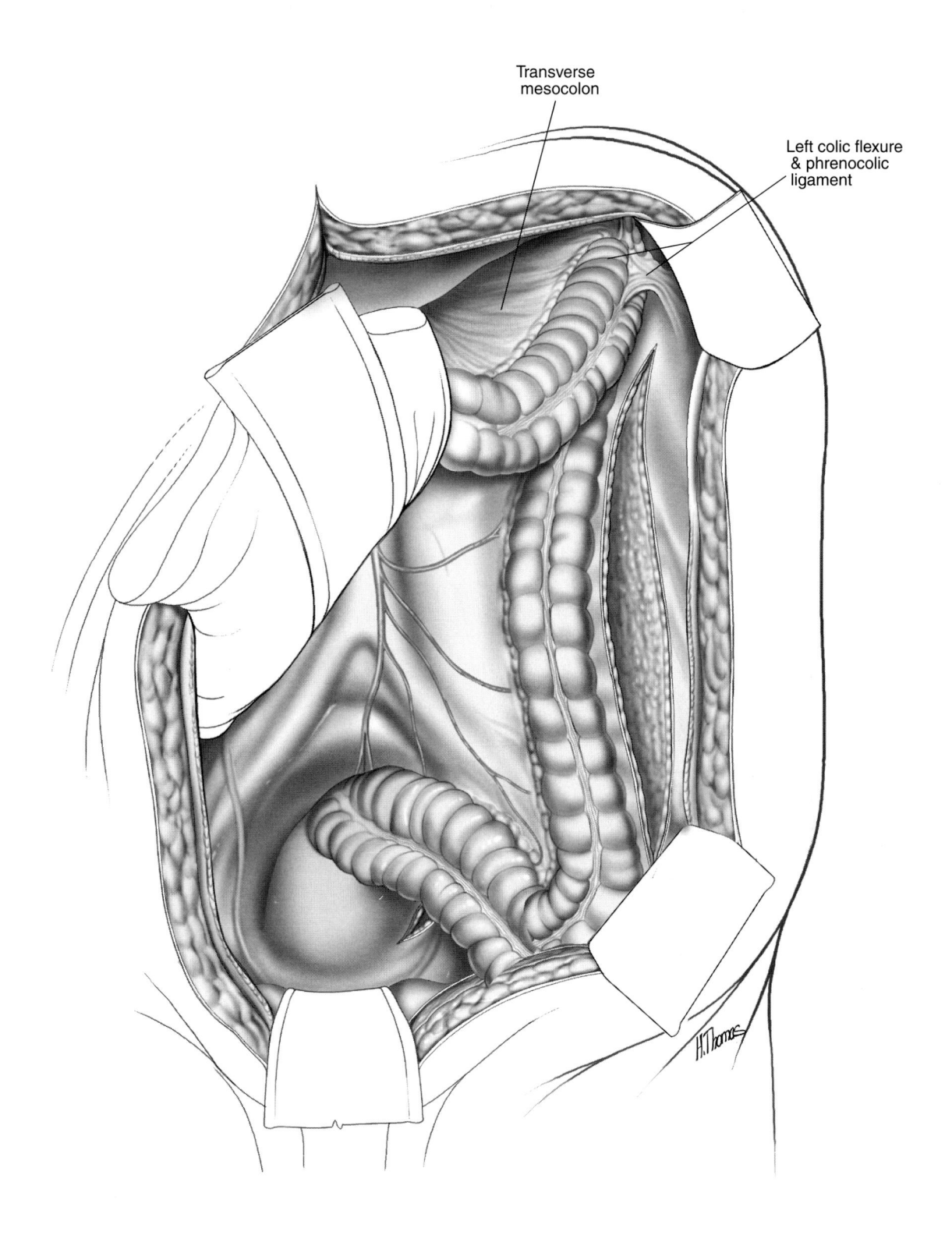

Figure 35–4 • The colon is mobilized to the splenic flexure and elevated medially off the psoas.

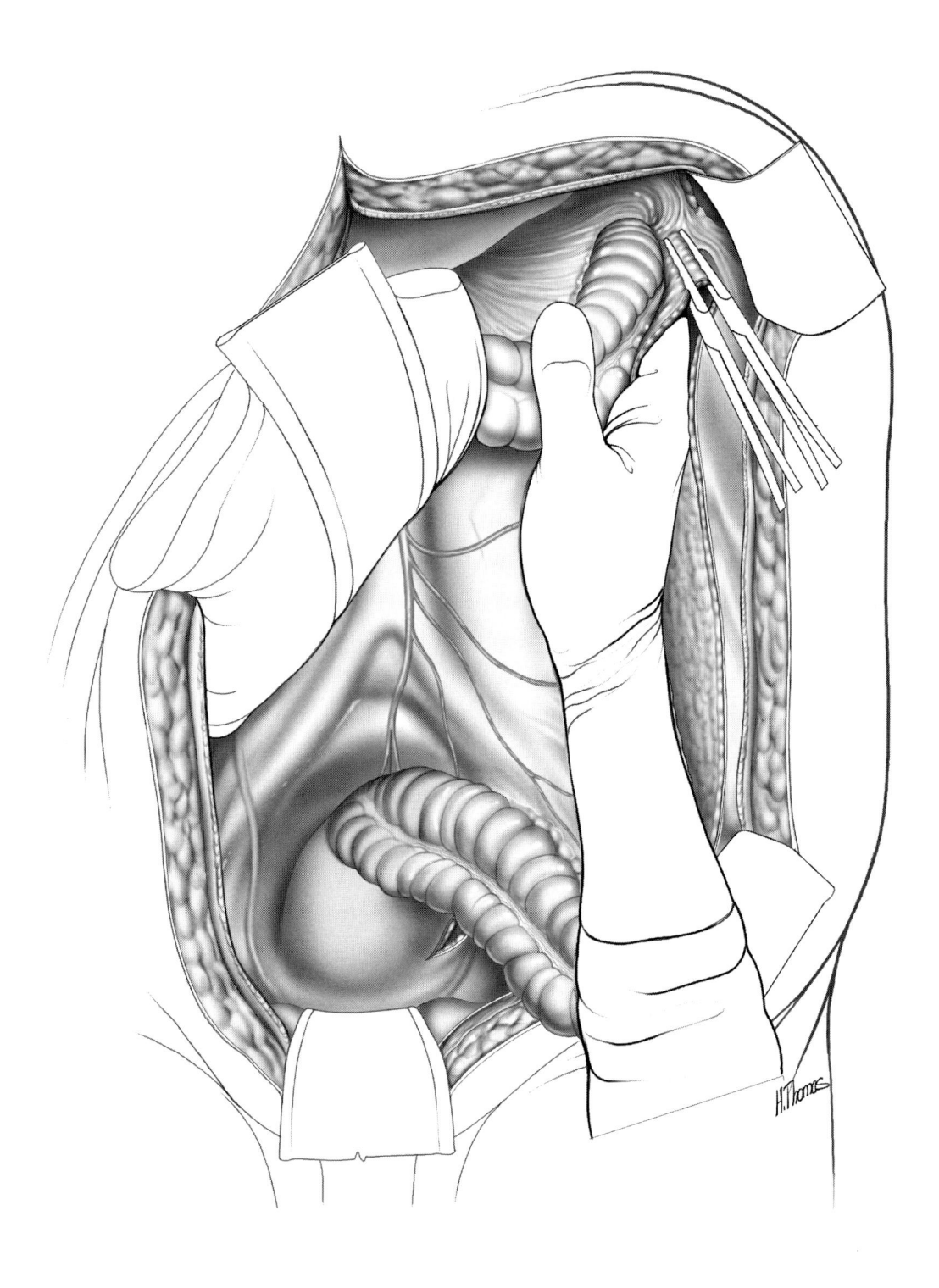

Figure 35–5 • The splenic flexure is mobilized.

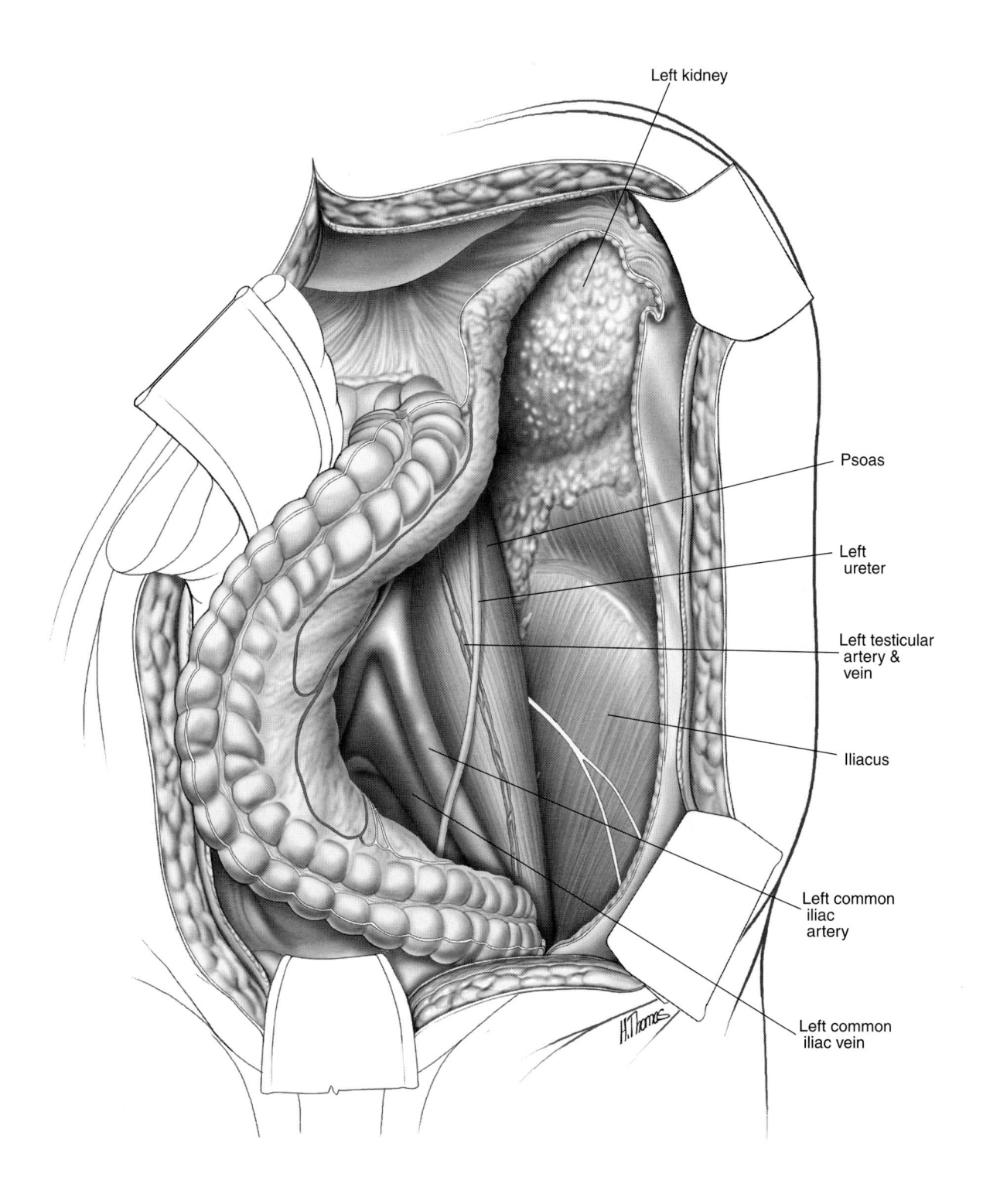

Figure 35–6 • The transverse mesocolon is divided to the middle colic vessels.

Left Hemicolectomy • 299

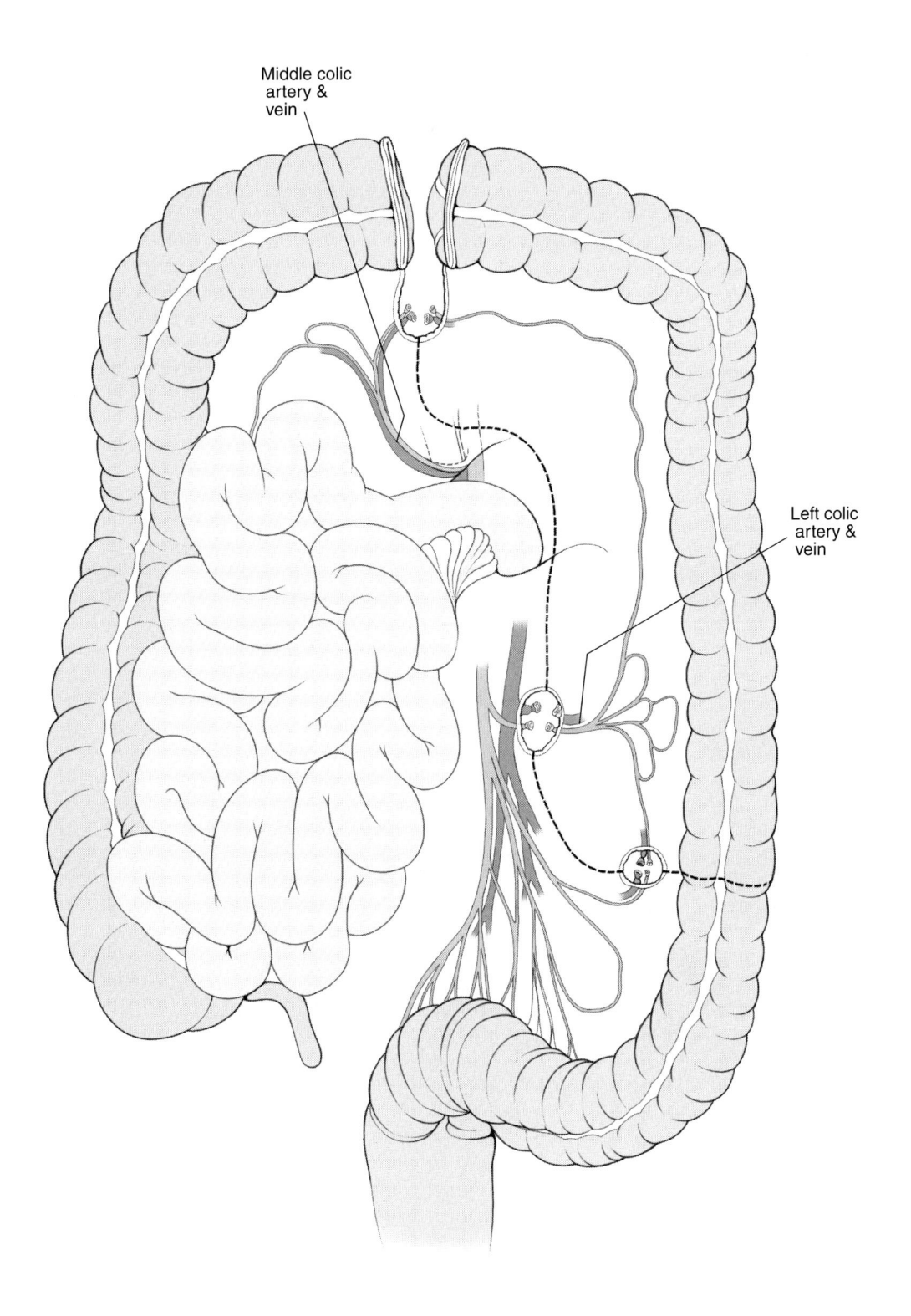

Figure 35–7 • Depicted is division of the middle colic and left colic arteries and veins and vessels forming the arcade, as well as the line of resection of the mesentery.

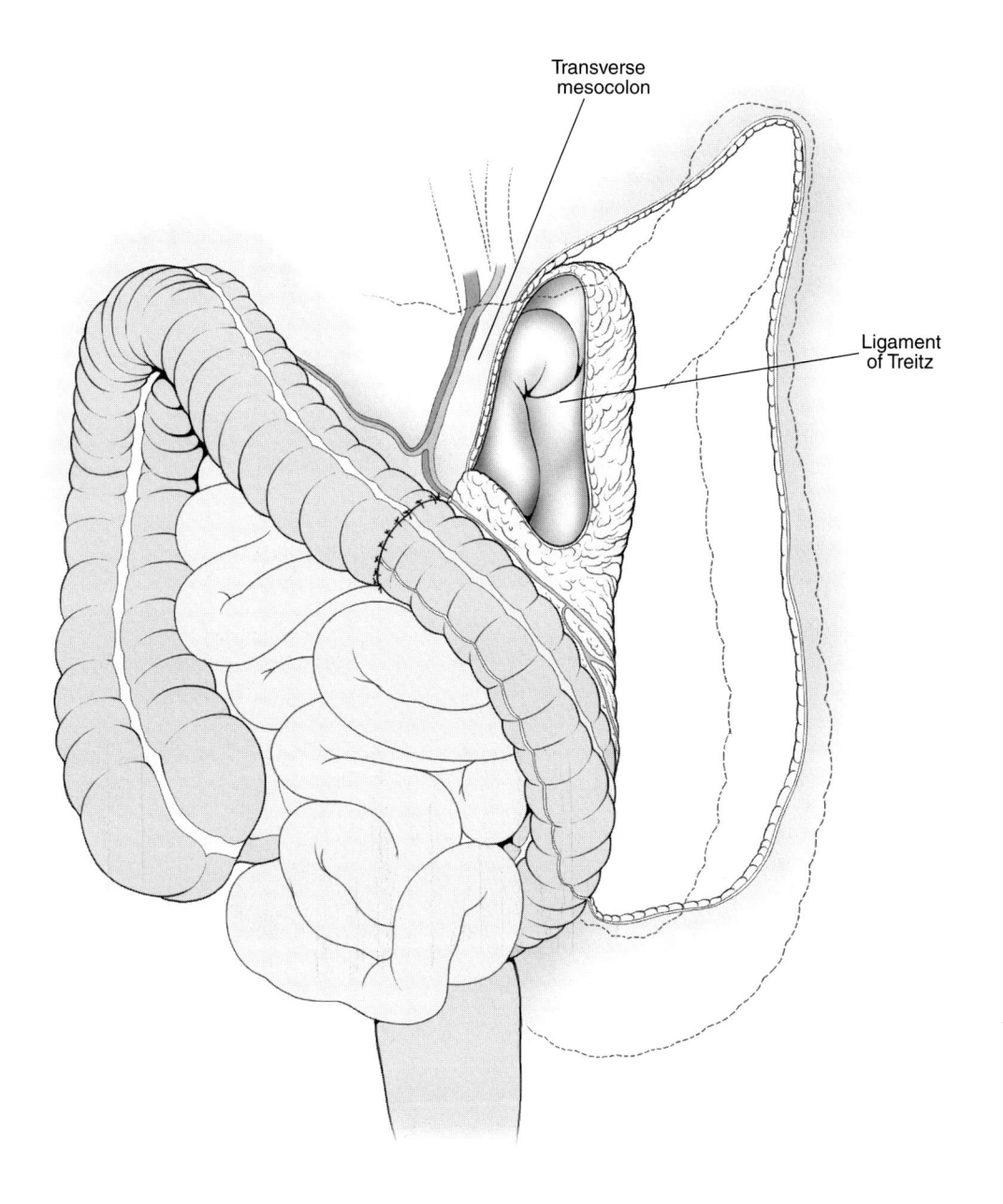

Figure 35–8 • The divided mesenteries are reapproximated, and the colonic anastomosis is performed.

Chapter 36
Transverse Colectomy

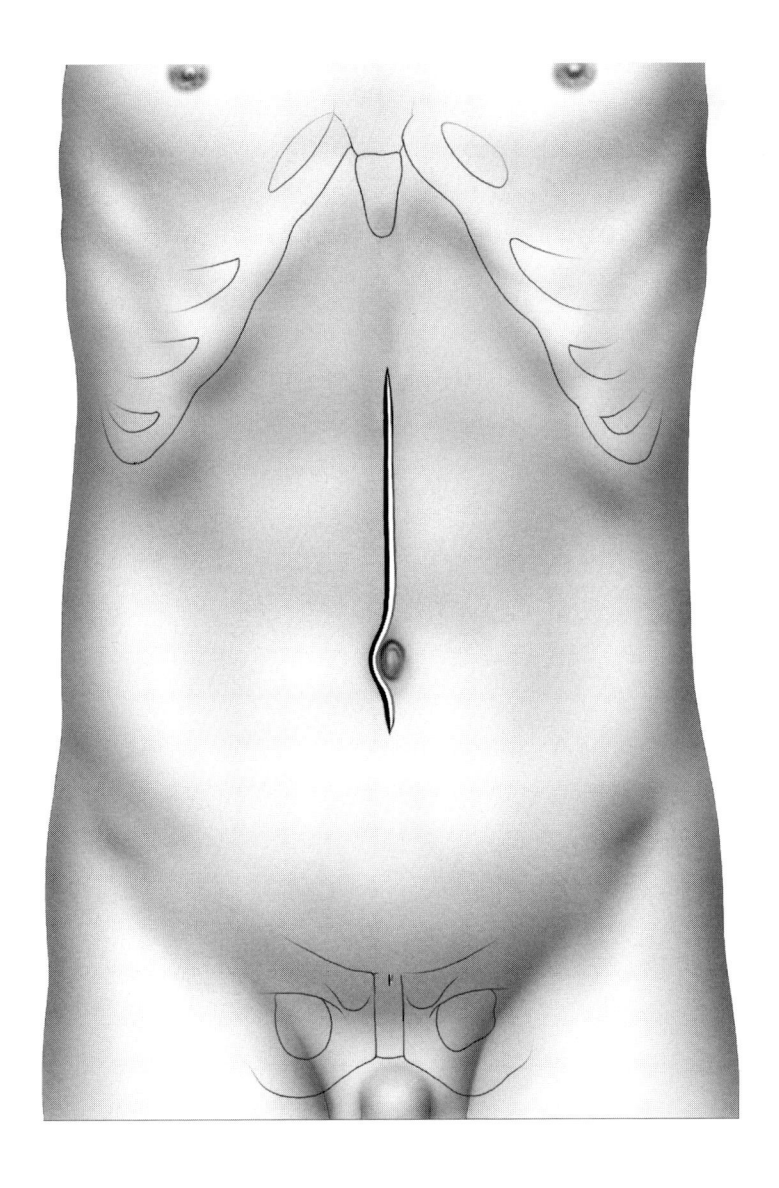

Figure 36–1 • A generous midline abdominal incision is performed.

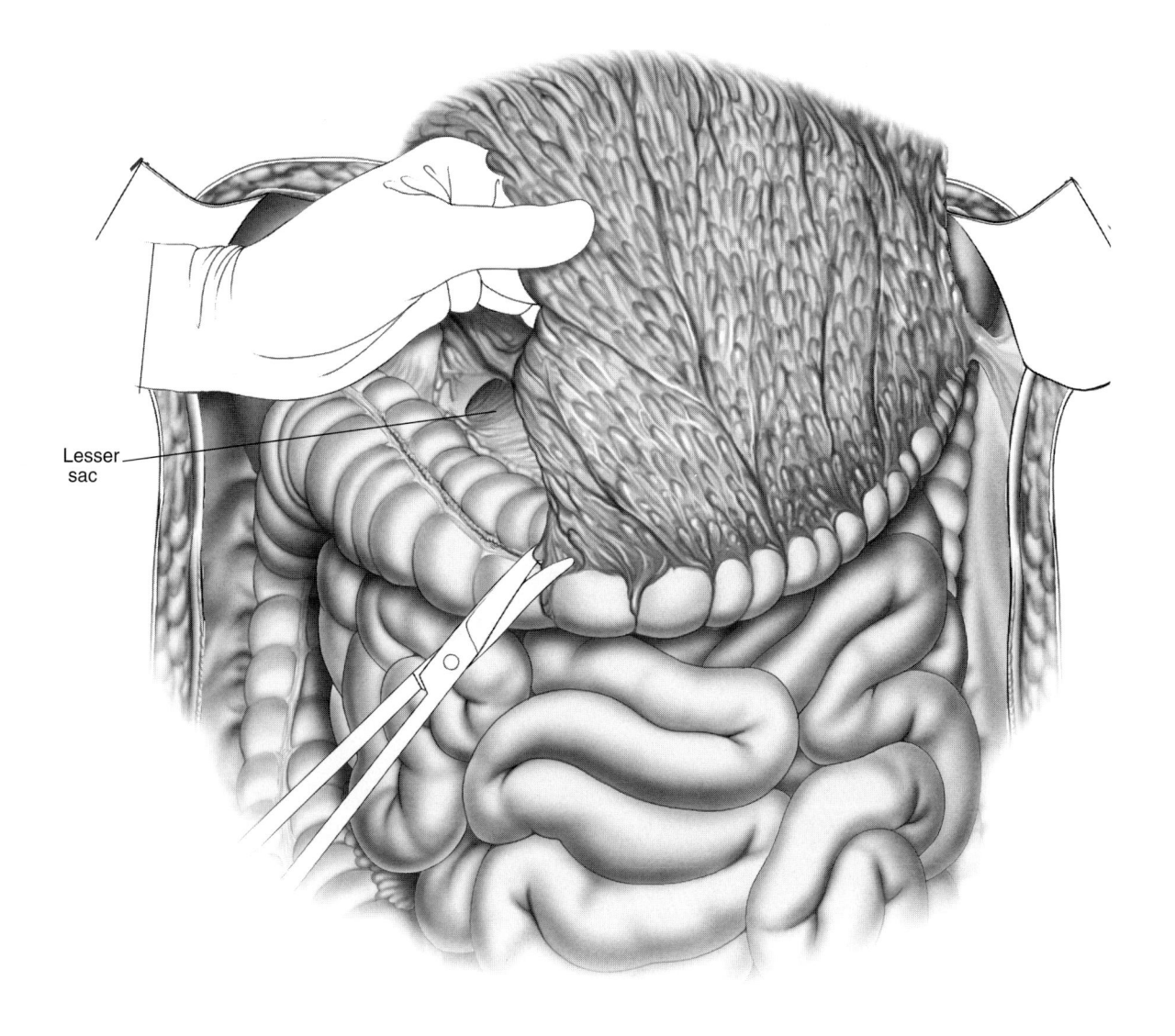

Figure 36–2 • The greater omentum is detached from the transverse colon along an avascular plane.

Transverse Colectomy • 303

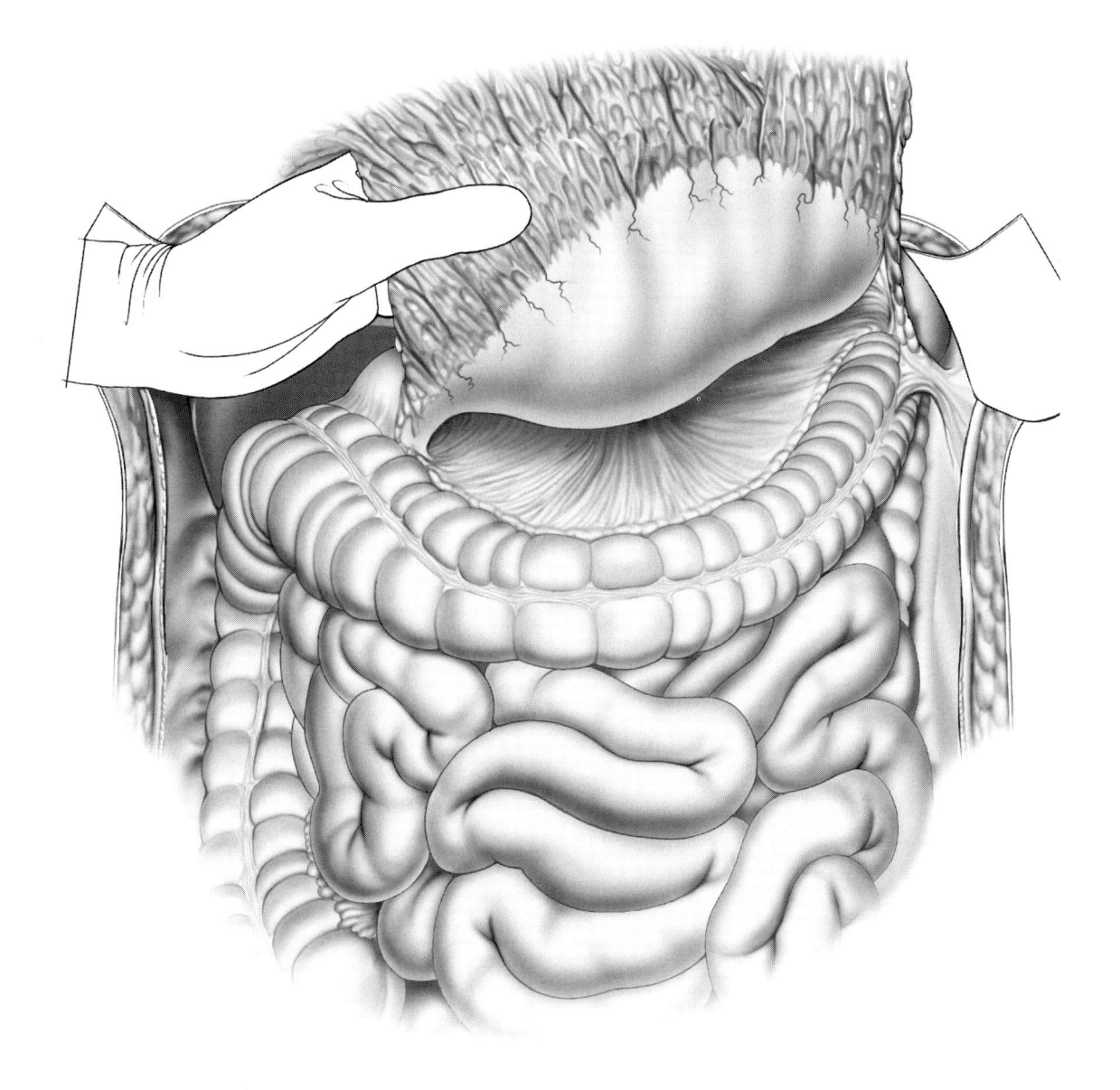

Figure 36–3 • The greater omentum is completely mobilized off the transverse colon and the lesser sac is entered.

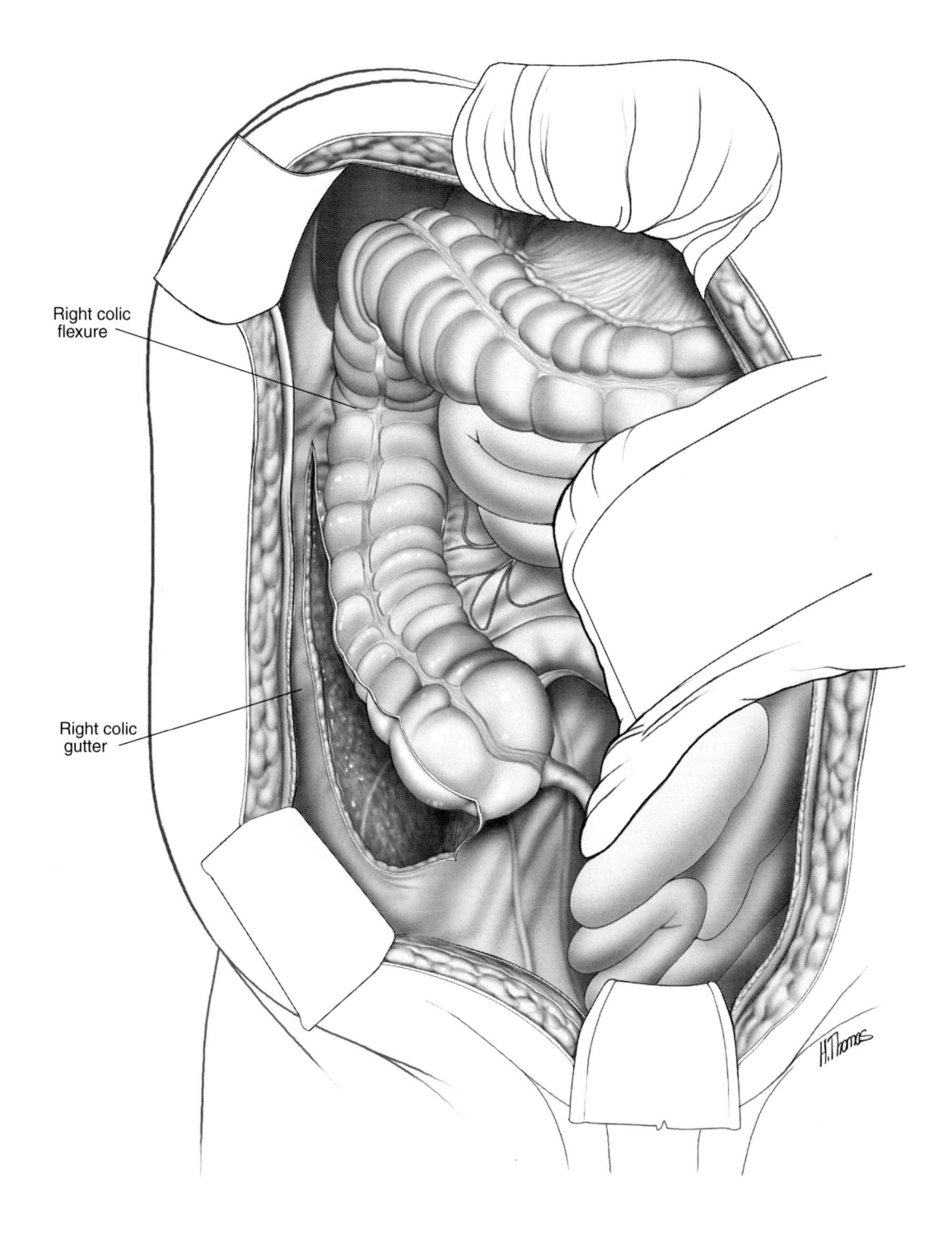

Figure 36–4 • The right colon is mobilized along the white line of Toldt.

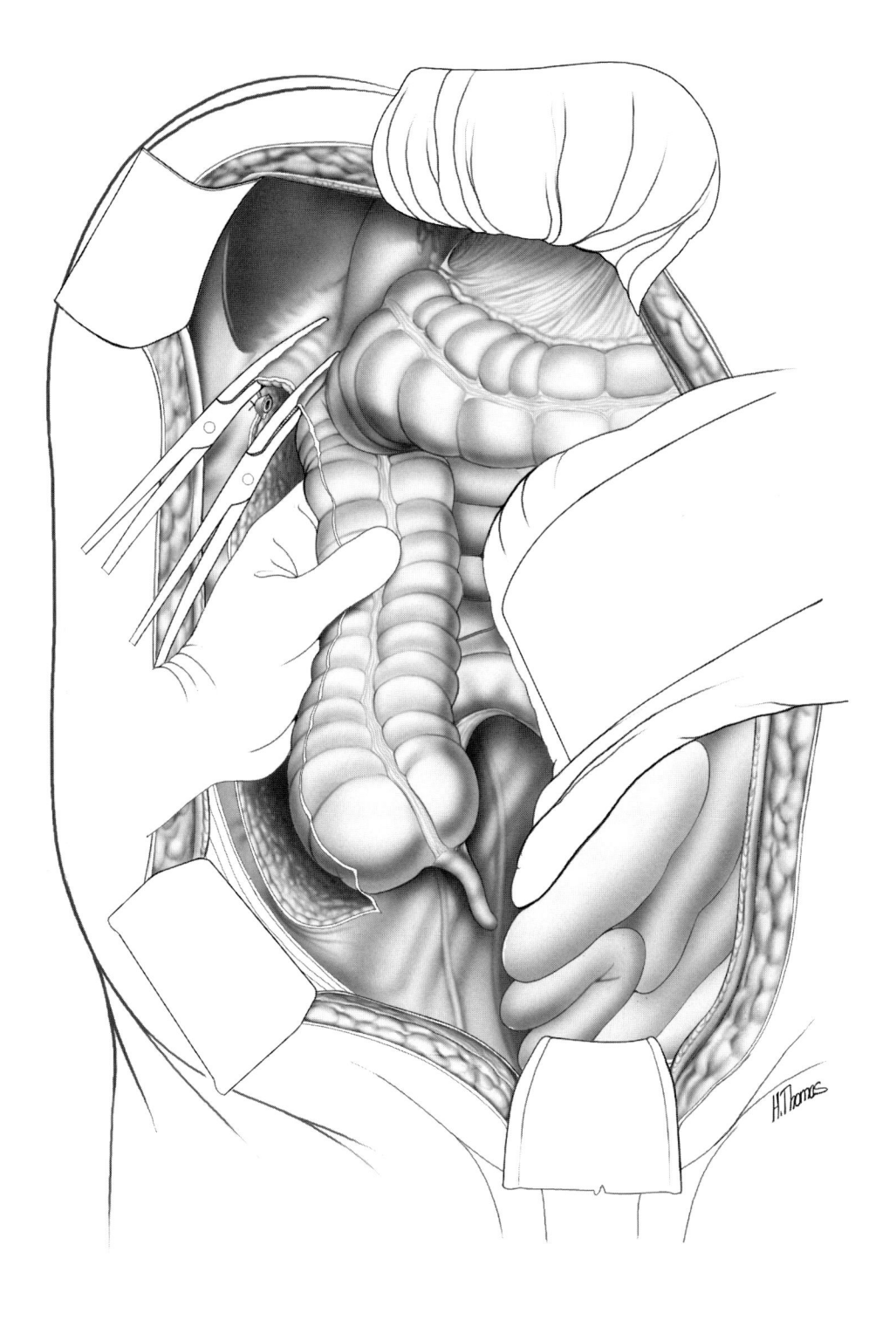

Figure 36–5 • The hepatic flexure is taken down between clamps.

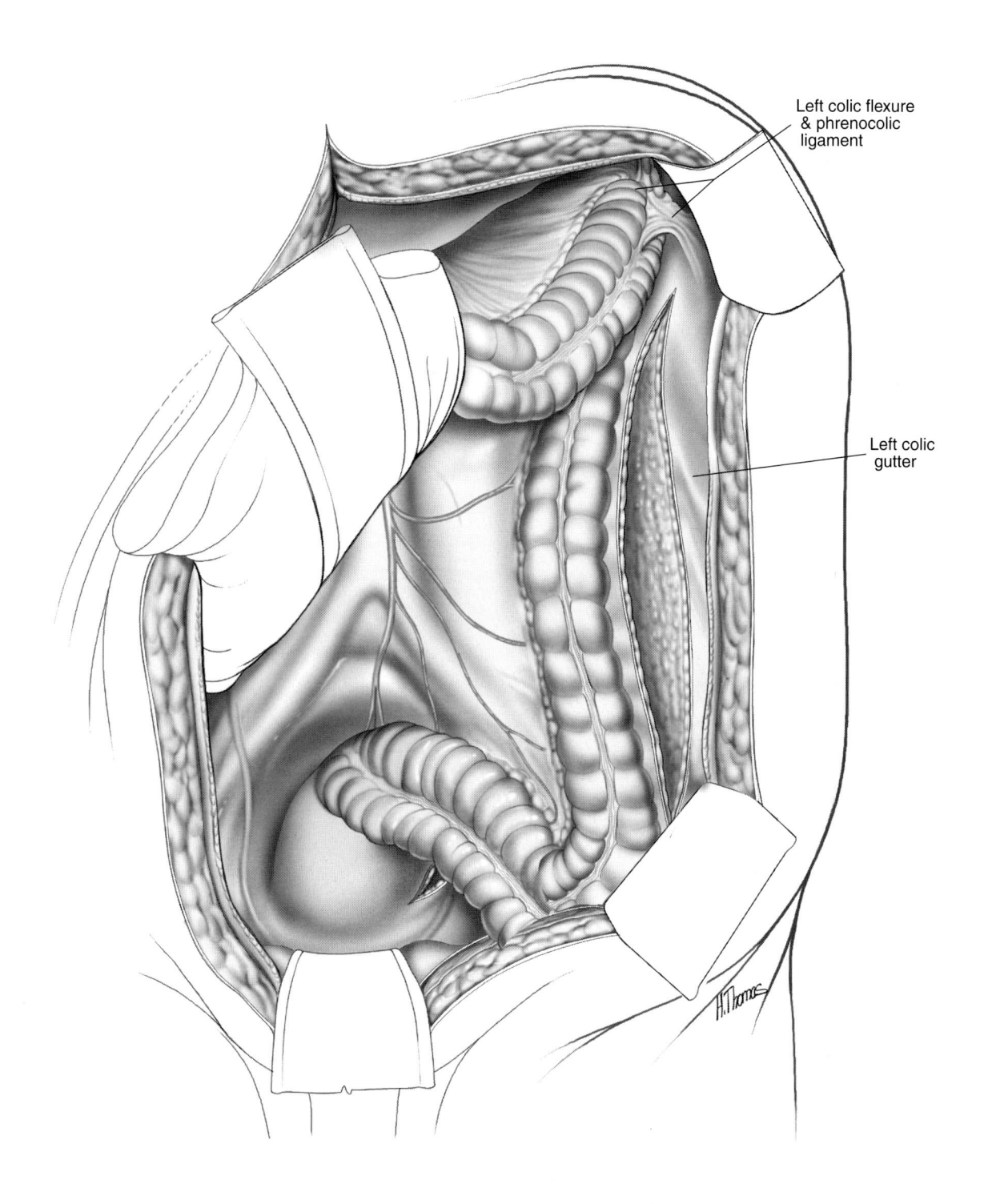

Figure 36–6 • The left colon is mobilized in a similar fashion.

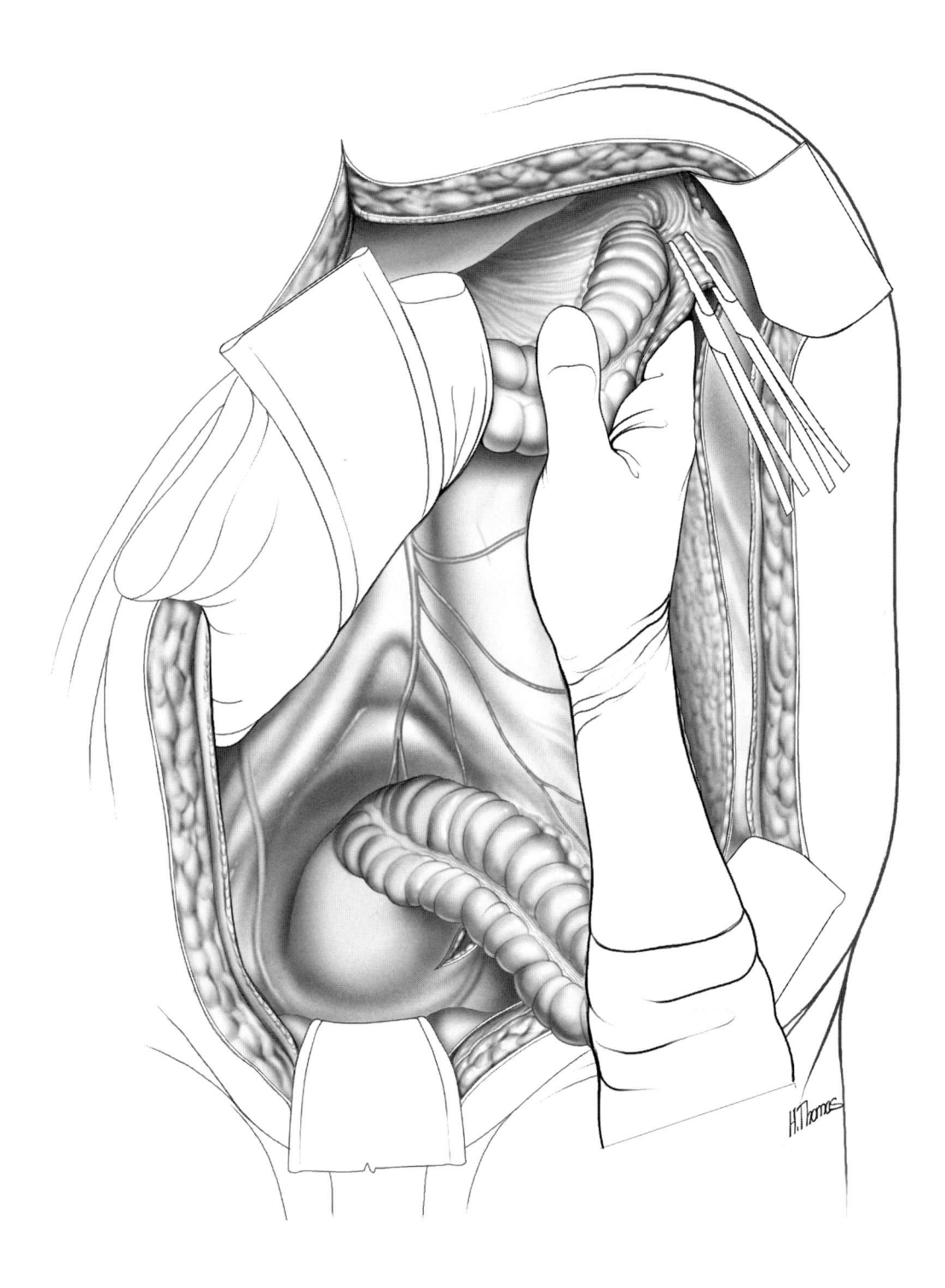

Figure 36-7 • The splenic flexure is taken down, and care is taken not to injure the spleen.

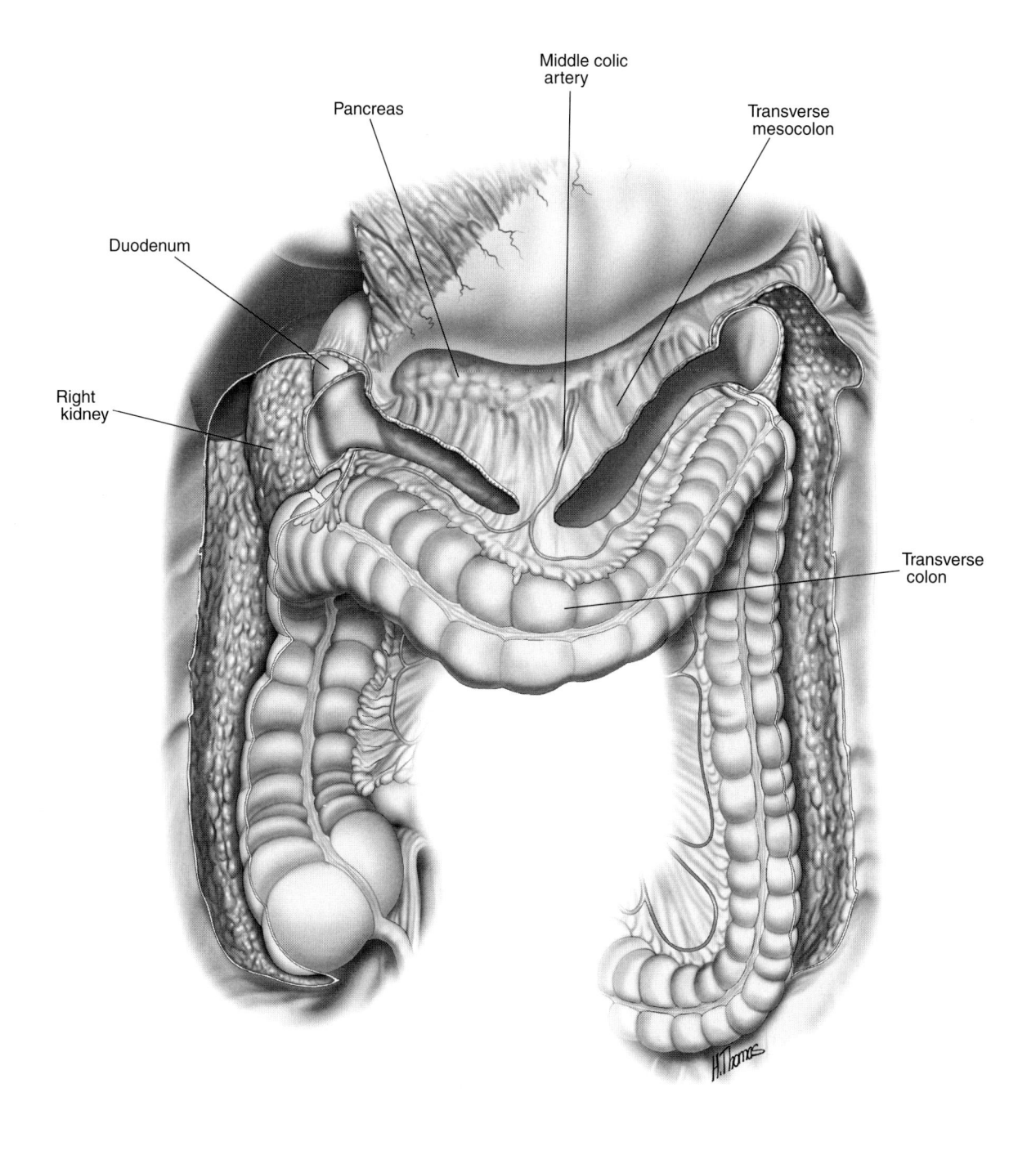

Figure 36–8 • The transverse mesocolon is divided, and the middle colic vessels are identified.

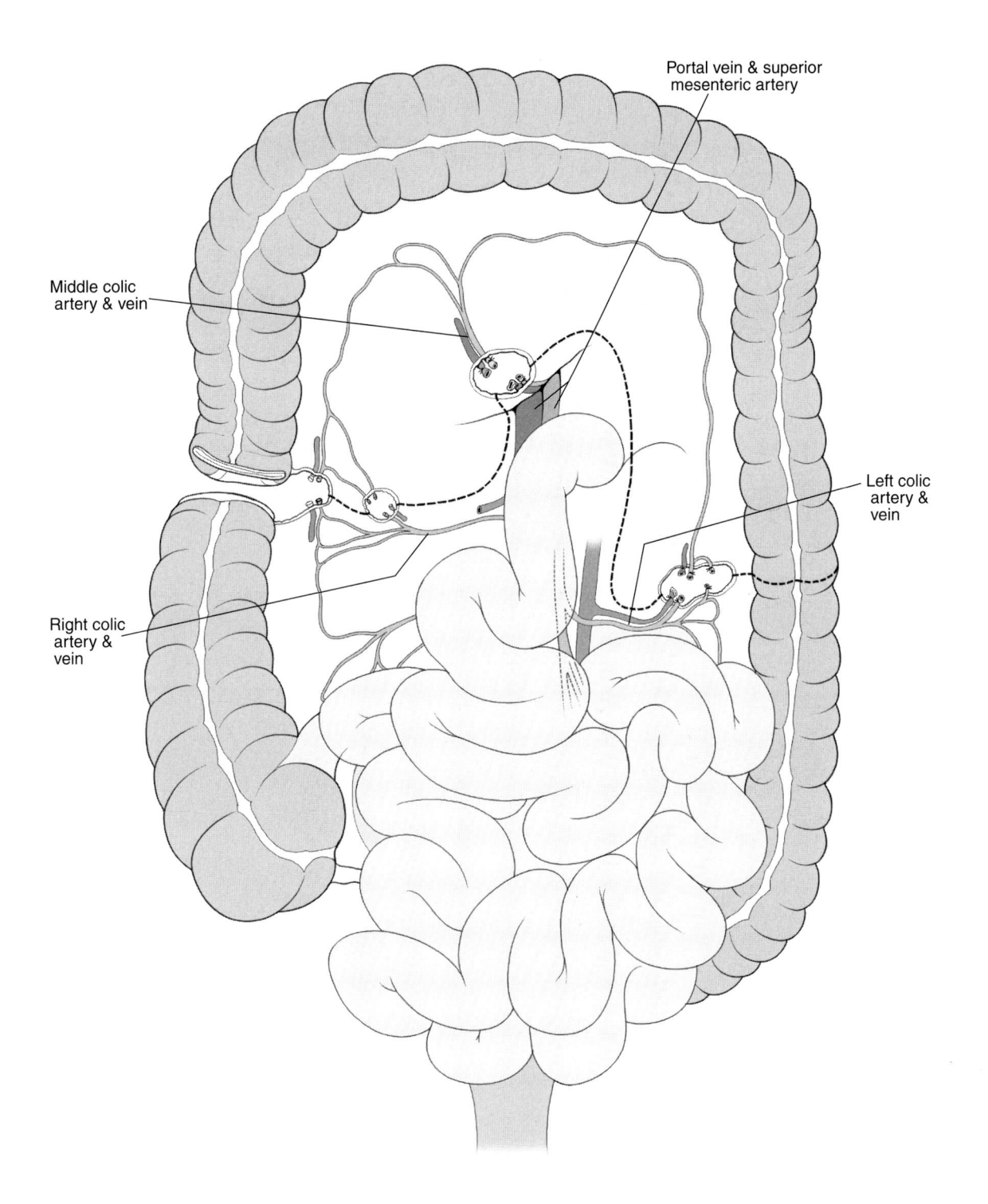

Figure 36-9 • The transverse colectomy is completed, taking into consideration the vascular supply to be preserved.

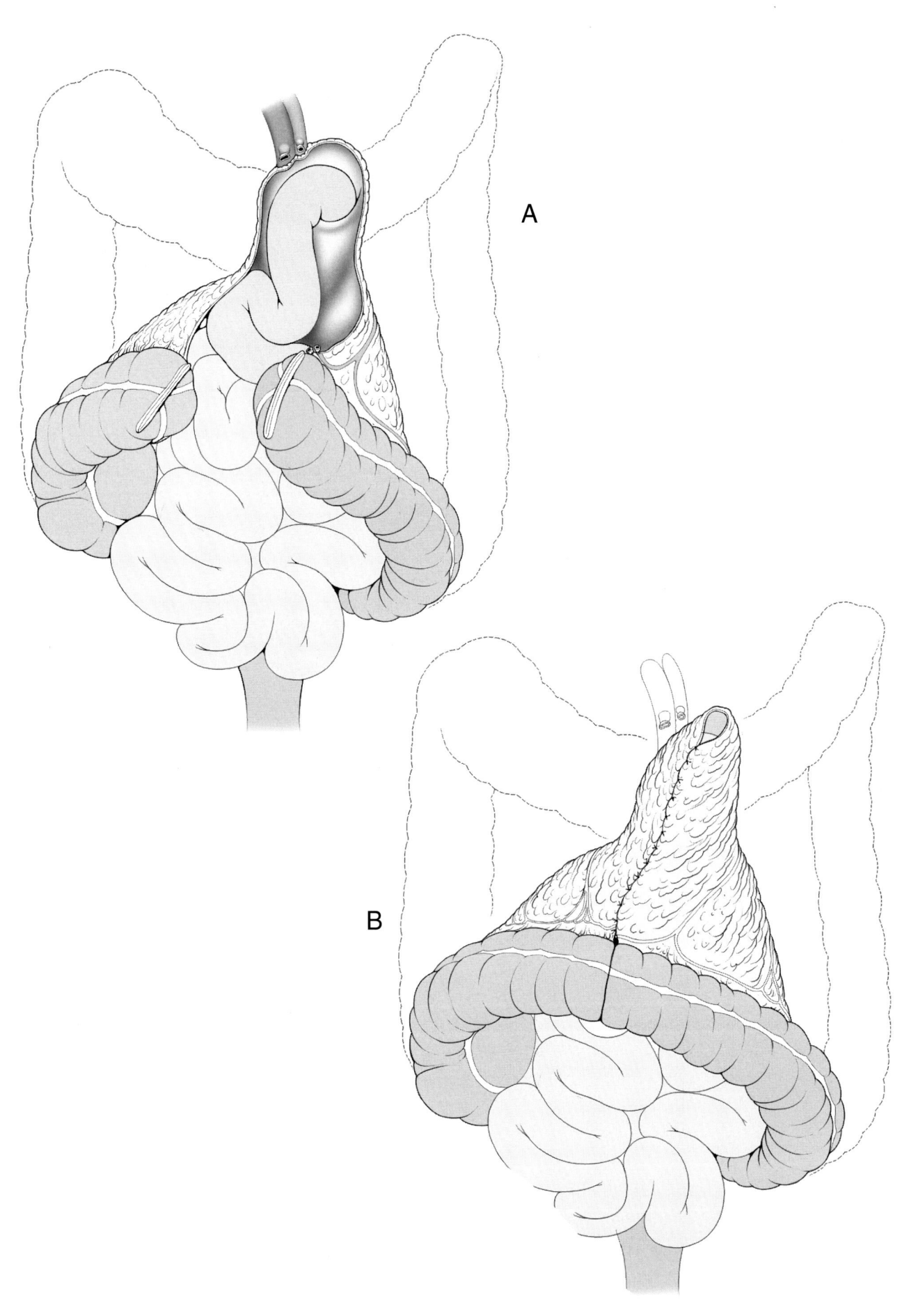

Figure 36–10 • **A**, The mesentery is reapproximated.
B, A colo-colic anastomosis is performed.

Chapter 37
Sigmoid Colectomy

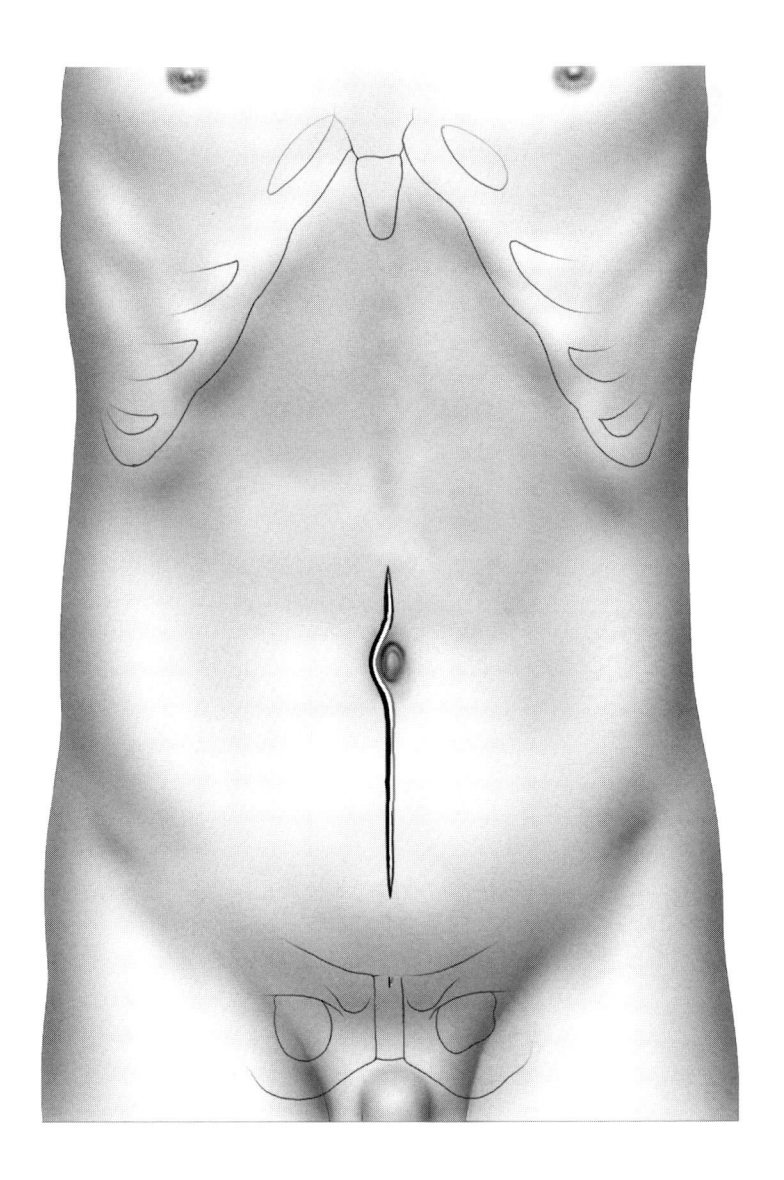

Figure 37–1 • A lower midline abdominal incision is performed.

312 • Part IV LOWER ABDOMEN

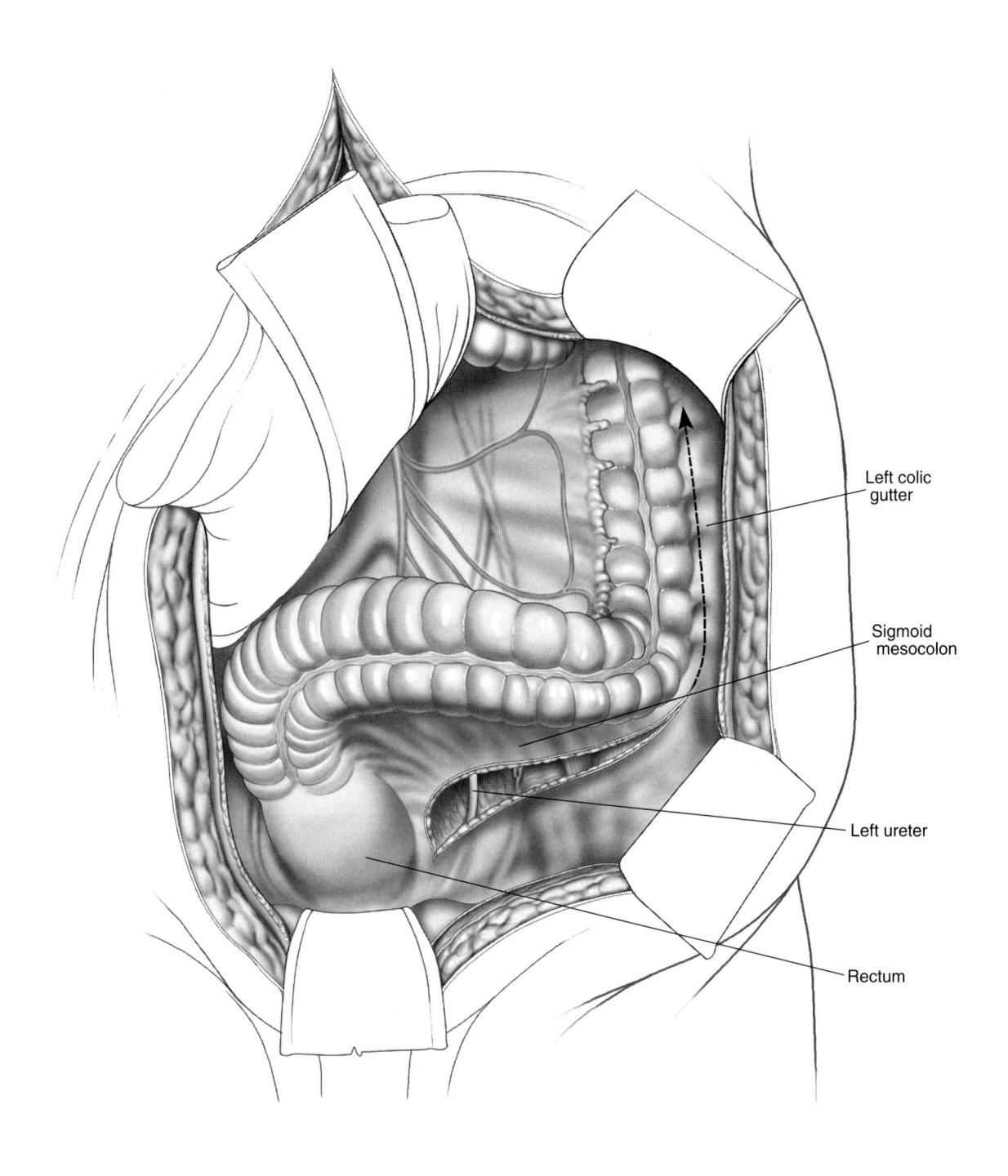

Figure 37-2 • An incision is made along the left colic gutter.

Sigmoid Colectomy • 313

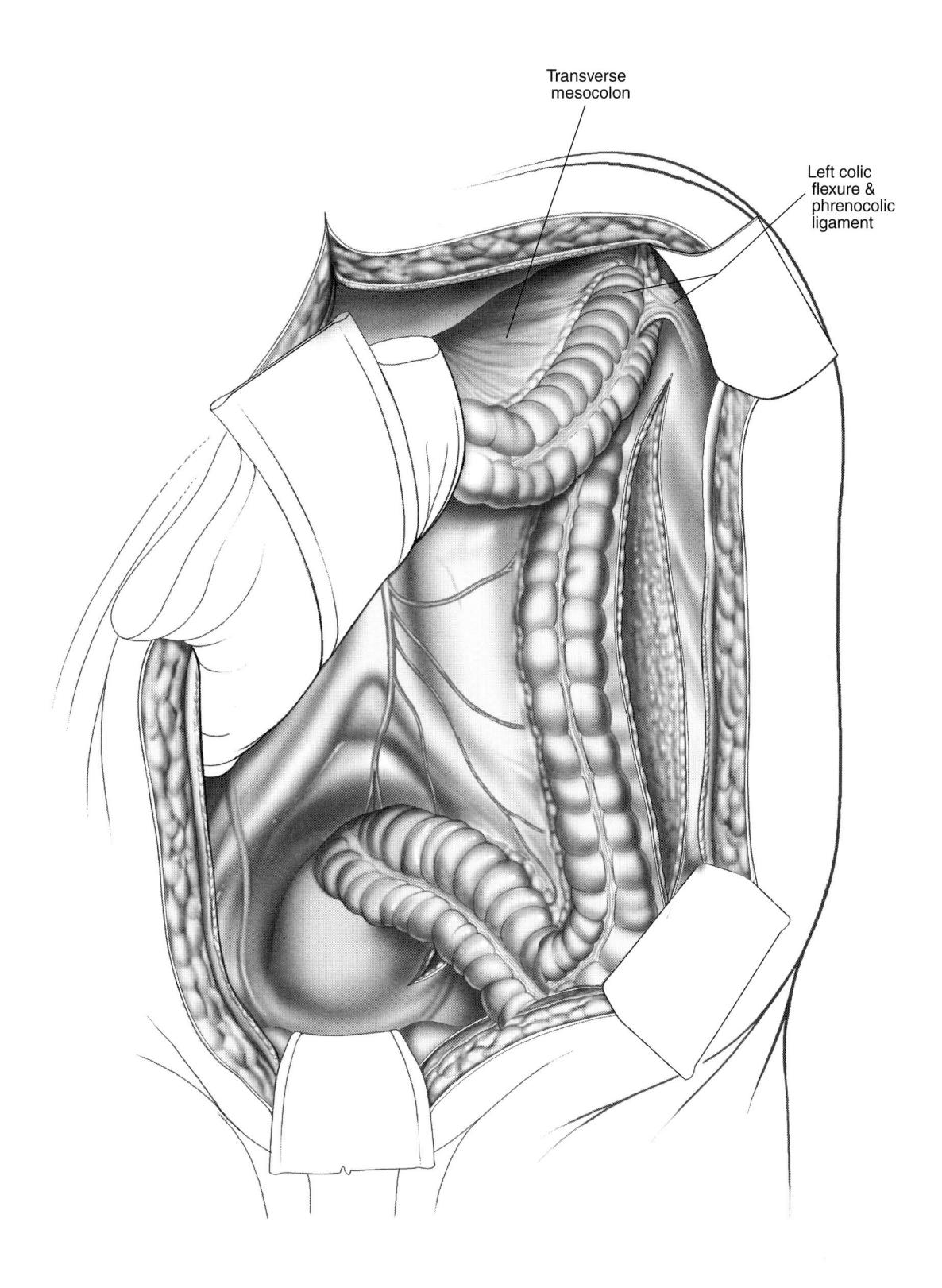

Figure 37–3 • The incision is carried along the white line of Toldt to the splenic flexure.

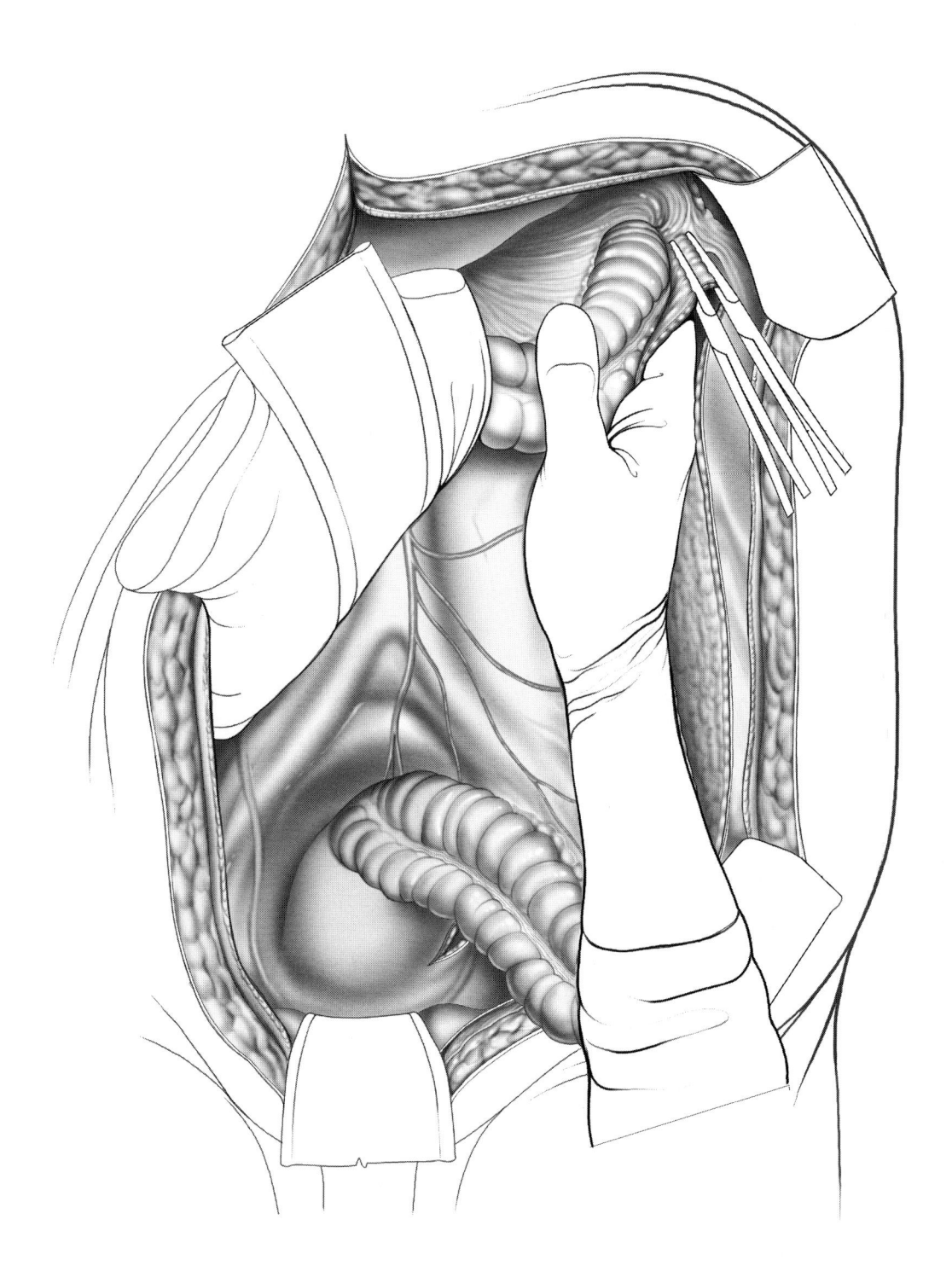

Figure 37–4 • The inferior mesenteric vessel and the sigmoid vessels are identified in the sigmoid mesocolon. The splenic flexure can be taken down if necessary.

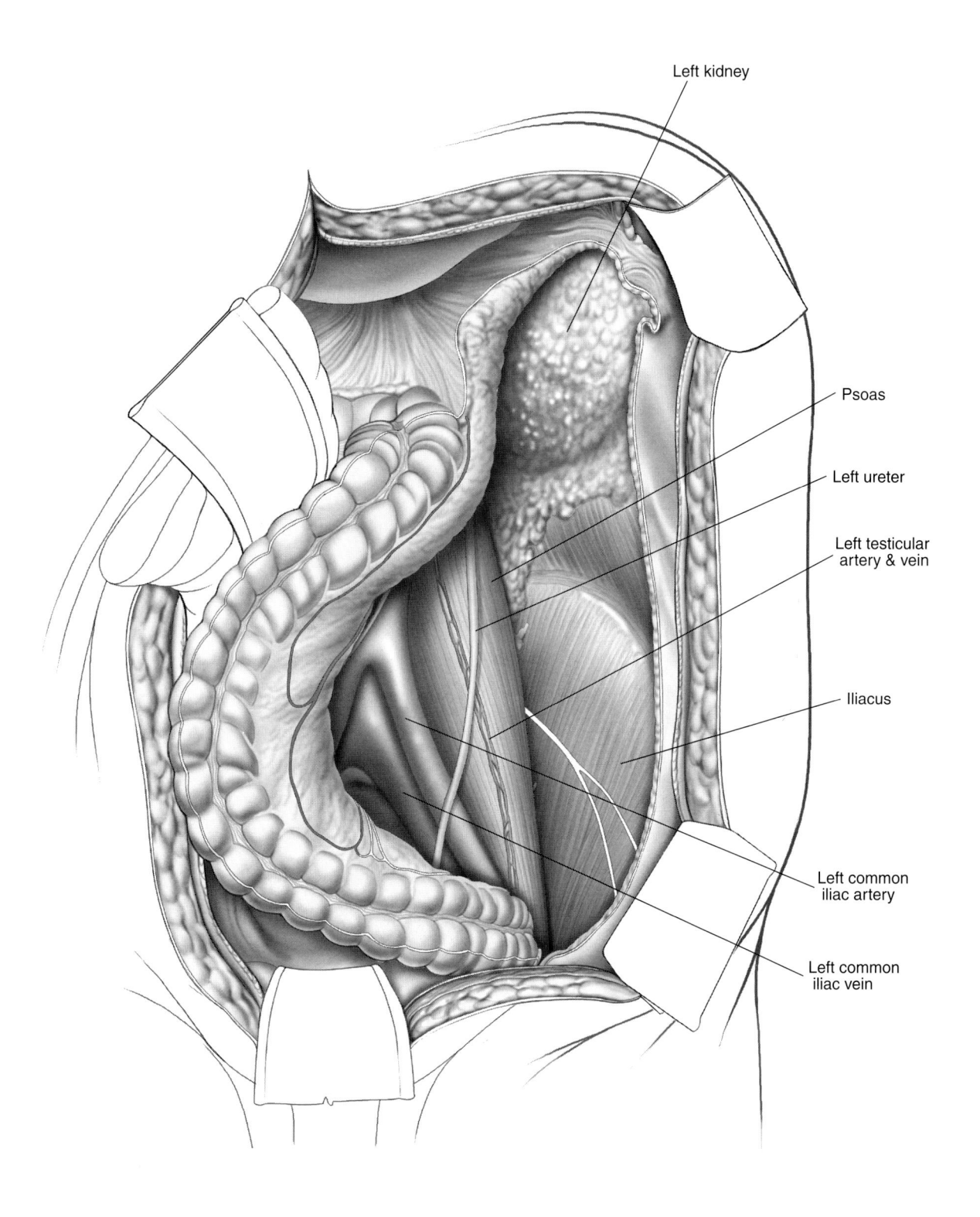

Figure 37–5 • The sigmoid is reflected medially and the ureter is identified.

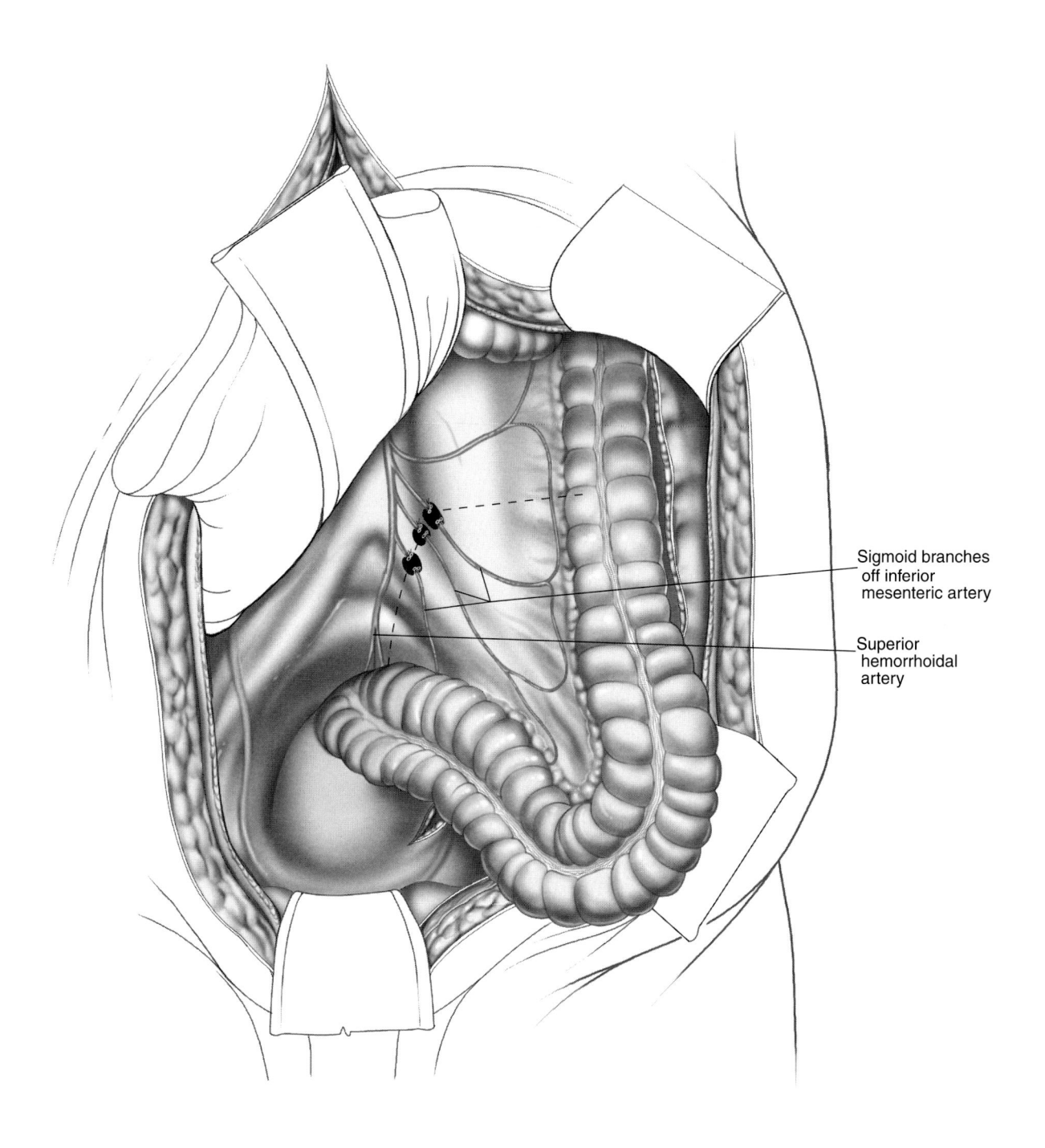

Figure 37–6 • The sigmoid branches are divided, leaving the superior hemorrhoidal artery intact. The line of resection along the mesentery is illustrated.

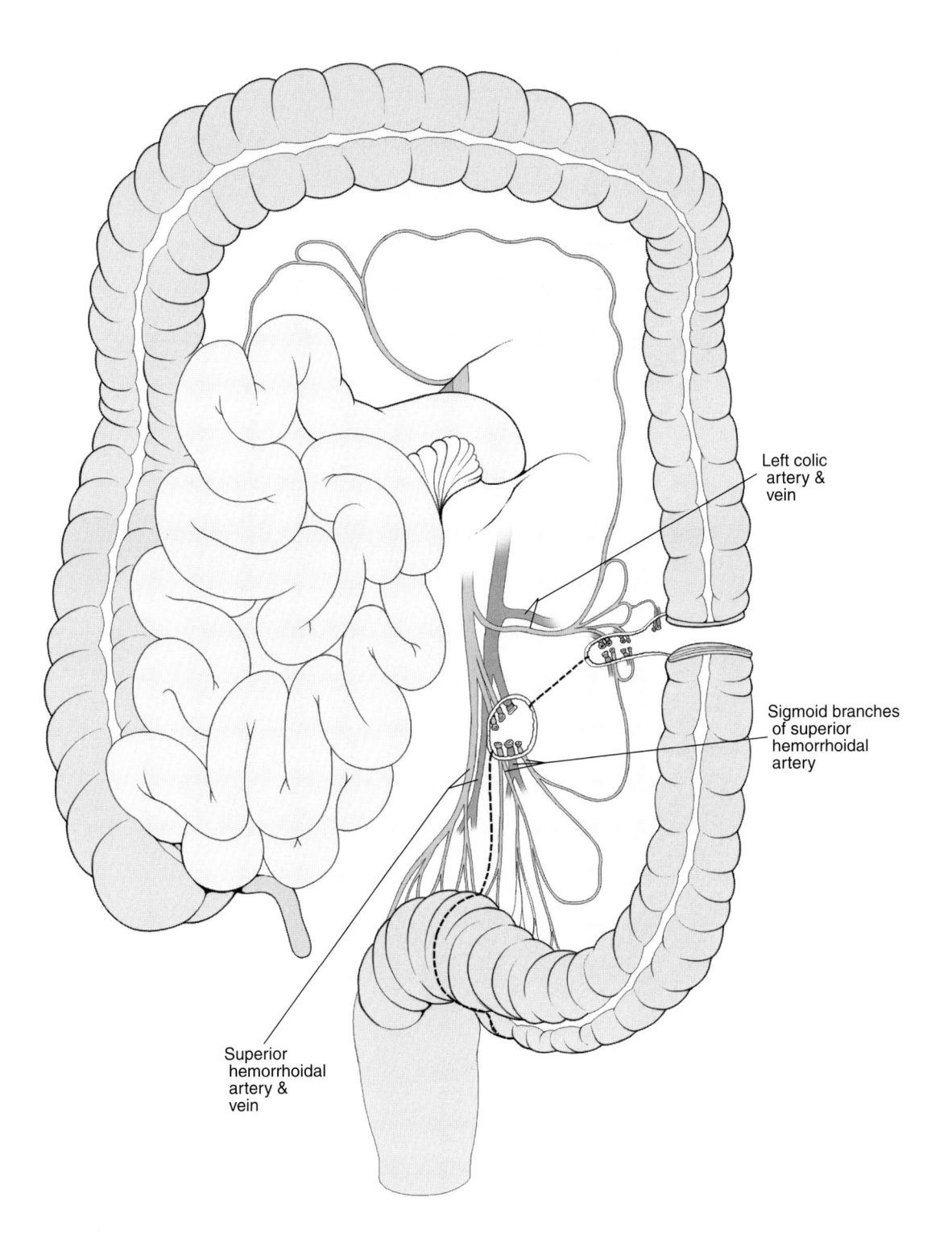

Figure 37–7 • The sigmoid branches supplying the segment of the colon to be removed are ligated flush with the inferior mesenteric artery, and the colon is removed.

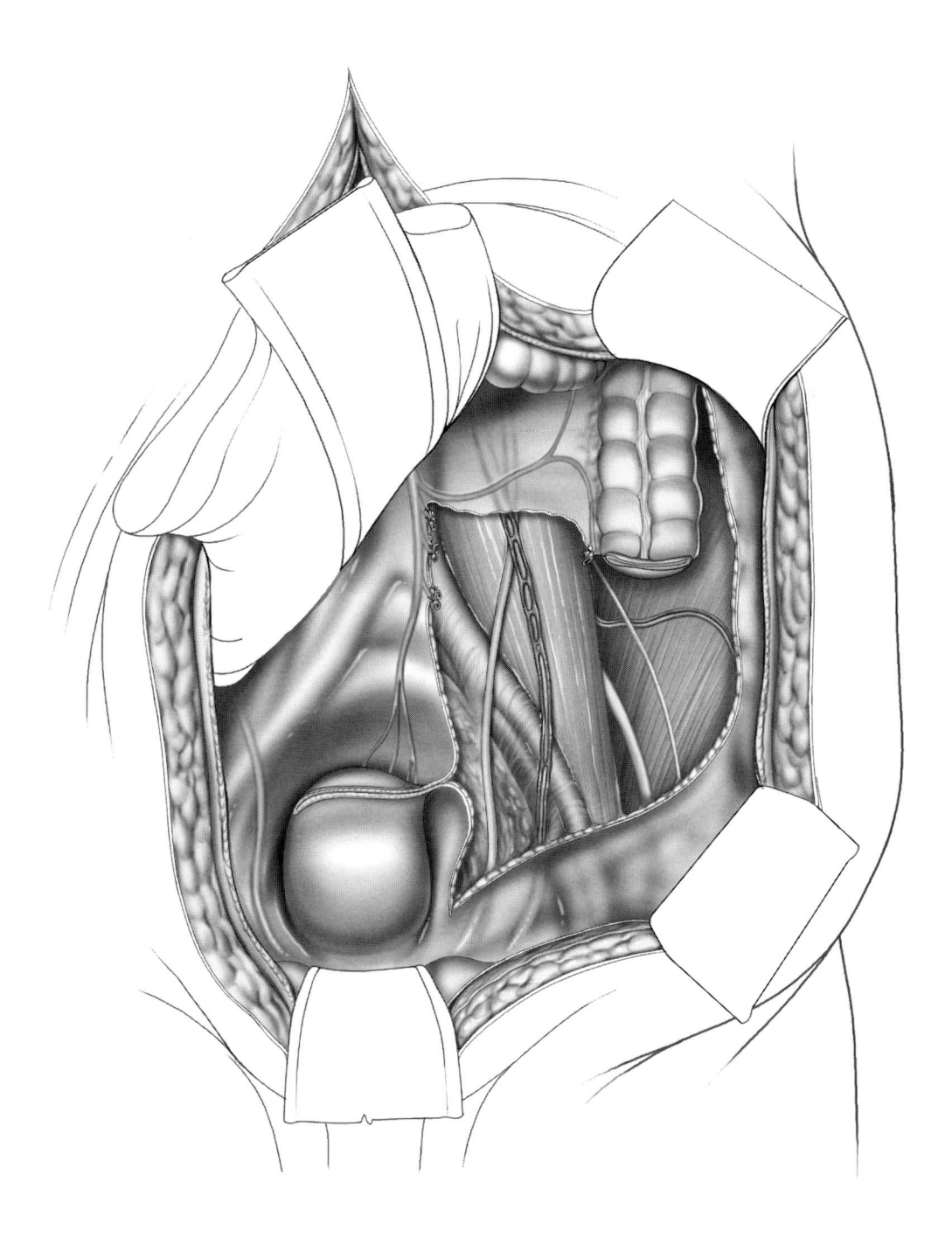

Figure 37–8 • The resection is completed.

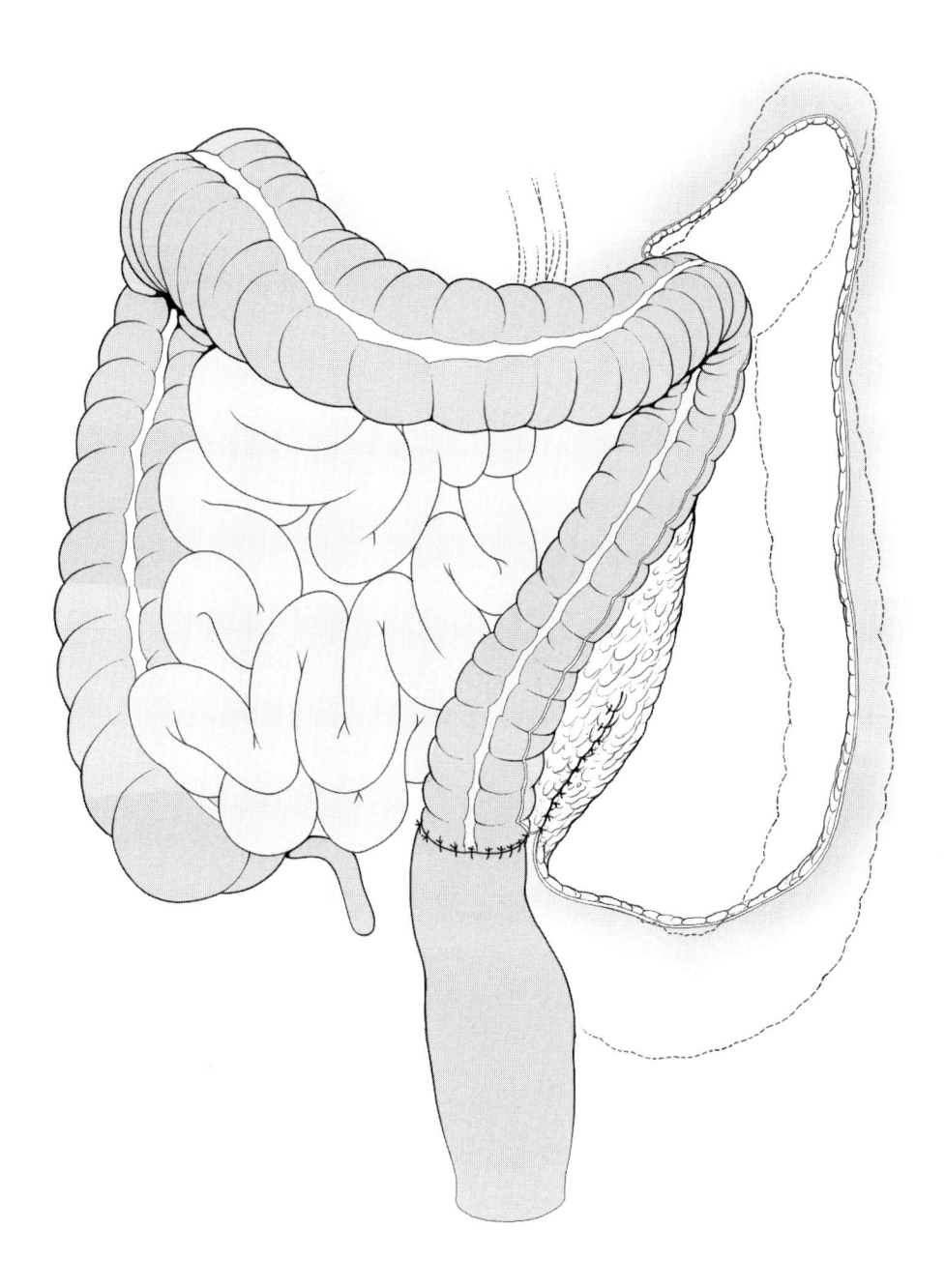

Figure 37–9 • The divided mesentery is closed. The splenic flexure is mobilized, if necessary, to create a tension-free anastomosis.

Chapter 38
Low Anterior Resection

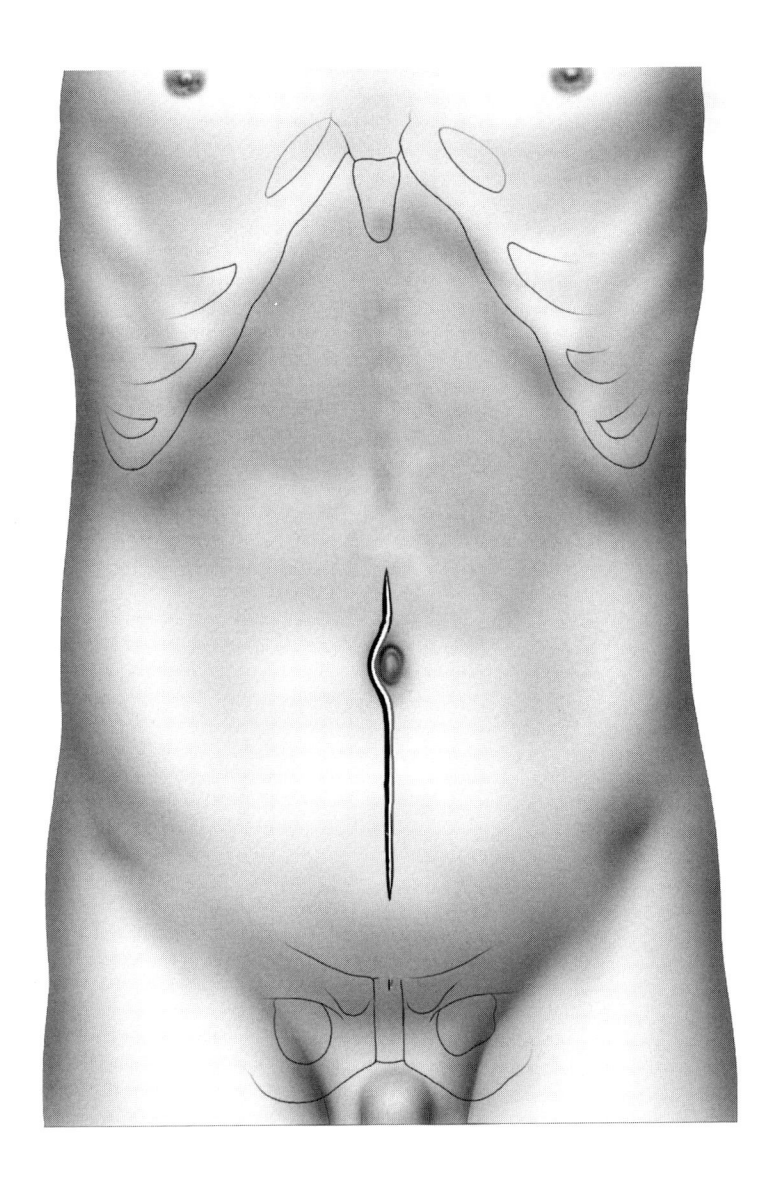

Figure 38–1 • A lower midline abdominal incision is performed.

322 • Part IV LOWER ABDOMEN

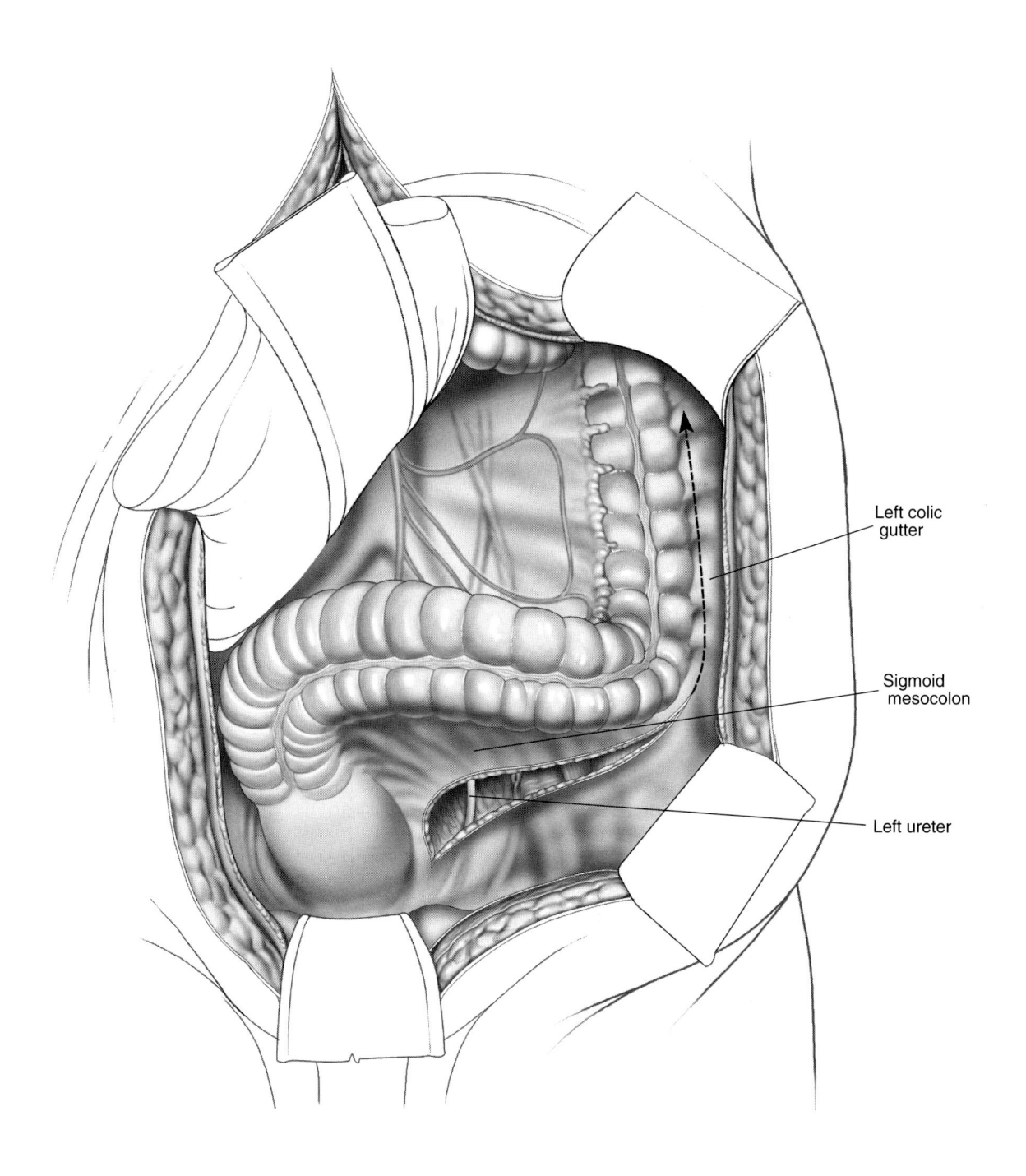

Figure 38–2 • The sigmoid and left colon are mobilized along the white line of Toldt.

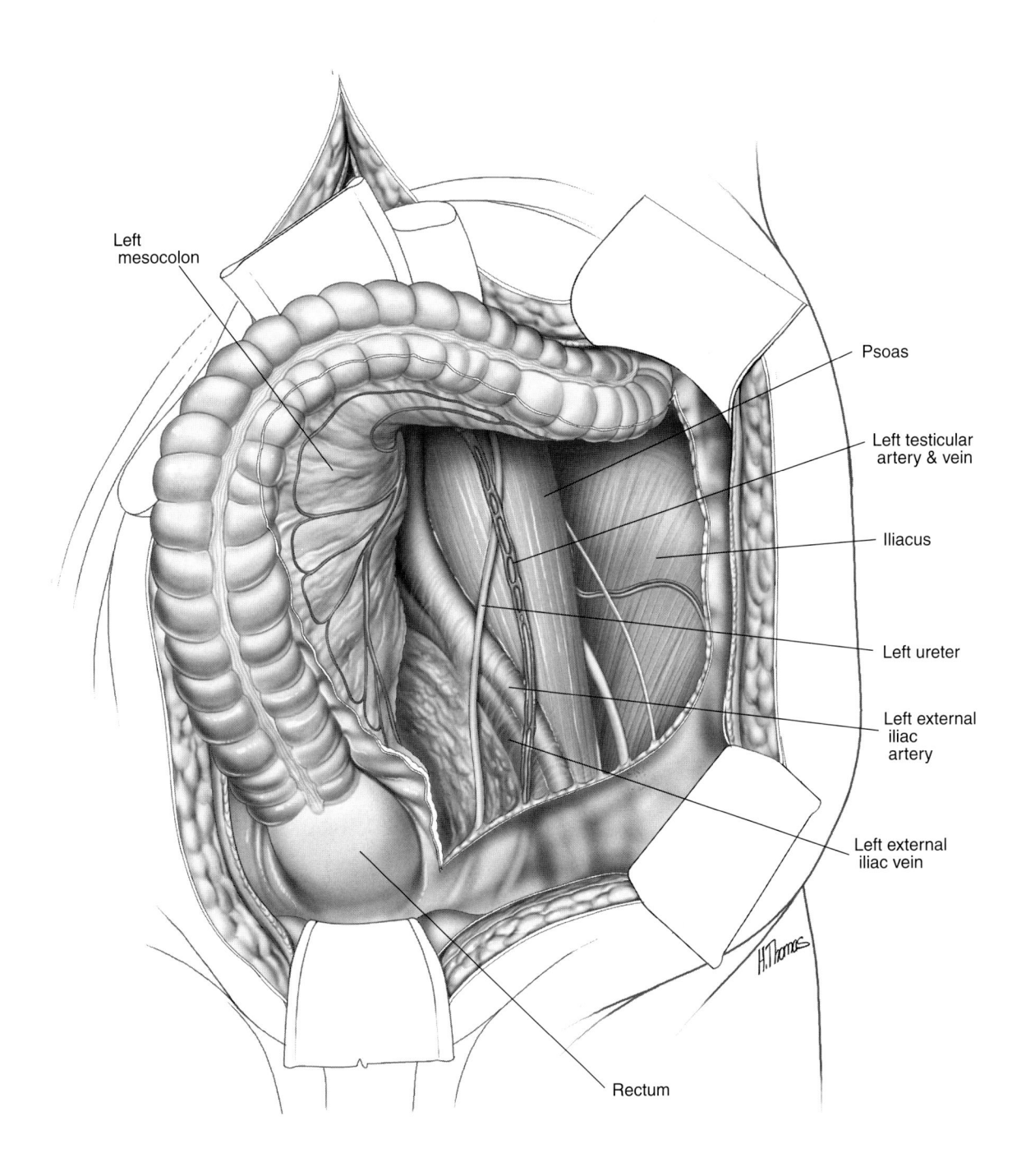

Figure 38–3 • The sigmoid colon is reflected medially, exposing the psoas and the ureter crossing the iliac vessels at the pelvic brim.

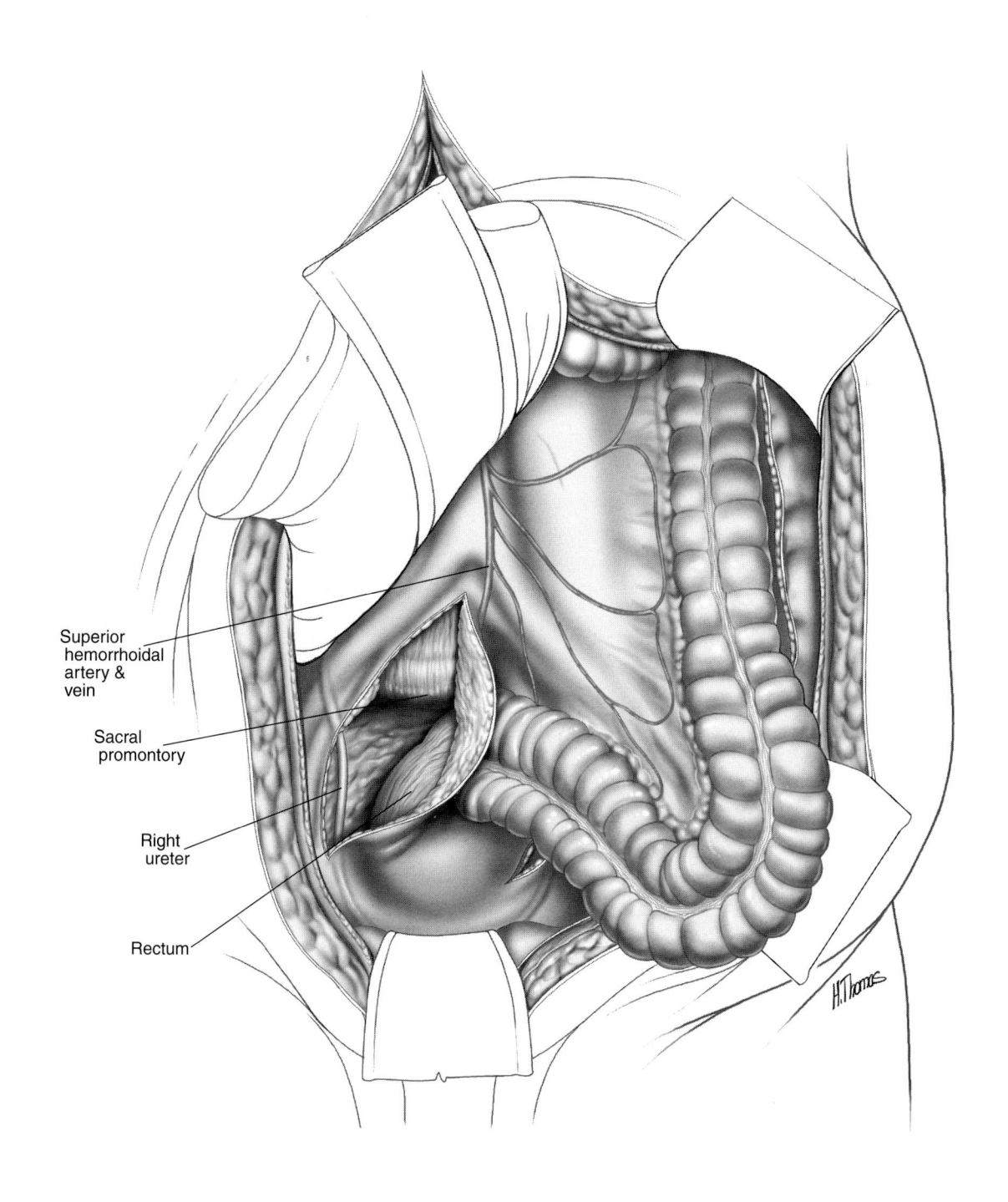

Figure 38–4 • The medial leaf of the sigmoid mesentery is incised from the sacral promontory along the right iliac vessels, identifying the right ureter.

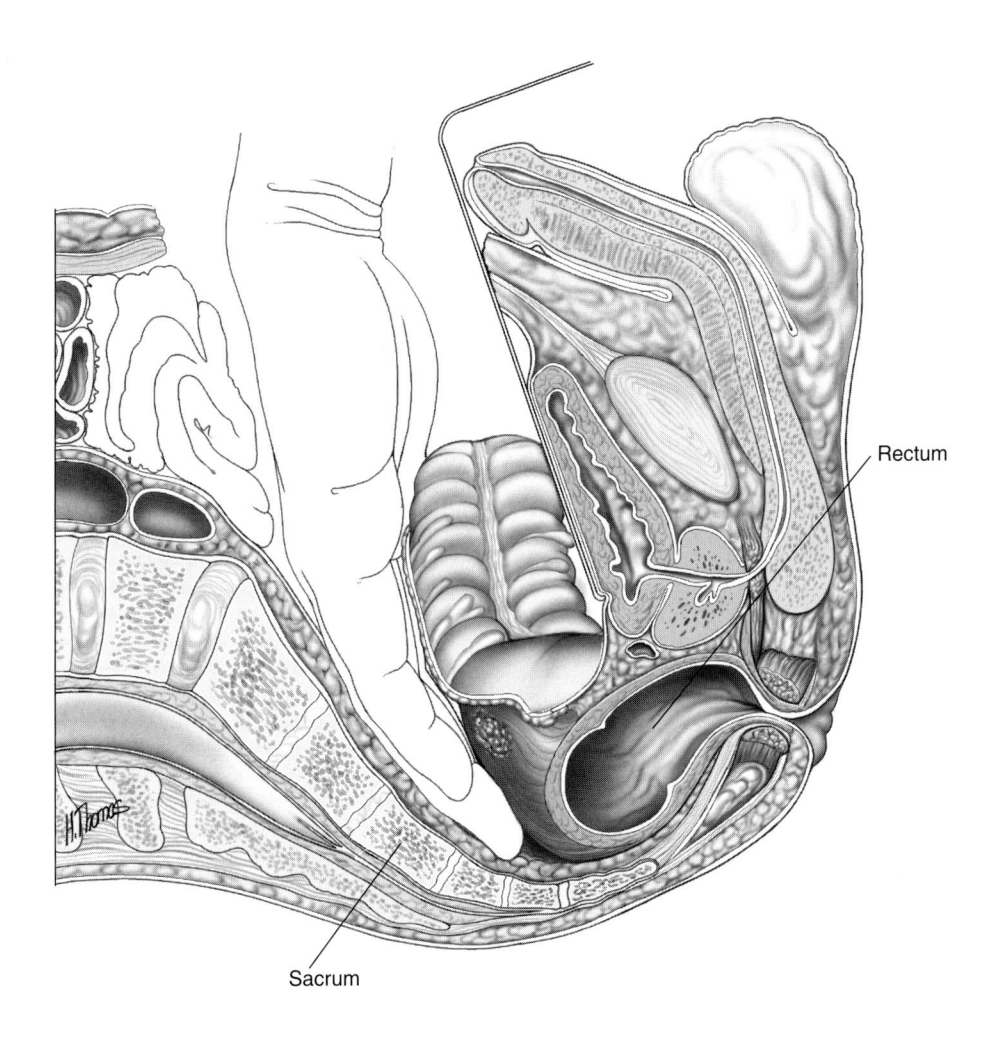

Figure 38–5 • The presacral space is entered, and the rectum is mobilized off the sacrum.

326 • Part IV LOWER ABDOMEN

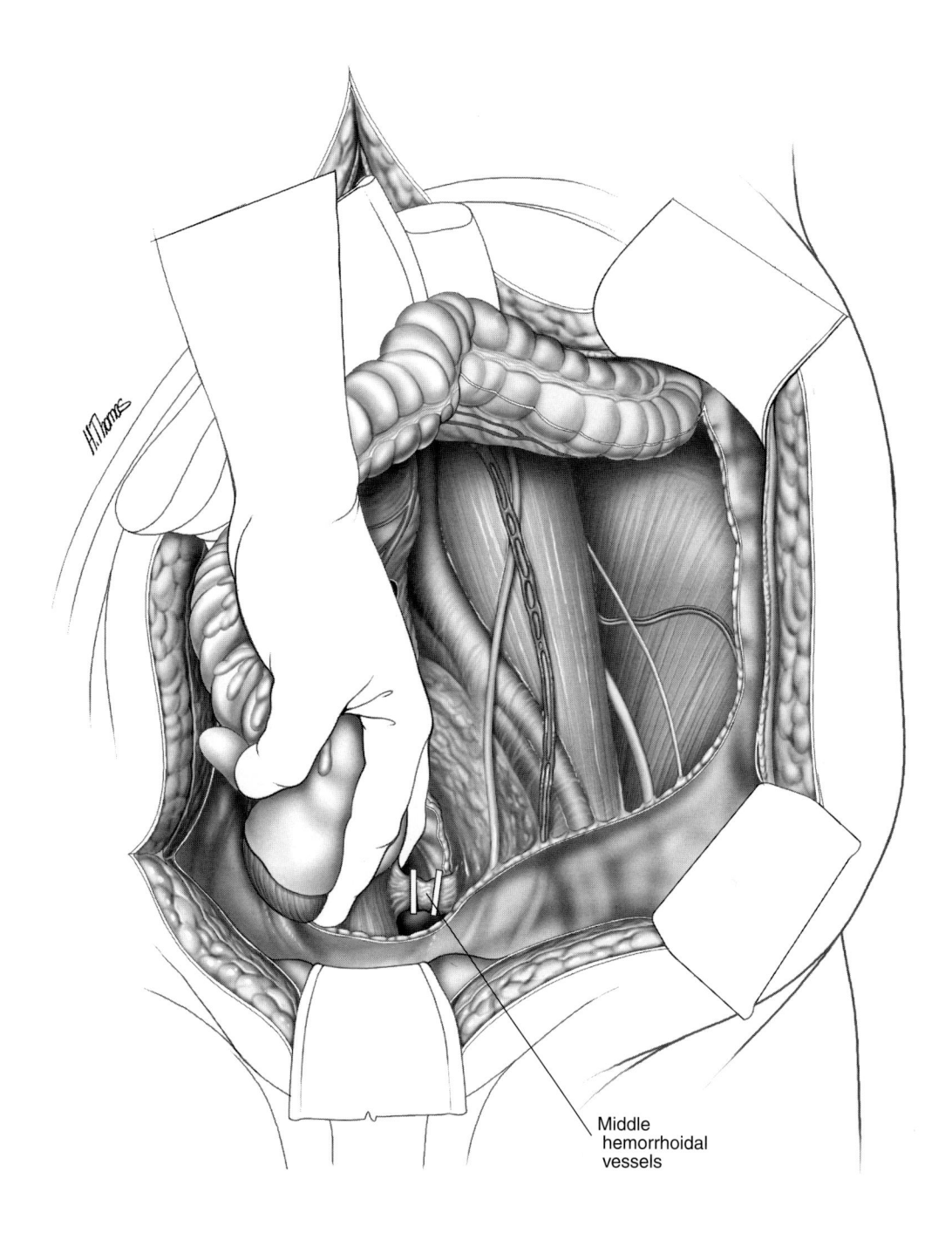

Figure 38–6 • On the left, the middle hemorrhoidal vessels are divided between clips.

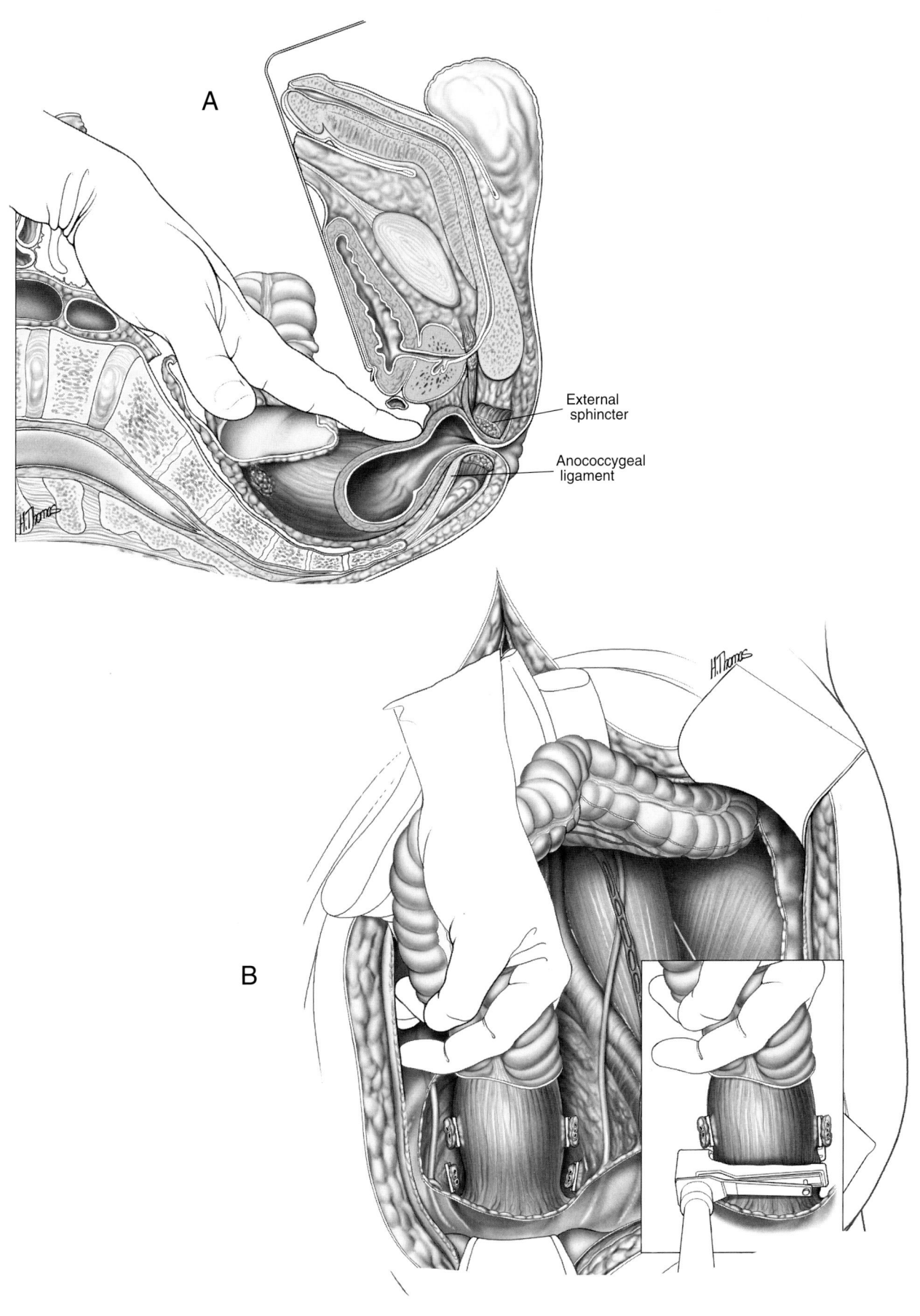

Figure 38–7 • **A,** In men, the vesicorectal space is mobilized by incising the peritoneal reflection between the posterior bladder and rectum.

B, A midrectal resection is illustrated after the middle hemorrhoidal vessels on the right are divided.

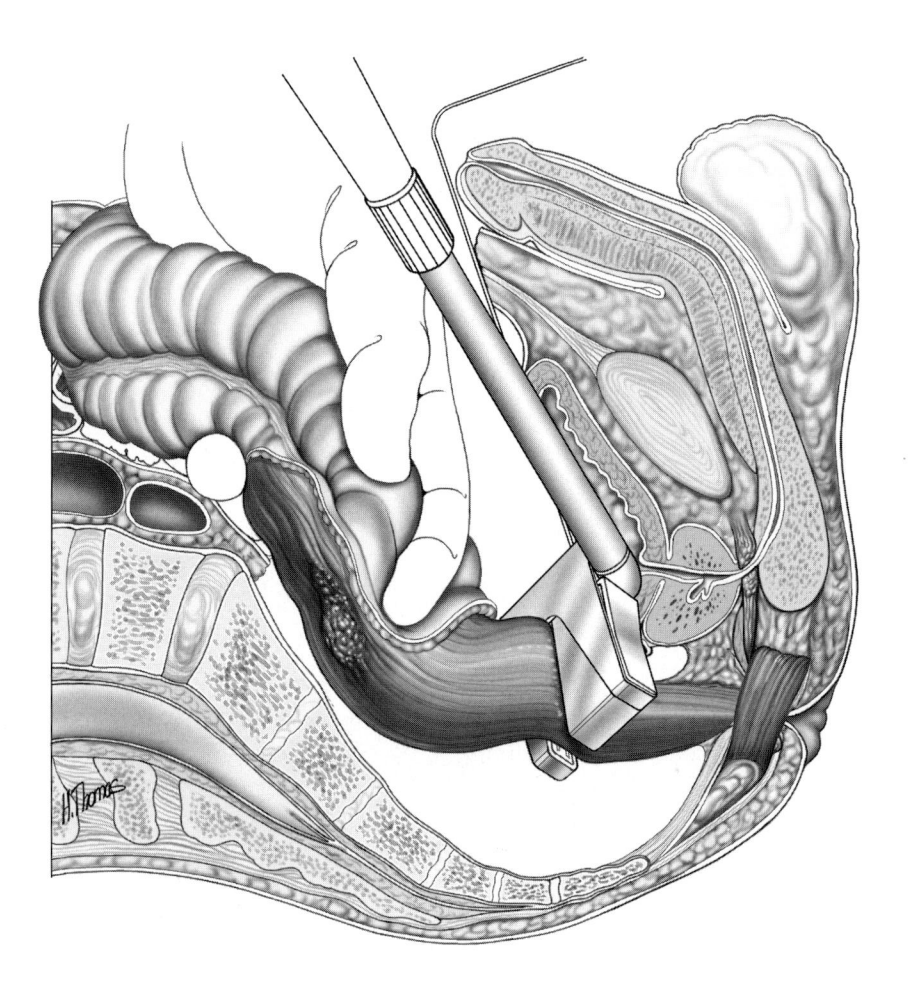

Figure 38–8 • A lateral view depicts the line of resection and the utility of a reticulated stapler.

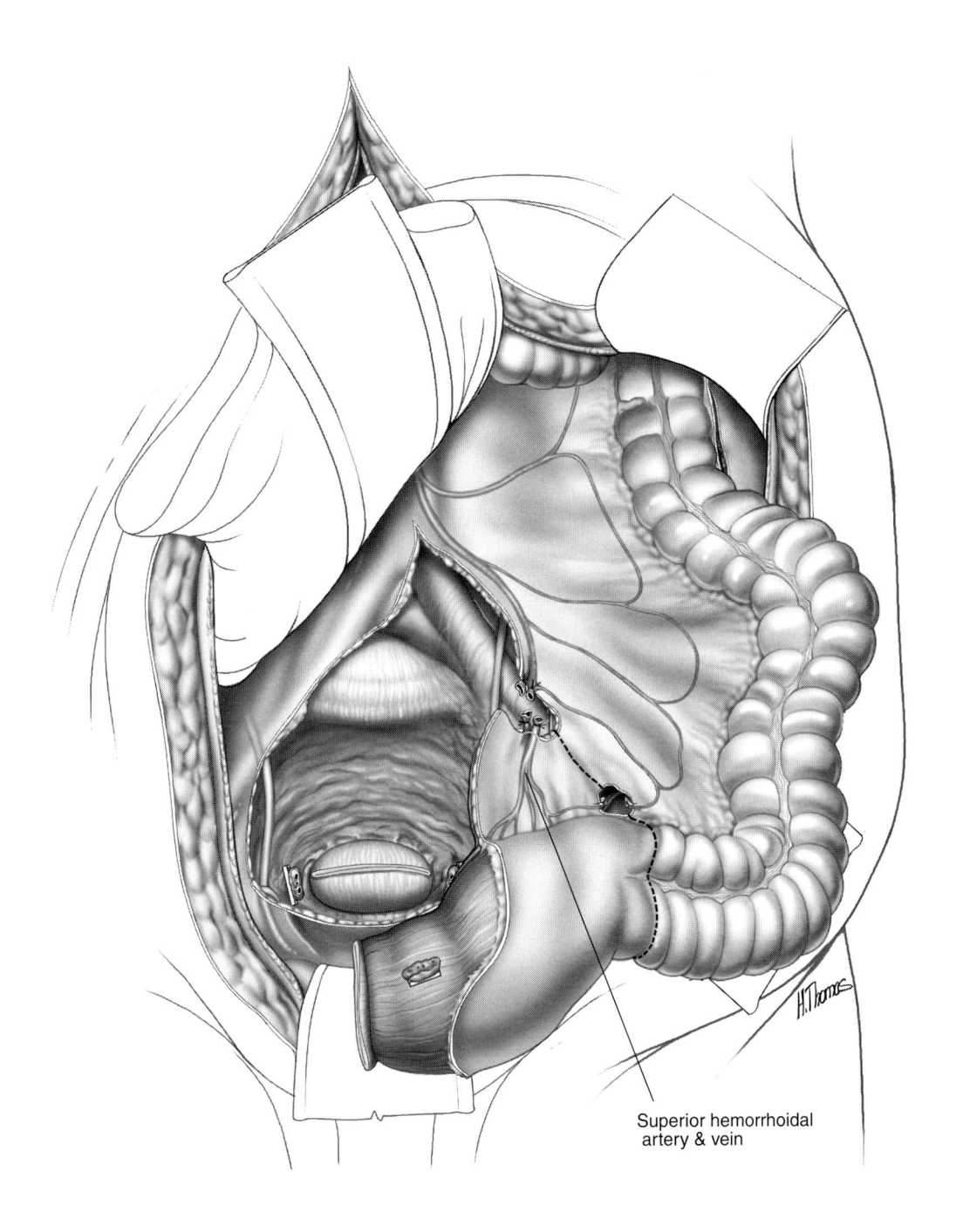

Figure 38–9 • The superior hemorrhoidal artery and vein are divided just distal to the last sigmoidal branch.

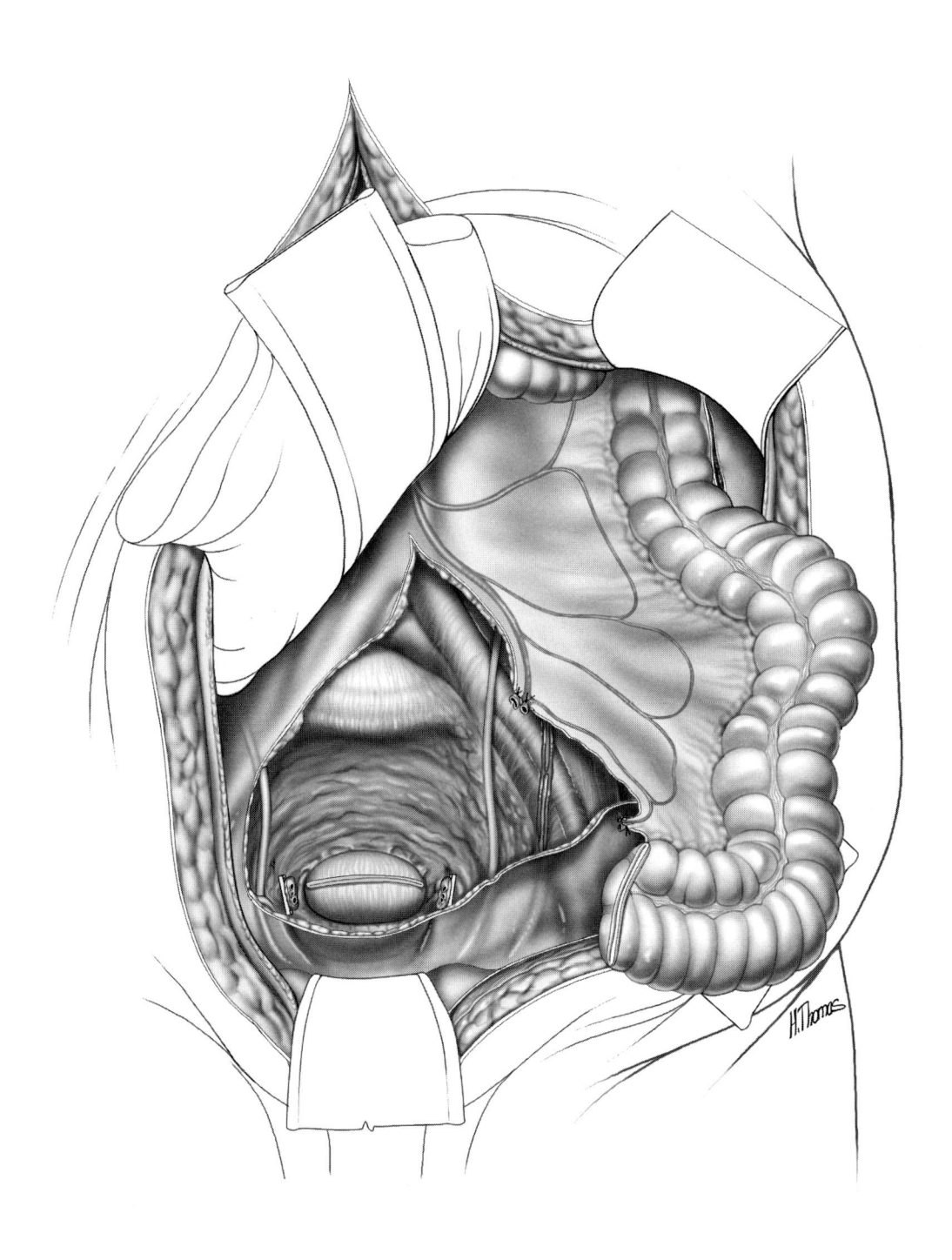

Figure 38–10 • The resected bowel and mesentery are depicted.

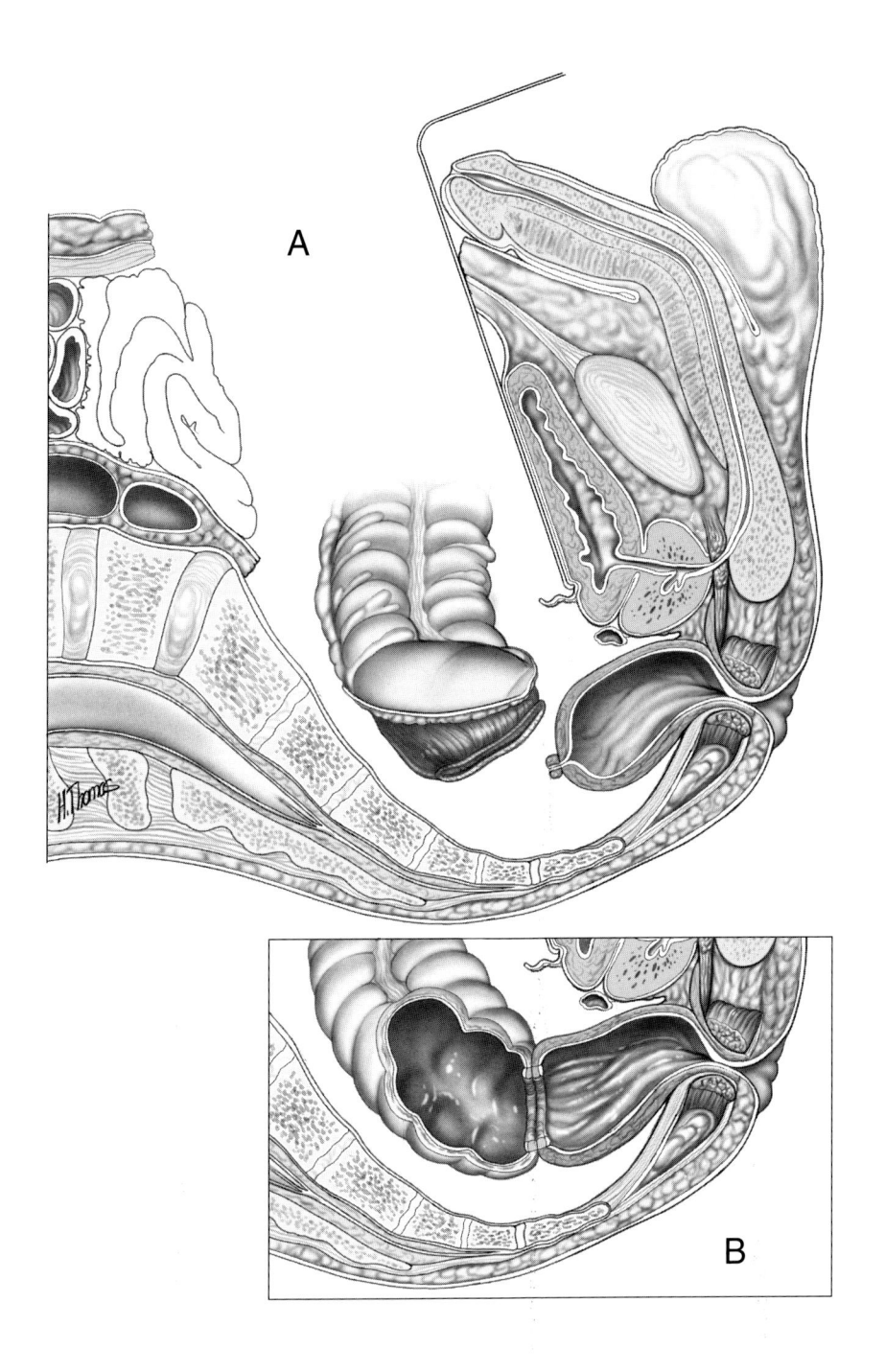

Figure 38–11 • **A,** A colorectal anastomosis can be accomplished via a handsewn or stapled anastomosis.
B, The completed anastomosis is depicted.

Chapter 39
Surgical Anatomy of the Perineum

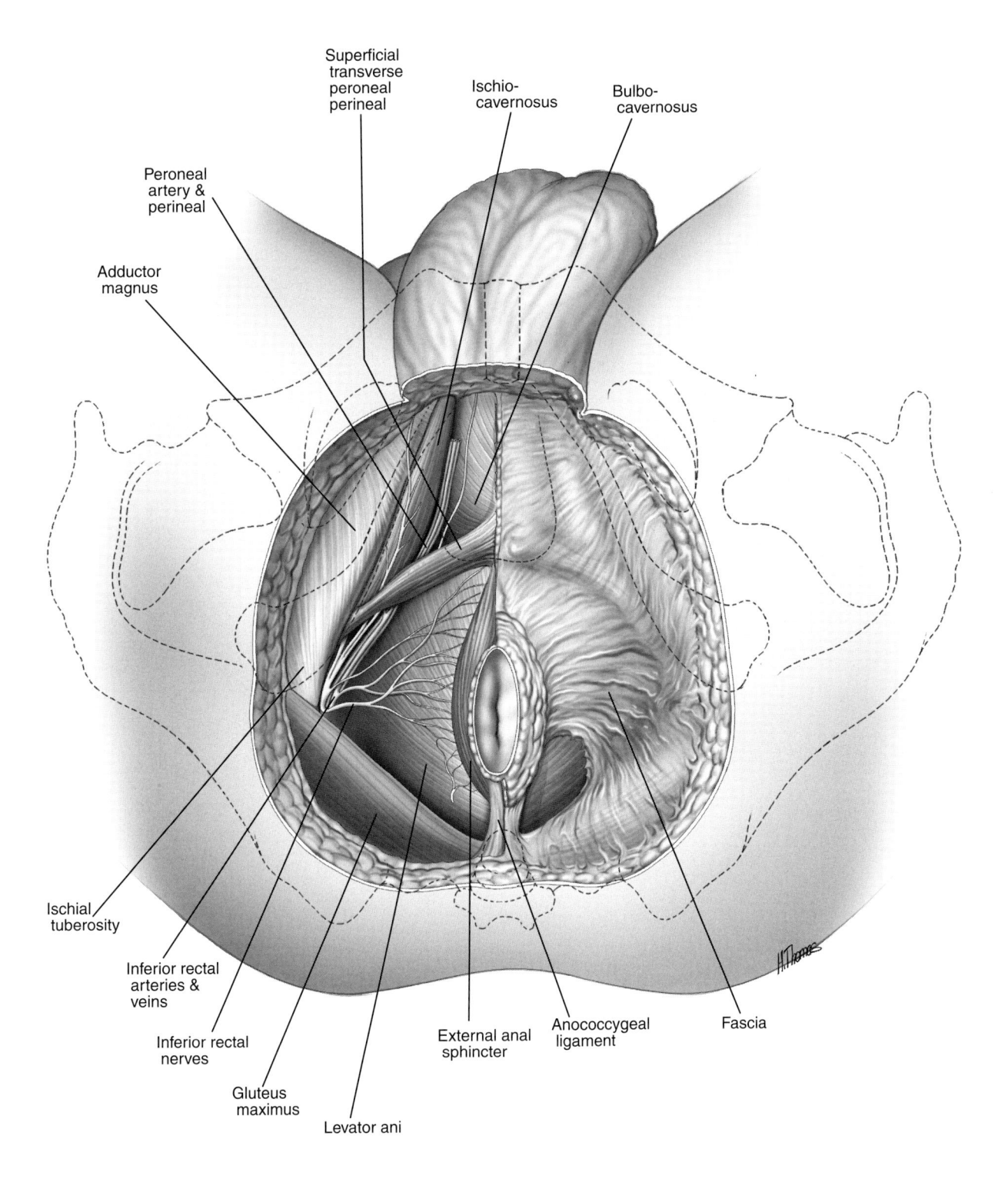

Figure 39–1 • In abdominal perineal resections, the procedure for the abdominal portion is identical to that of a low anterior resection. The anatomy of the perineum is depicted.

Chapter 40
Abdominal Perineal Resection

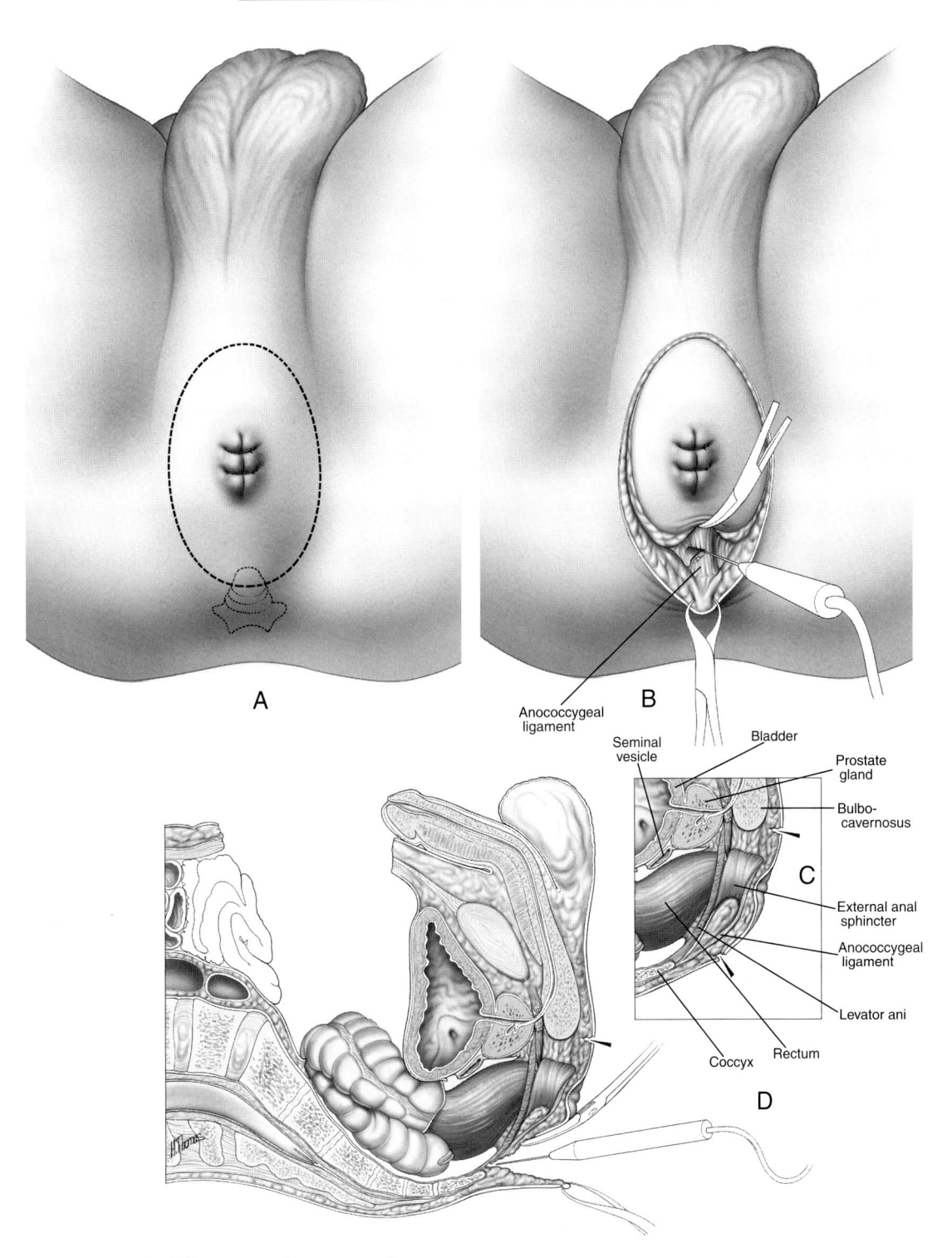

Figure 40–1 • **A,** The anus is sewn shut.

B, A circumferential incision around the anus from ischial tuberosity to ischial tuberosity is performed. The posterior portion of the incision is completed first.

C, A lateral view defines the superior and inferior extents of the incision.

D, Inferiorly, the abdominal cavity is entered above the coccyx in the presacral space.

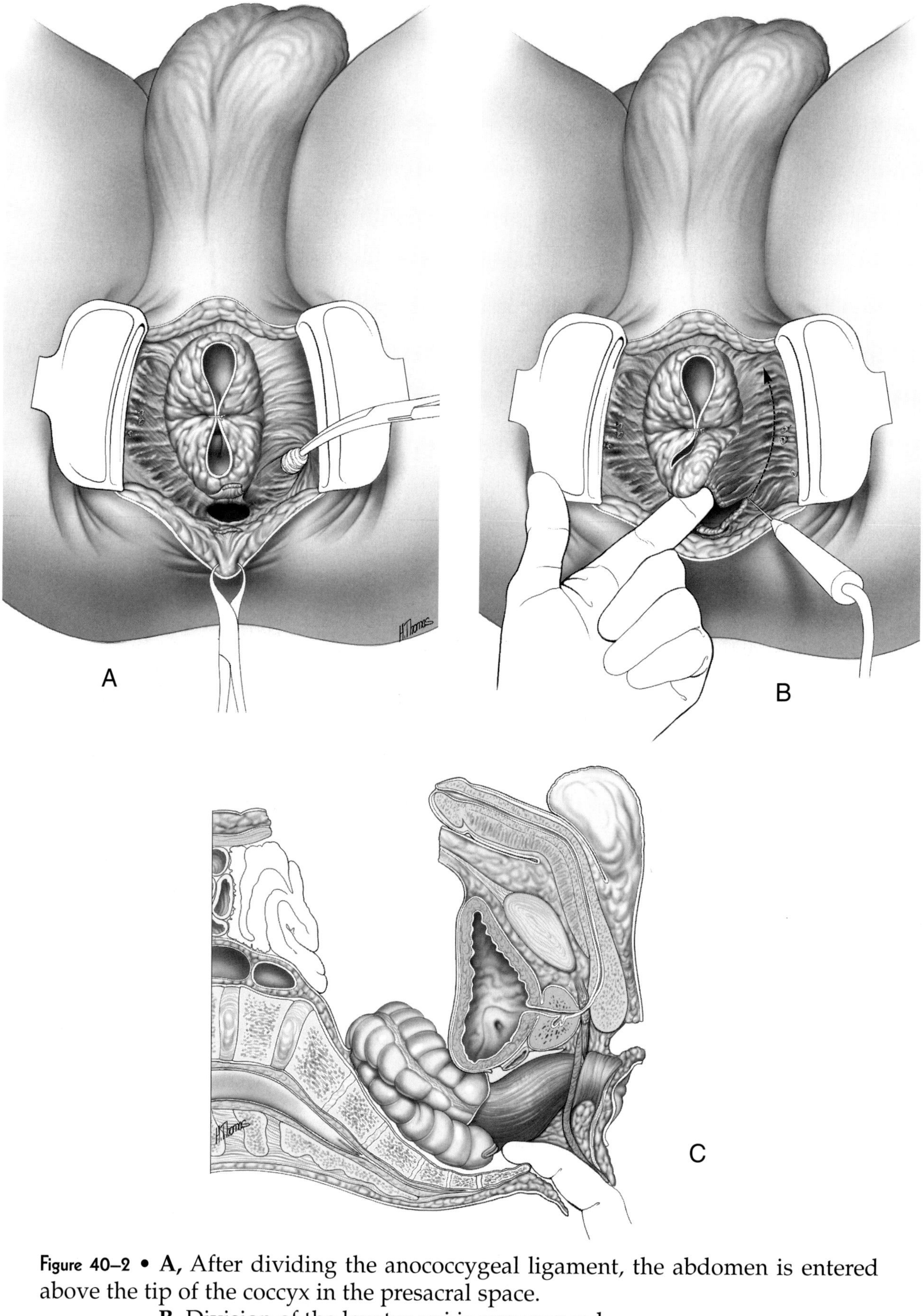

336 • Part IV LOWER ABDOMEN

Figure 40–2 • **A,** After dividing the anococcygeal ligament, the abdomen is entered above the tip of the coccyx in the presacral space.
B, Division of the levator ani is commenced.
C, A lateral view, showing access into the presacral space.

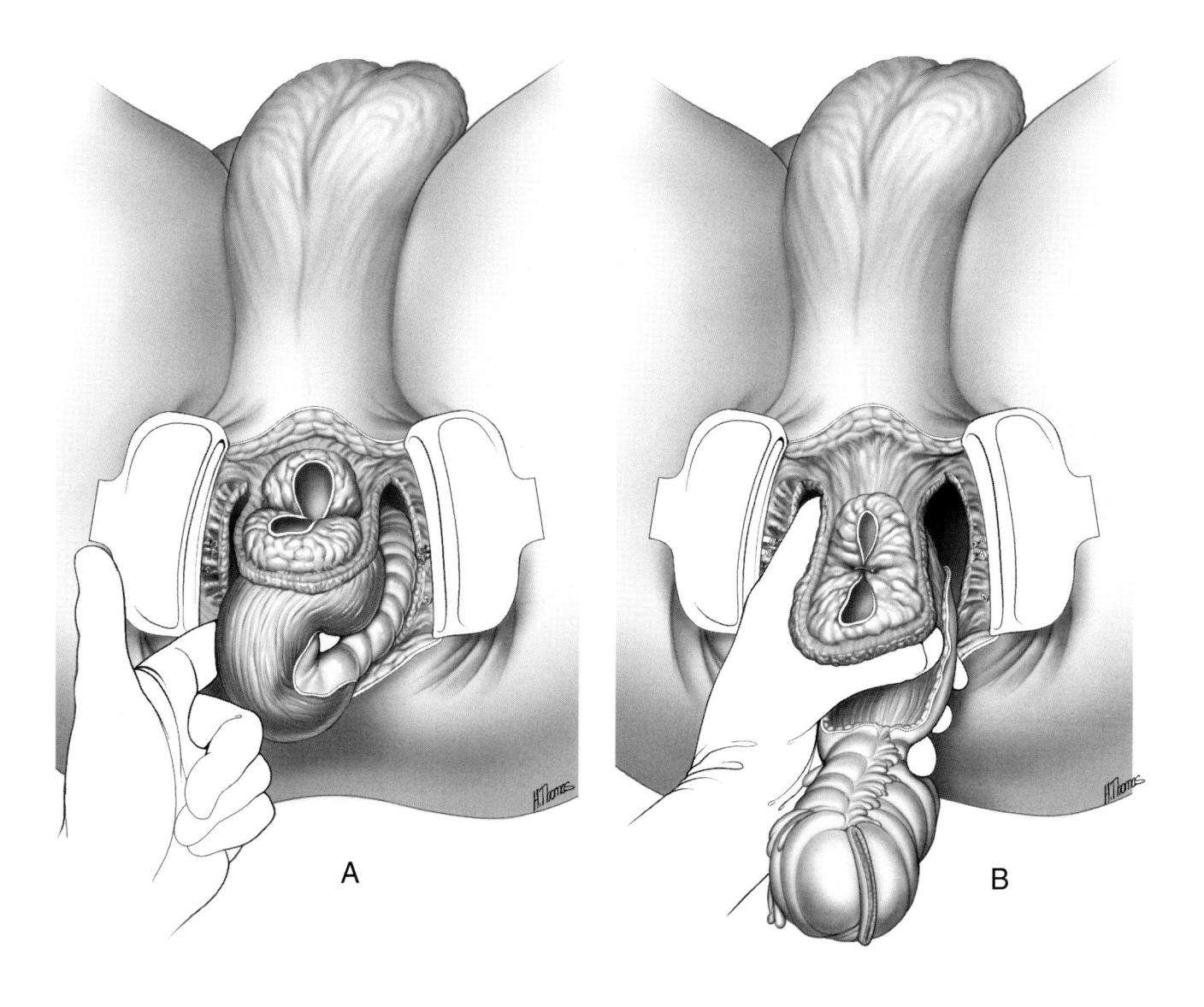

Figure 40-3 • **A,** The levator ani are divided laterally.
B, The specimen is delivered through the perineum.

338 • Part IV LOWER ABDOMEN

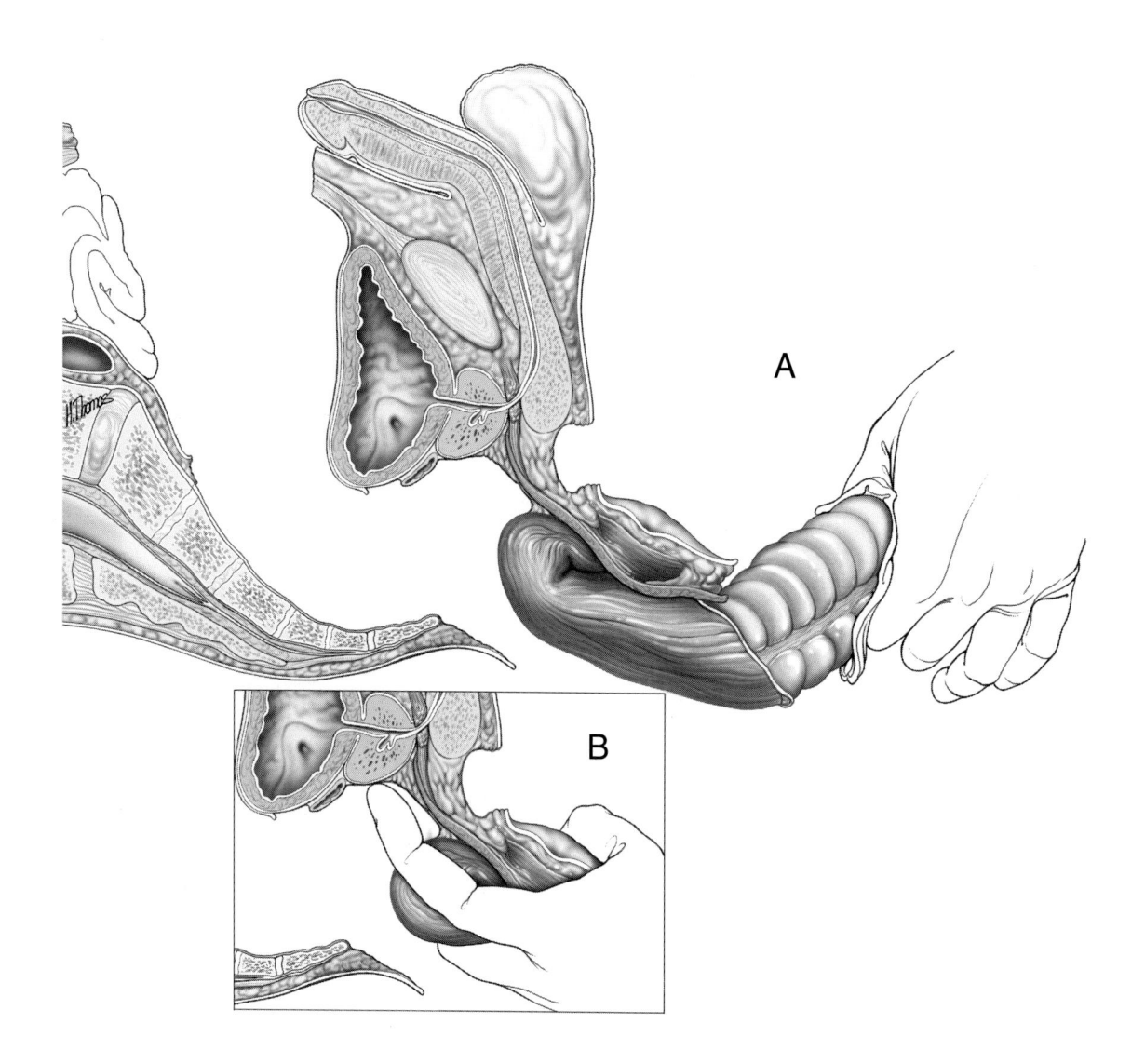

Figure 40-4 • **A,** The anterior attachments are divided last. Following delivery of the specimen, only anterior attachments to the prostate and urethra remain.
B, By placing a hand around the specimen with a finger on the prostate the remaining attachments can be safely removed.

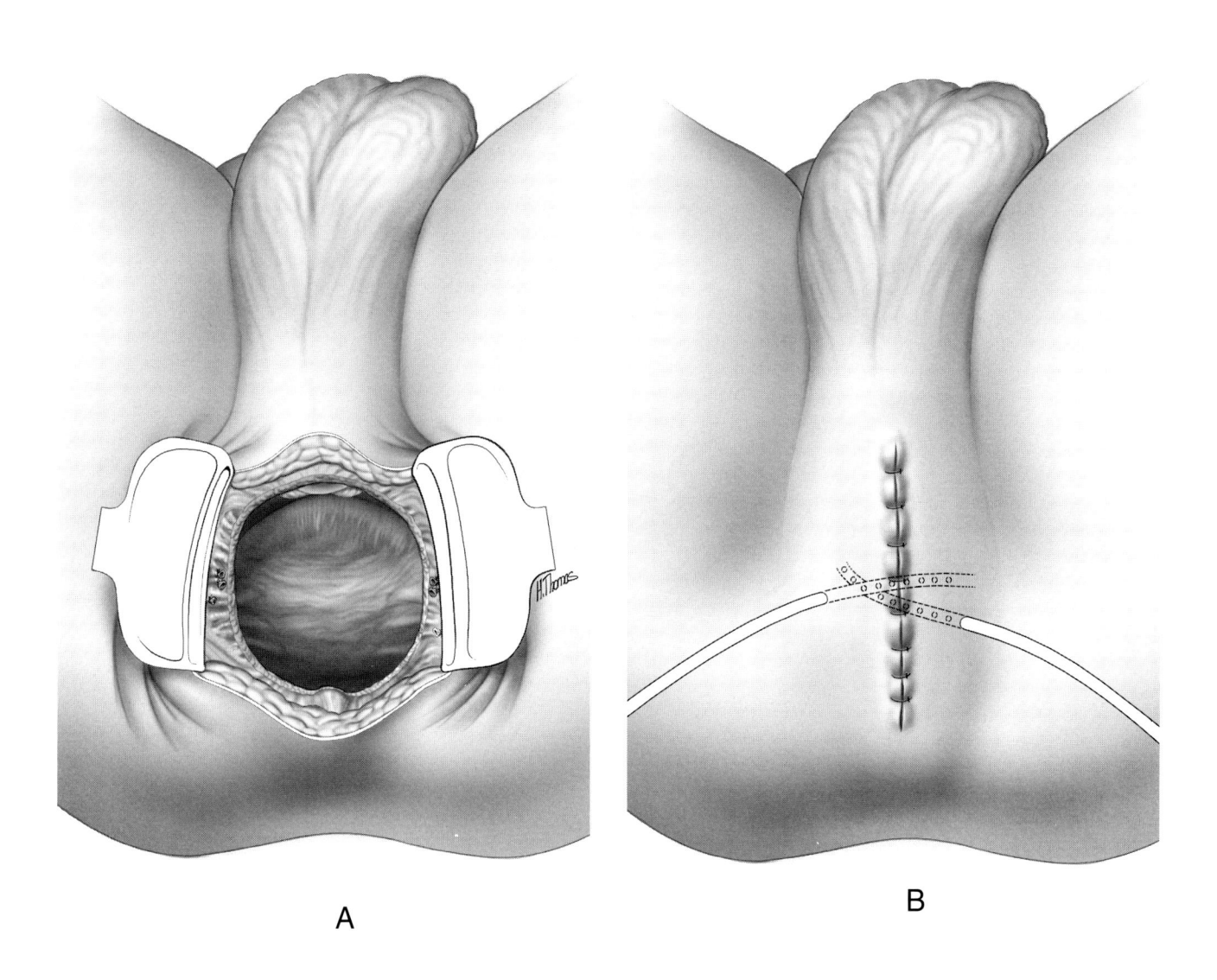

Figure 40–5 • **A,** The perineal defect is shown.
B, The perineal defect is closed over drains.

Chapter 41
Surgical Anatomy for Pelvic Exenteration (Female)

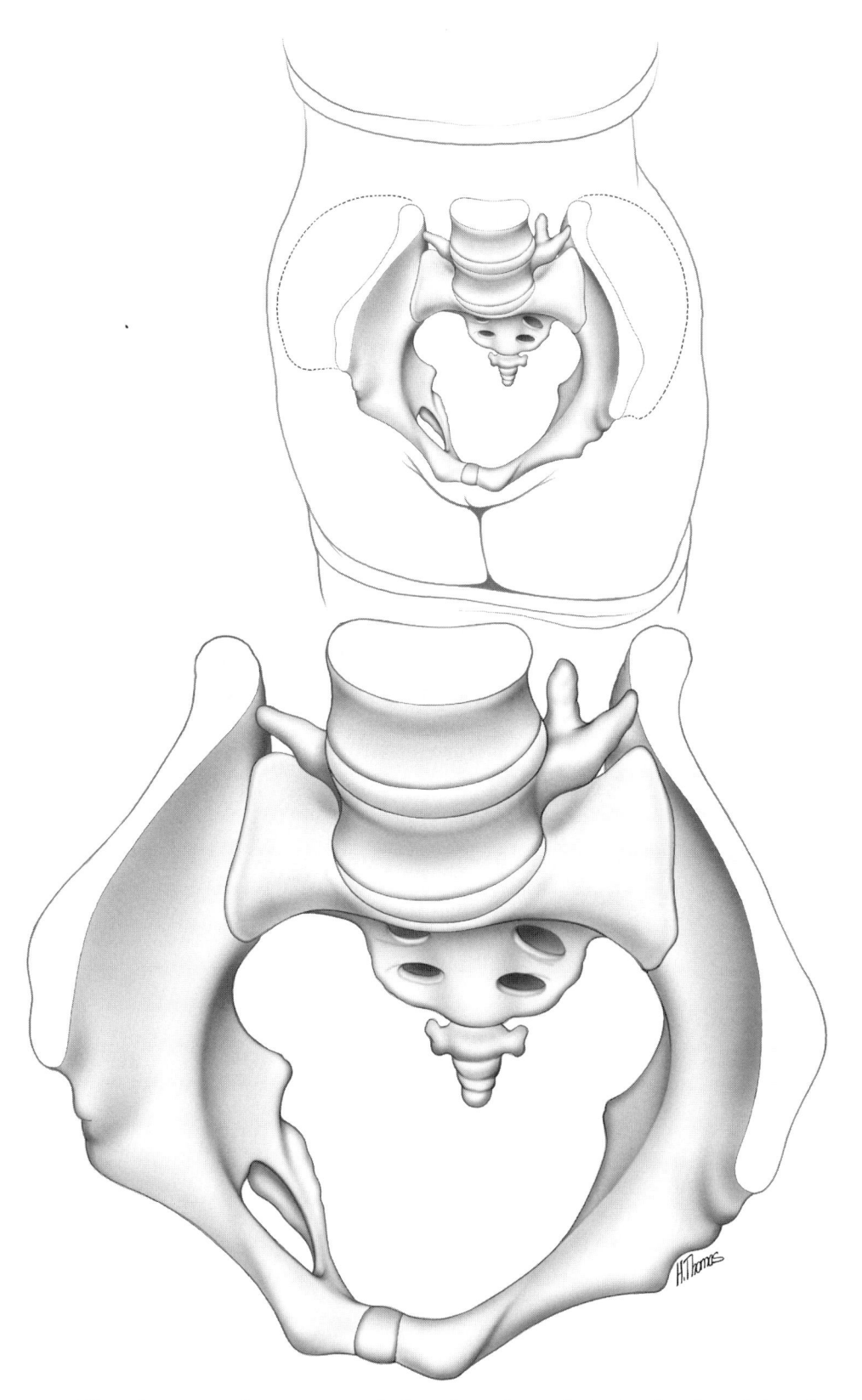

Figure 41–1 • The bony architecture of the female pelvis is depicted in the same orientation as the surgeon's view in performing this operation.

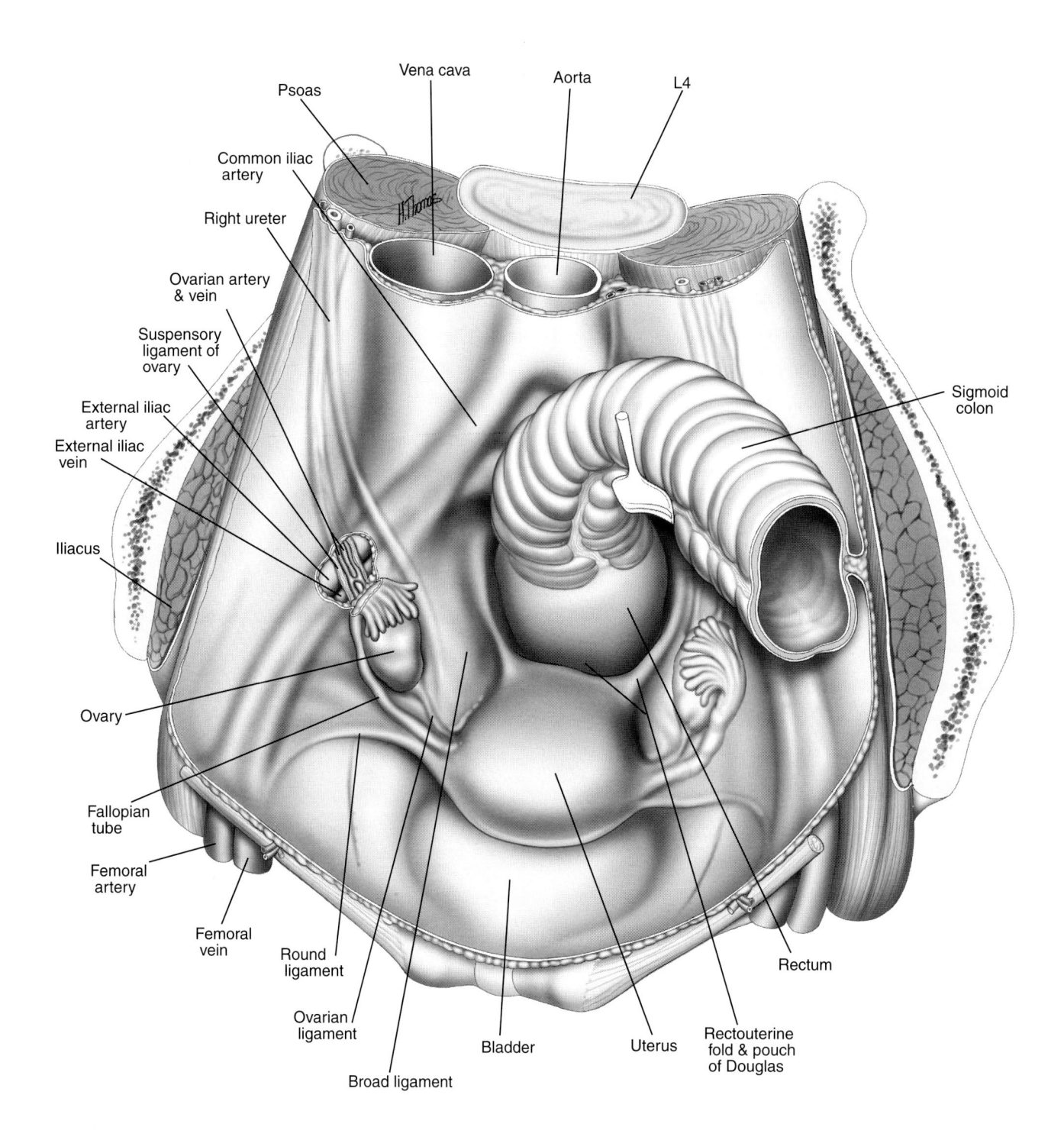

Figure 41–2 • The pelvic anatomy is depicted from the lower lumbar region downward.

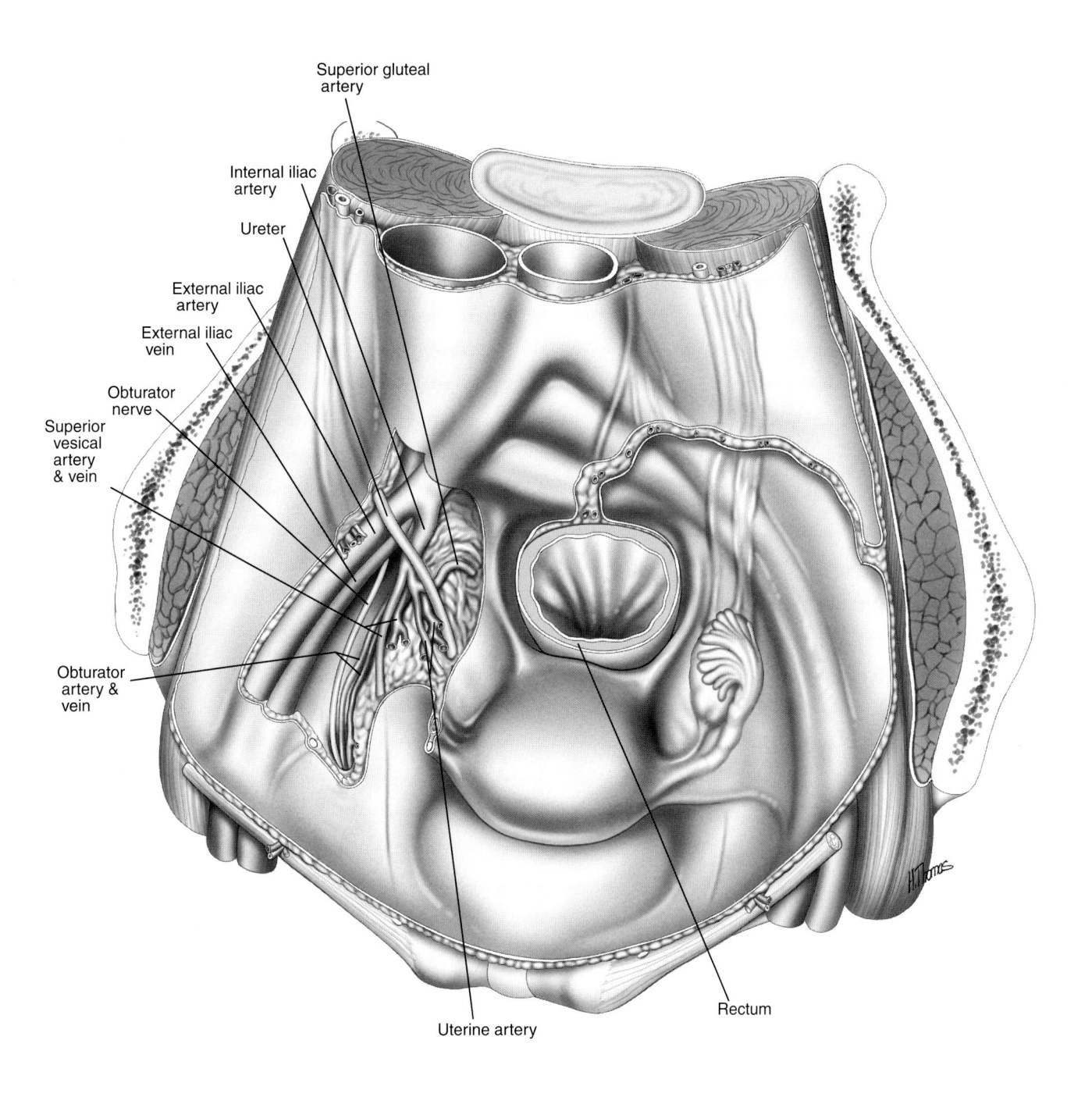

Figure 41–3 • The pelvic sidewall vascular anatomy is highlighted.

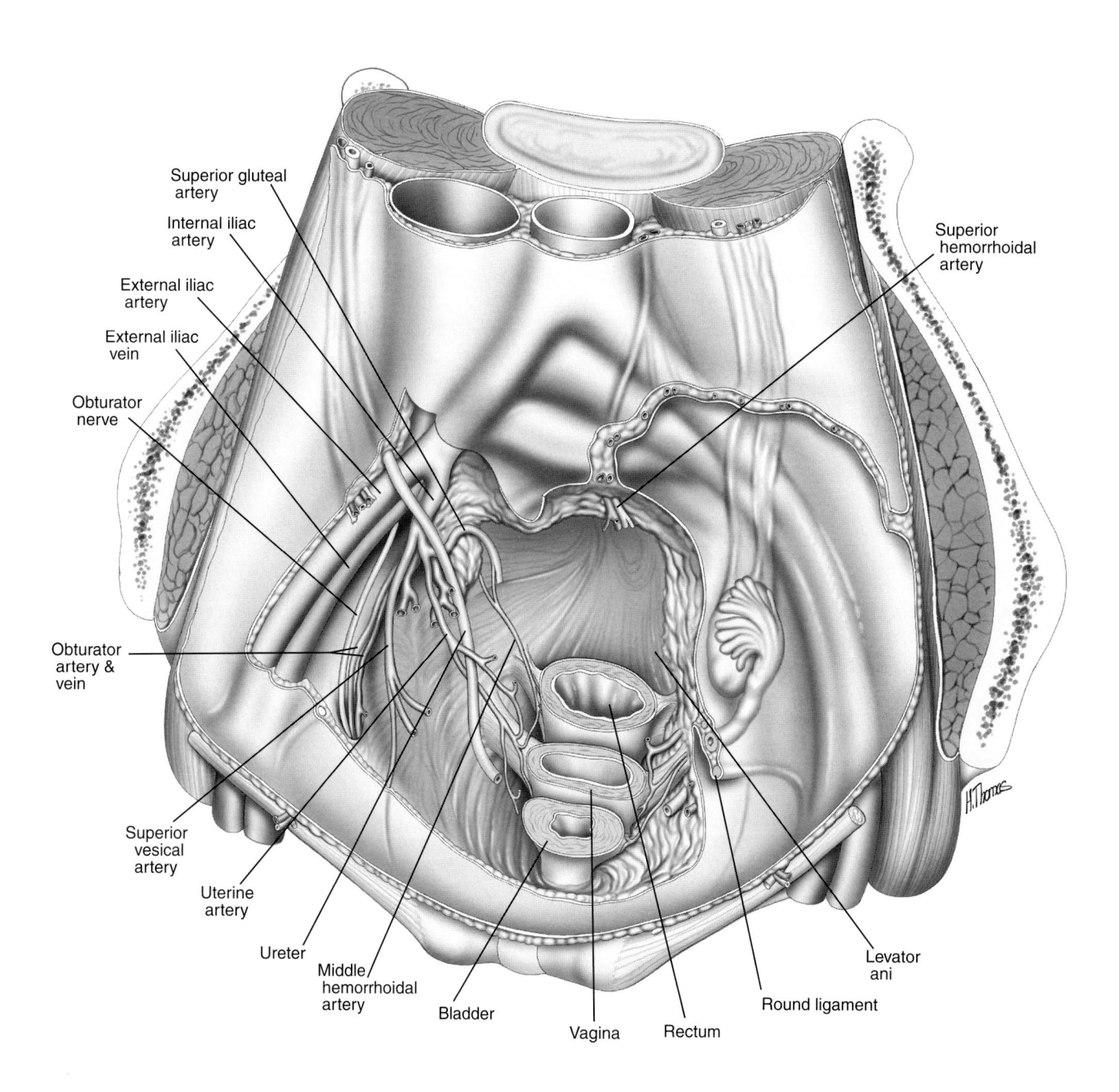

Figure 41–4 • The anatomy of the pelvis is depicted, with the bladder, rectum, and uterus removed.

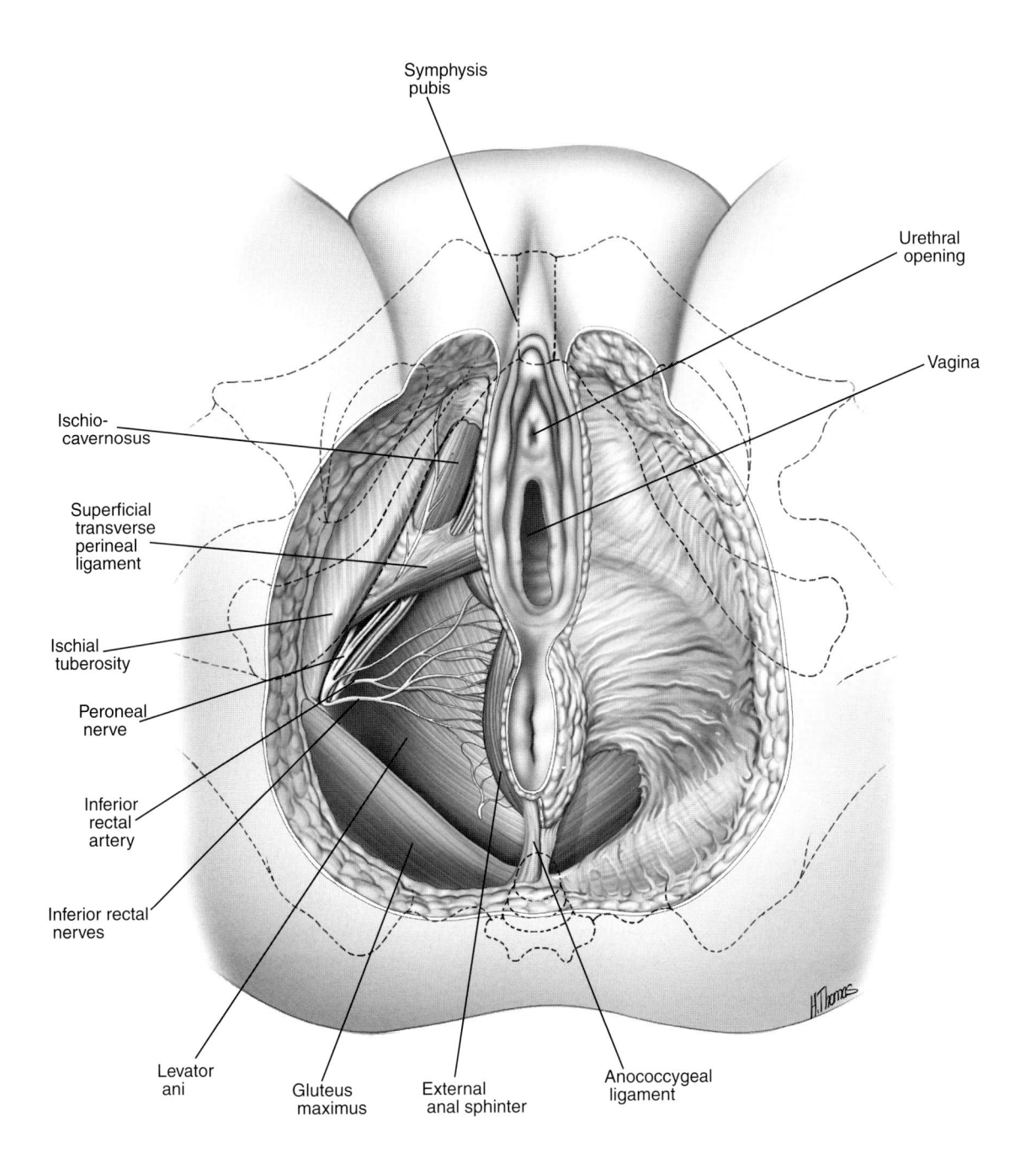

Figure 41–5 • The female perineal anatomy is illustrated.

Chapter 42
Pelvic Exenteration (Female)

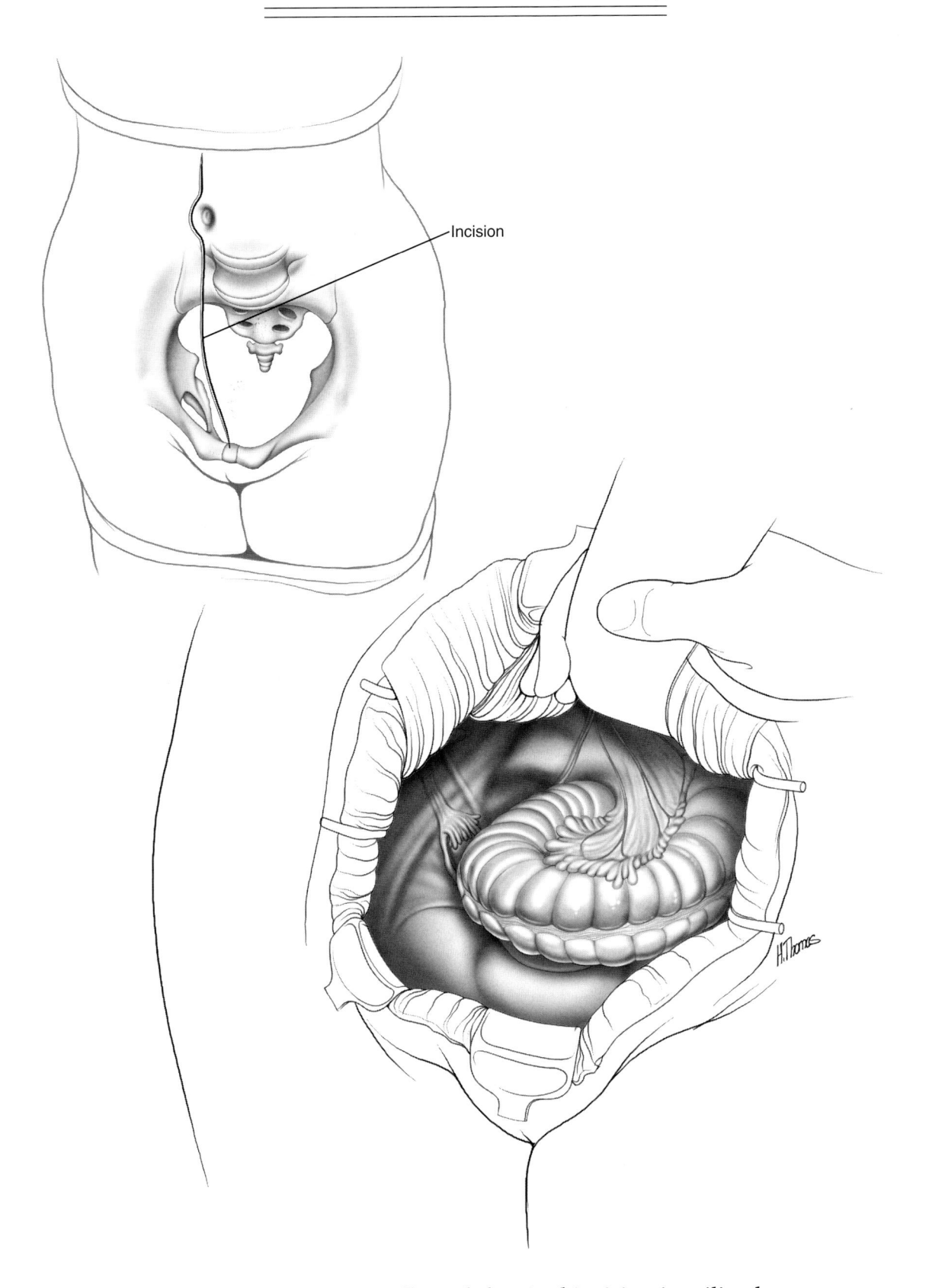

Figure 42–1 • A lower midline abdominal incision is utilized.

348 • Part IV LOWER ABDOMEN

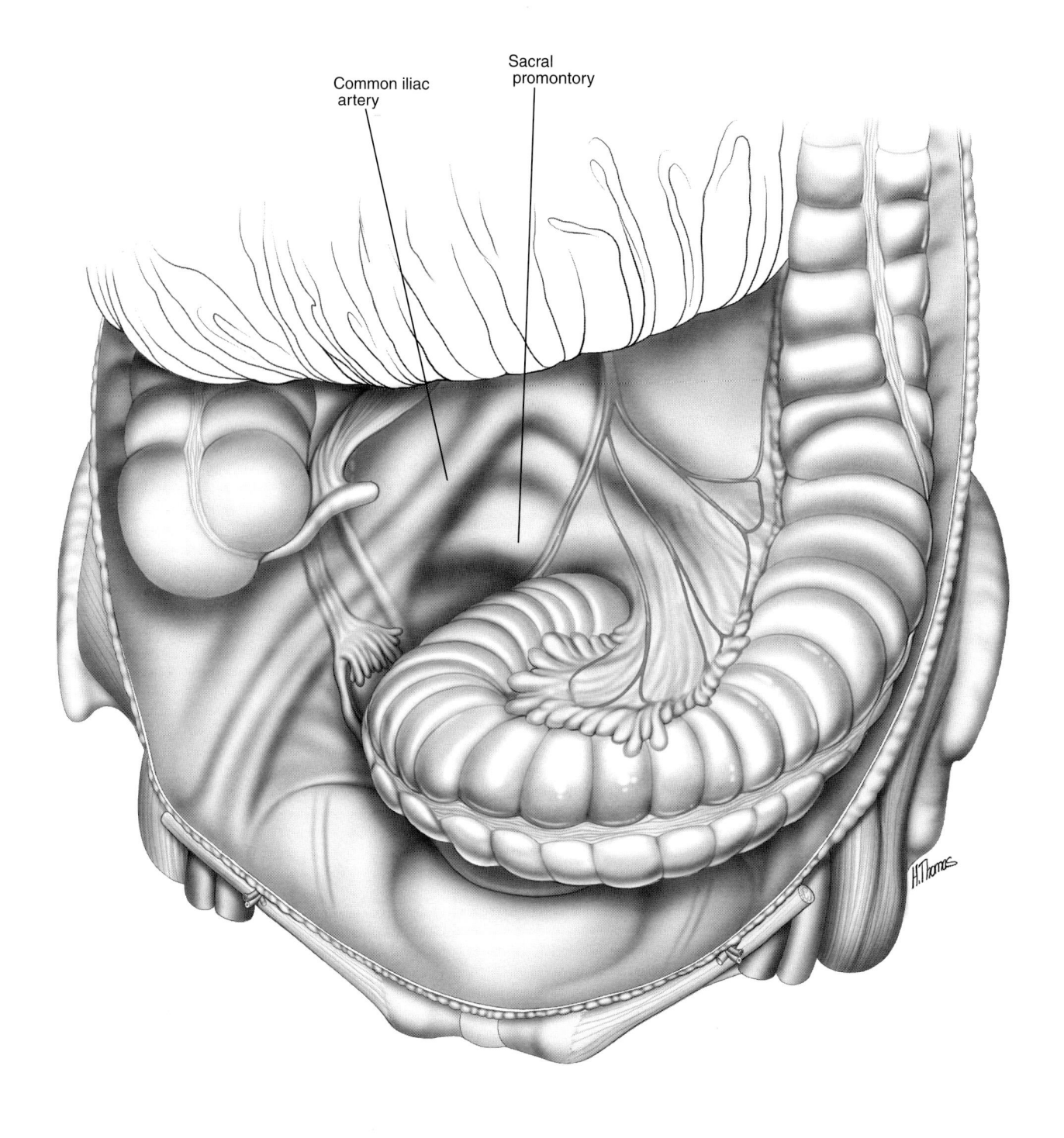

Figure 42–2 • The small bowel is mobilized out of the pelvis.

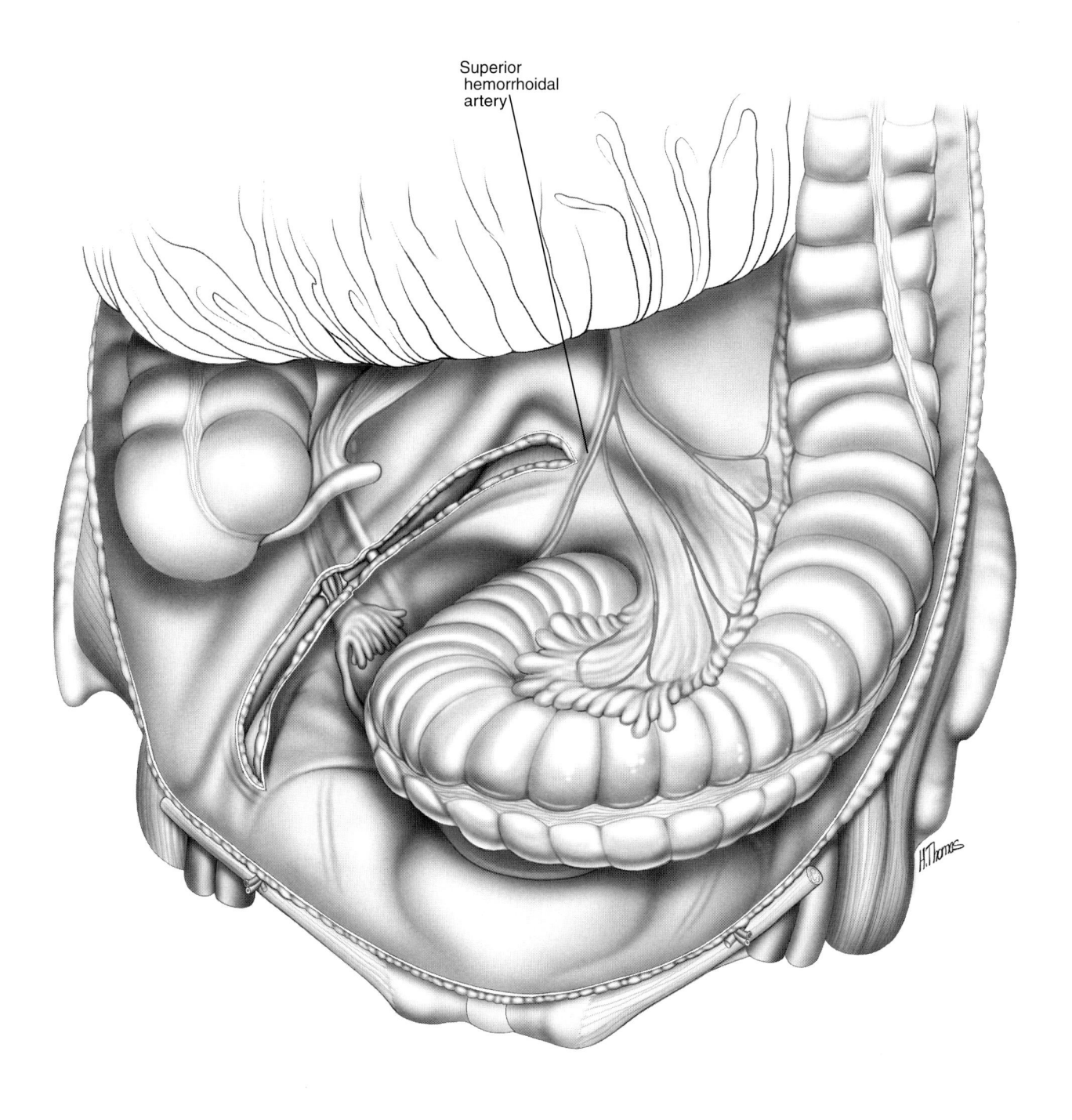

Figure 42–3 • The medial leaf of the sigmoid mesentery is incised, and the peritoneum is incised along the right common iliac vessels.

350 • Part IV LOWER ABDOMEN

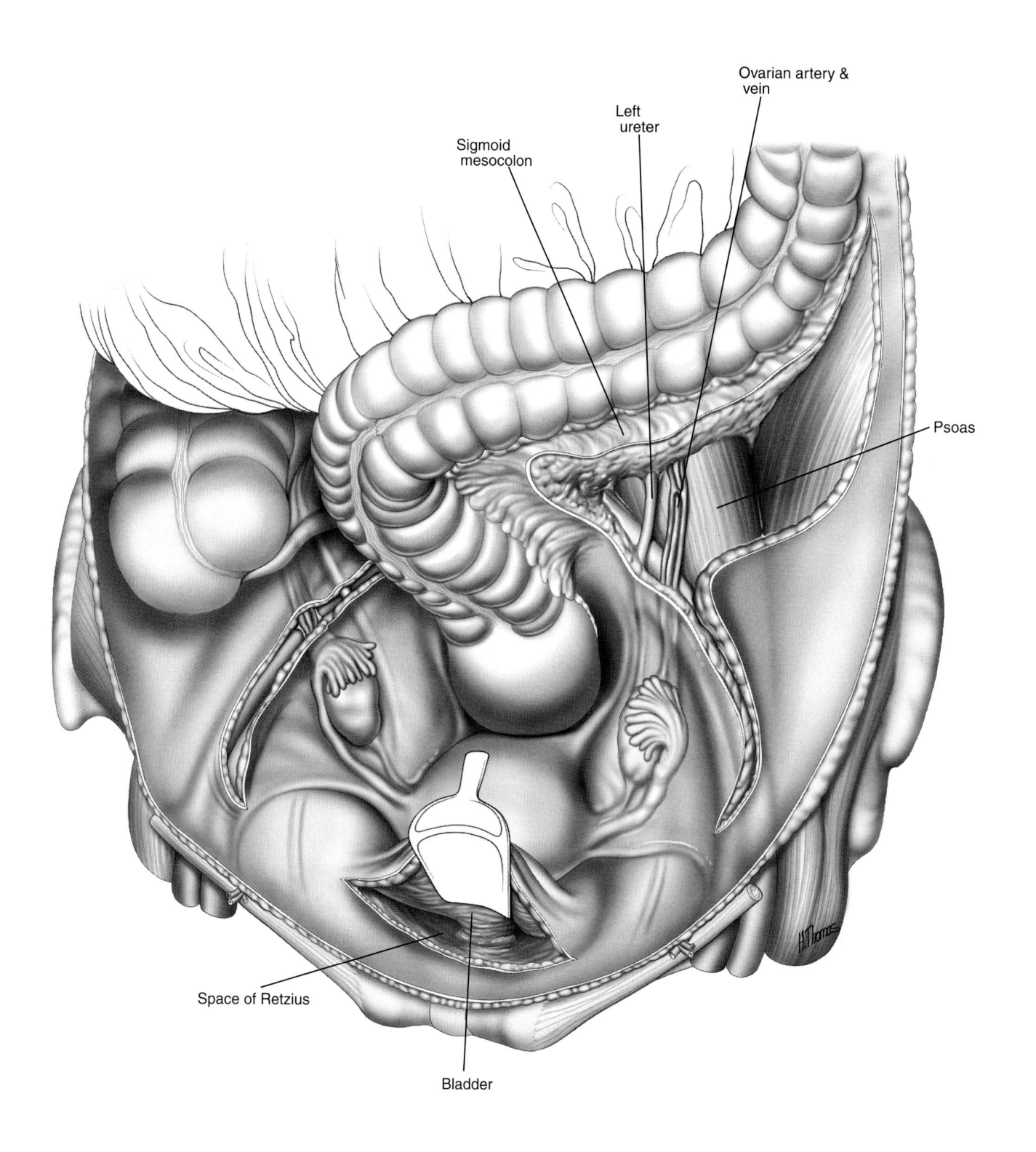

Figure 42-4 • The sigmoid colon is mobilized, and the peritoneum over the left common iliac vessels is incised, as well as the peritoneal reflection over the bladder.

Pelvic Exenteration (Female) • 351

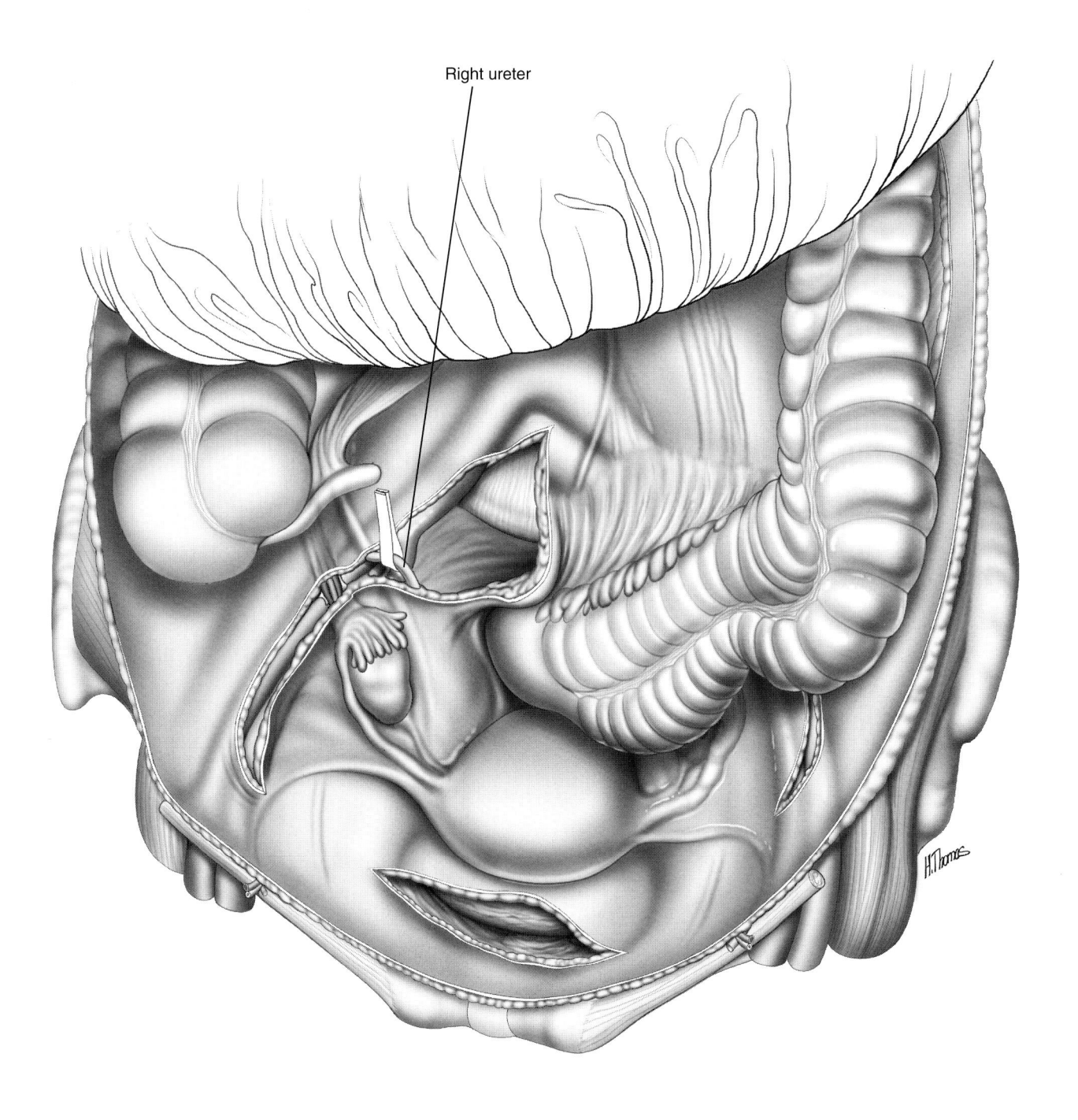

Figure 42–5 • The right ureter is identified.

352 • Part IV LOWER ABDOMEN

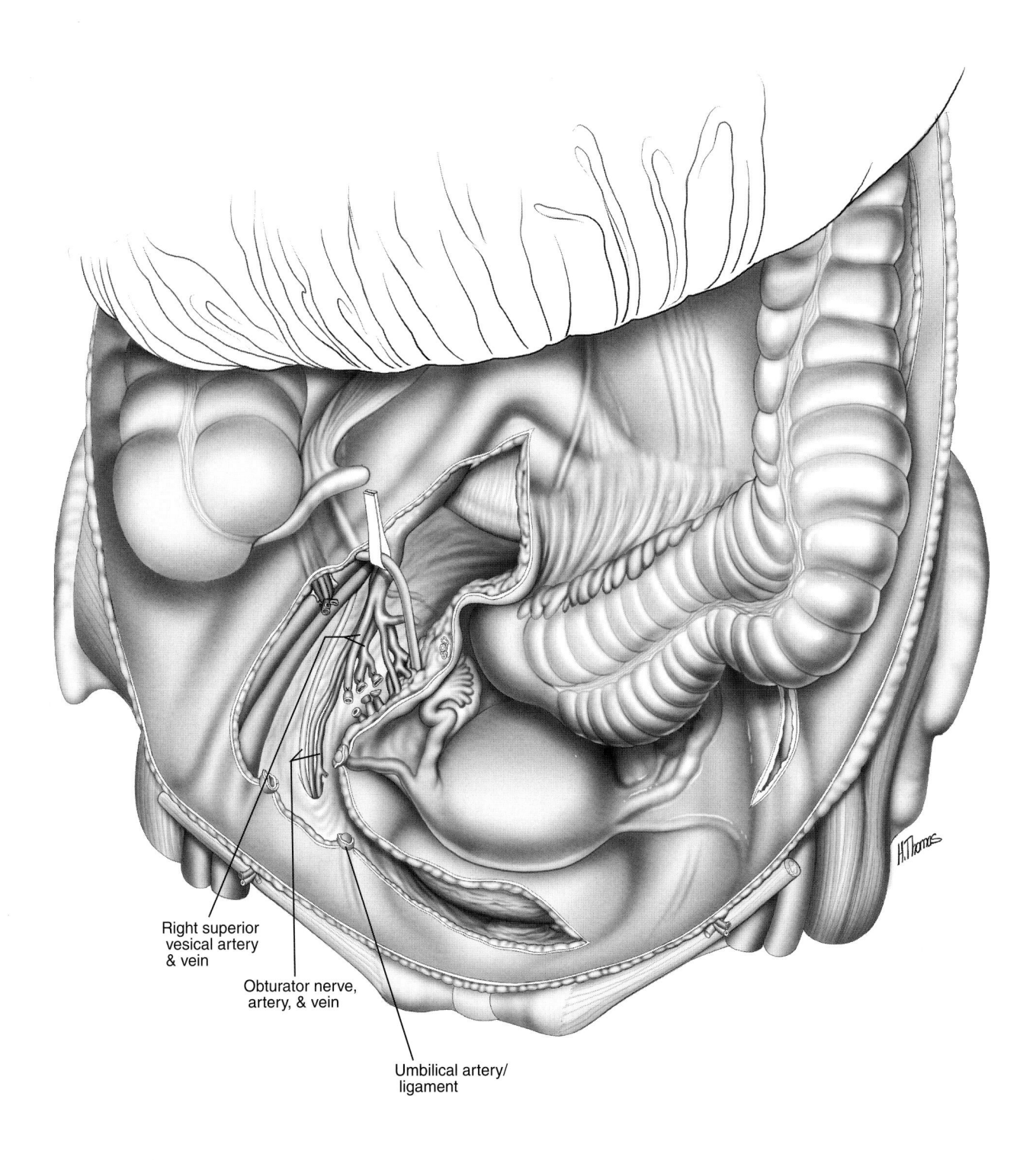

Figure 42-6 • The ovarian vessels are divided initially and then the branches off the right hypogastric to the bladder and uterus. The obturator nerve, artery, and vein are preserved. The ureter is divided.

Pelvic Exenteration (Female) • 353

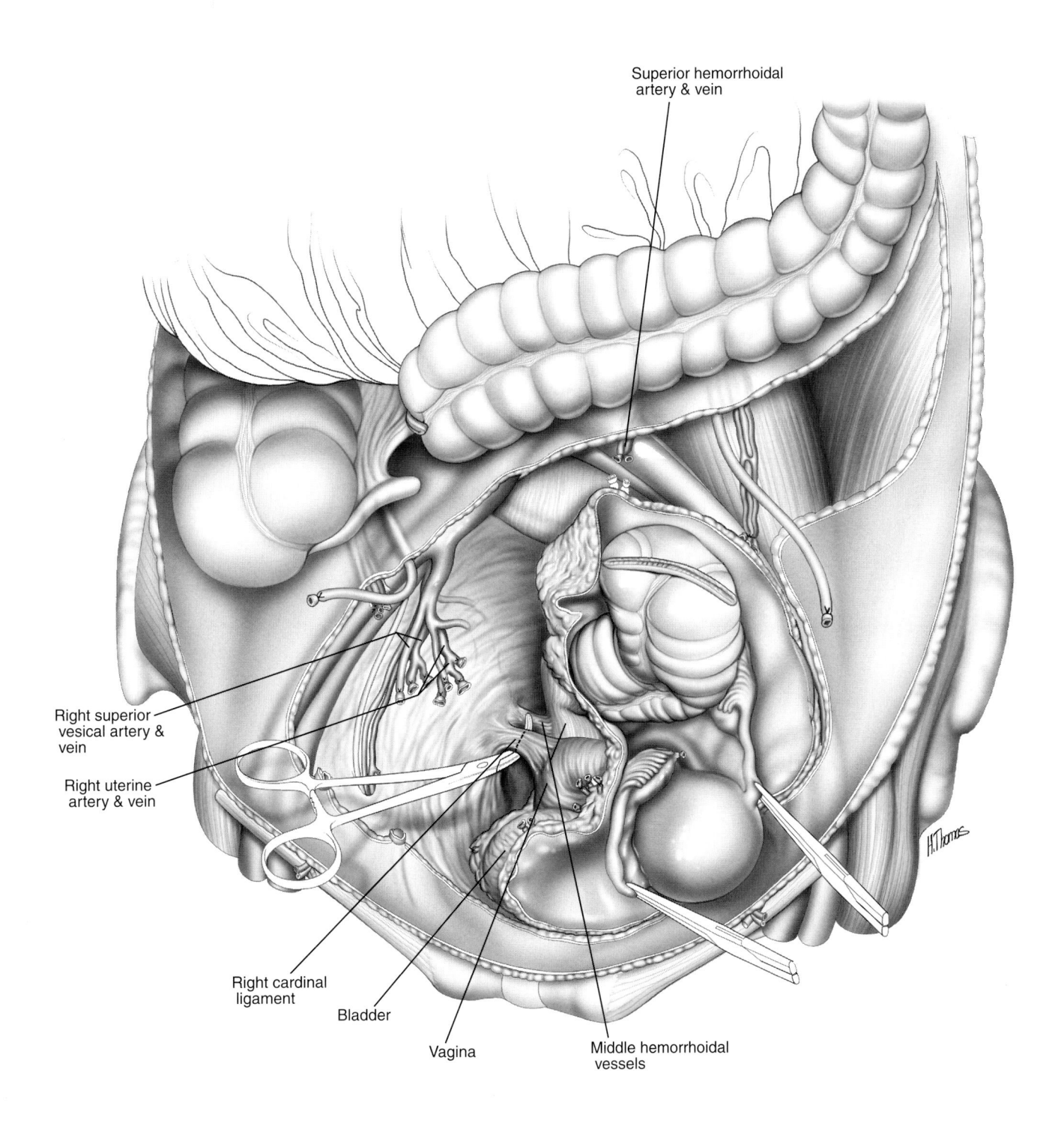

Figure 42–7 • The cardinal ligament and superior hemorrhoidal vessels are divided. The sigmoid mesentery is divided, as is the sigmoid colon and the left ureter.

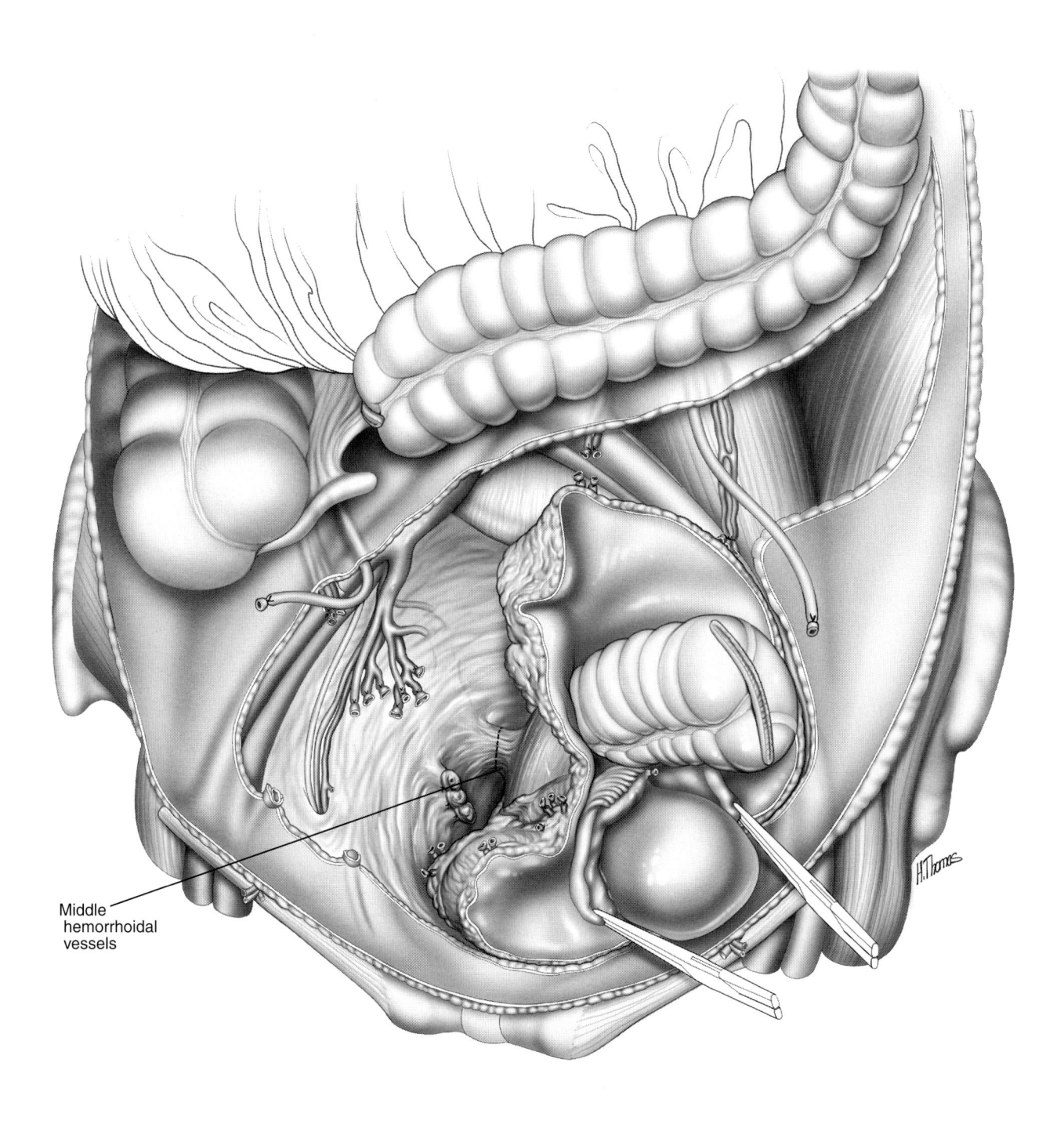

Figure 42–8 • The middle hemorrhoidal vessels are divided, and the mobilization of the rectum is completed on the right side.

Pelvic Exenteration (Female) • 355

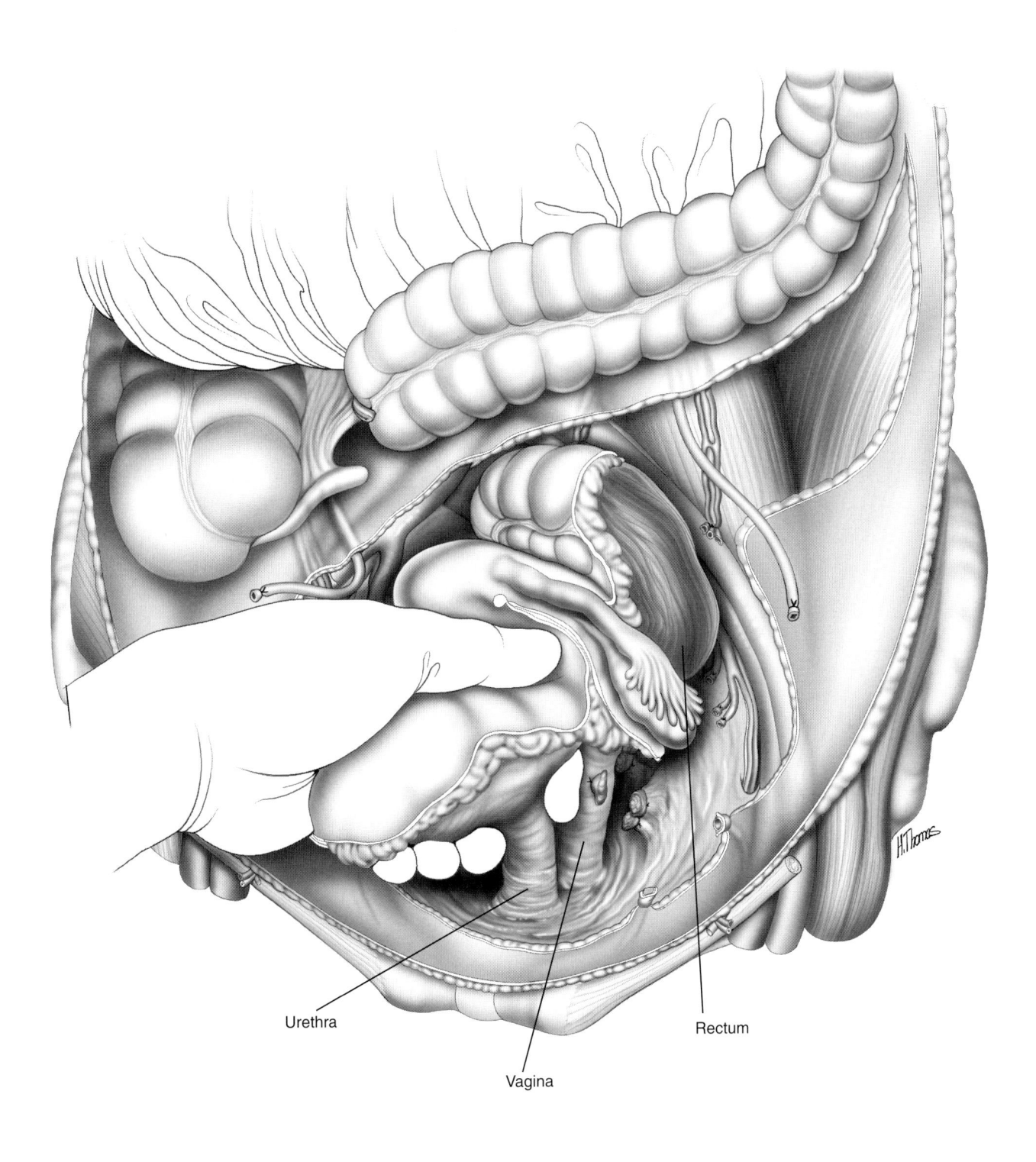

Figure 42–9 • The branches off the left hypogastric are divided in a similar fashion. The left ureter is divided.

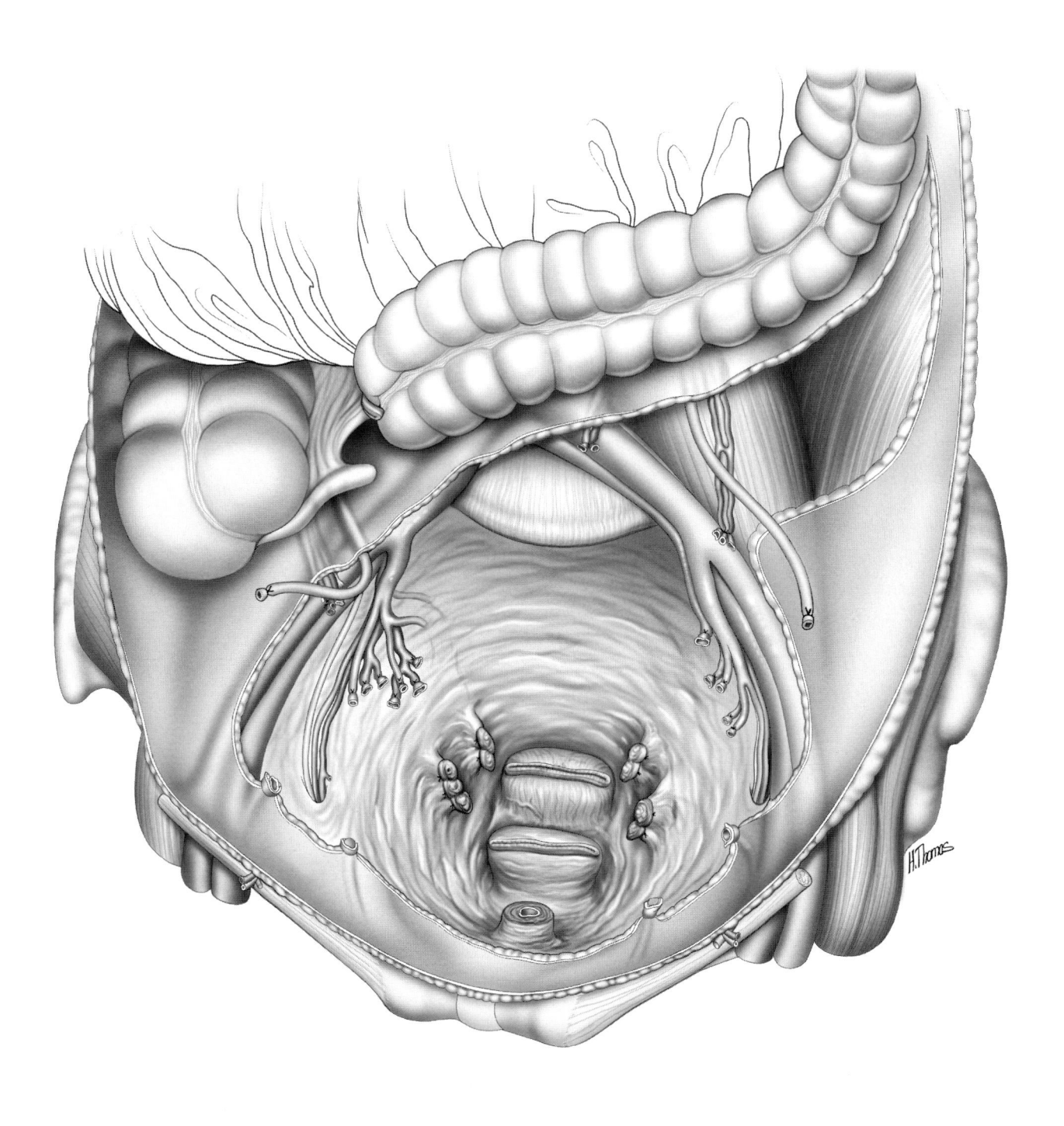

Figure 42–10 • If the perineum is not to be resected, the urethra, vagina, and distal rectum are divided and the specimen is removed.

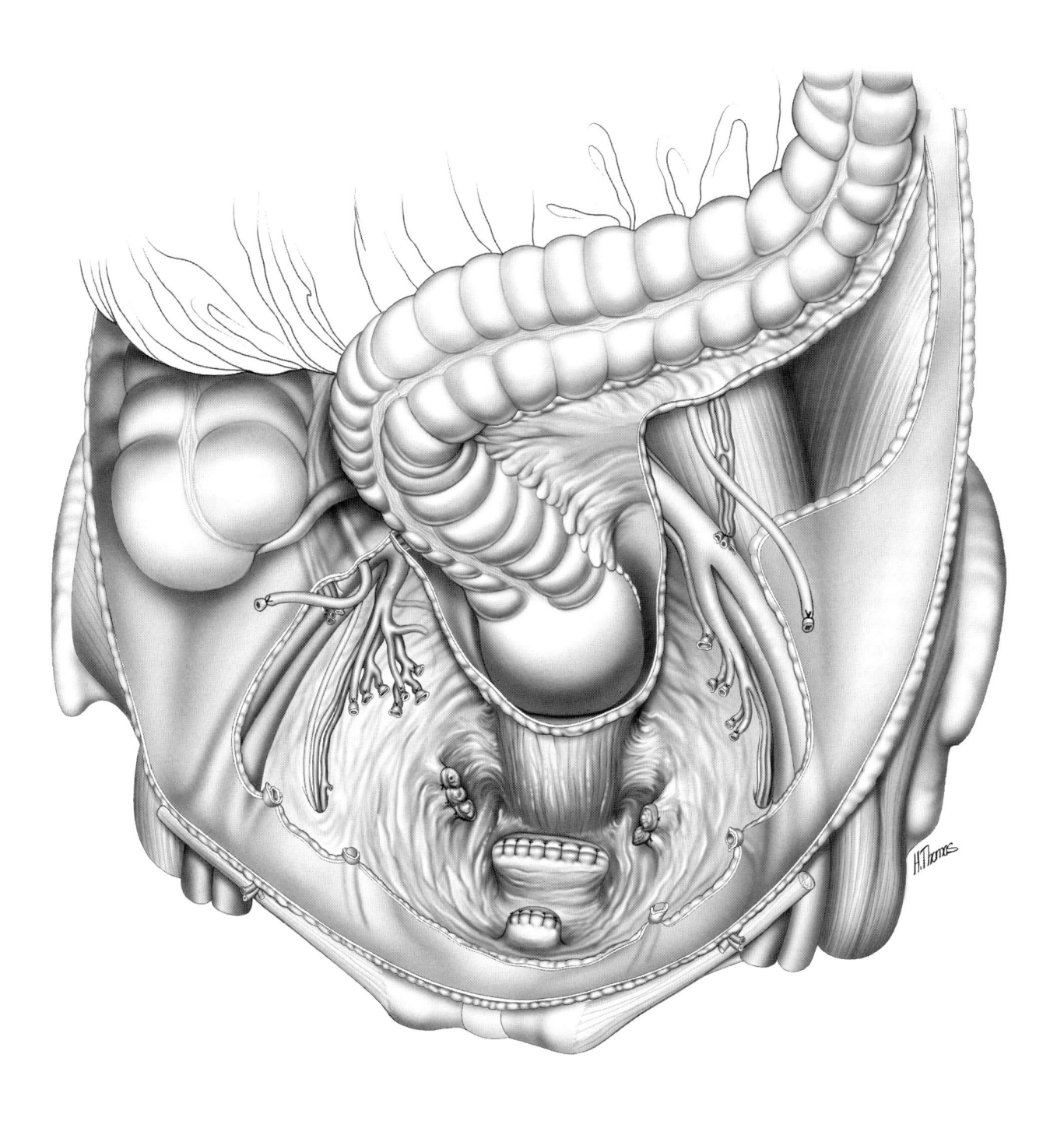

Figure 42–11 • A low rectal anastomosis is performed.

358 • Part IV LOWER ABDOMEN

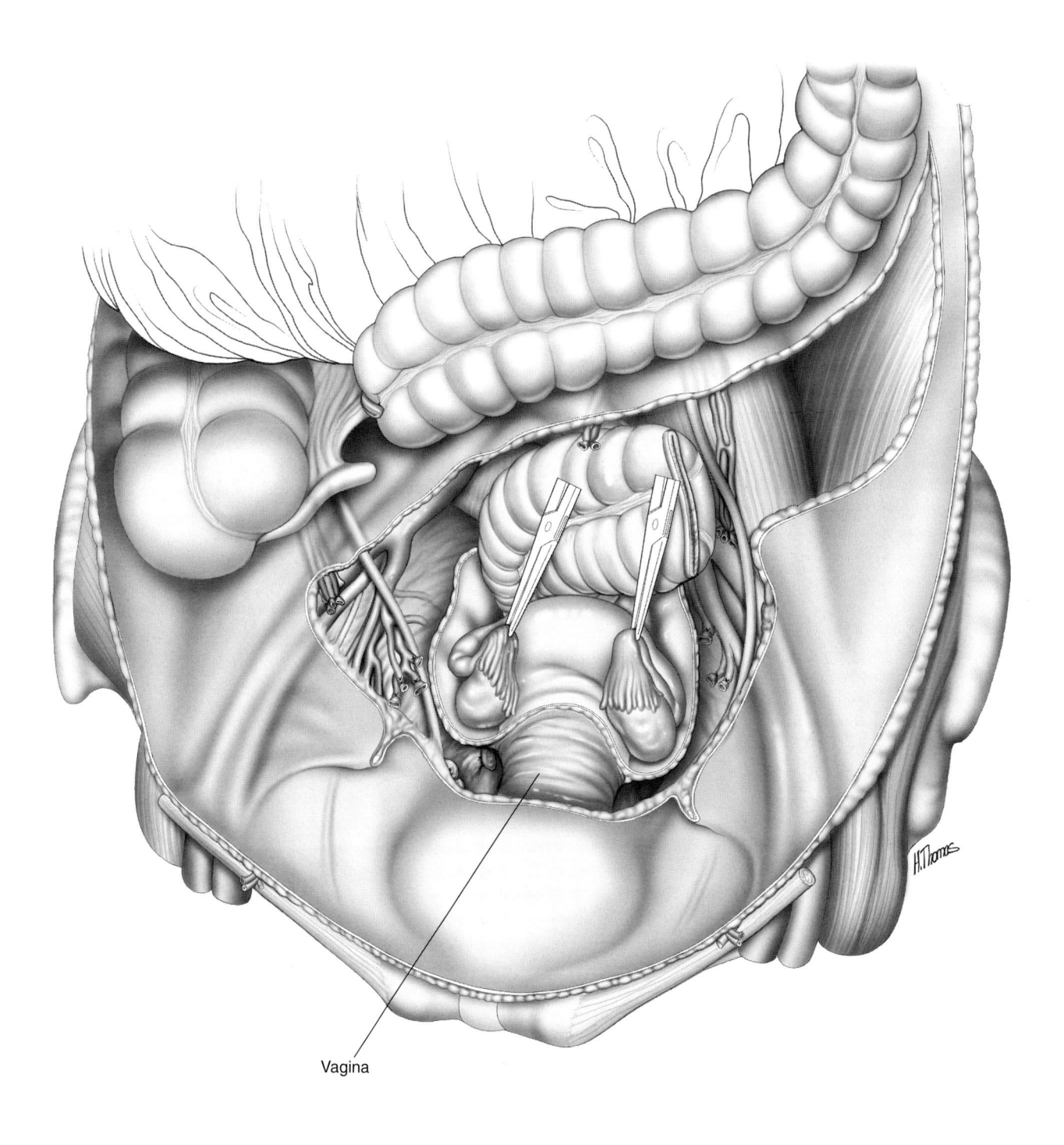

Vagina

Figure 42–12 • If a posterior exenteration is to be performed, only the peritoneal reflection in the pouch of Douglas is incised, and the ureters and superior vesical vessels are preserved.

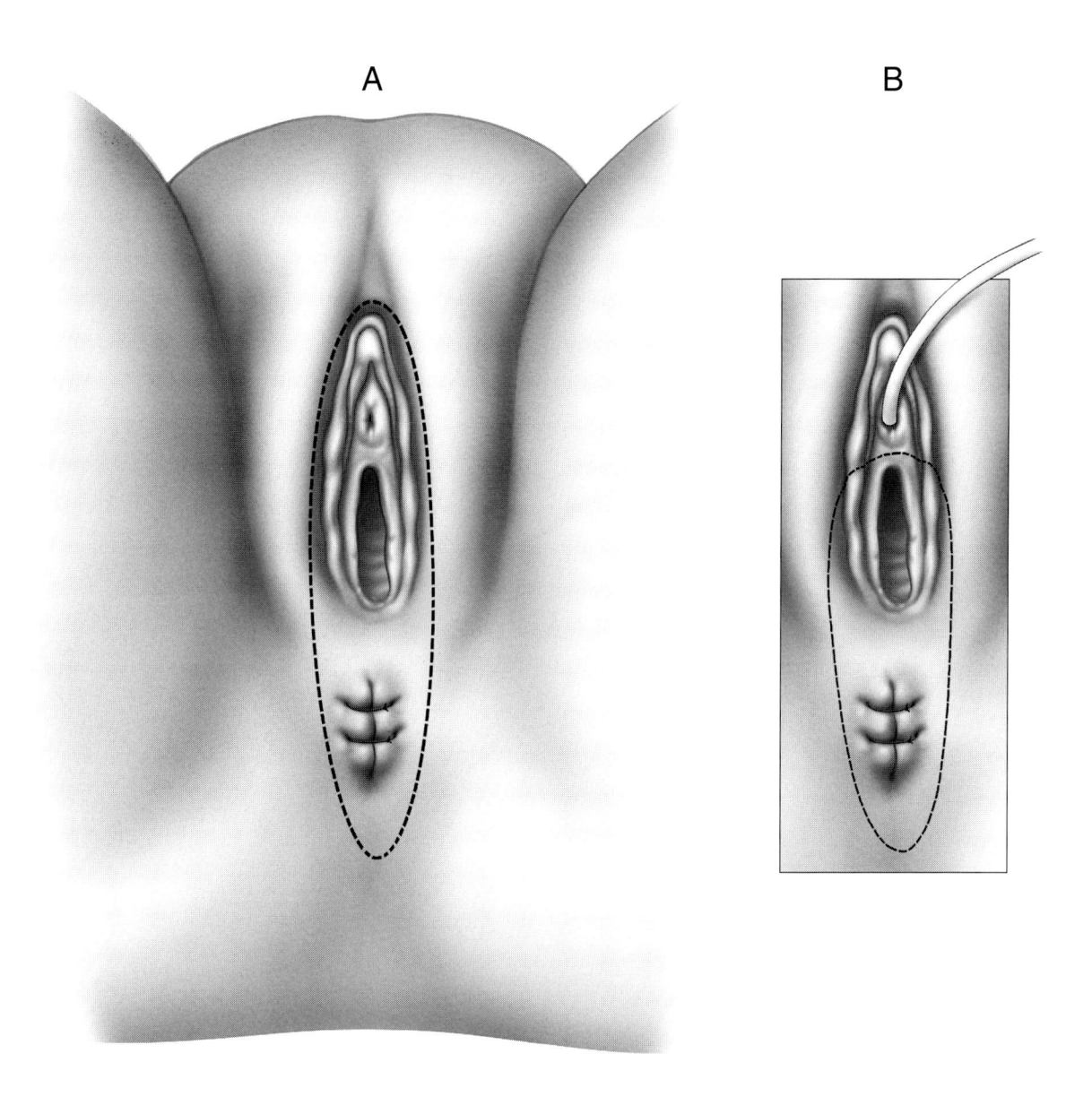

Figure 42–13 • **A,** The perineal incision for a total pelvic exenteration and perineal resection is depicted.
B, The perineal incision for a posterior exenteration is depicted.

360 • Part IV LOWER ABDOMEN

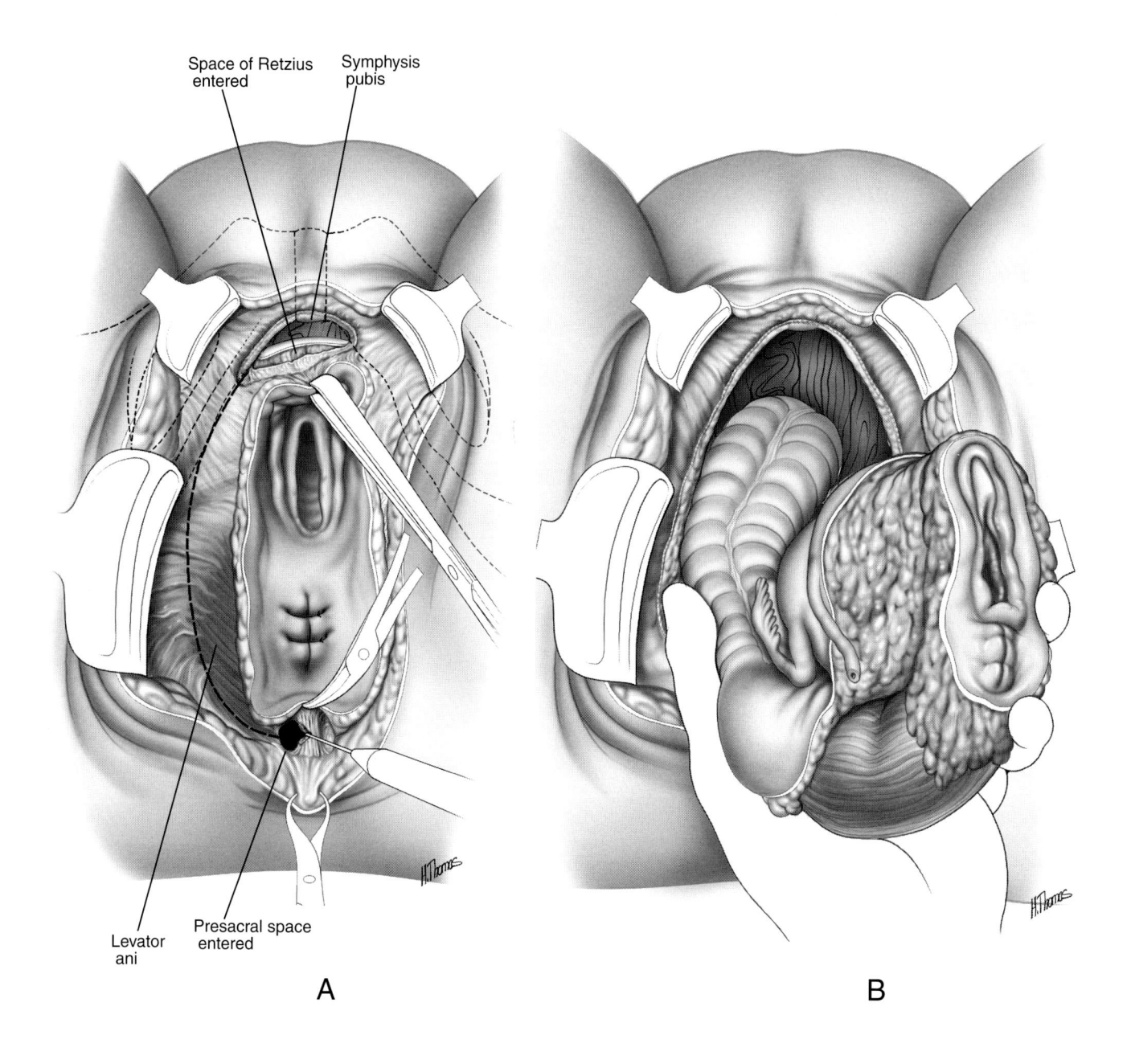

Figure 42–14 • **A,** As depicted in greater detail in Chapter 40, the perineal resection is initially completed inferiorly, gaining access into the abdominal cavity in the presacral space. Anteriorly, the space of Retzius is entered just below the symphysis pubis.

B, The entire specimen is delivered through the perineum.

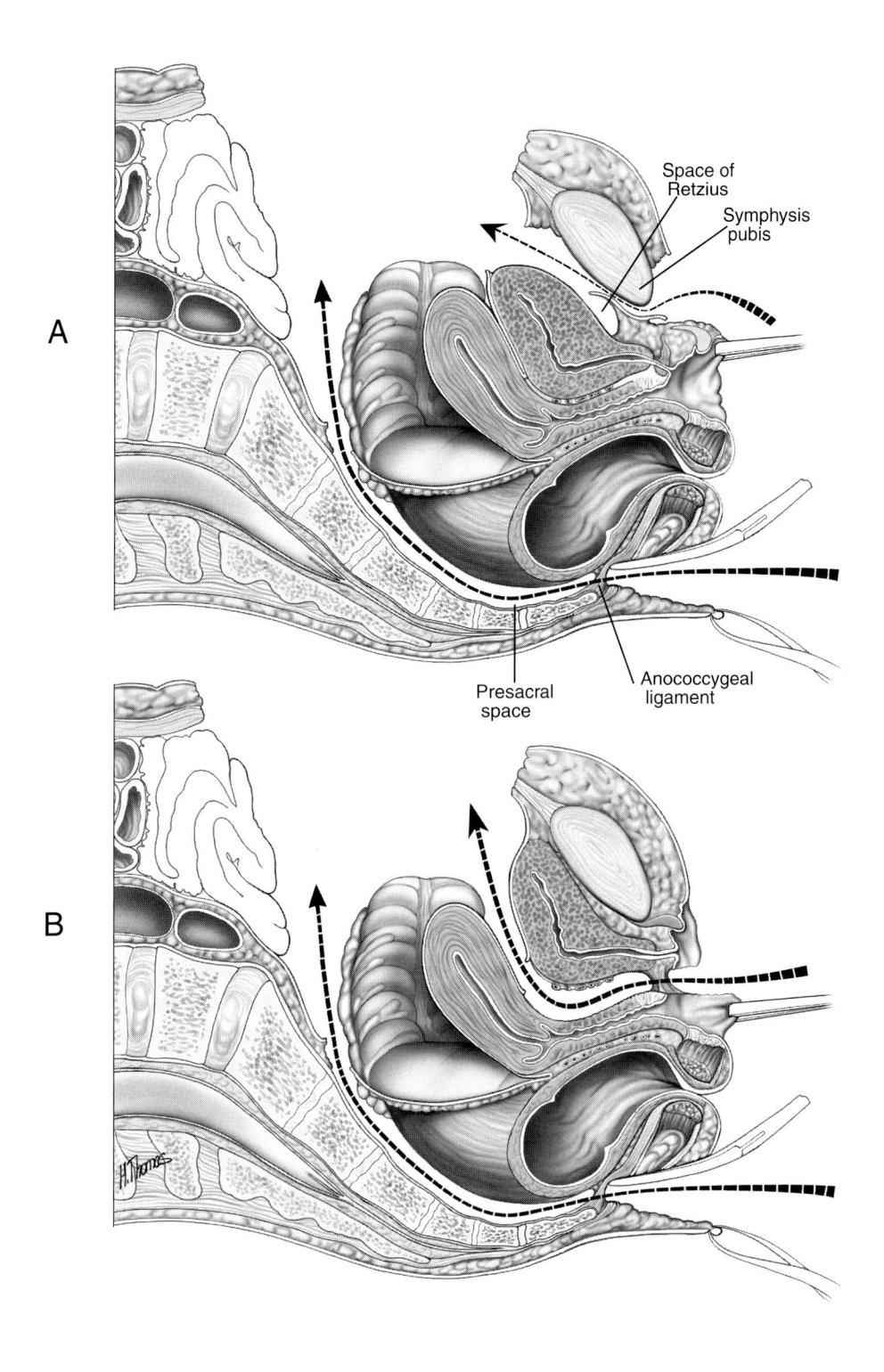

Figure 42–15 • **A,** A lateral view depicting the superior and inferior lines of resection for a total pelvic exenteration.
B, A lateral view depicting the posterior exenteration.

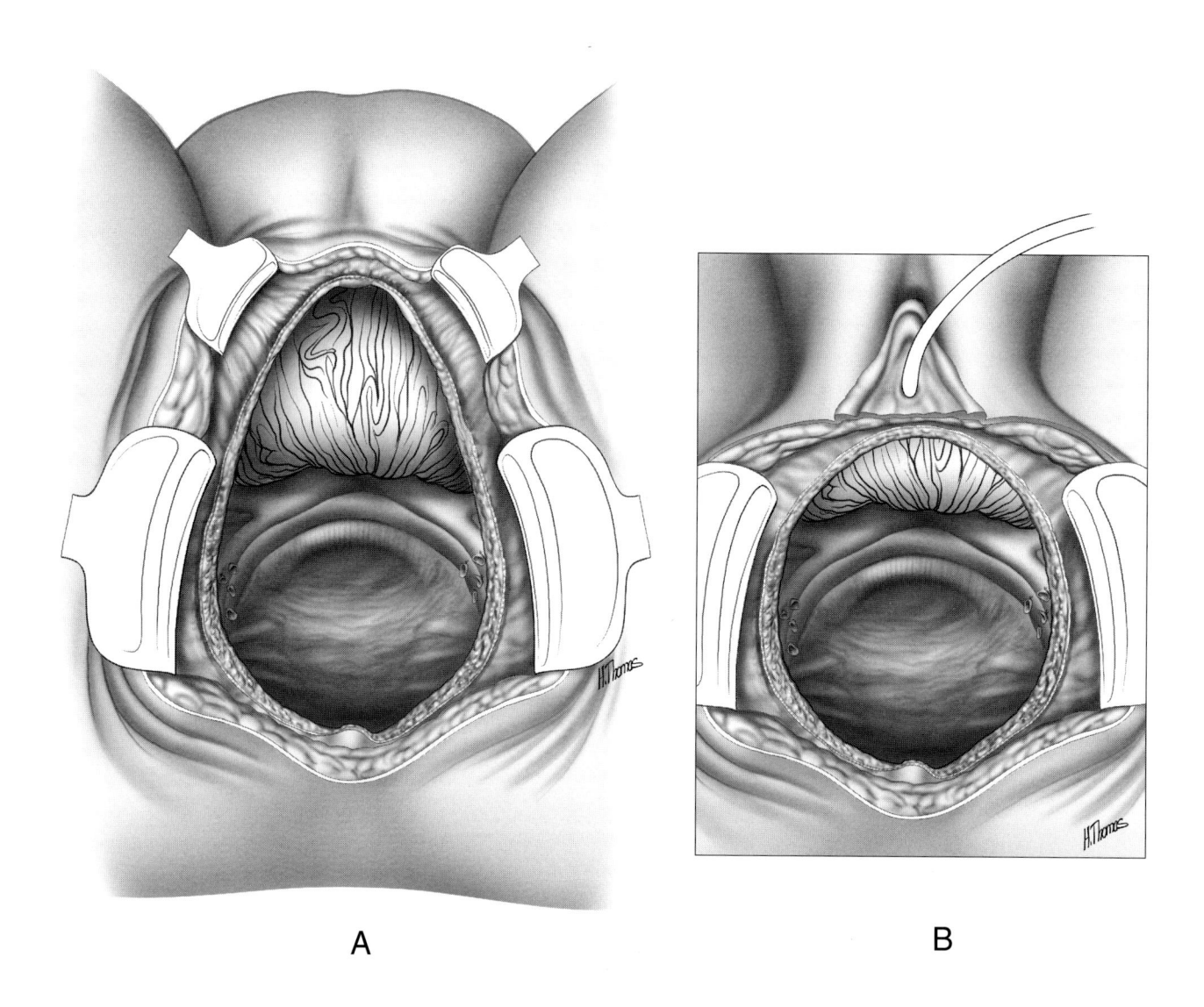

Figure 42–16 • **A,** The perineal defects following the exenterative procedures. Total exenteration.

B, Posterior exenteration.

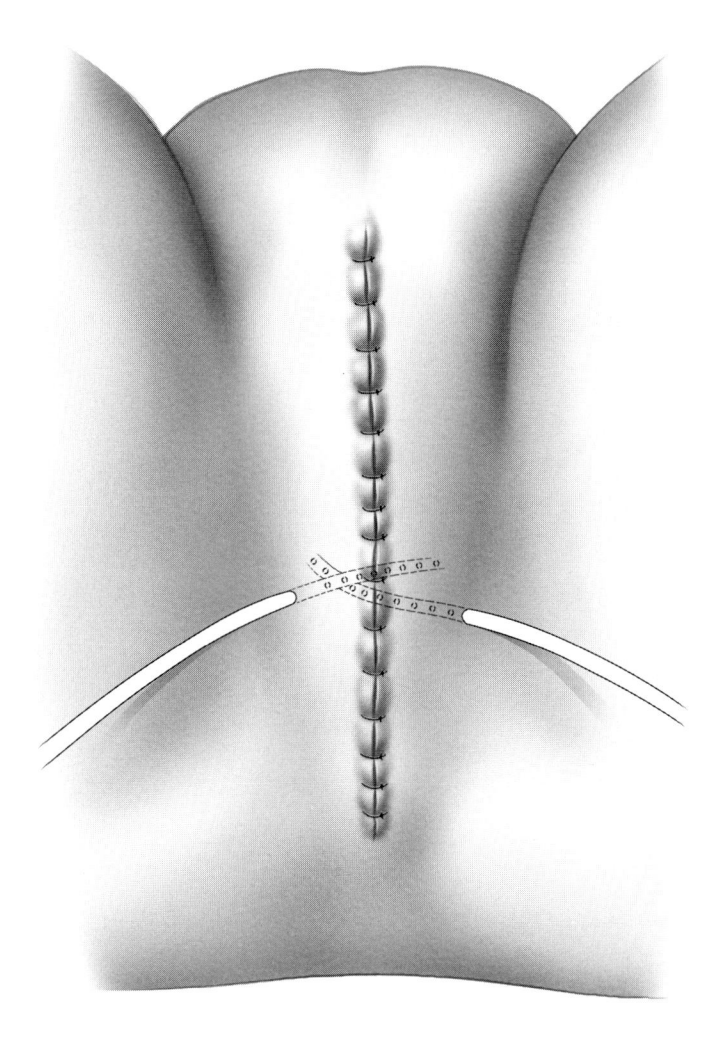

Figure 42–17 • The perineum is closed over suction drains. A Gore-Tex patch can be used below the perineal skin closure.

Chapter 43
Urinary Diversion

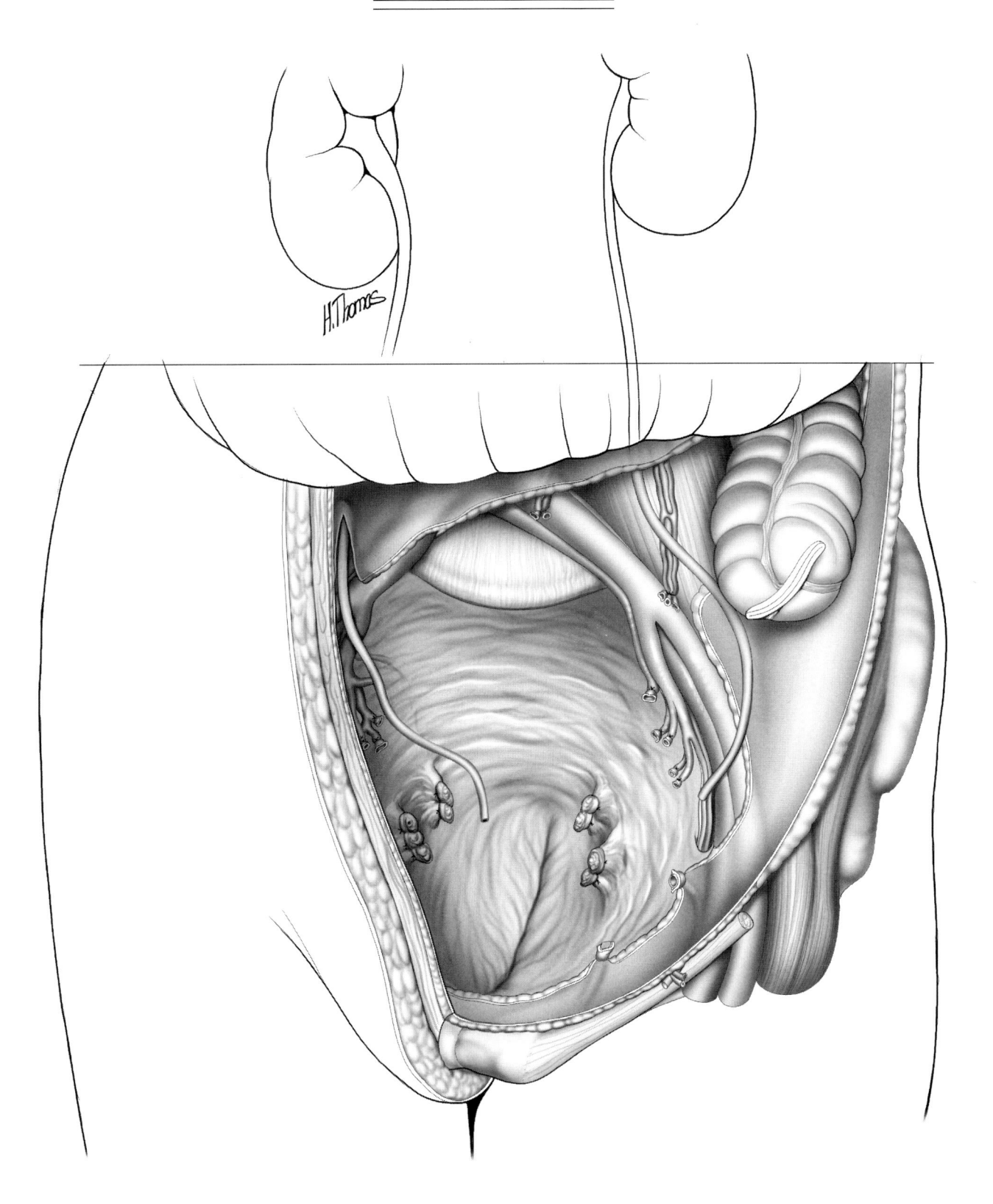

Figure 43–1 • An ileal conduit is created following the completion of a total pelvic exenteration and prior to the creation of an end sigmoid colostomy.

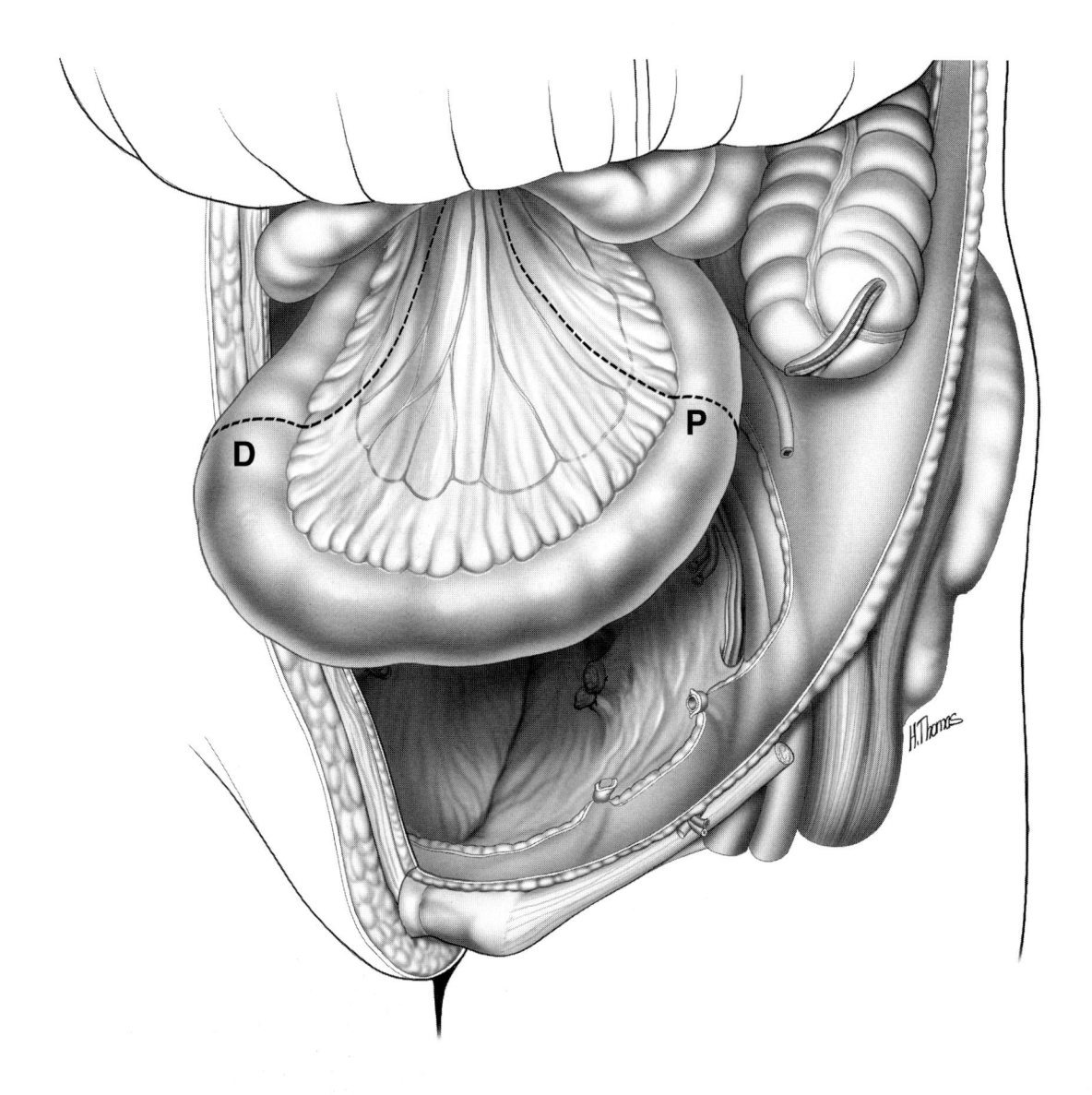

Figure 43–2 • The segment of ileum to be utilized is identified. (D, distal; P, proximal.)

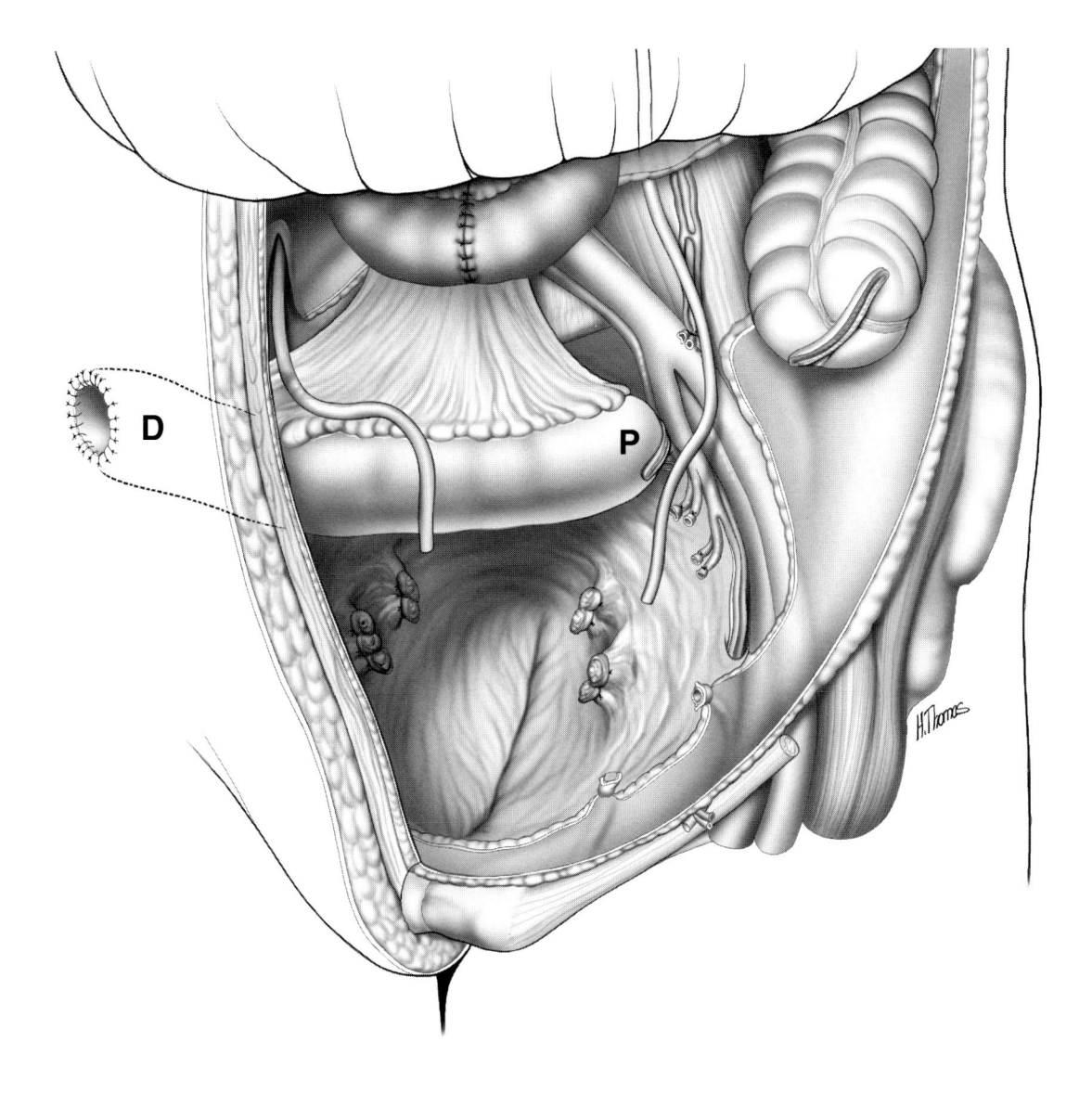

Figure 43–3 • After isolating the ileal loop, the remaining ileum is reanastomosed. The closed-off proximal end of the ileal loop is tacked to the presacral fascia, and the stoma is created in the right lower quadrant.

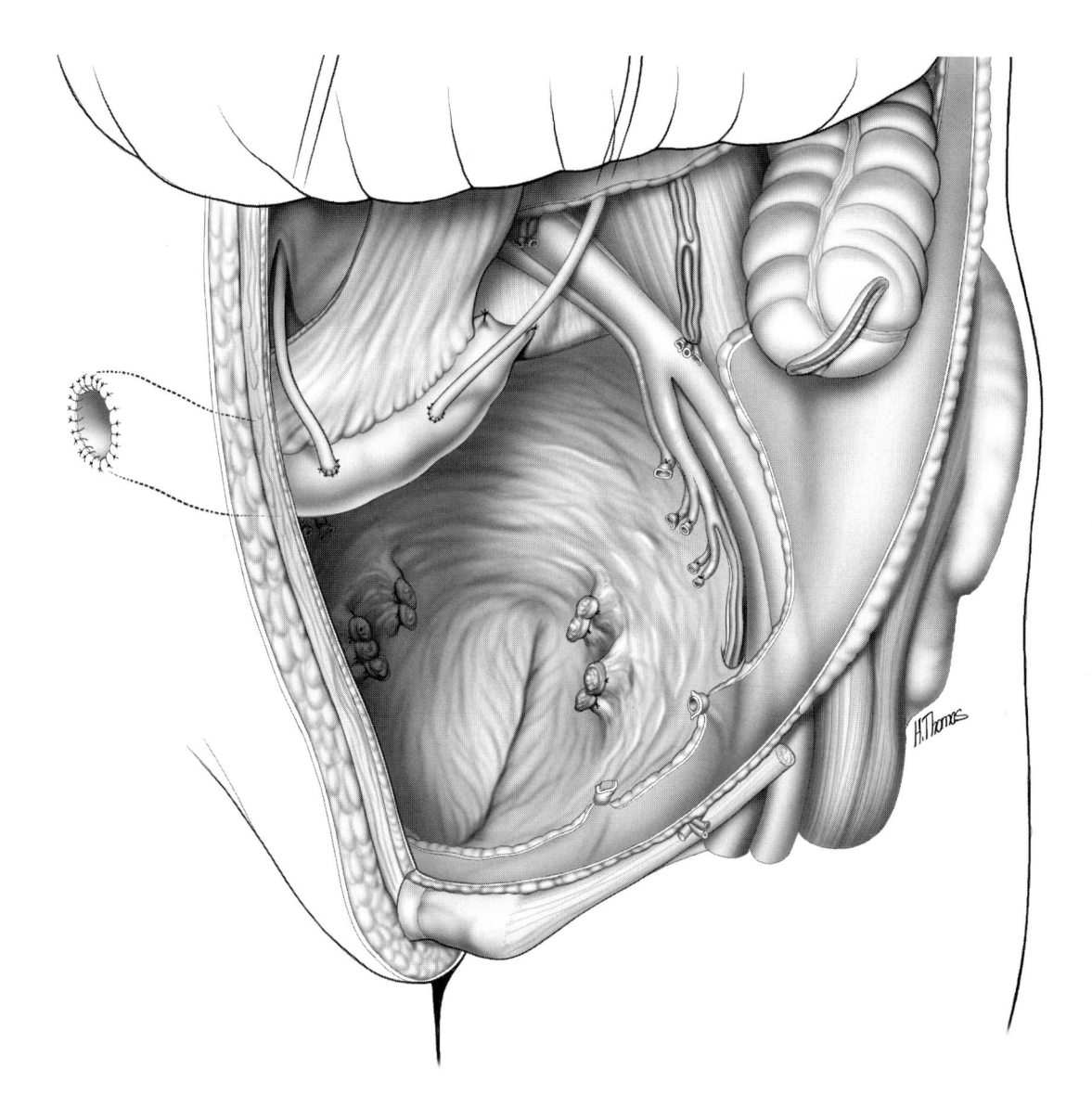

Figure 43-4 • The right and left ureters are then implanted into the ileal loop by creating two mucosa-to-mucosa anastomoses. Stents placed into the ureters to protect the anastomoses are brought out through the stoma.

Chapter 44
Surgical Anatomy for Pelvic Exenteration (Male)

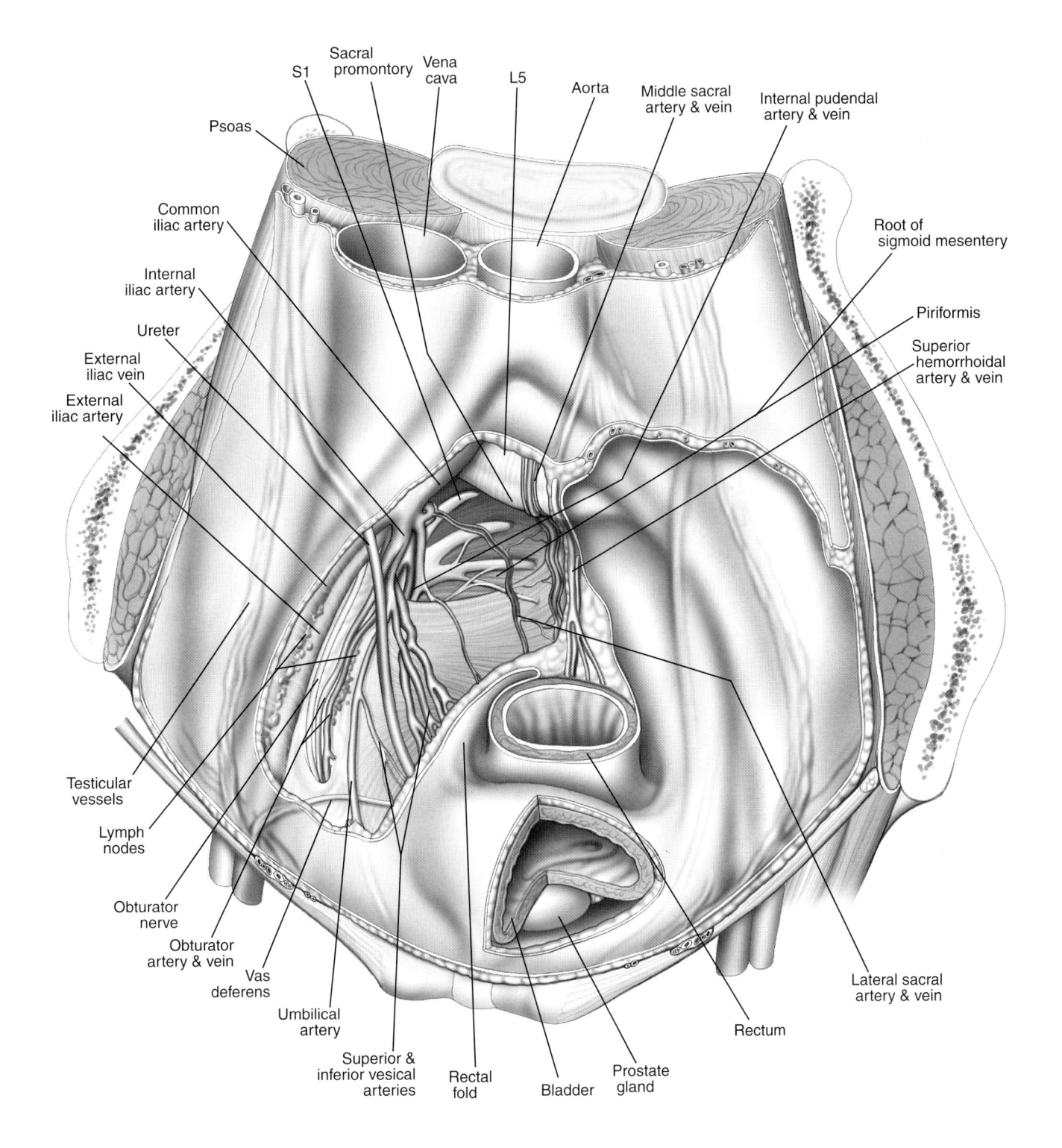

Figure 44–1 • The cross-sectional anatomy of the male pelvis is depicted.

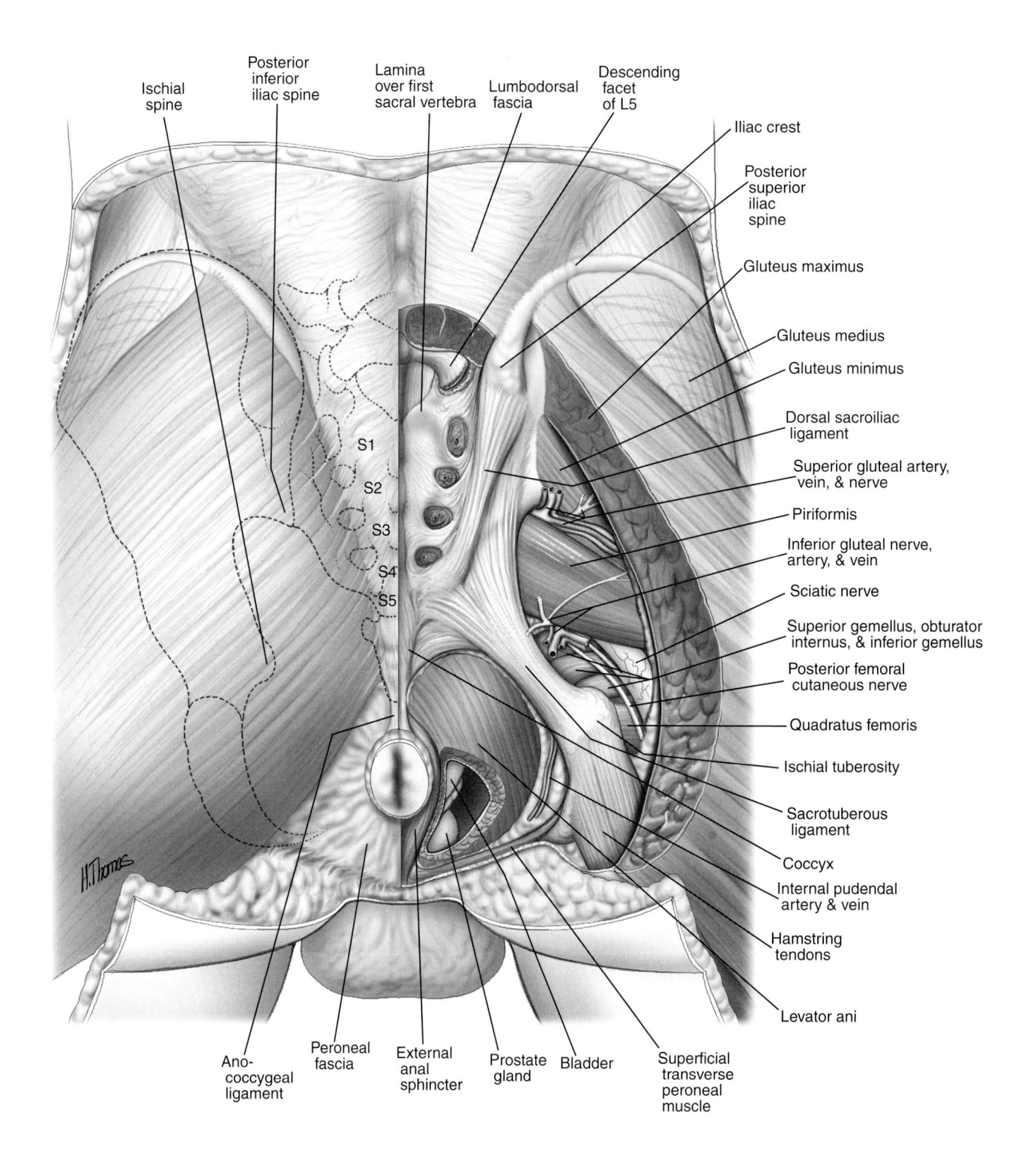

Figure 44–2 • The anatomy of the male perineum and sacrum is depicted in detail.

Chapter 45
Pelvic Exenteration—Male

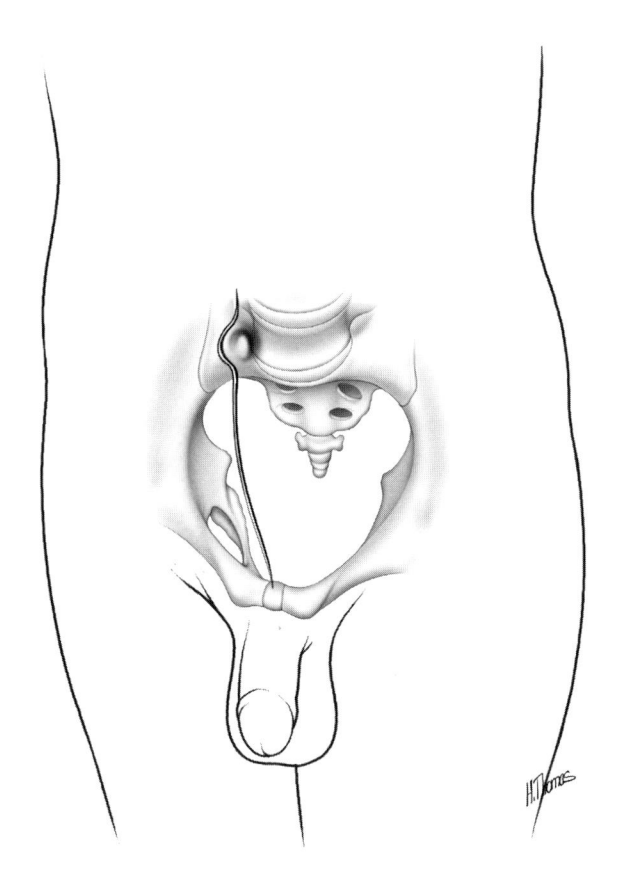

Figure 45–1 • A lower midline abdominal incision is utilized in the performance of a pelvic exenteration.

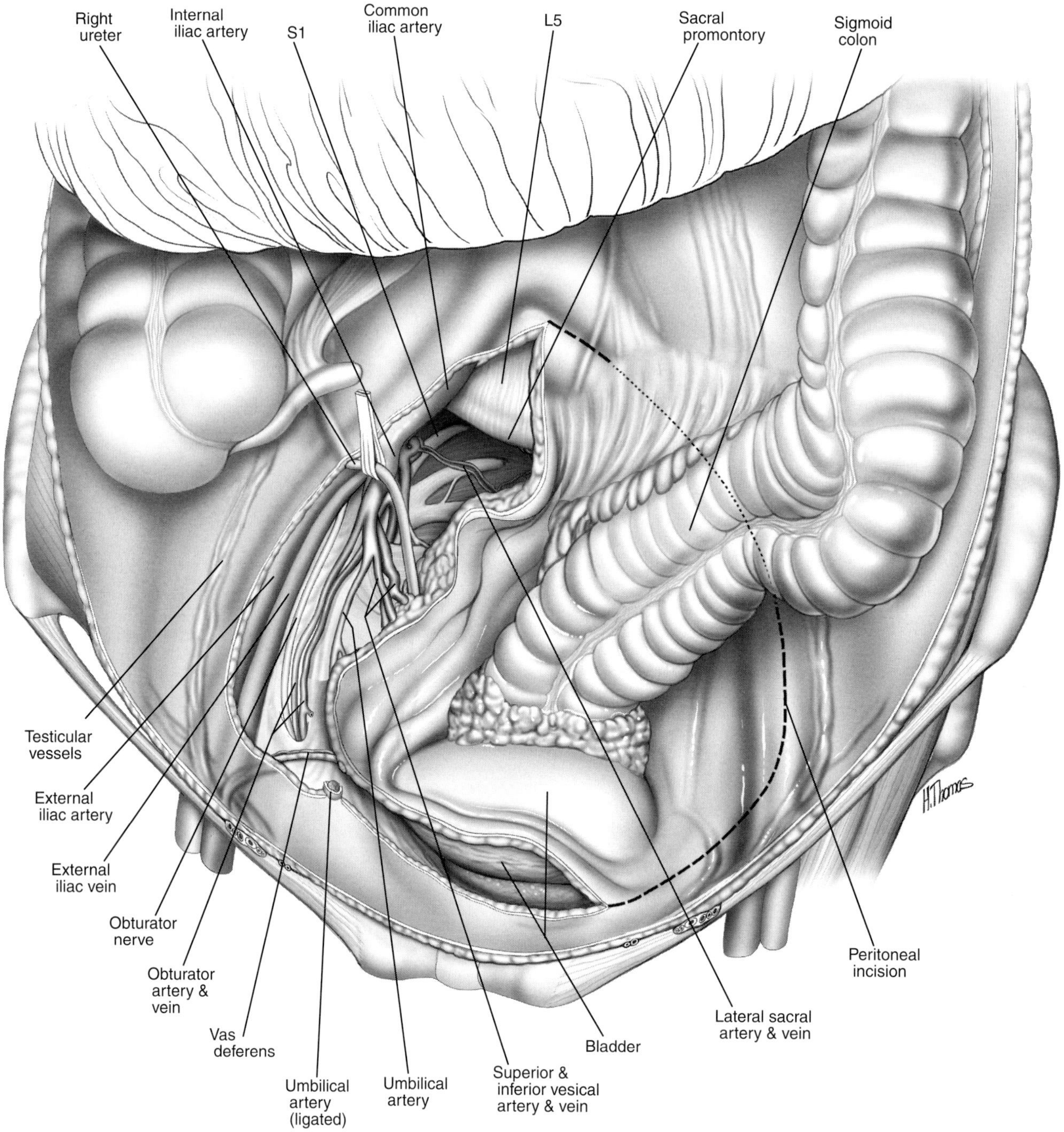

Figure 45–2 • On the right, the parietal peritoneum is incised, along the common iliac vessels from the sacral promontory to the area where the vas deferens can be identified. The dissection is then carried across the prevesical space and onto the left side of the pelvis.

Pelvic Exenteration—Male • 373

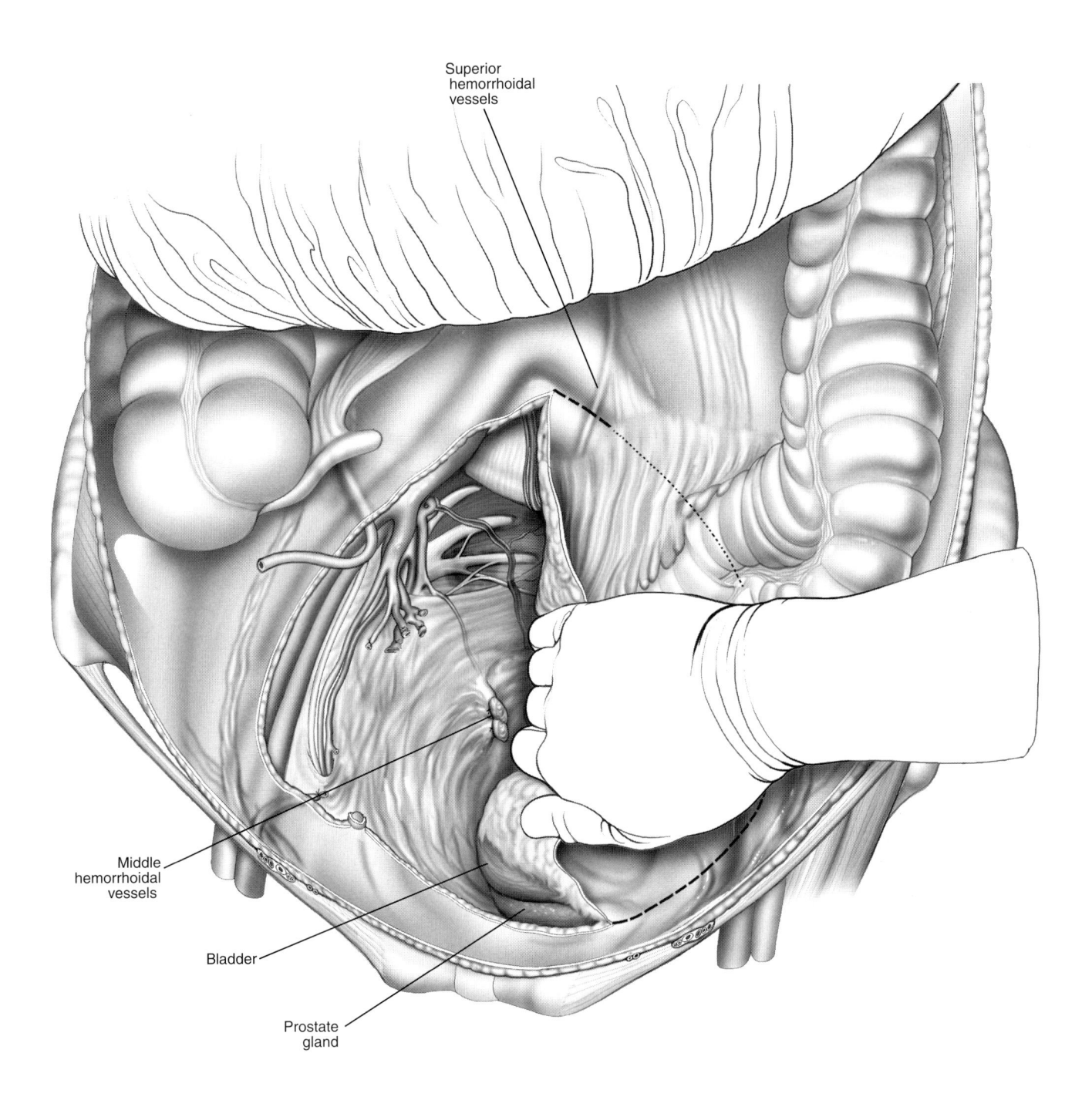

Figure 45–3 • The ureters and major vessels off the hypogastrics are divided, as is the middle hemorrhoidal vessel. The obturator nerve and vessels are preserved.

374 • Part IV LOWER ABDOMEN

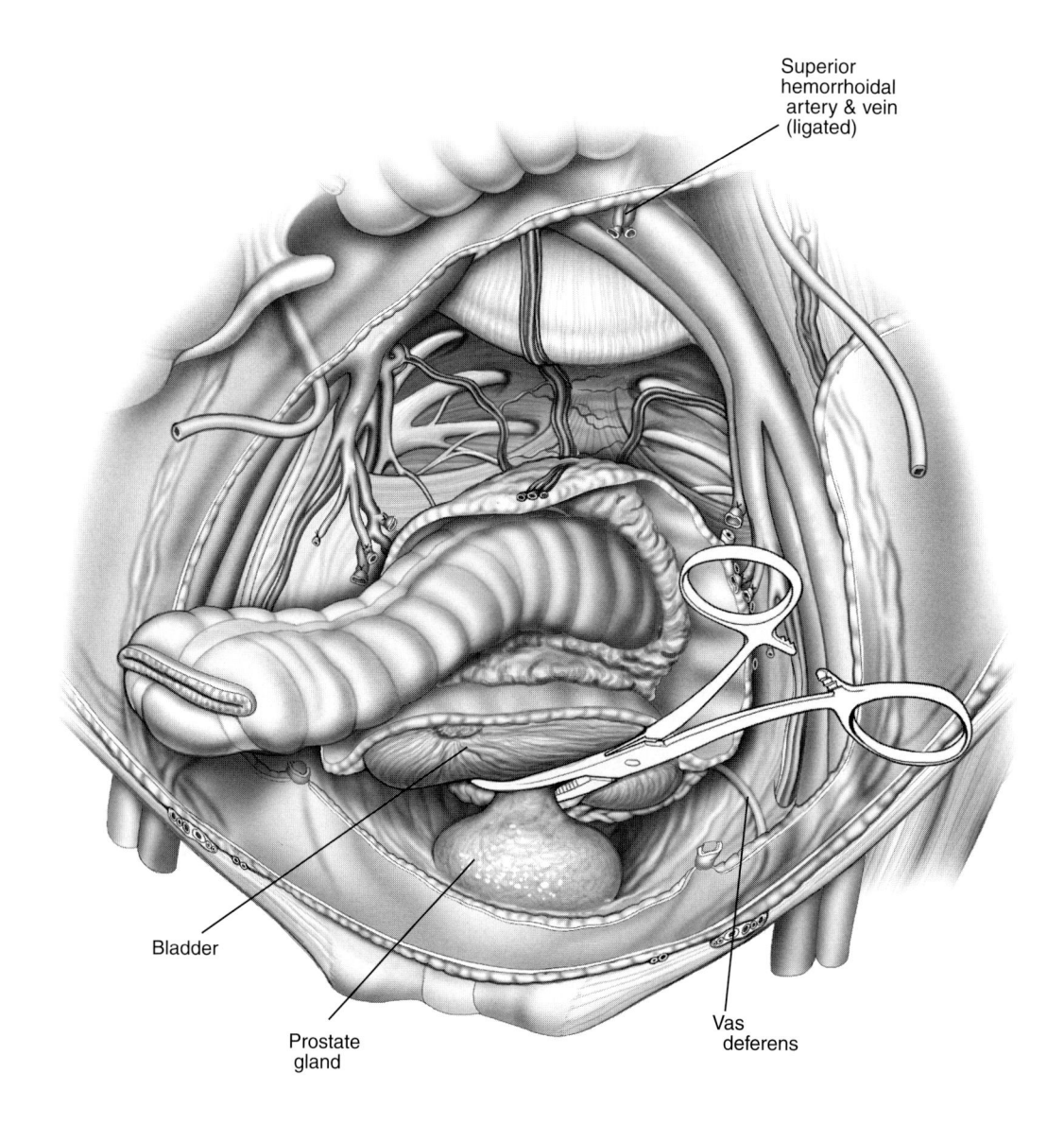

Figure 45–4 • The sigmoid colon is divided, and the left side of the pelvis is mobilized. The bladder neck is divided, exposing the anterior wall of the rectum.

Pelvic Exenteration—Male • 375

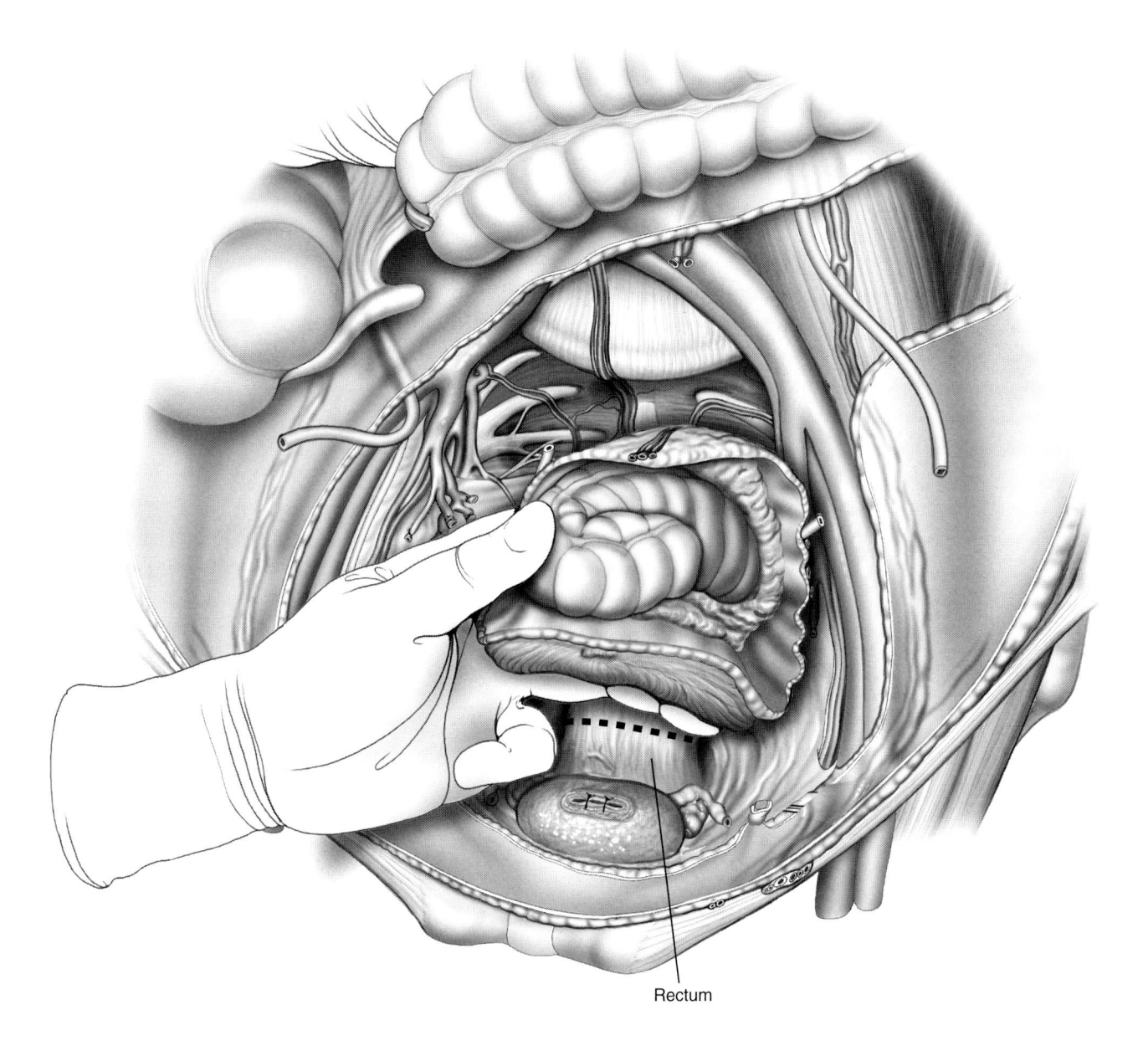

Rectum

Figure 45–5 • The rectum is transected and the specimen is removed.

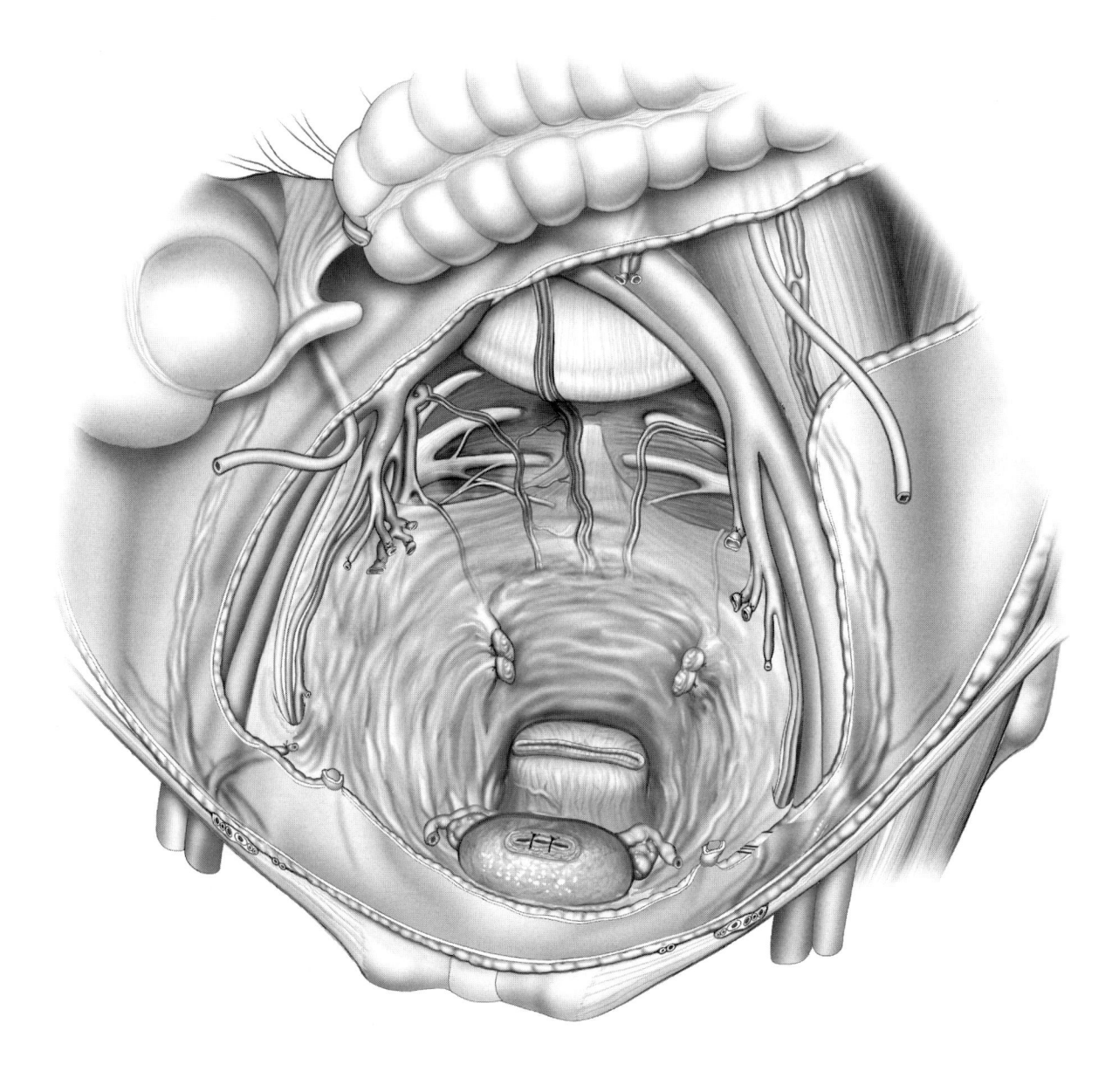

Figure 45-6 • The resulting pelvic defect is depicted. An ileal conduit and colorectal anastomosis will be created before closing the abdomen.

Chapter 46
Clinical Case: Abdominosacral Resection

Harold Wanebo

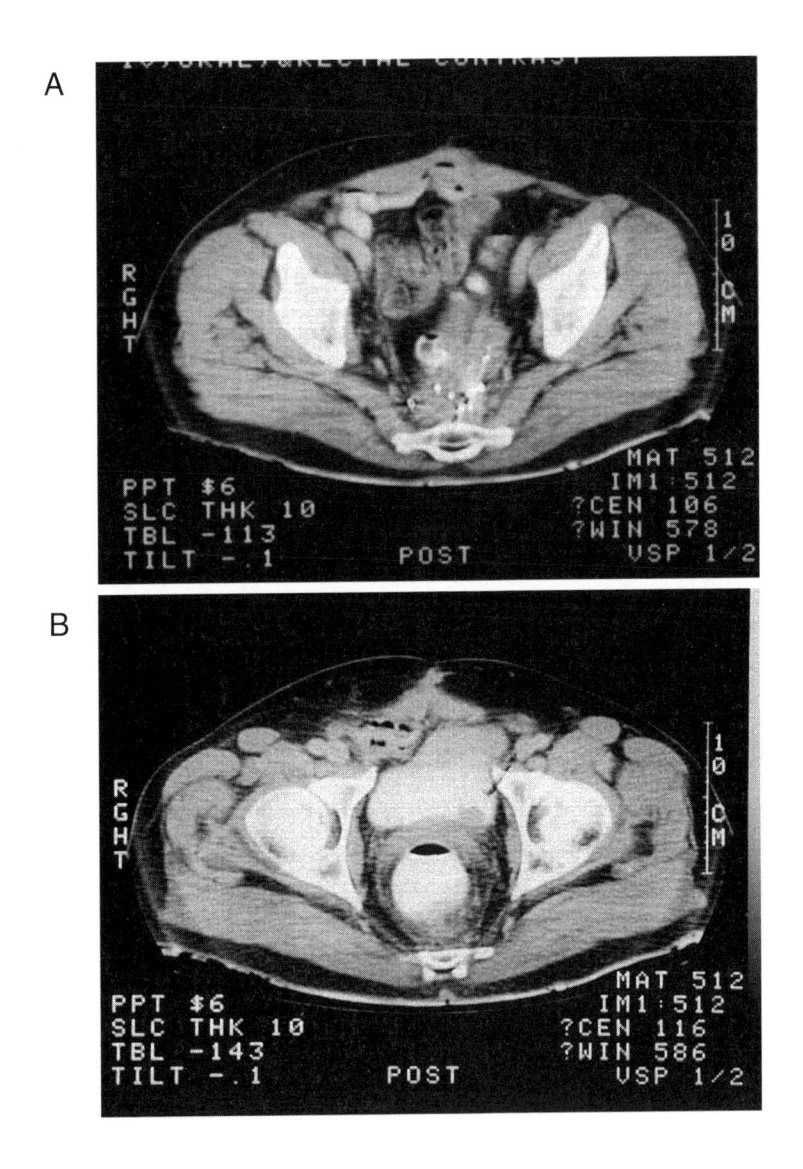

Figure 46–1 • A 58-year-old man presented with a rectal recurrence 2 years after a low anterior resection for a Dukes' BII carcinoma. The recurrence invaded the sacrum posteriorly (**A**) and the bladder anteriorly (**B**).

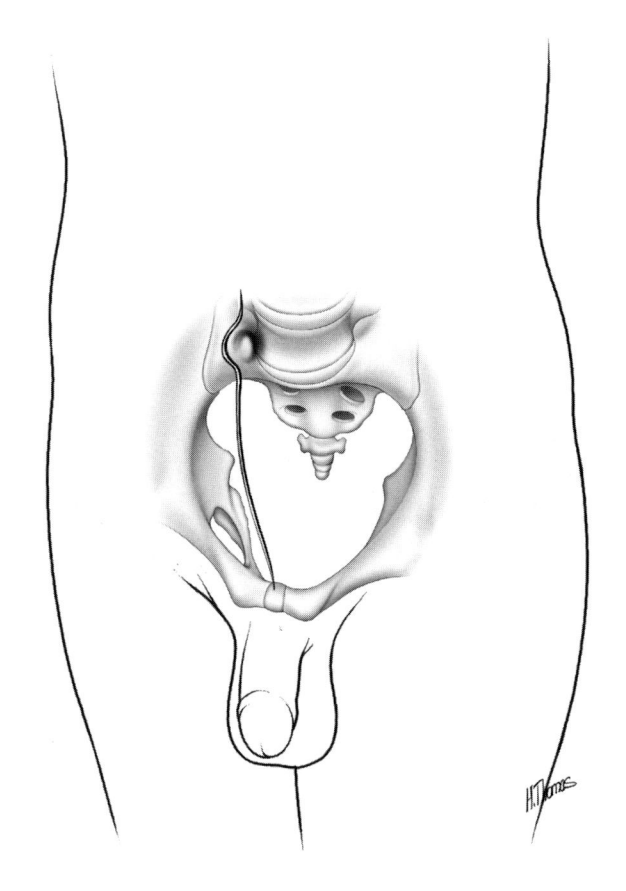

Figure 46–2 • A generous lower midline abdominal incision is made.

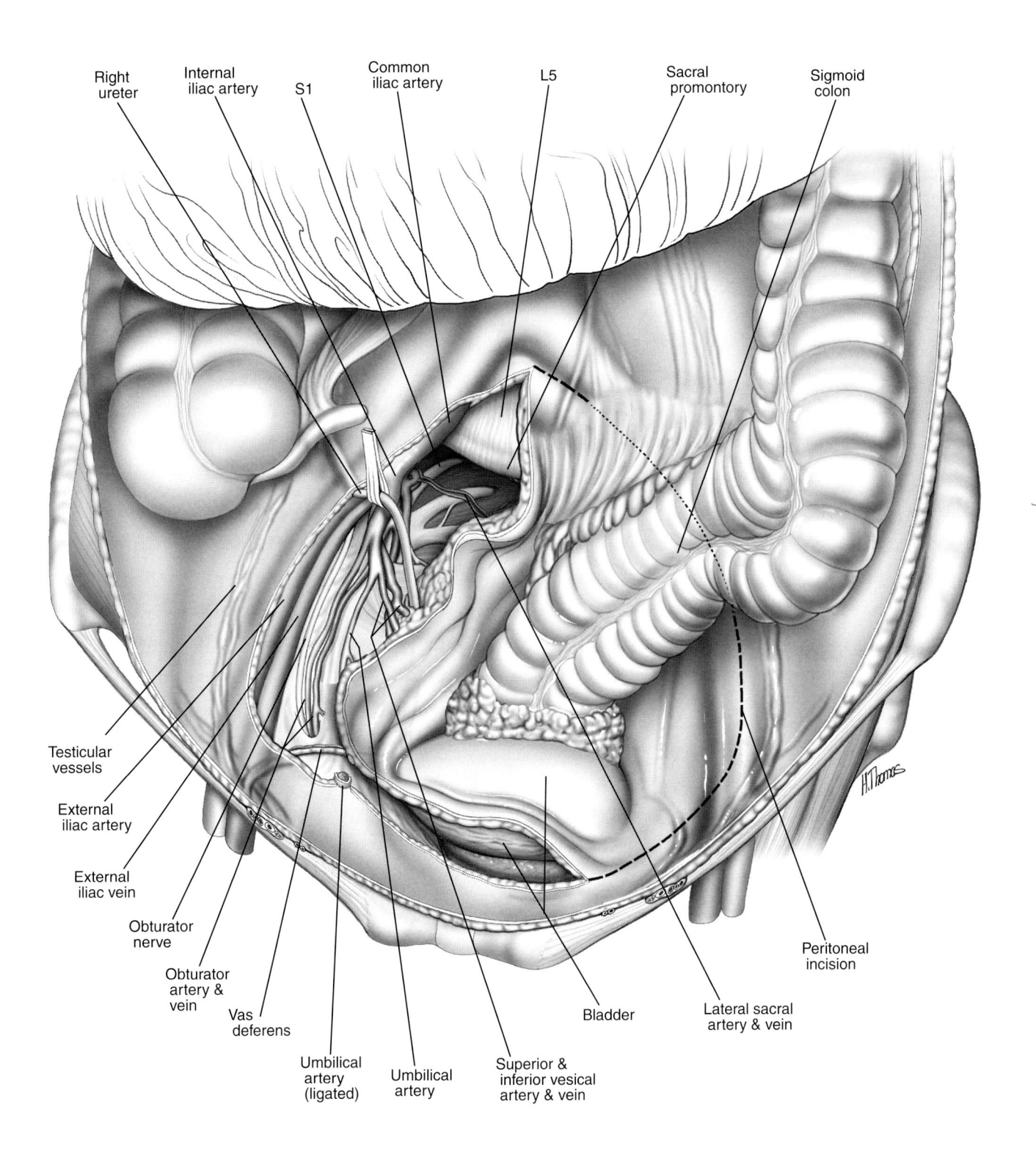

Figure 46–3 • The peritoneal incision on the right is completed; the iliac and obturator nodes are dissected and the ureter is identified. The remainder of the peritoneal incision is indicated.

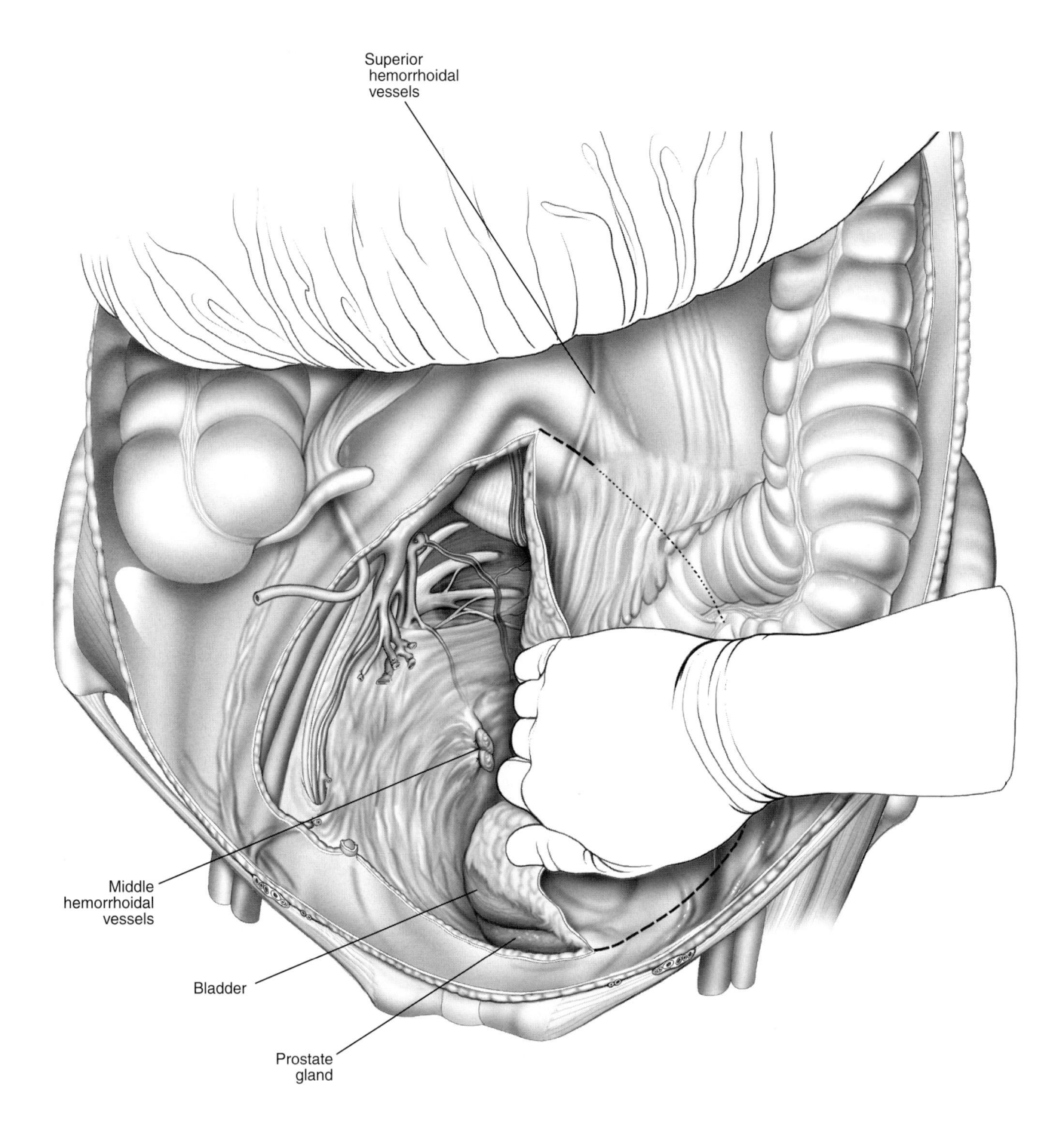

Figure 46–4 • The sigmoid and rectum are mobilized to the area of recurrence.

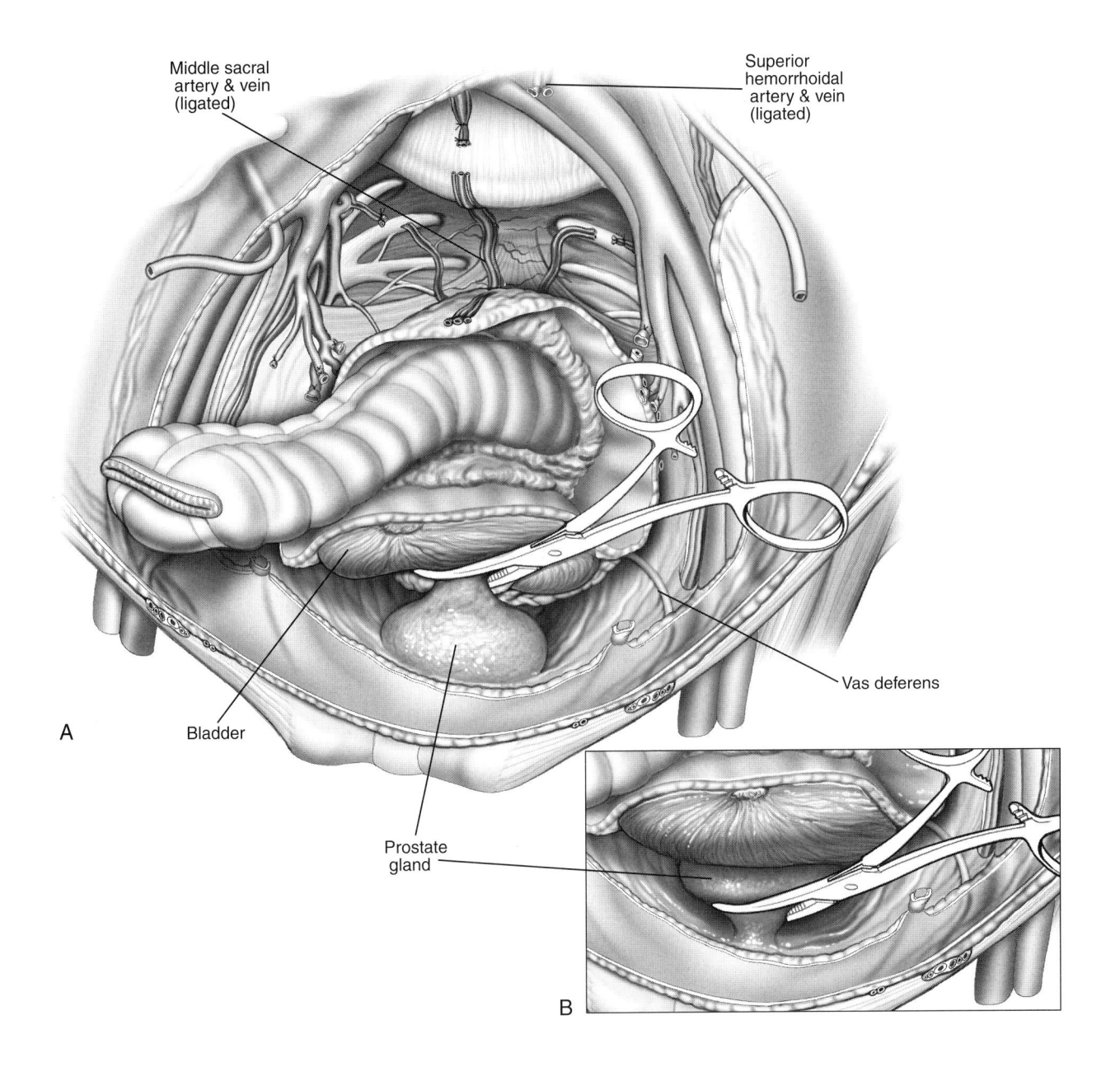

Figure 46–5 • **A,** The ureters are divided, as are the hypogastrics on the right side. The middle sacral vessels are divided and the sacral promontory and SI level are identified.

B, The urethra is divided above the prostate, but if the latter is involved, the prostate can be included.

382 • Part IV LOWER ABDOMEN

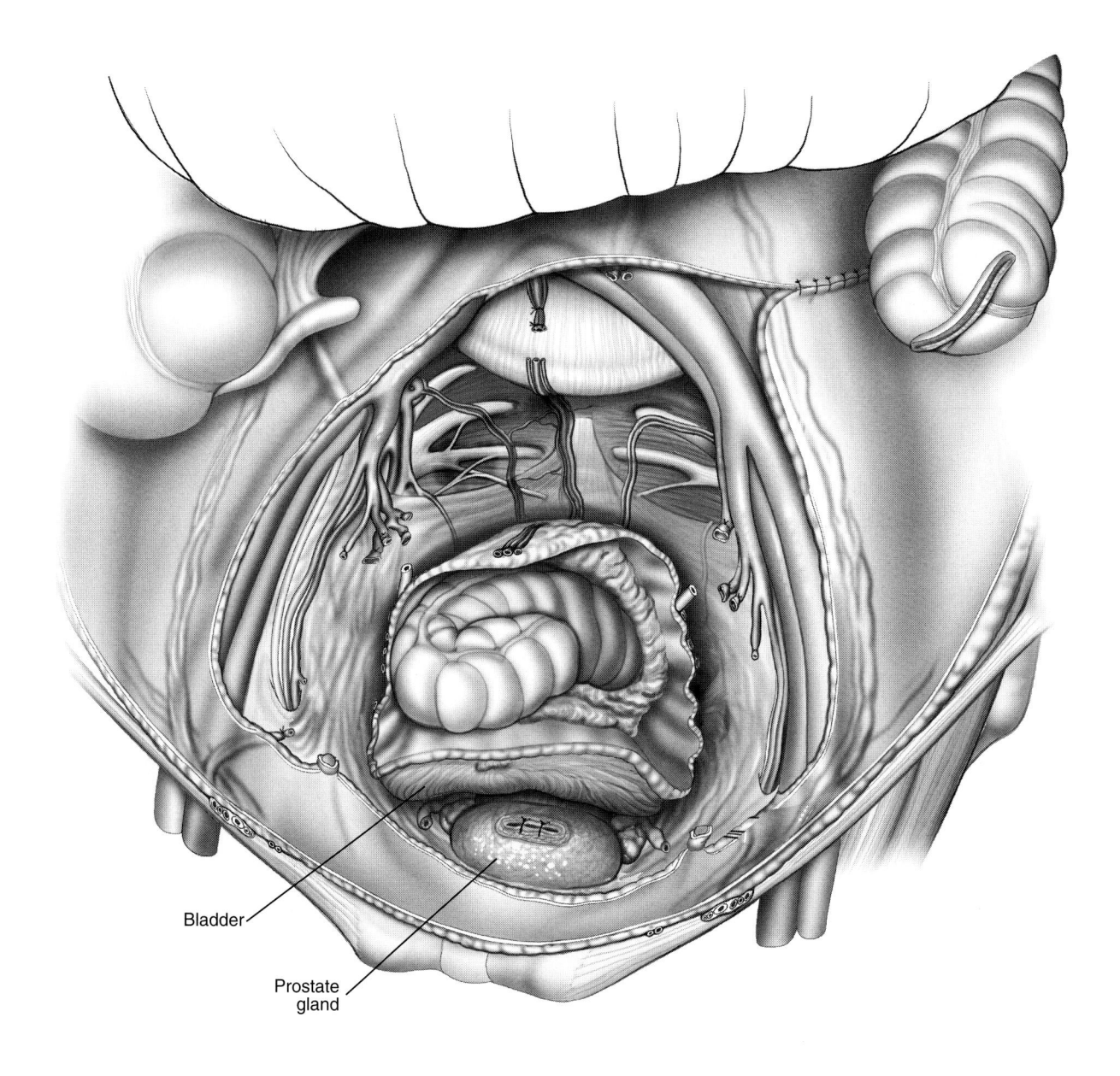

Figure 46–6 • If a staged procedure is to be performed, the abdomen is closed without any packing.

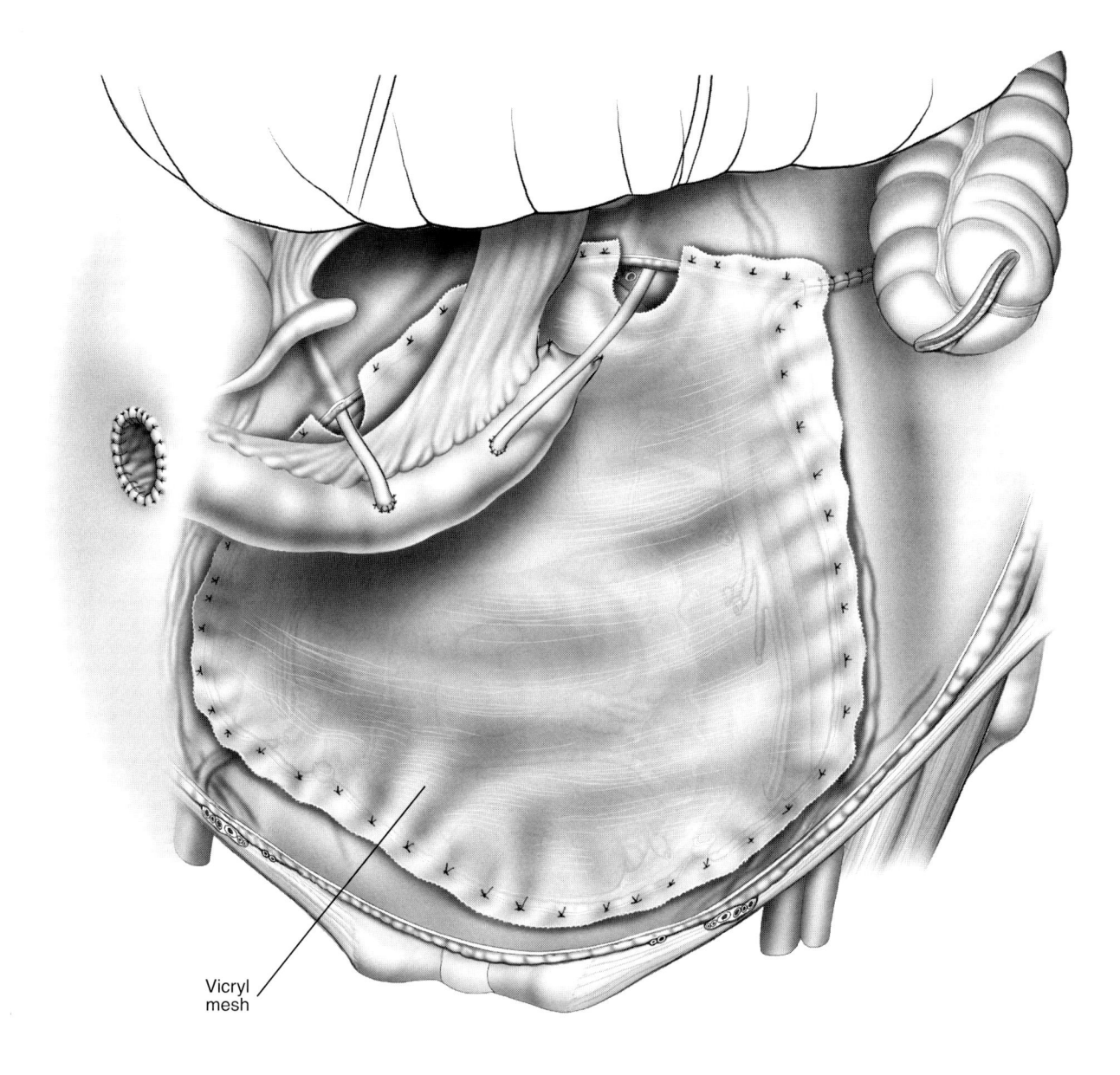

Figure 46–7 • A Vicryl mesh can be utilized to exclude the small bowel from the pelvis. An ileal conduit is created, as well as a colostomy, prior to closure of the abdomen.

384 • Part IV LOWER ABDOMEN

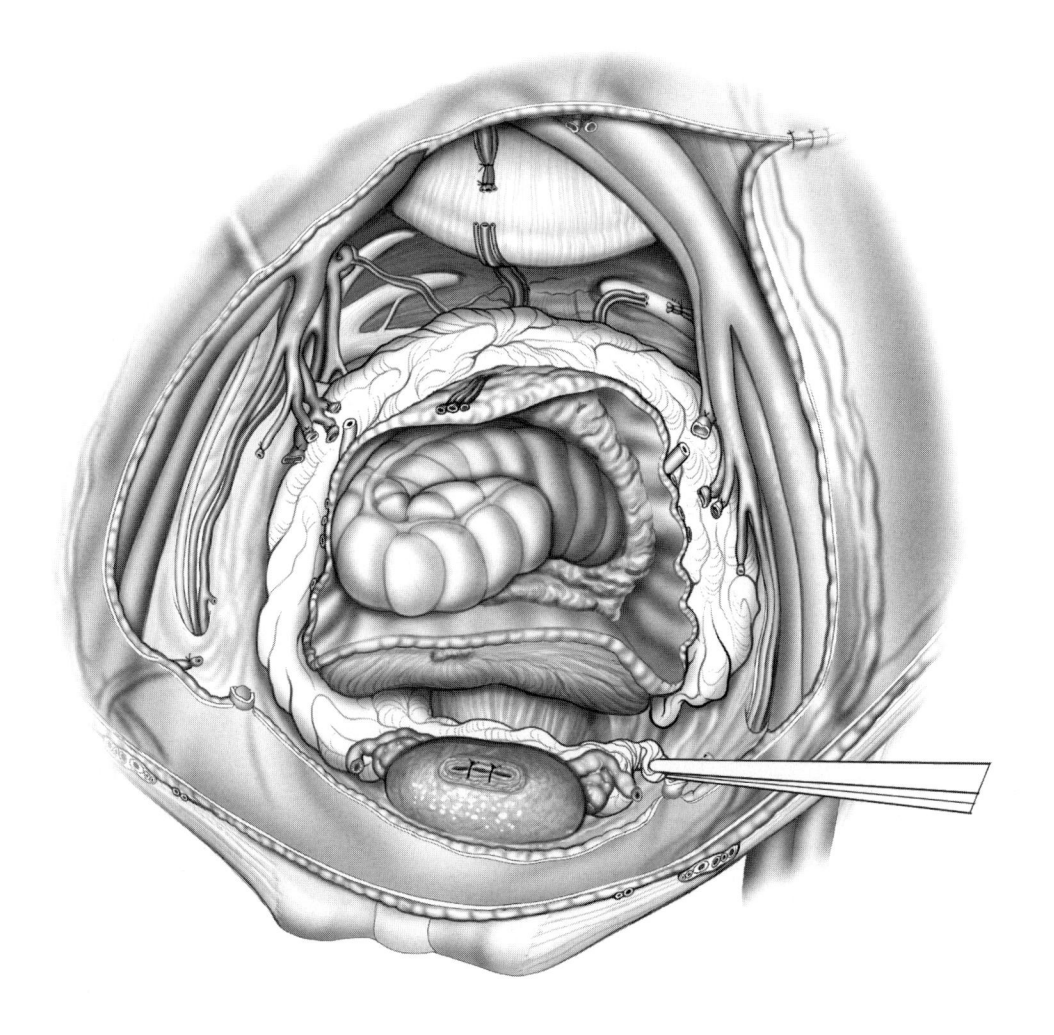

Figure 46–8 • If the perineal portion of the procedure is to take place as part of a one-stage procedure, lap pads can be placed behind the mobilized bowel prior to the placement of a Vicryl mesh and the creation of the stoma.

Clinical Case: Abdominosacral Resection • 385

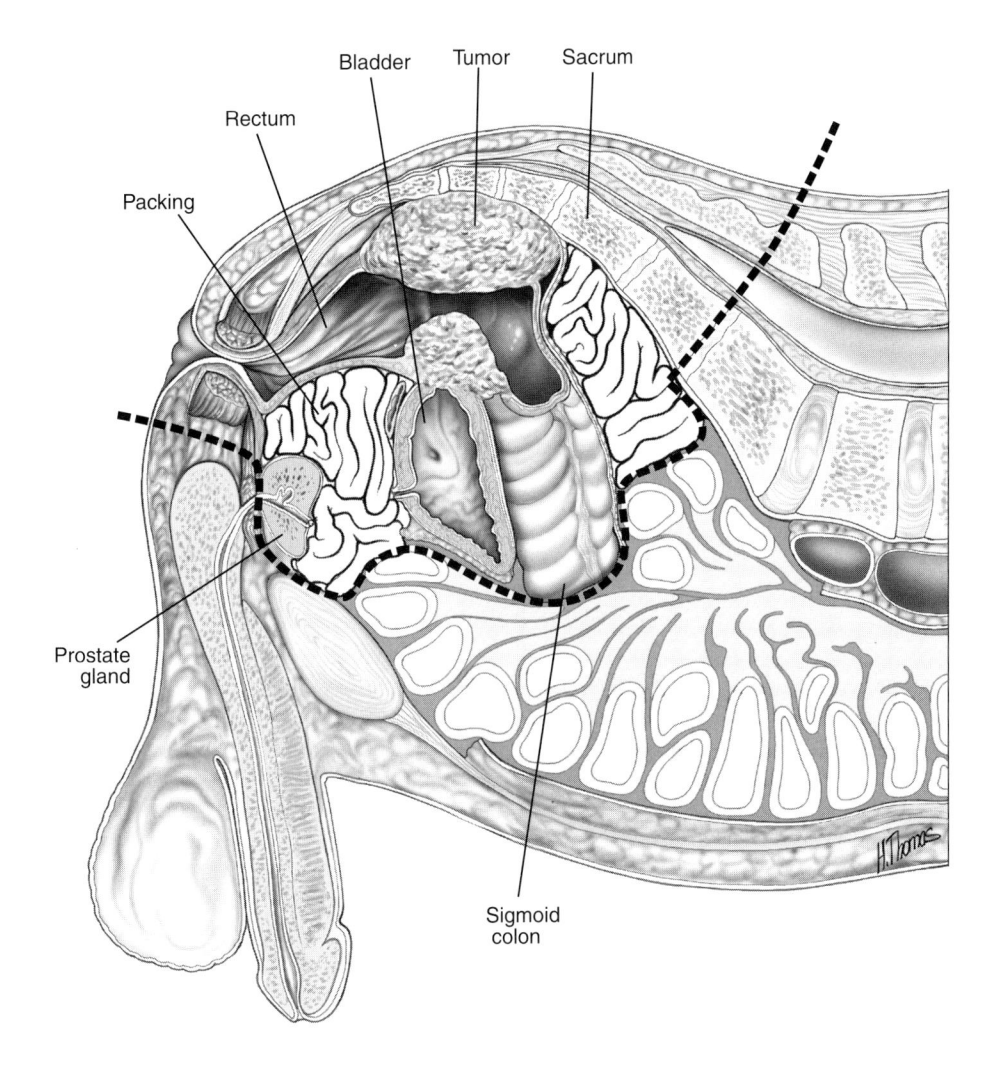

Figure 46–9 • A lateral view defining the line of resection. Posteriorly, the sacrum is divided at the S1 or S2 level. Anteriorly, the retropubic space is entered, and the prostate and the urethra are included in the resection.

386 • Part IV LOWER ABDOMEN

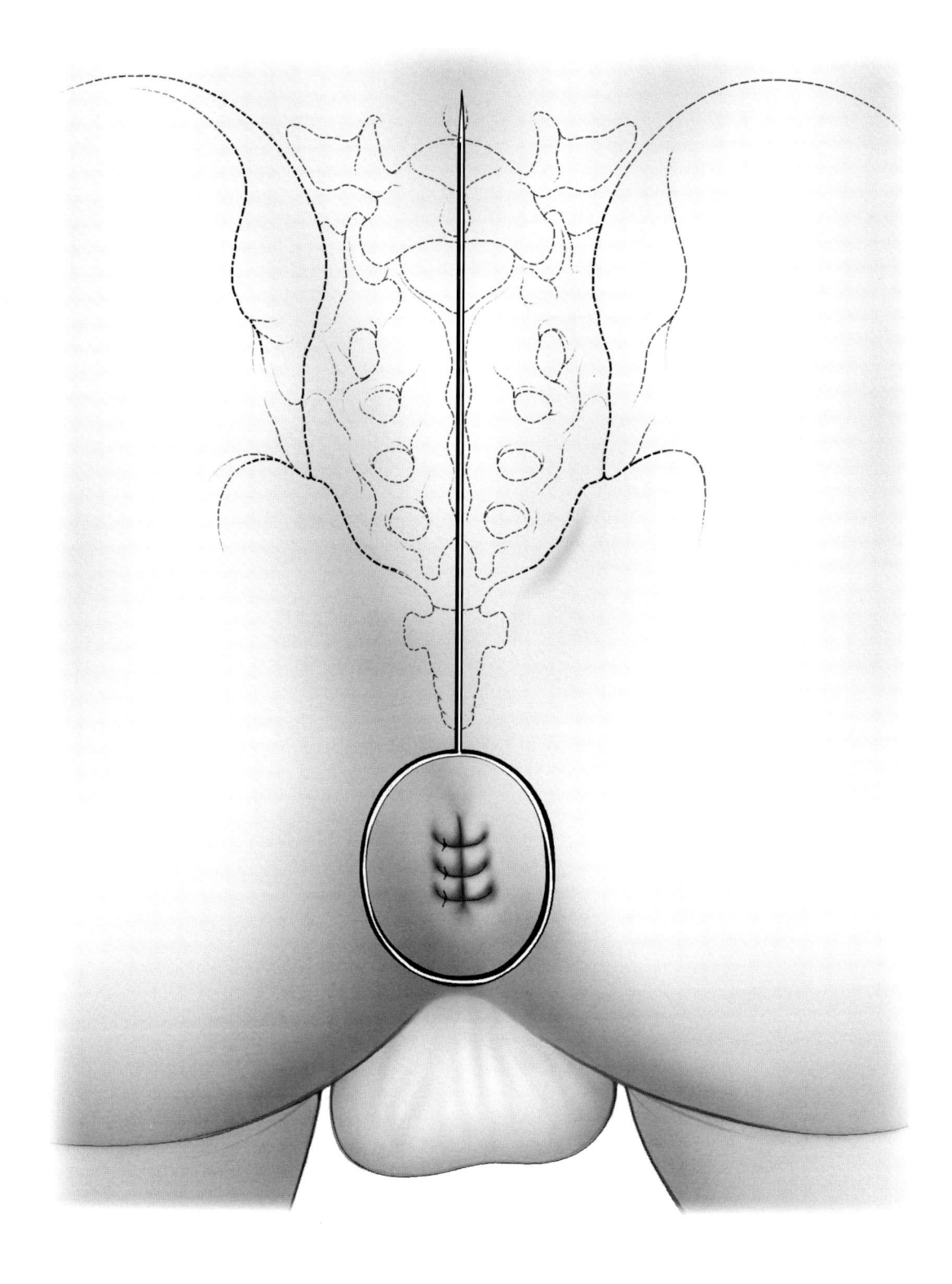

Figure 46–10 • The posterior incision is depicted.

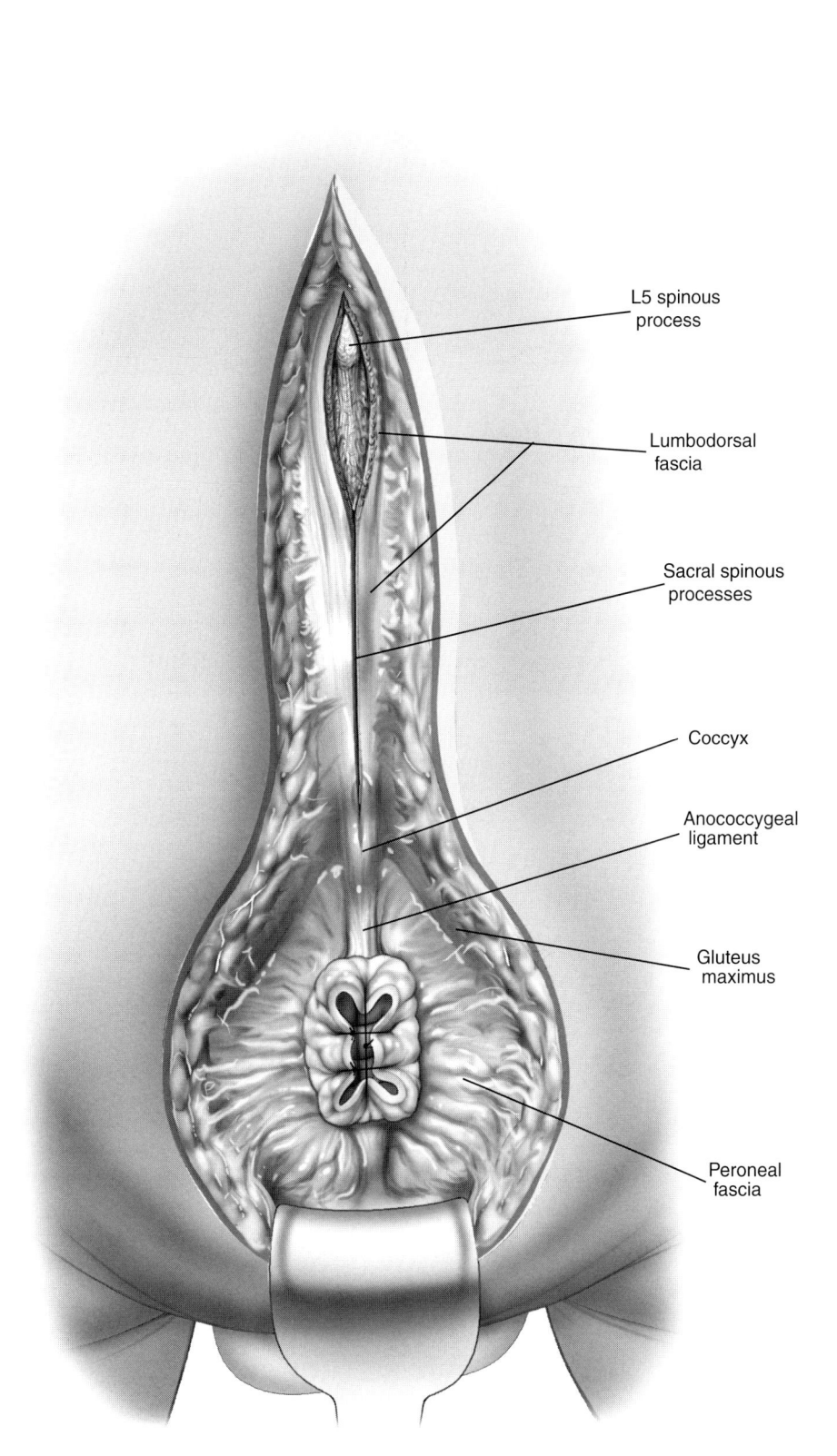

Figure 46–11 • The incision is carried in the midline down to the lumbodorsal fascia.

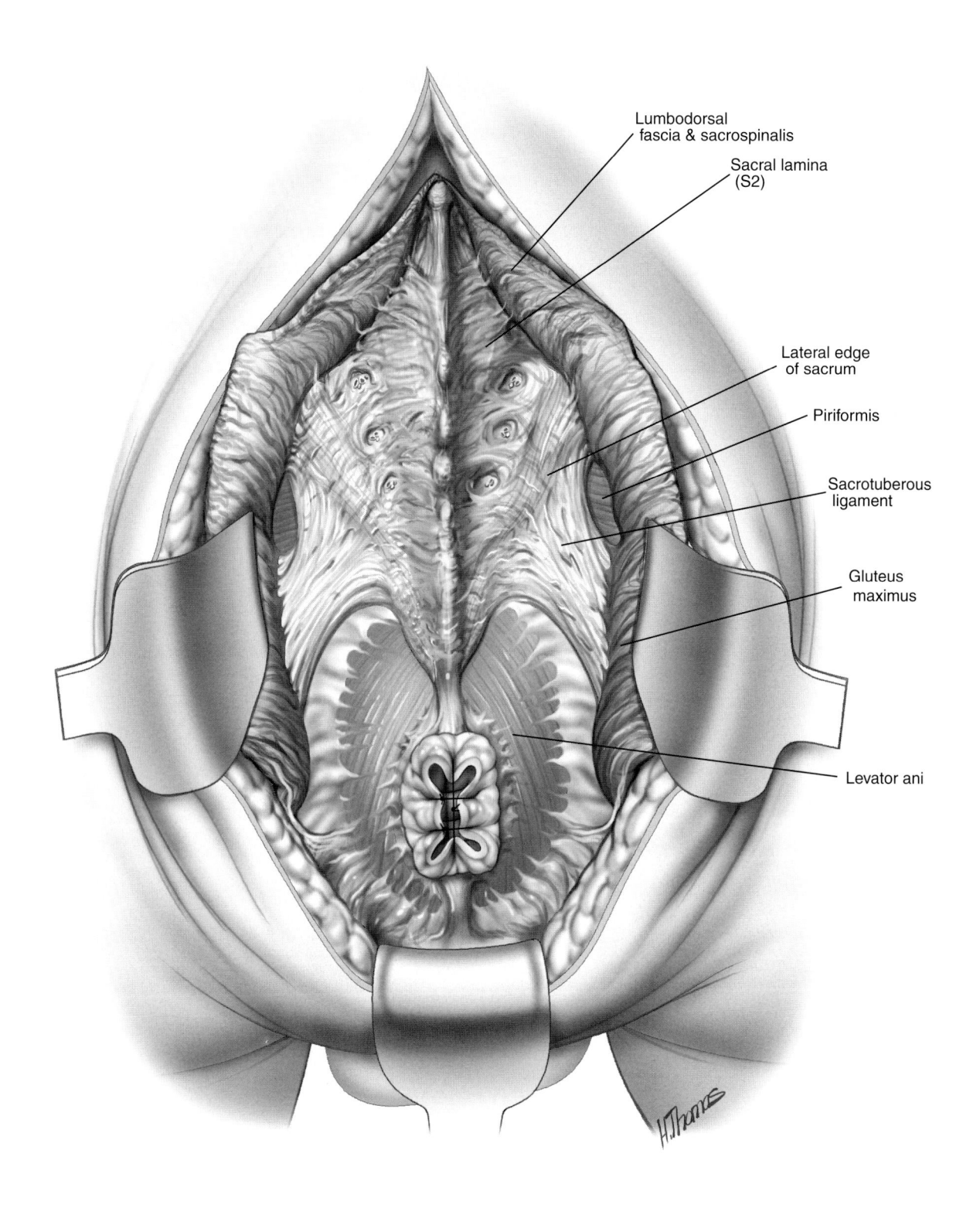

Figure 46–12 • Full thickness flaps are formed from L5 to the coccyx and lateral to the sacrospinous and sacrotuberous ligaments.

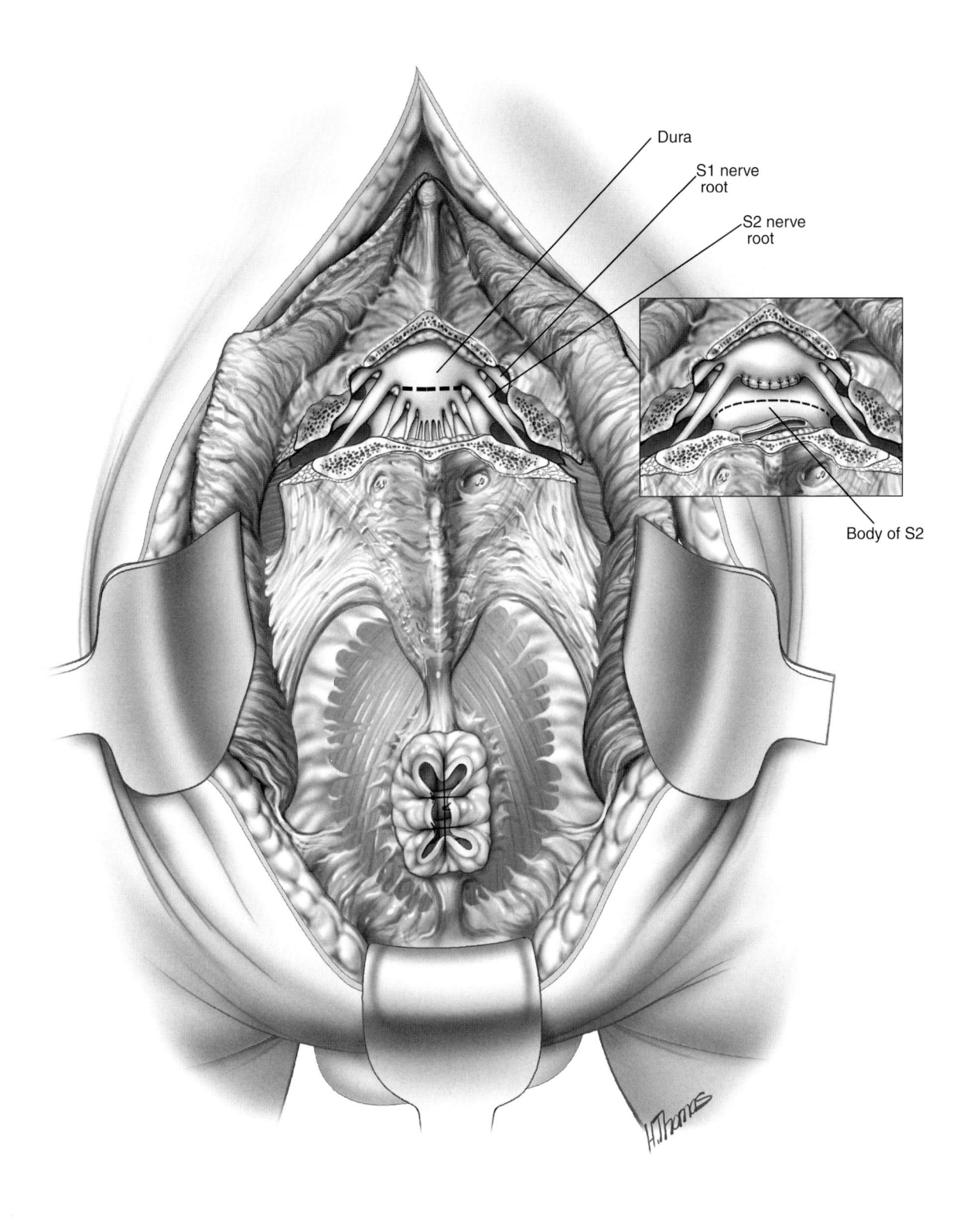

Figure 46-13 • A laminectomy is performed. The dural sac is divided below S2, the S1 nerve root is preserved, and the dural sac is closed (*inset*). If a higher level resection is to be performed, the S2 and S1 roots can be sacrificed as well and the dural sac closed at a higher level.

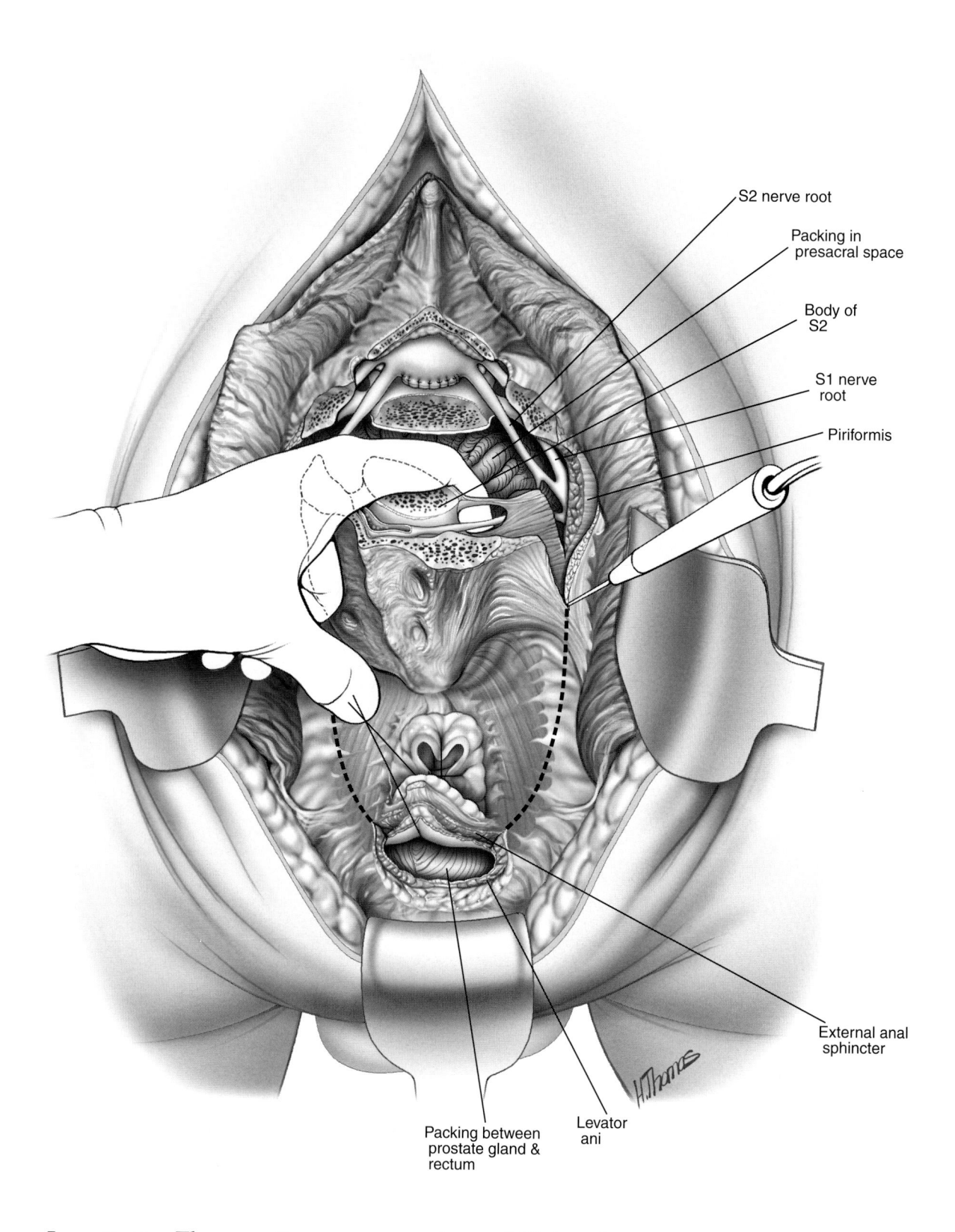

Figure 46–14 • The resection progresses by mobilizing the sacrum after dividing it and entering the peritoneal cavity. The lateral attachments, the S3 and S4 roots, the sacrospinous process, and the sacrotuberous ligaments are divided. The ischiorectal fossa and lateral attachments of the pelvic diaphragm are incised.

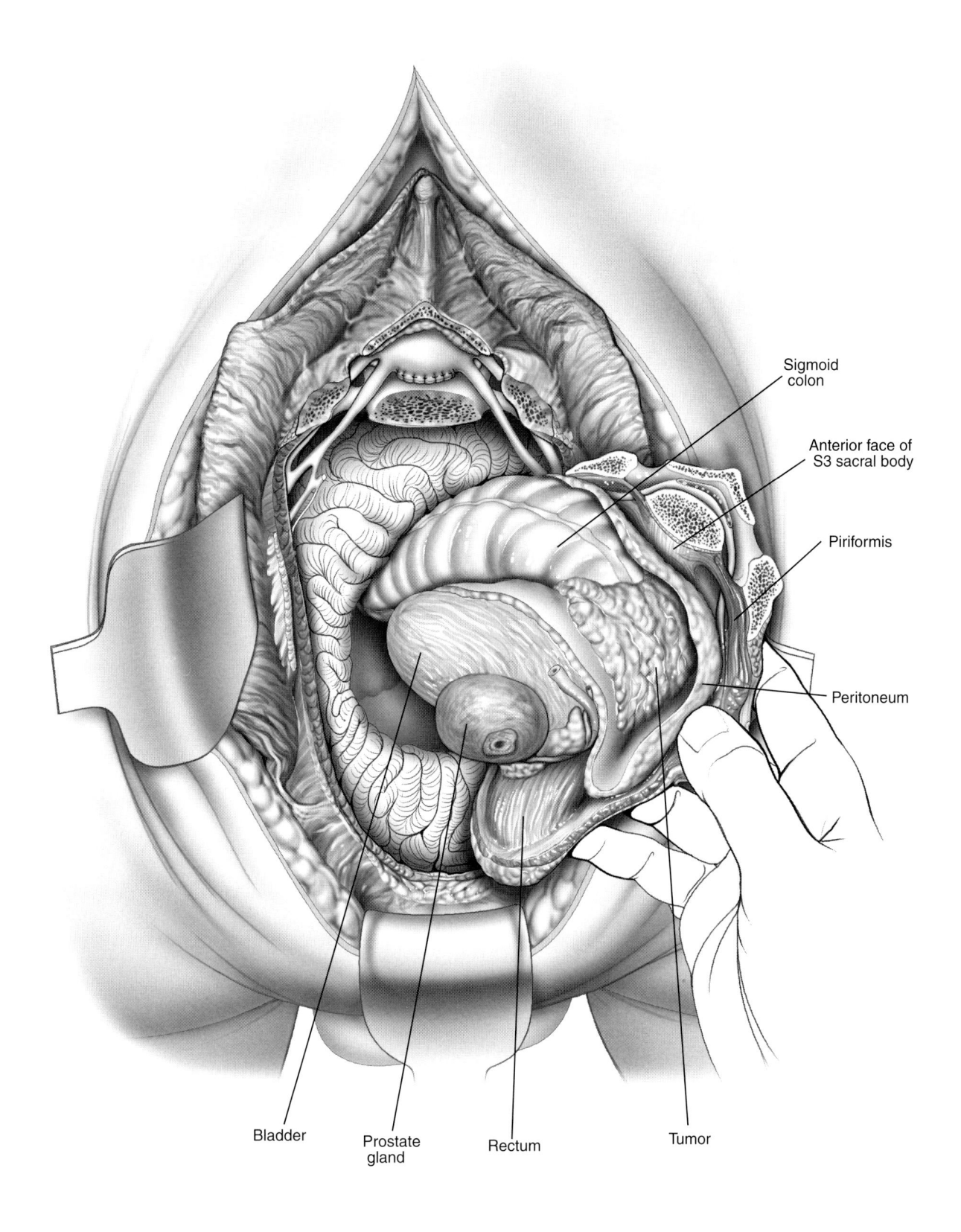

Figure 46–15 • The entire specimen is taken, including the sacrum, lateral sacral attachments, and attached anterior structures: rectum, bladder, prostate, and urethra.

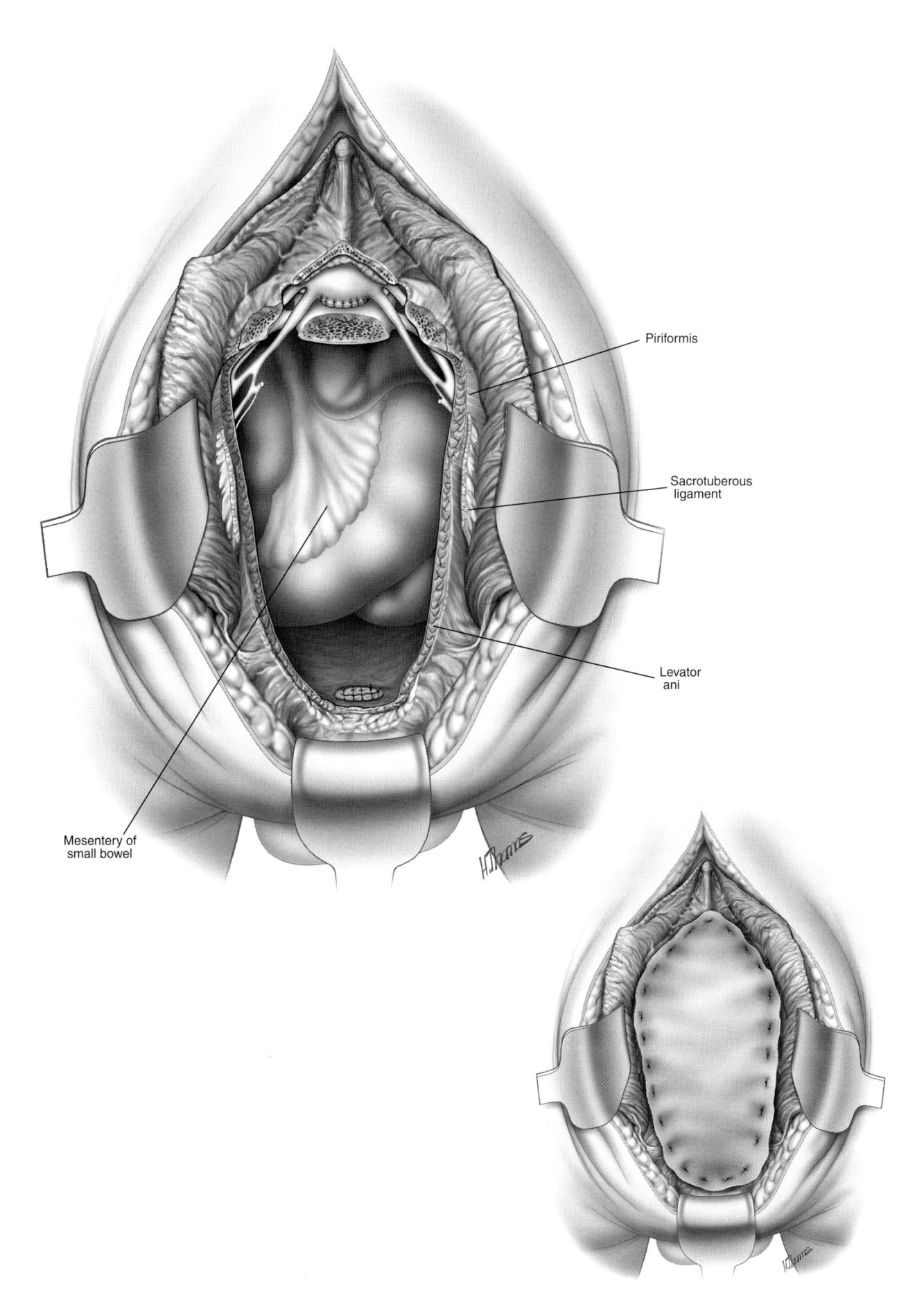

Figure 46–16 • Following the completed resection, the pelvic floor can be reconstructed by placing a Gore-Tex patch across the sacral defect.

Clinical Case: Abdominosacral Resection • 393

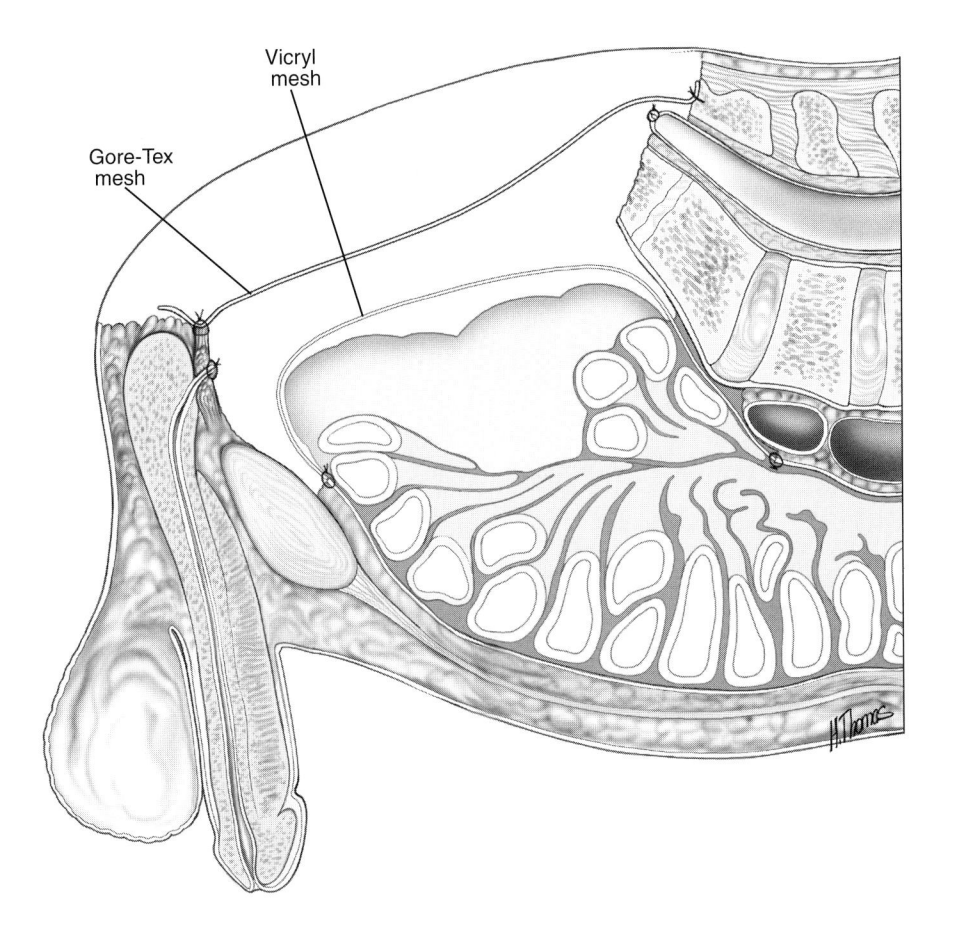

Figure 46–17 • A lateral view of the composite resection.

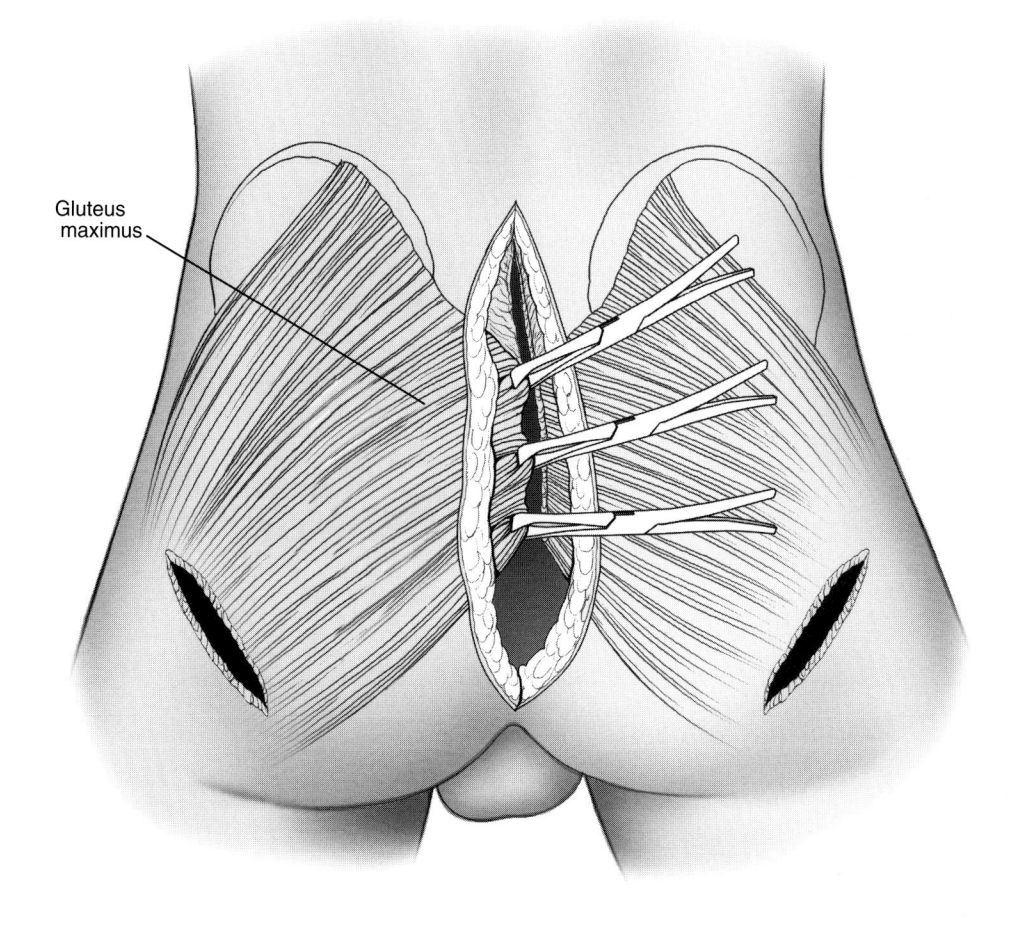

Figure 46–18 • The gluteus muscles are advanced to close the midline defect by making a relaxing incision laterally.

Part V

RADICAL AMPUTATIONS

Chapter 47
Surgical Anatomy for Radical Resections of the Upper Extremity

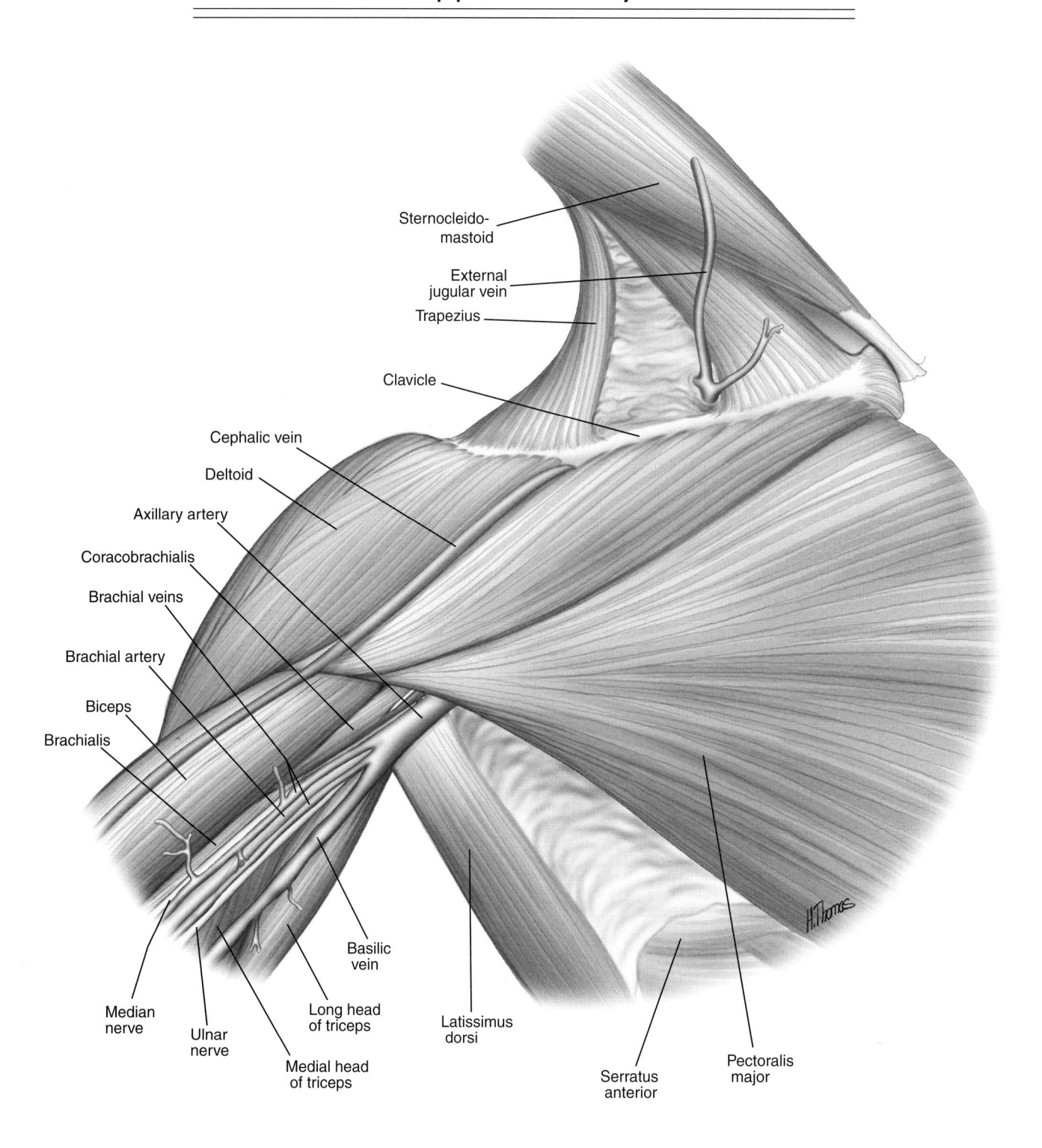

Figure 47–1 • An understanding of the complex anatomy in the shoulder girdle area provides a solid basis for mastering the operative techniques employed in resections of tumors here.

Surgical Anatomy for Radical Resections of the Upper Extremity • 397

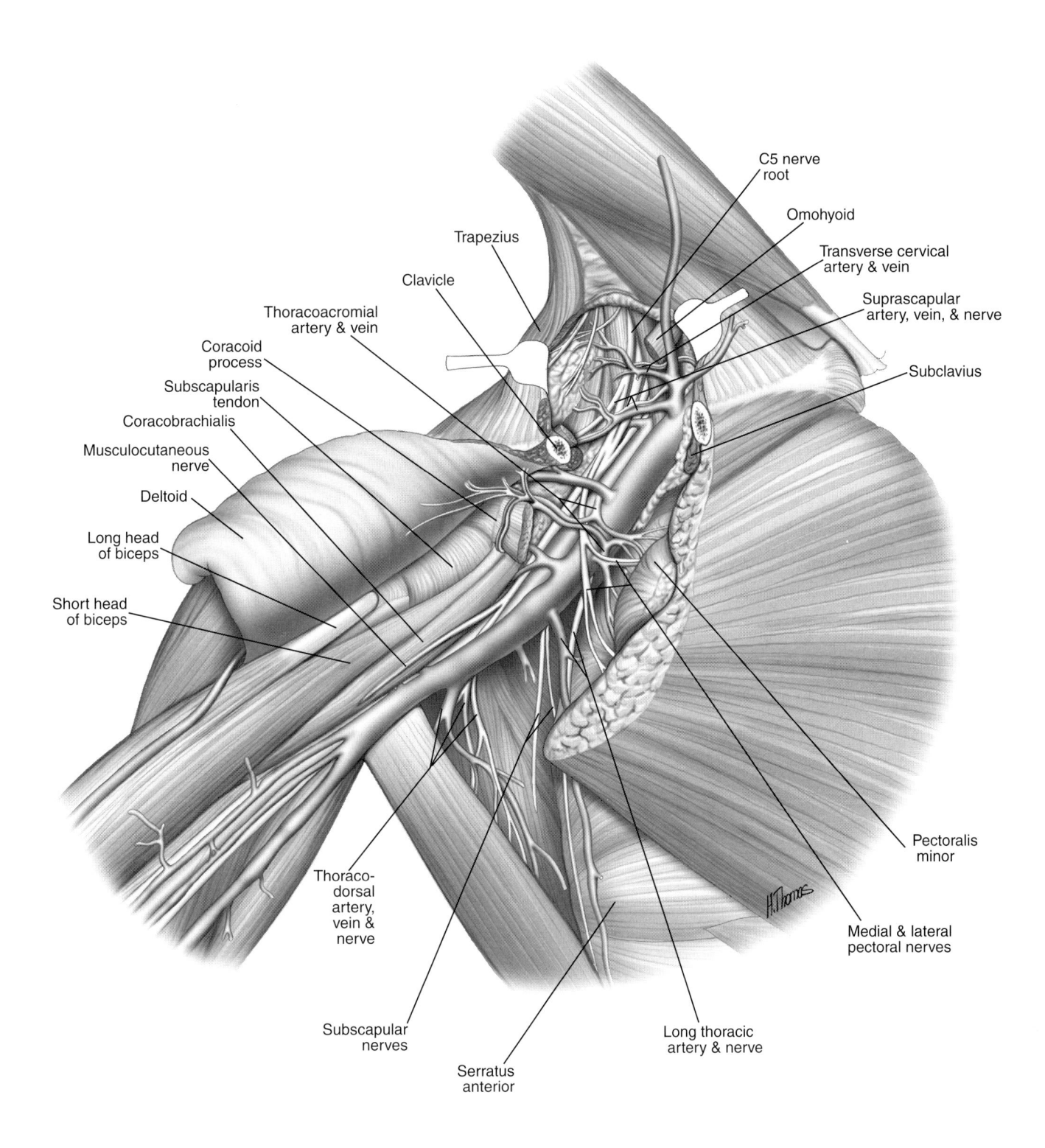

Figure 47–2 • The vascular anatomy and neural anatomy are depicted after division of the pectoralis major and minor and the clavicle.

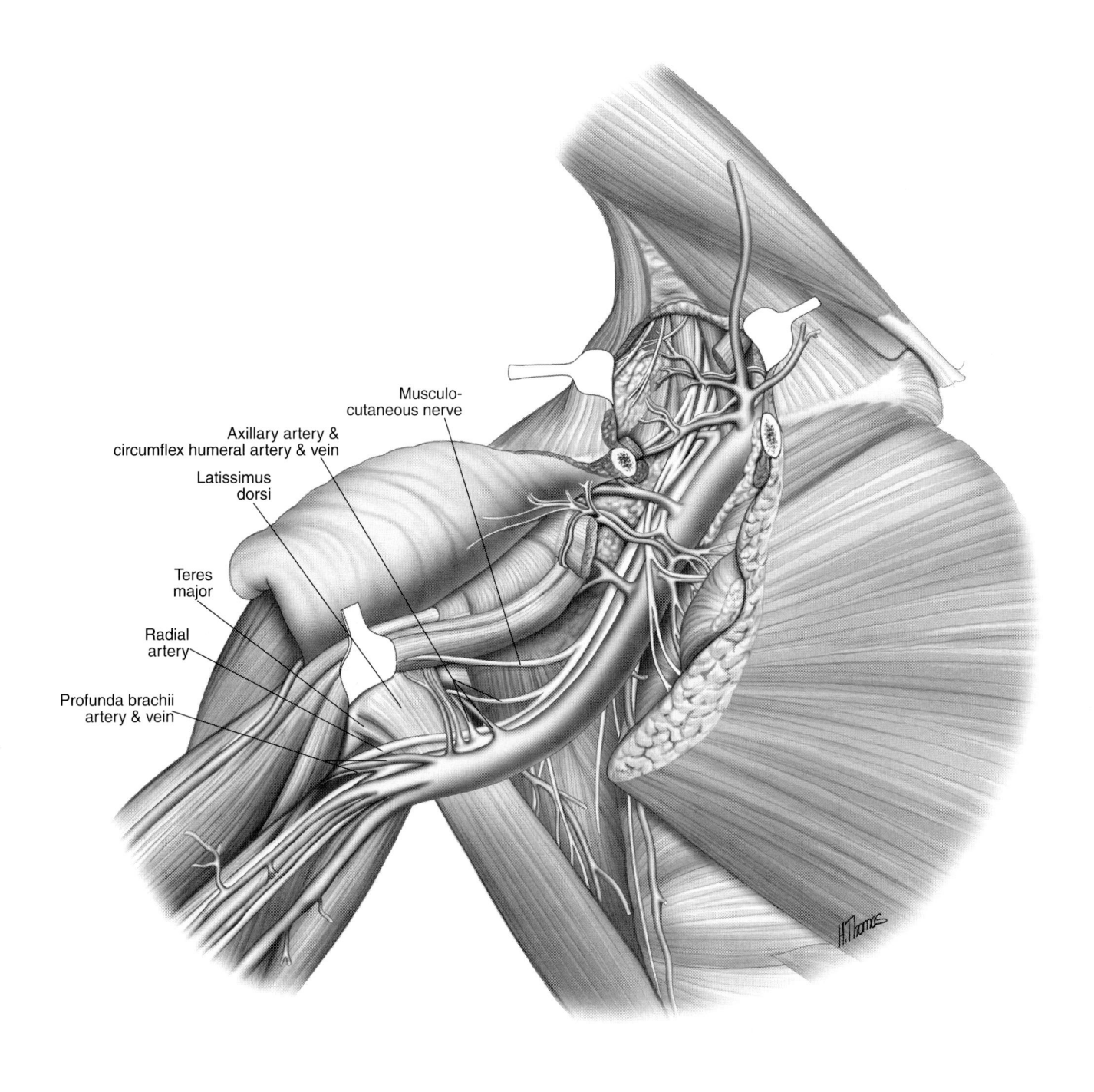

Figure 47–3 • The axillary anatomy is depicted.

Surgical Anatomy for Radical Resections of the Upper Extremity • 399

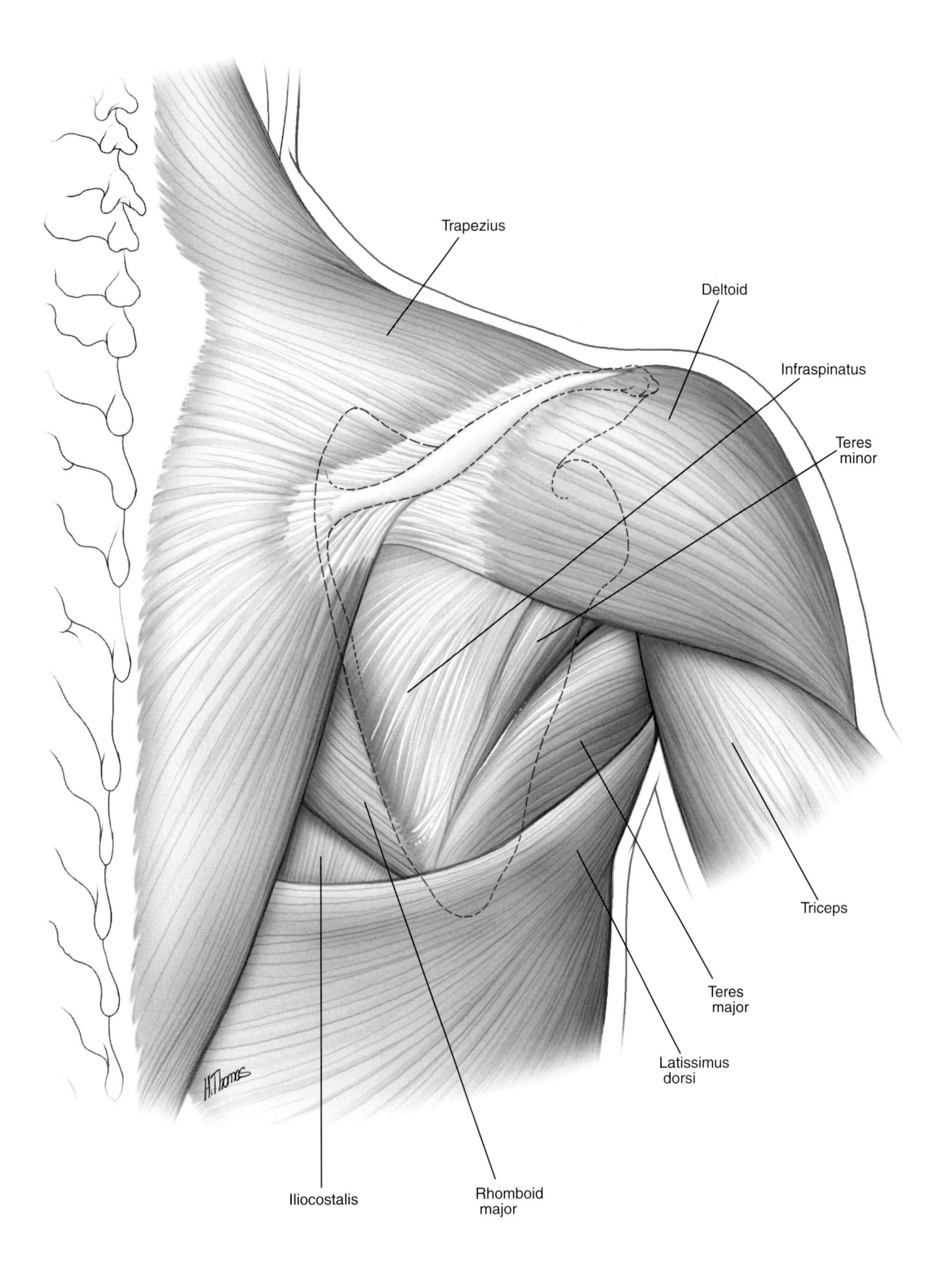

Figure 47–4 • The muscular anatomy of the posterior shoulder girdle is depicted.

Chapter 48
Forequarter Amputation

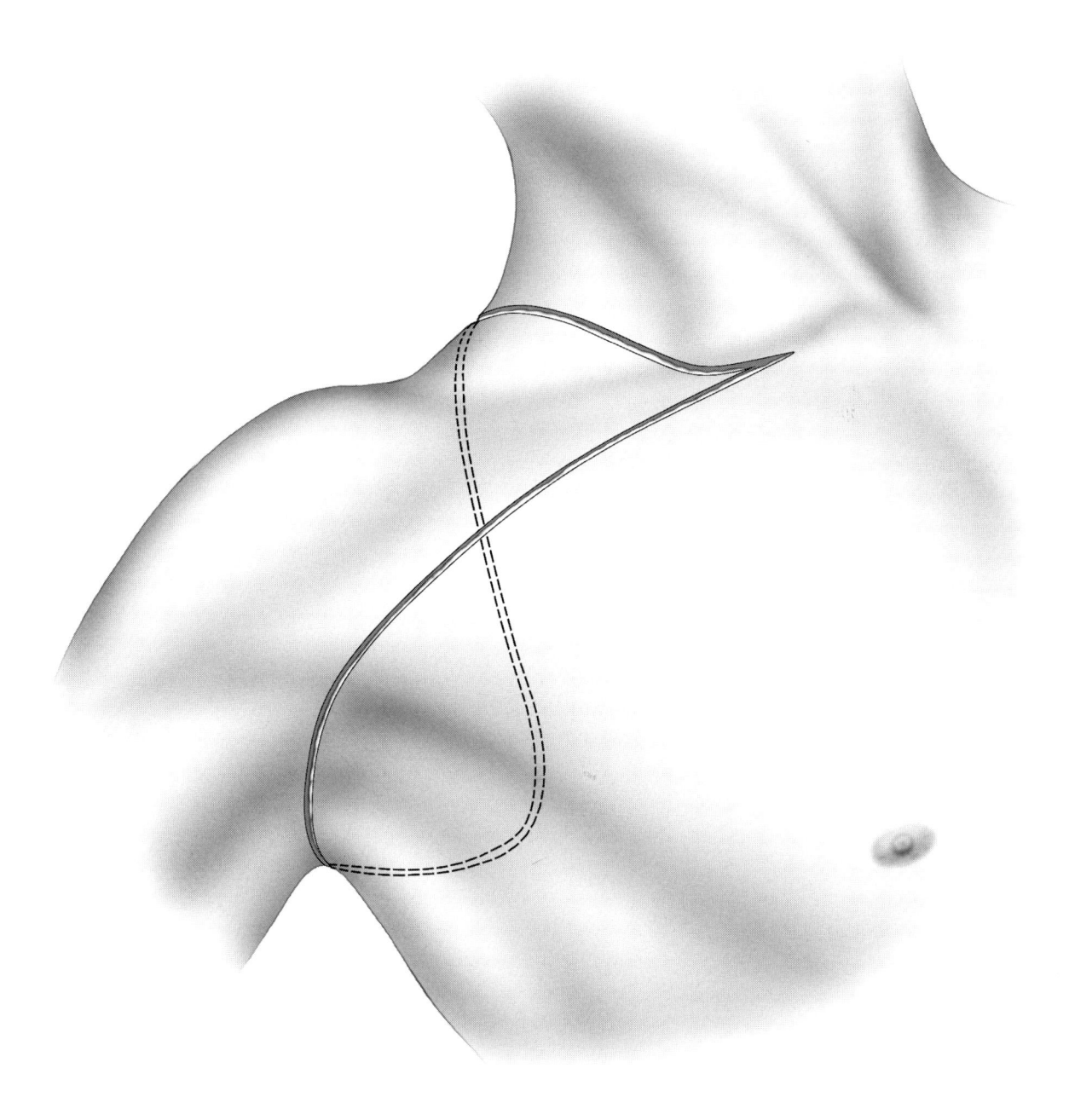

Figure 48–1 • The anterior (solid line) and posterior skin incisions are performed.

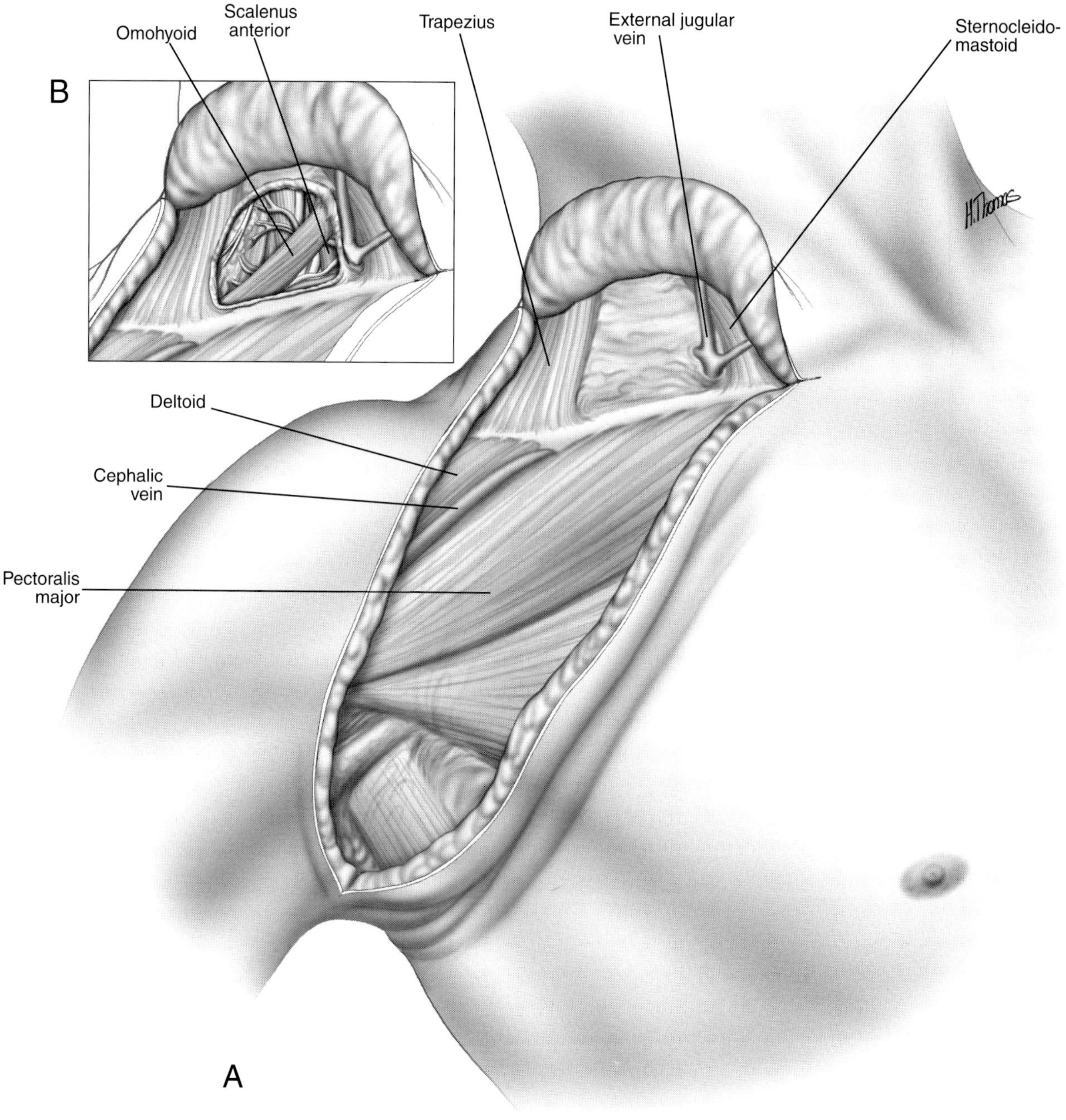

402 • Part V RADICAL AMPUTATIONS

Figure 48–2 • **A,** The skin flaps are elevated, exposing the pectoralis major muscles and the root of the neck.

B, Dissecting the fat in the posterior triangle of the neck identifies the omohyoid.

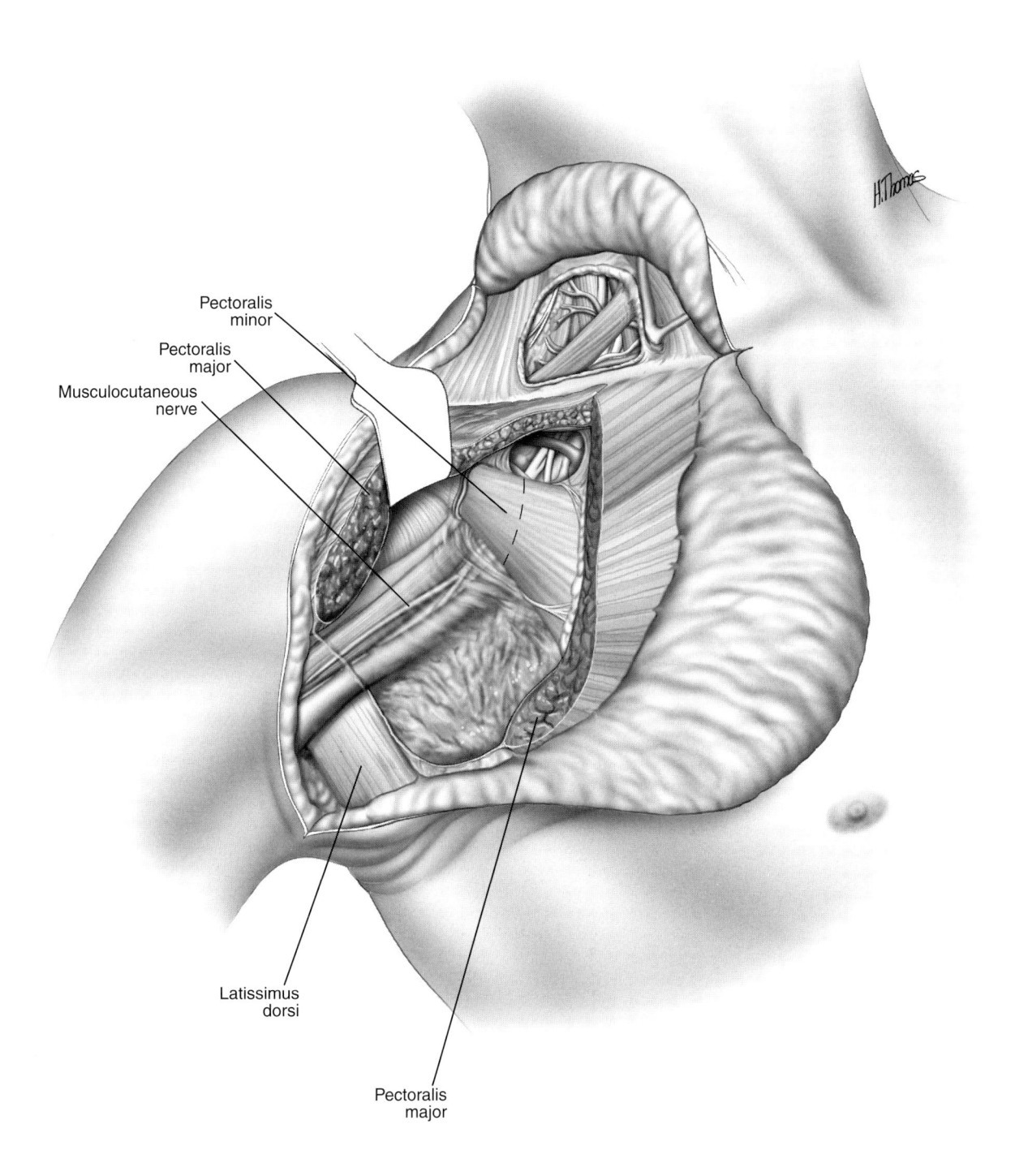

Figure 48–3 • The pectoralis major and minor muscles are divided.

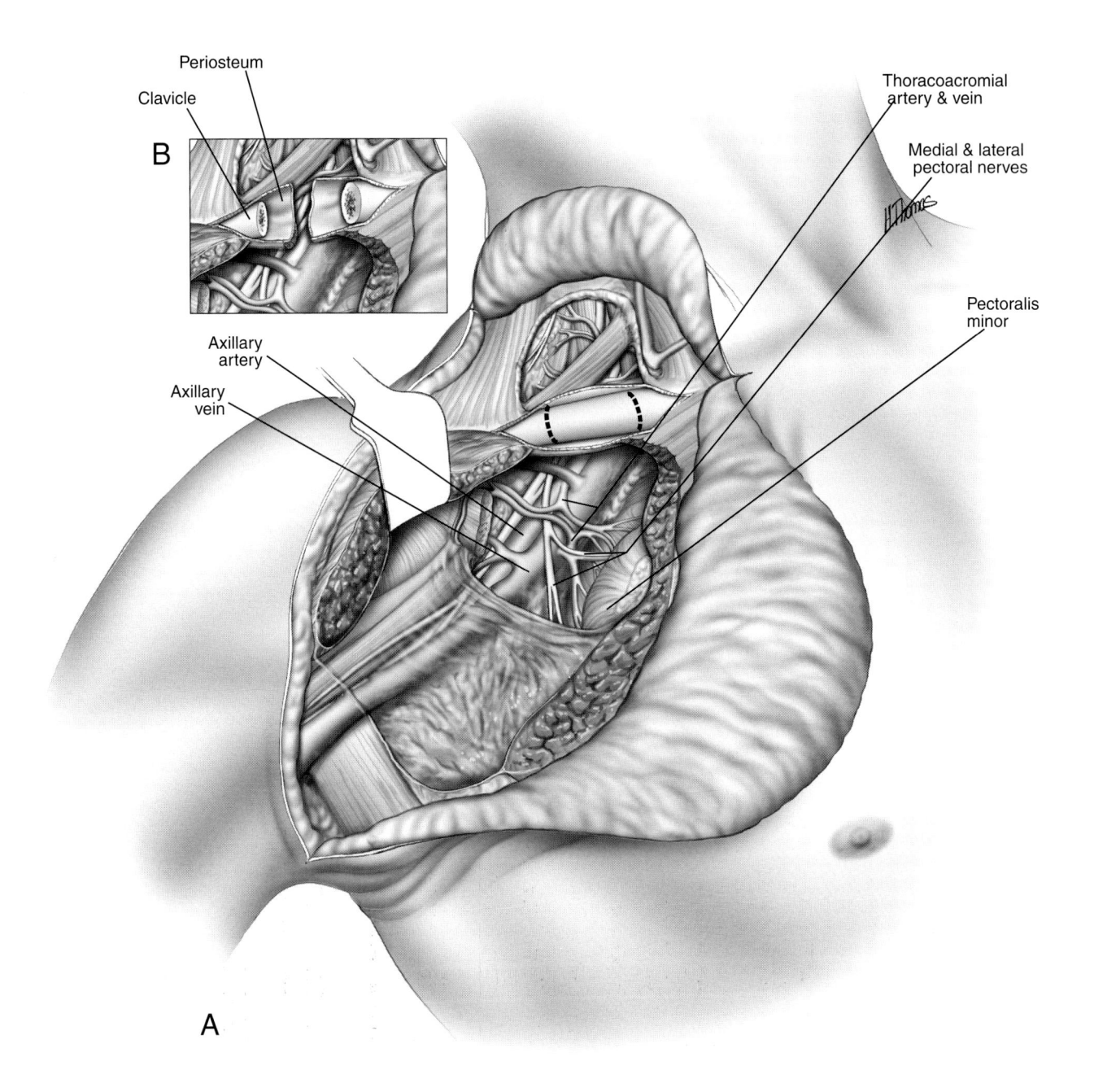

Figure 48–4 • **A,** The periosteum overlying the middle portion of the clavicle is incised.

B, The clavicle is removed with a Gigli saw, exposing the subclavius muscle.

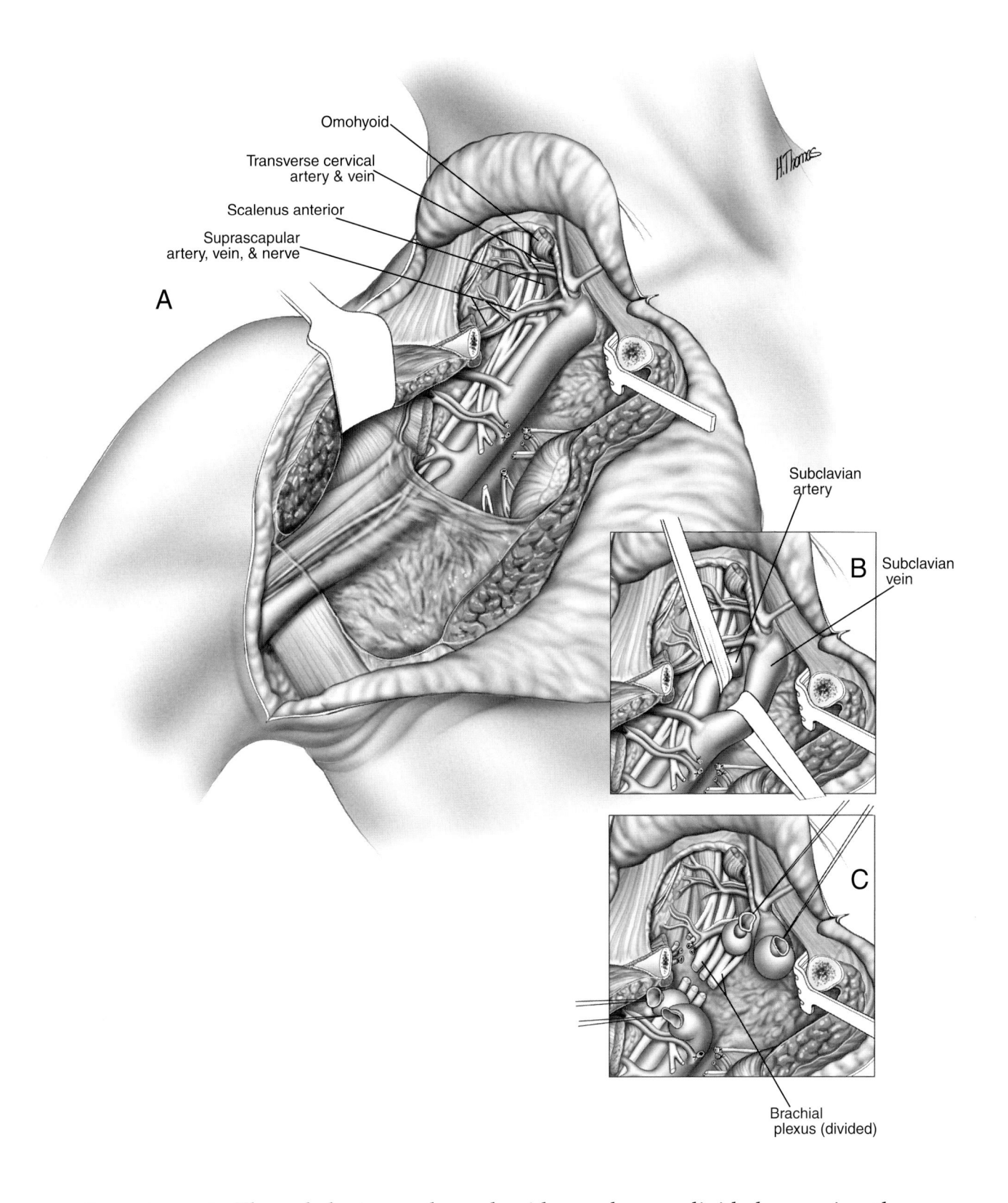

Figure 48–5 • **A,** The subclavius and omohyoid muscles are divided, exposing the subclavian artery and vein.

B, The artery and vein are mobilized.

C, The artery, vein, and main chords of the brachial plexus are divided.

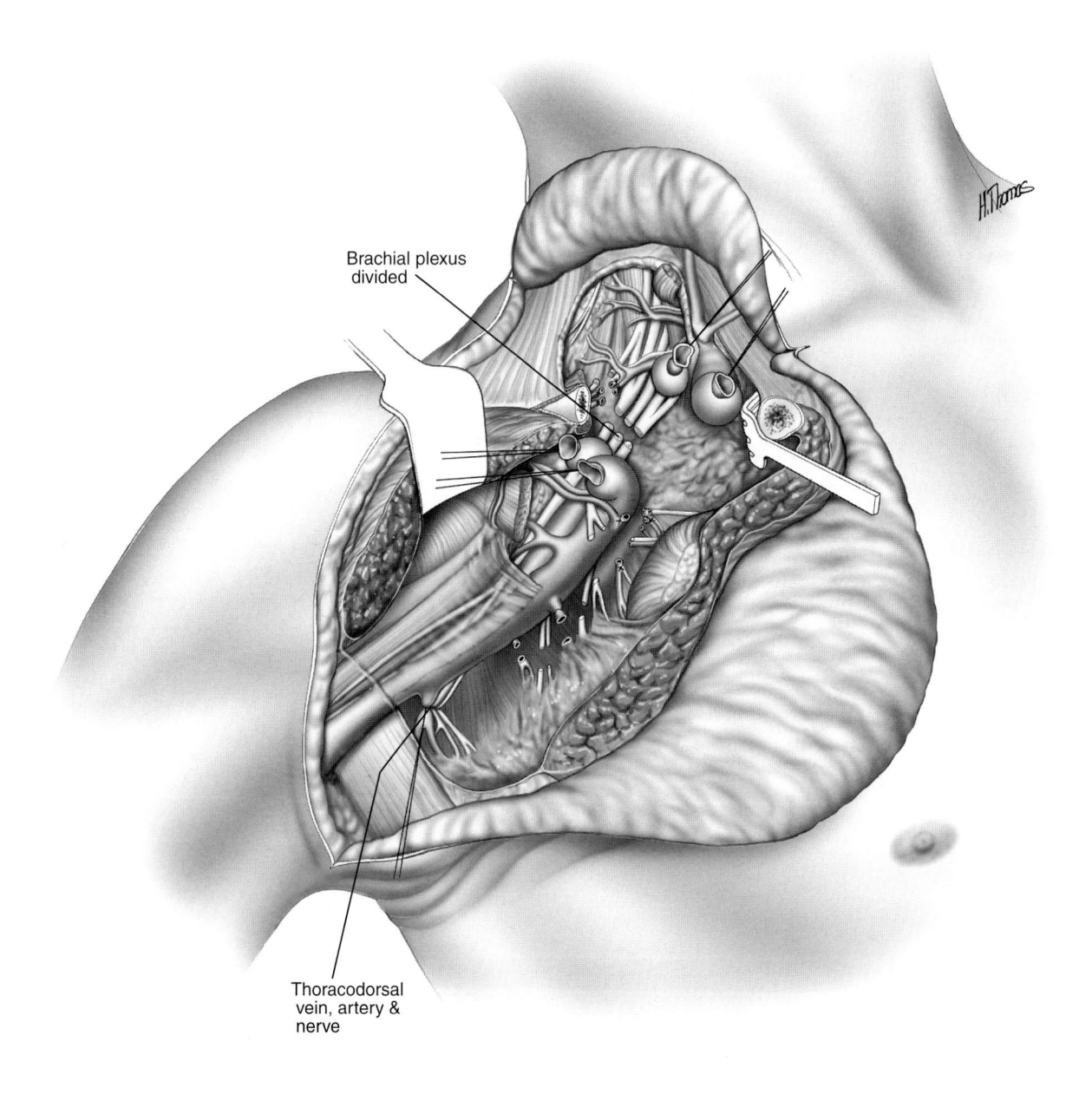

Figure 48–6 • Mobilization of the vessels distally is completed by dividing all the branches off the axillary artery and vein to the thoracodorsal vessels.

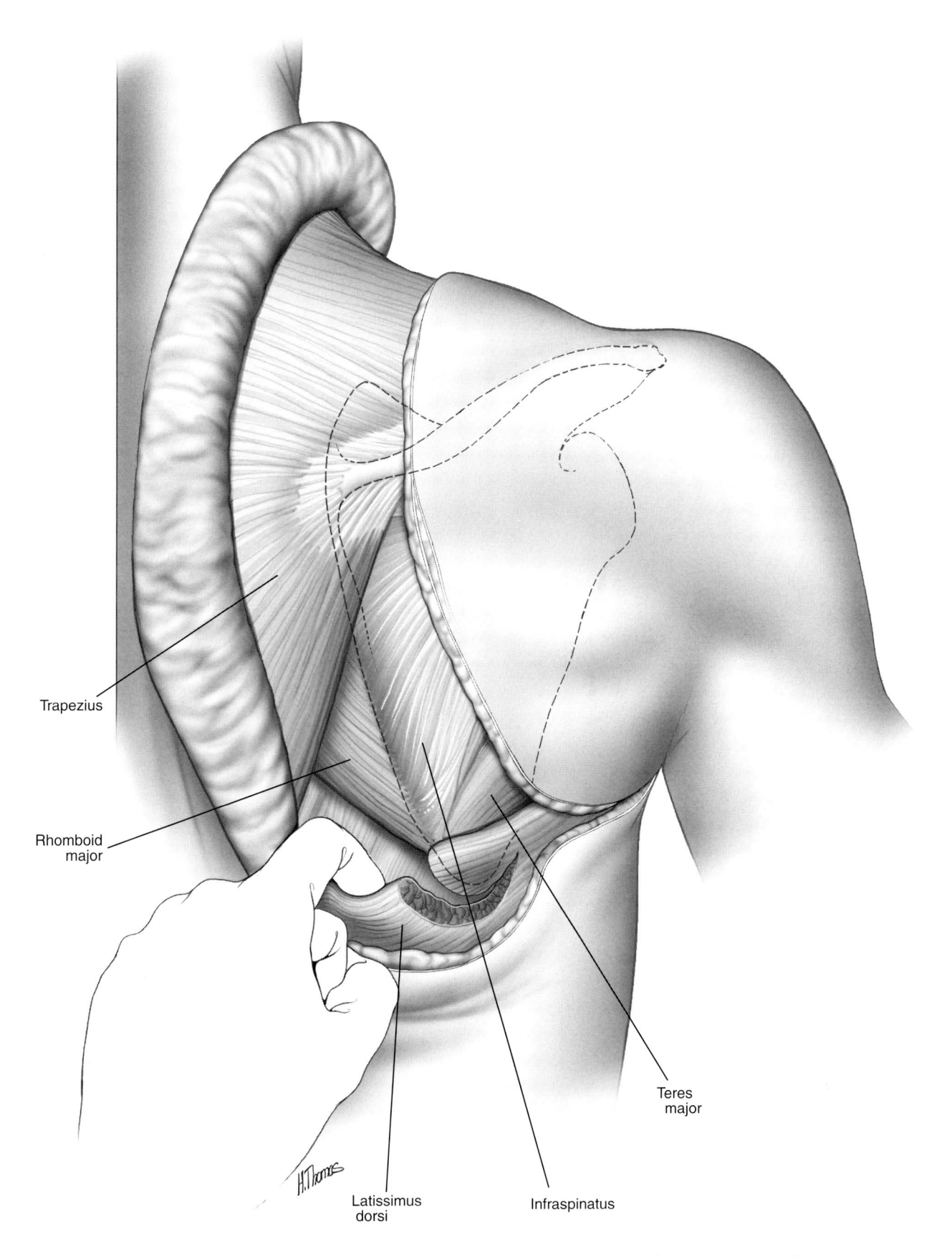

Figure 48–7 • The posterior skin flaps are completed. The latissimus and serratus anterior are divided lateral to the auscultatory triangle.

408 • Part V RADICAL AMPUTATIONS

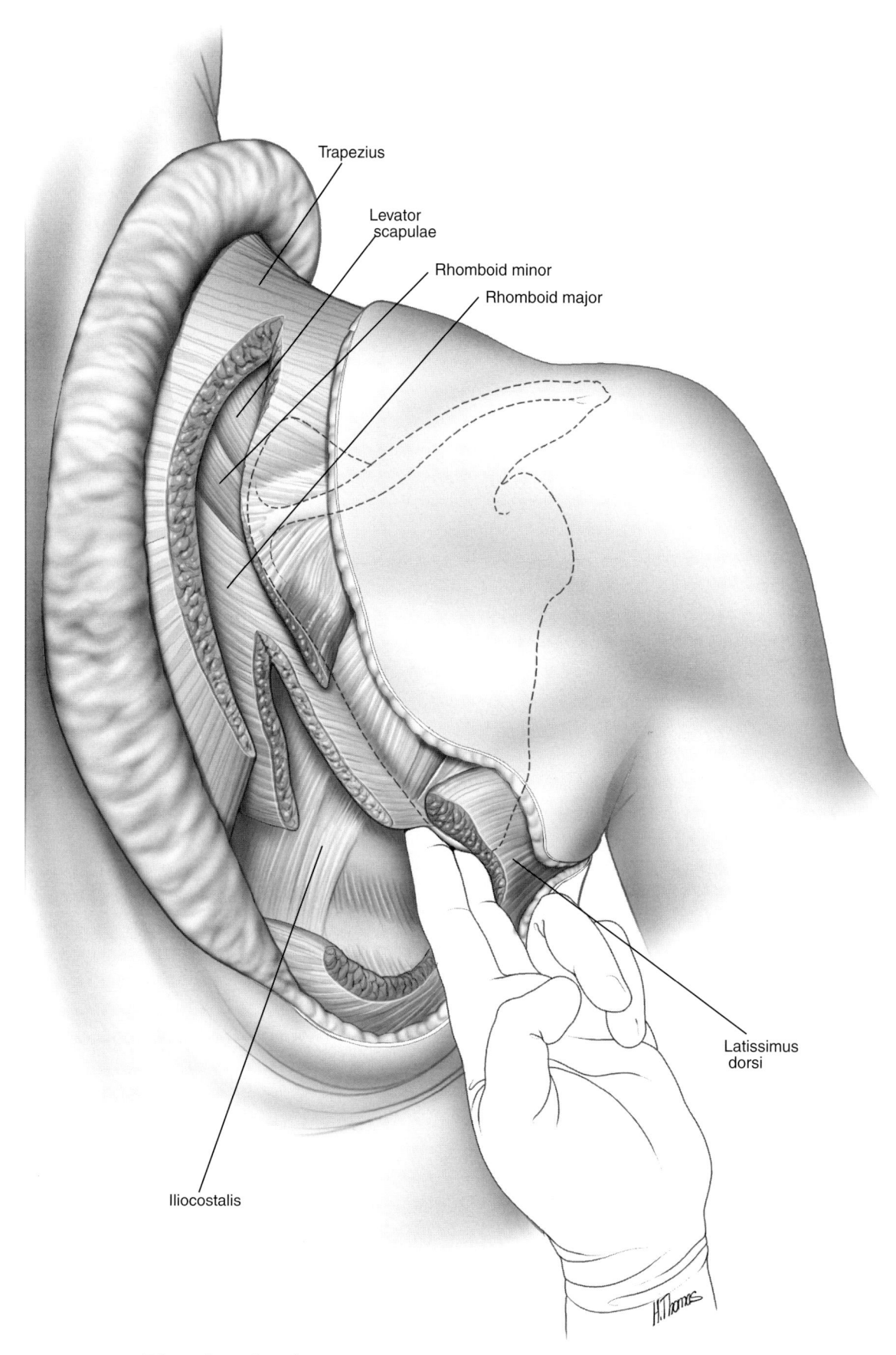

Figure 48–8 • The rhomboids, teres major and teres minor, levator scapulae and trapezius are divided.

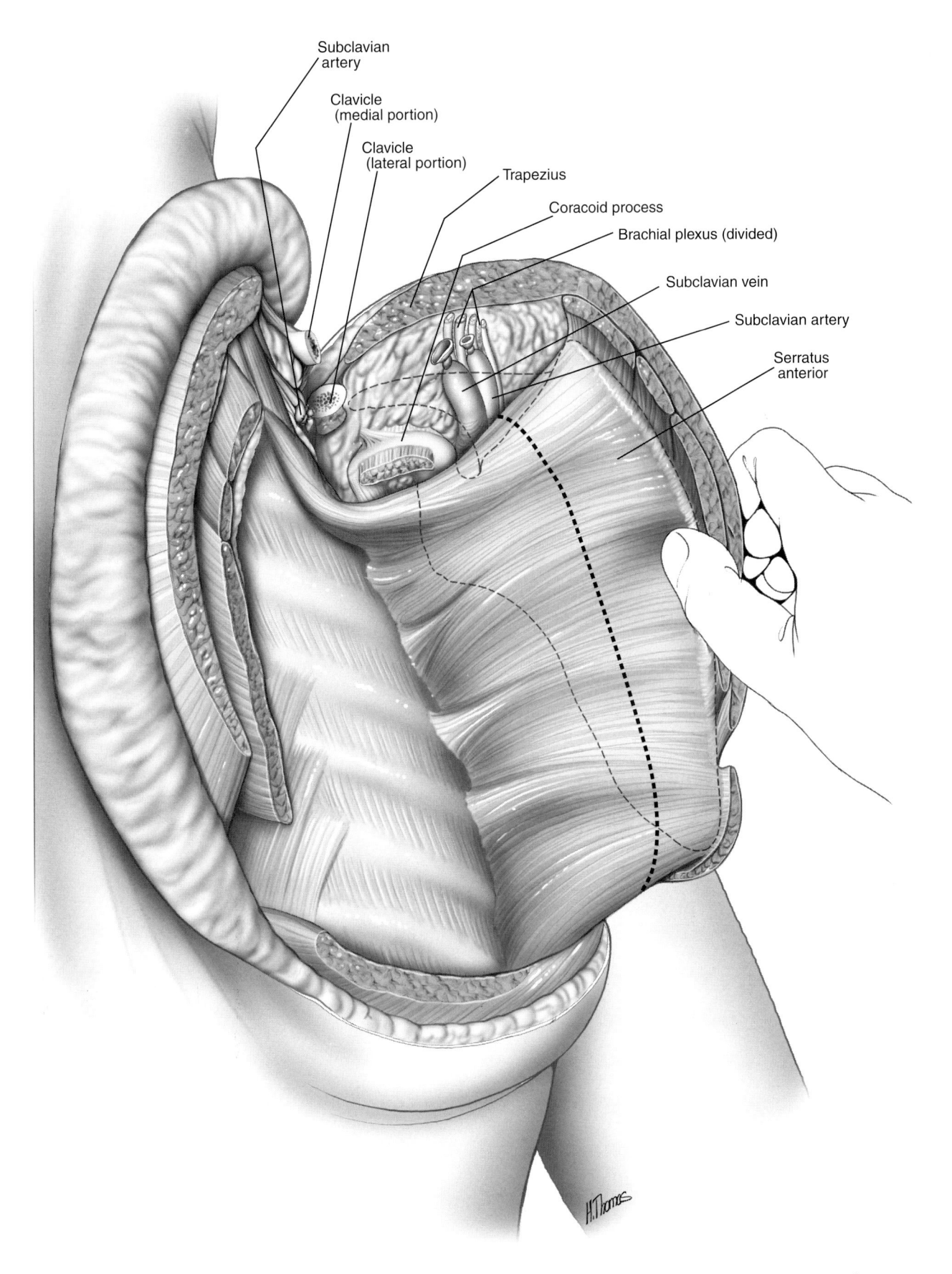

Figure 48-9 • The serratus is divided posteriorly. If a chest wall resection is to be included, the posterior line of resection of the ribs is noted.

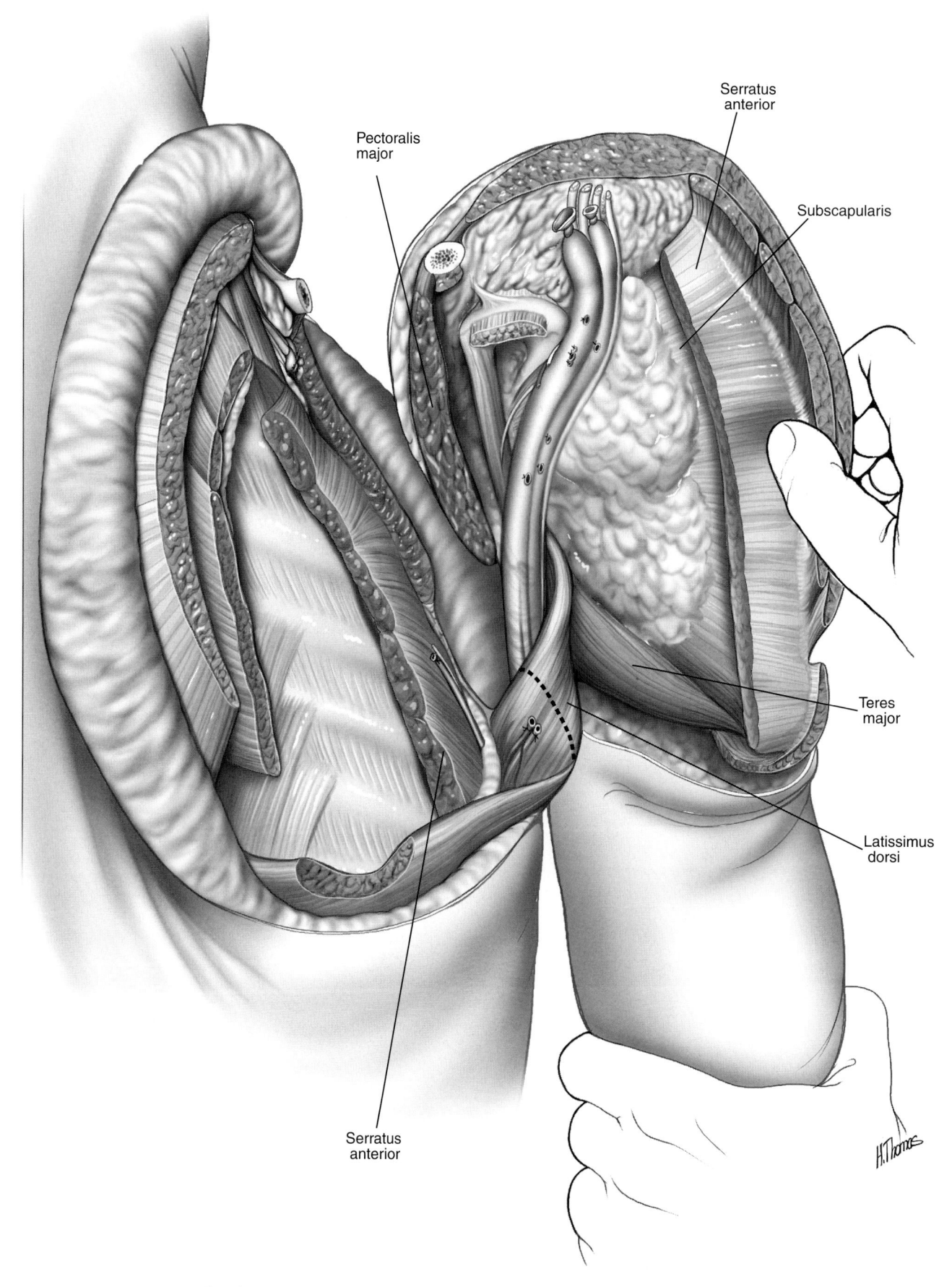

Figure 48–10 • The latissimus dorsi is divided, and the entire specimen is removed.

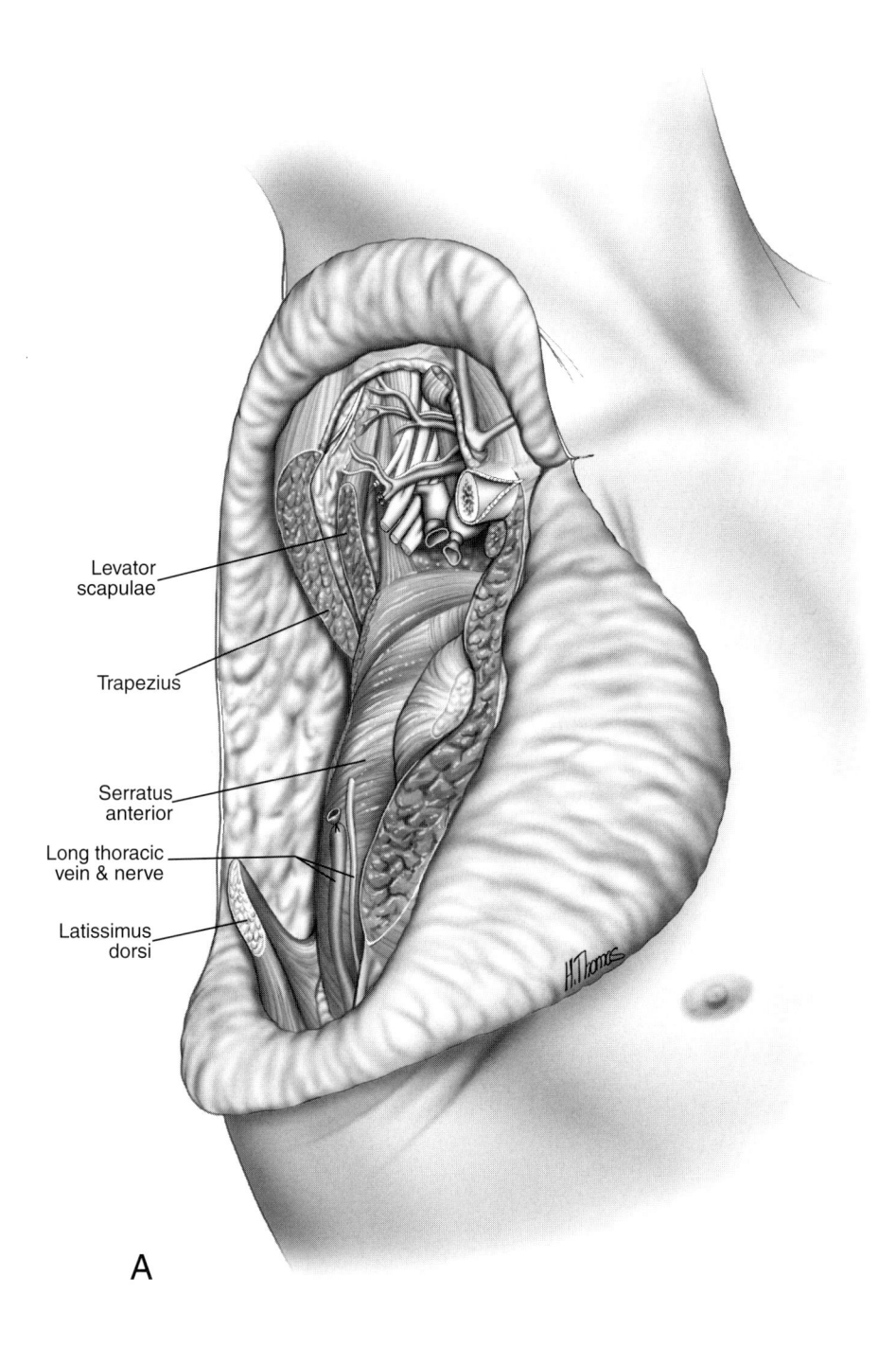

Figure 48–11 • **A**, Anterior and
B, posterior views of the resected specimen are depicted.
Illustration continued on following page

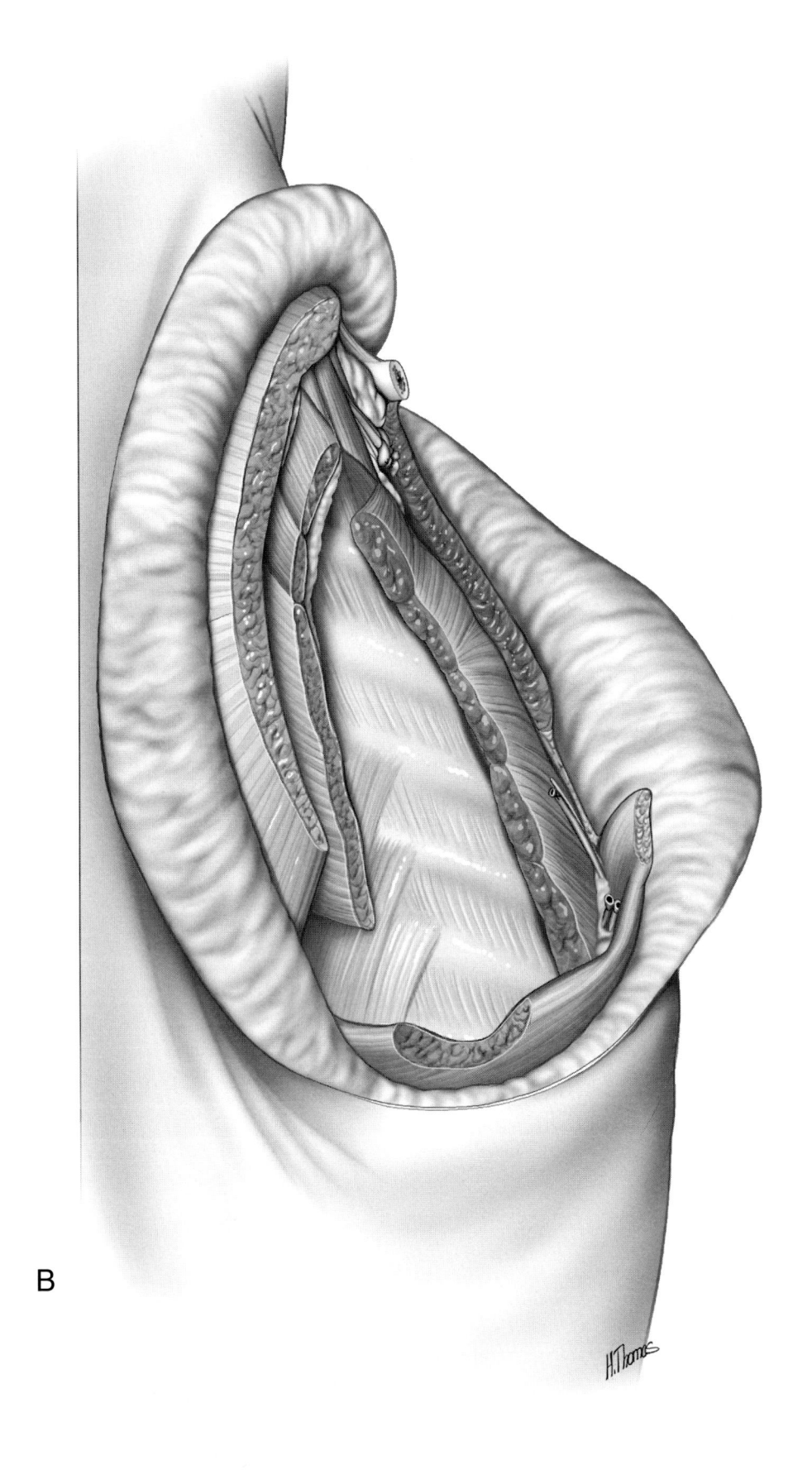

Figure 48–11B • *Continued*

Forequarter Amputation • 413

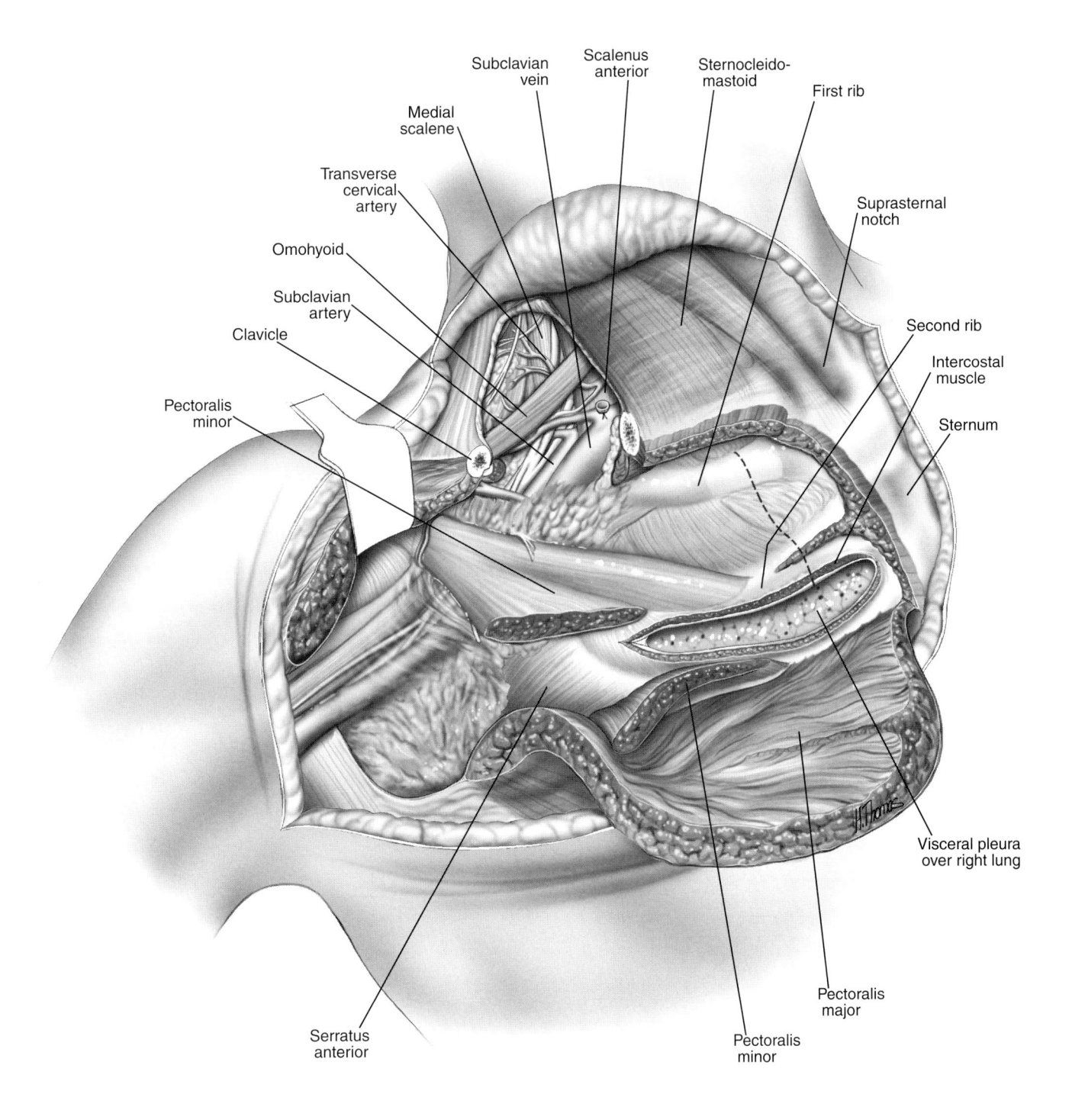

Figure 48–12 • If an intrathoracic forequarter amputation is to be performed because of inaccessibility of the subclavian vessels at the thoracic inlet caused by tumor, the second and third ribs are exposed by taking down the pectoralis major and minor medially. The chest cavity is usually entered in the second interspace.

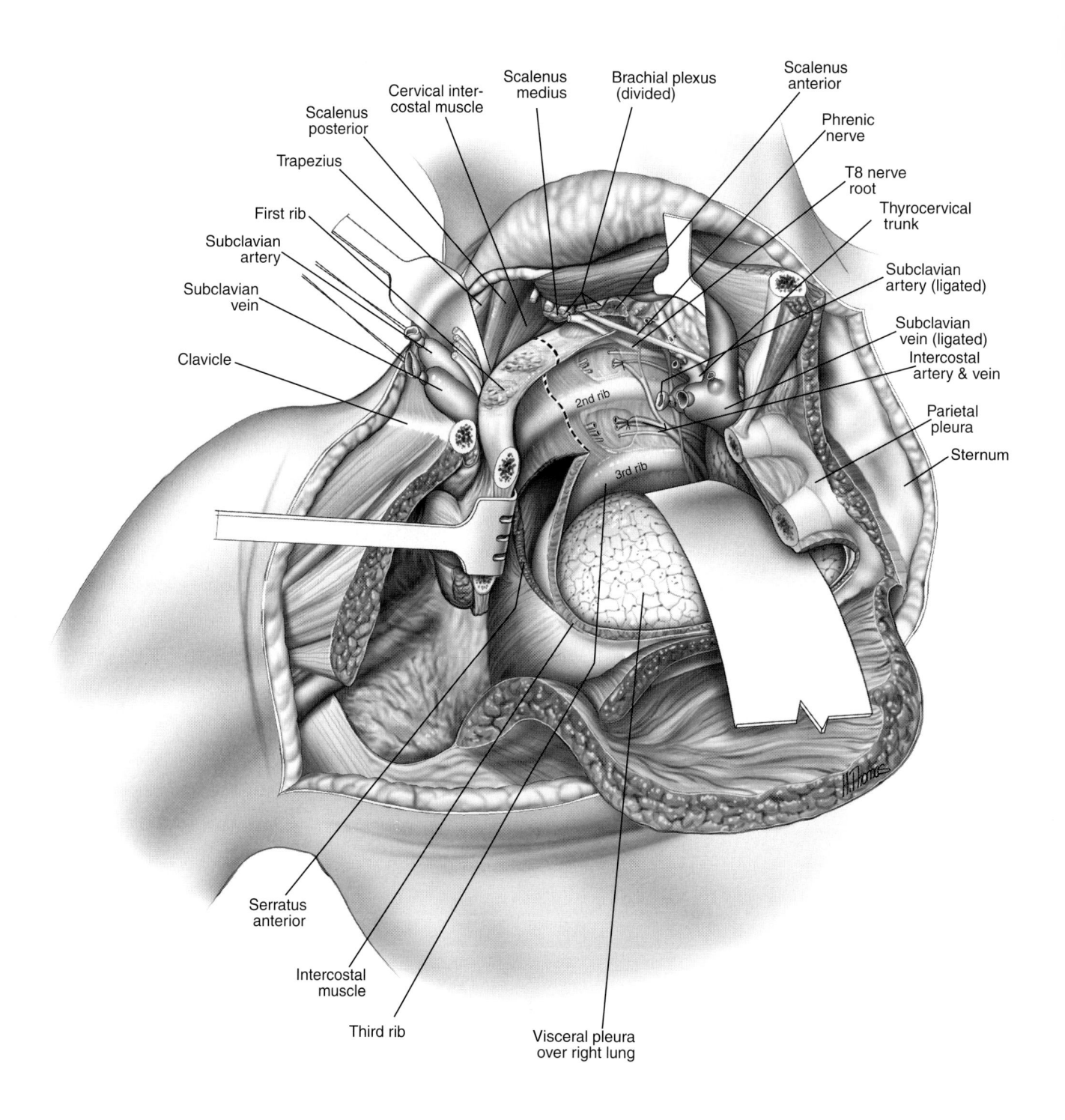

Figure 48–13 • The subclavian vessels are ligated in the chest, and the chest wall resection is completed. Marlex mesh is used to close the defect in the chest wall.

Chapter 49
Tikoff-Lindberg Procedure

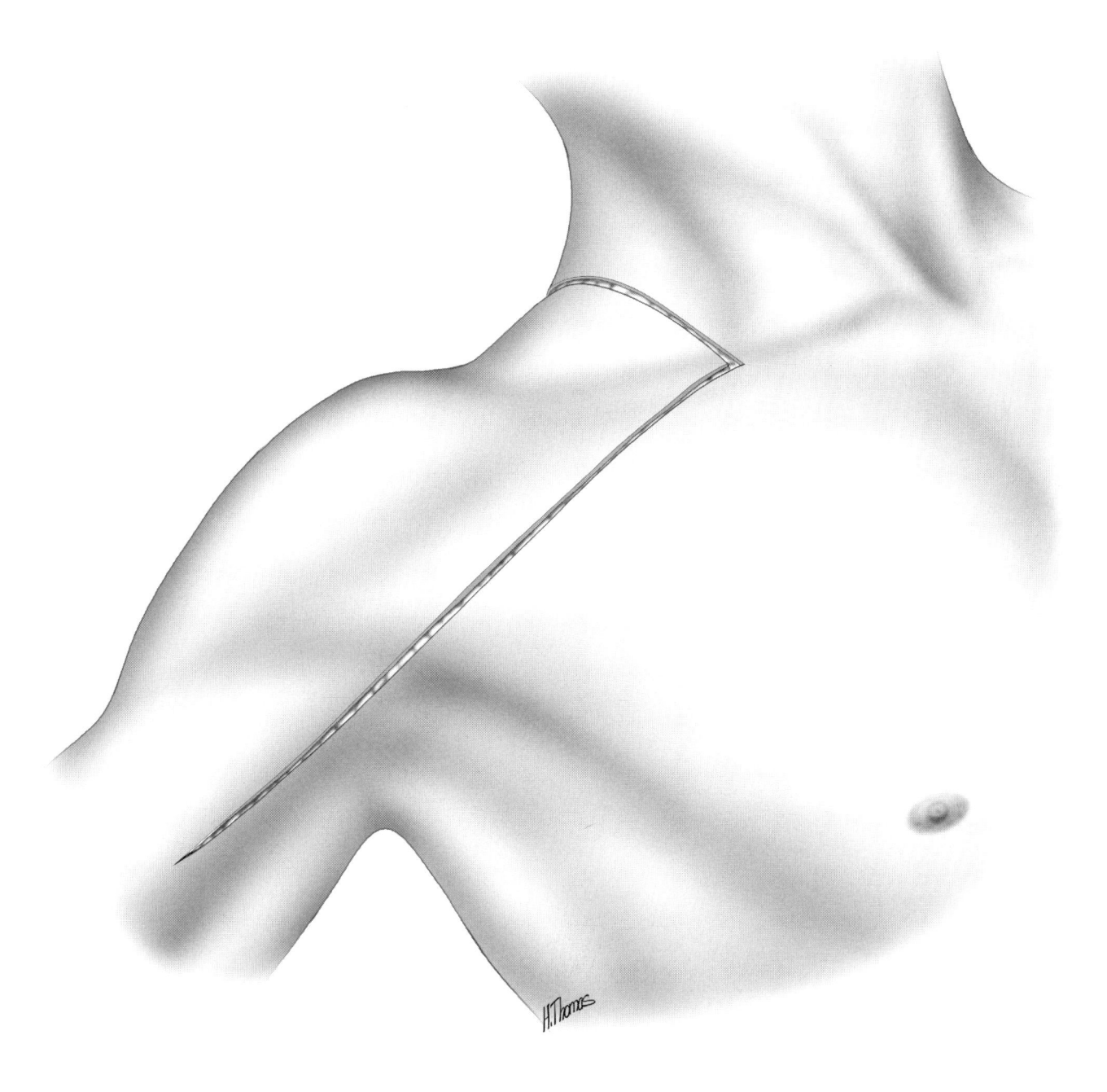

Figure 49–1 • In most situations a Tikoff-Lindberg procedure can be performed in lieu of a forequarter amputation. The skin incision is placed parallel to the cephalic vein to a point on the clavicle where the sternocleidomastoid muscle inserts.

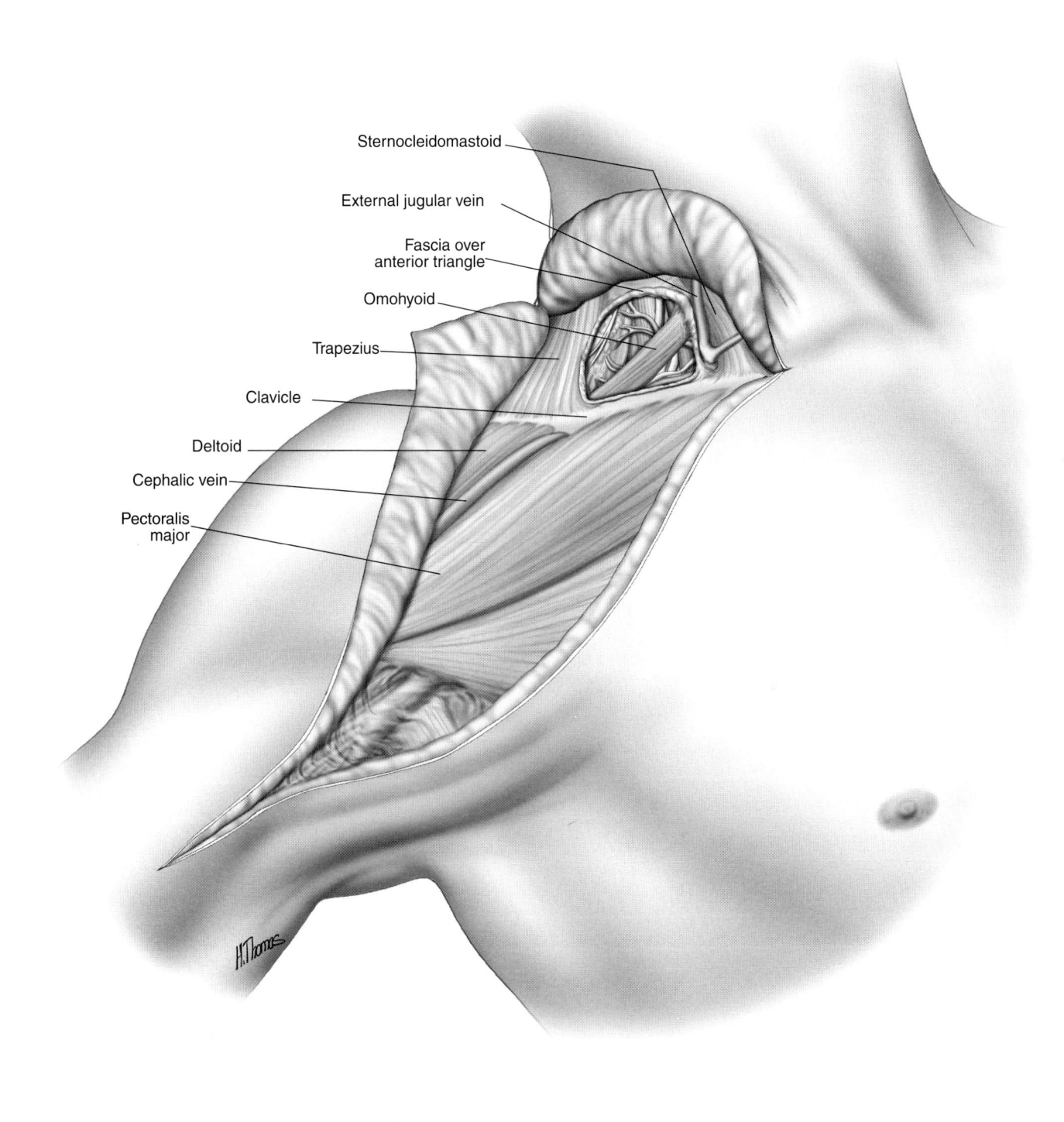

Figure 49-2 • The skin flaps are elevated, exposing the pectoralis major muscles and the root of the neck.

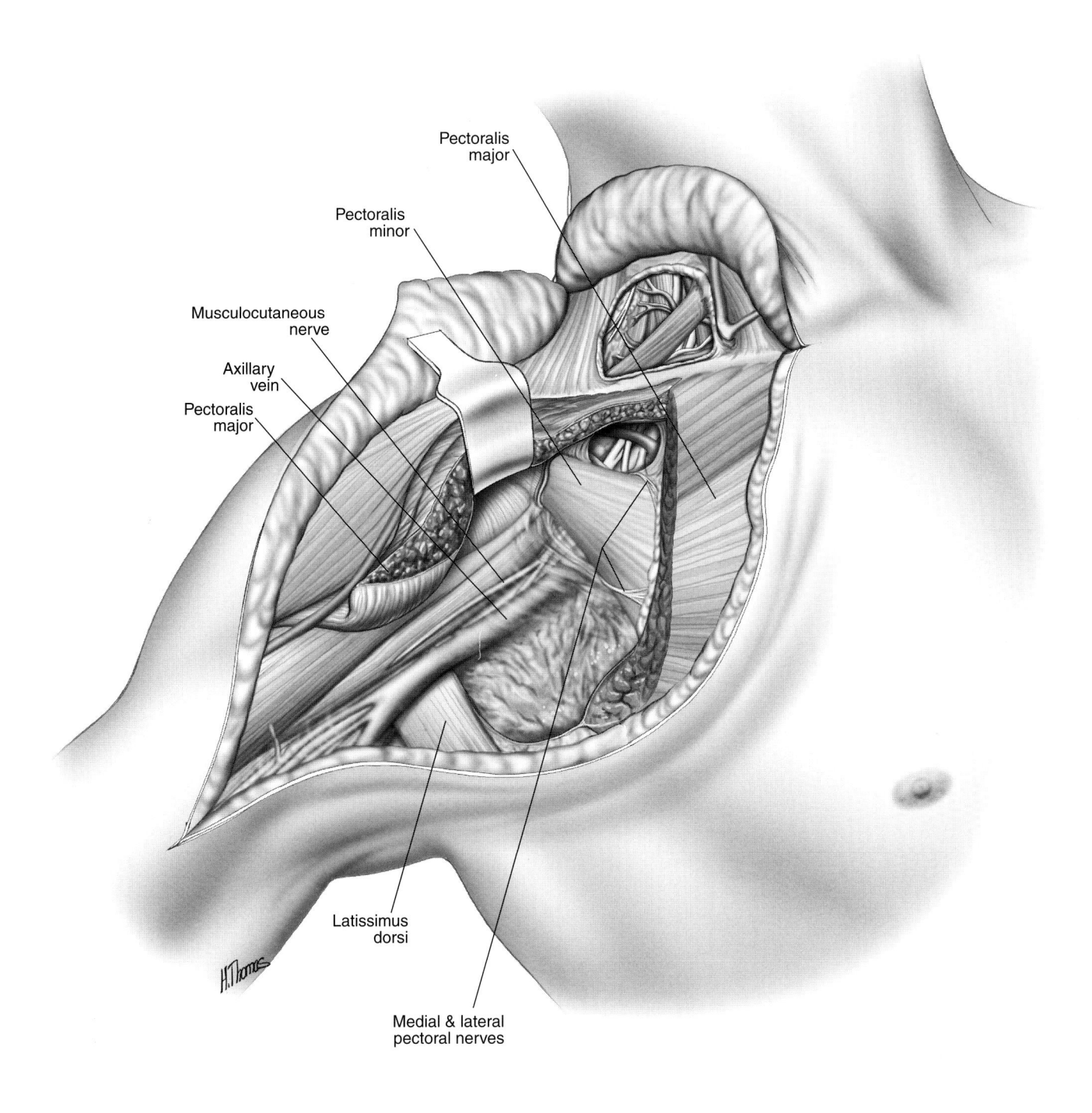

Figure 49–3 • The pectoralis major and minor muscles are divided as indicated.

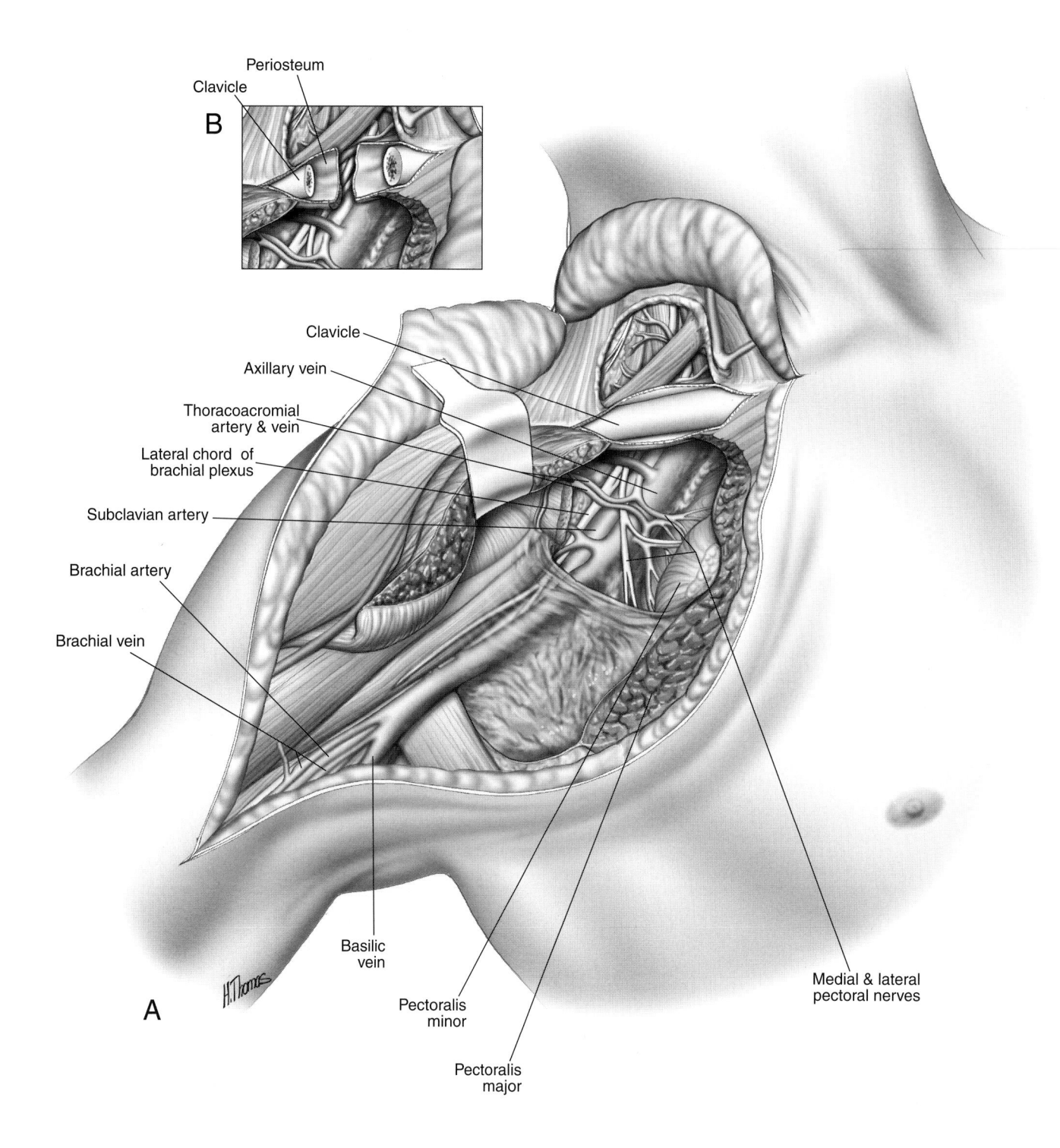

Figure 49–4 • **A,** The clavipectoral fascia is incised along the superior edge of the neurovascular bundle, and the periosteum overlying the midportion of the clavicle is incised.

B, The medial third of the clavicle is removed, utilizing a Gigli or power saw, and the subclavius muscle is divided.

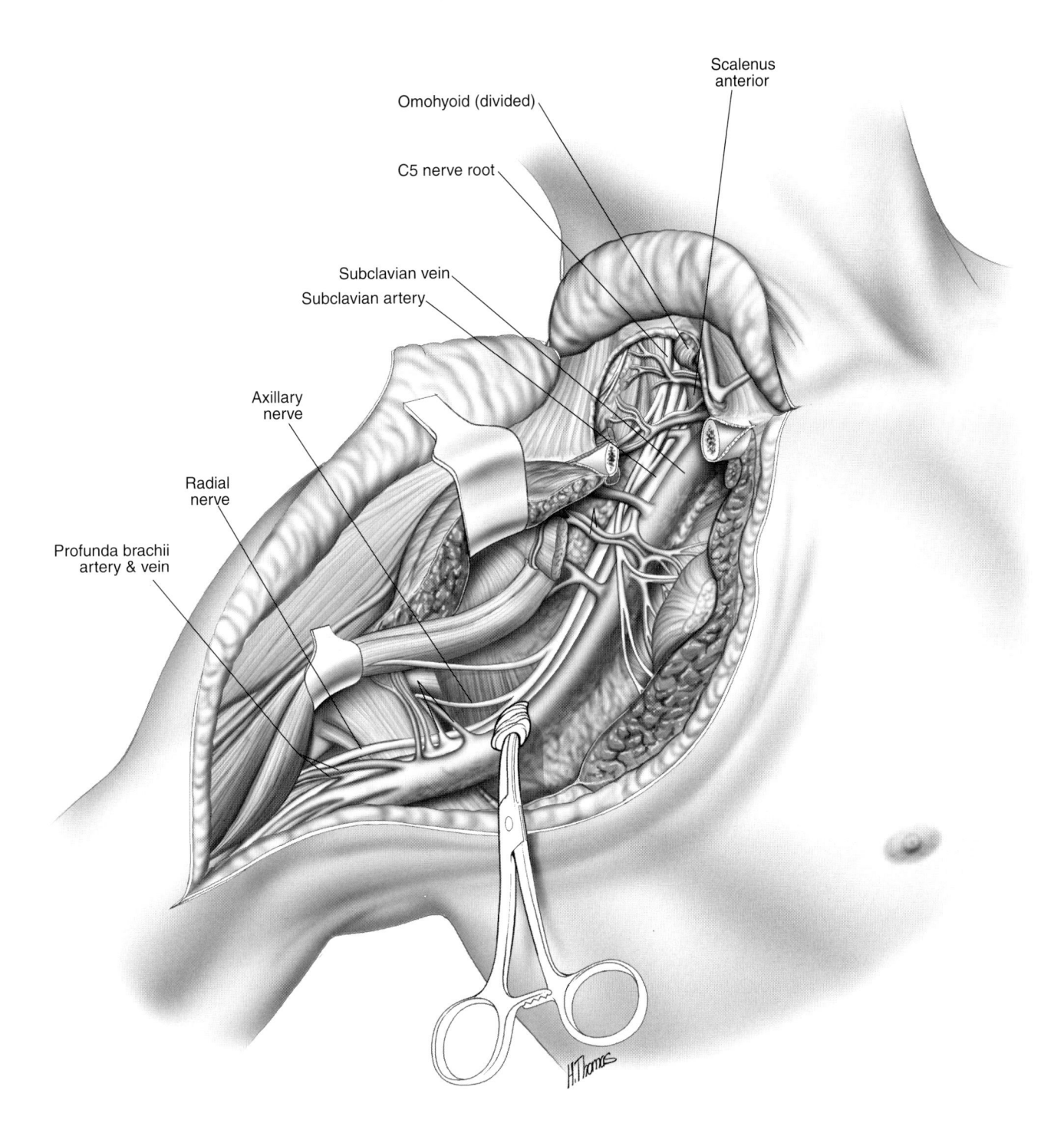

Figure 49-5 • The neurovascular bundle is mobilized distally along its entire length, exposing the vascular and nerve branches to be divided as indicated.

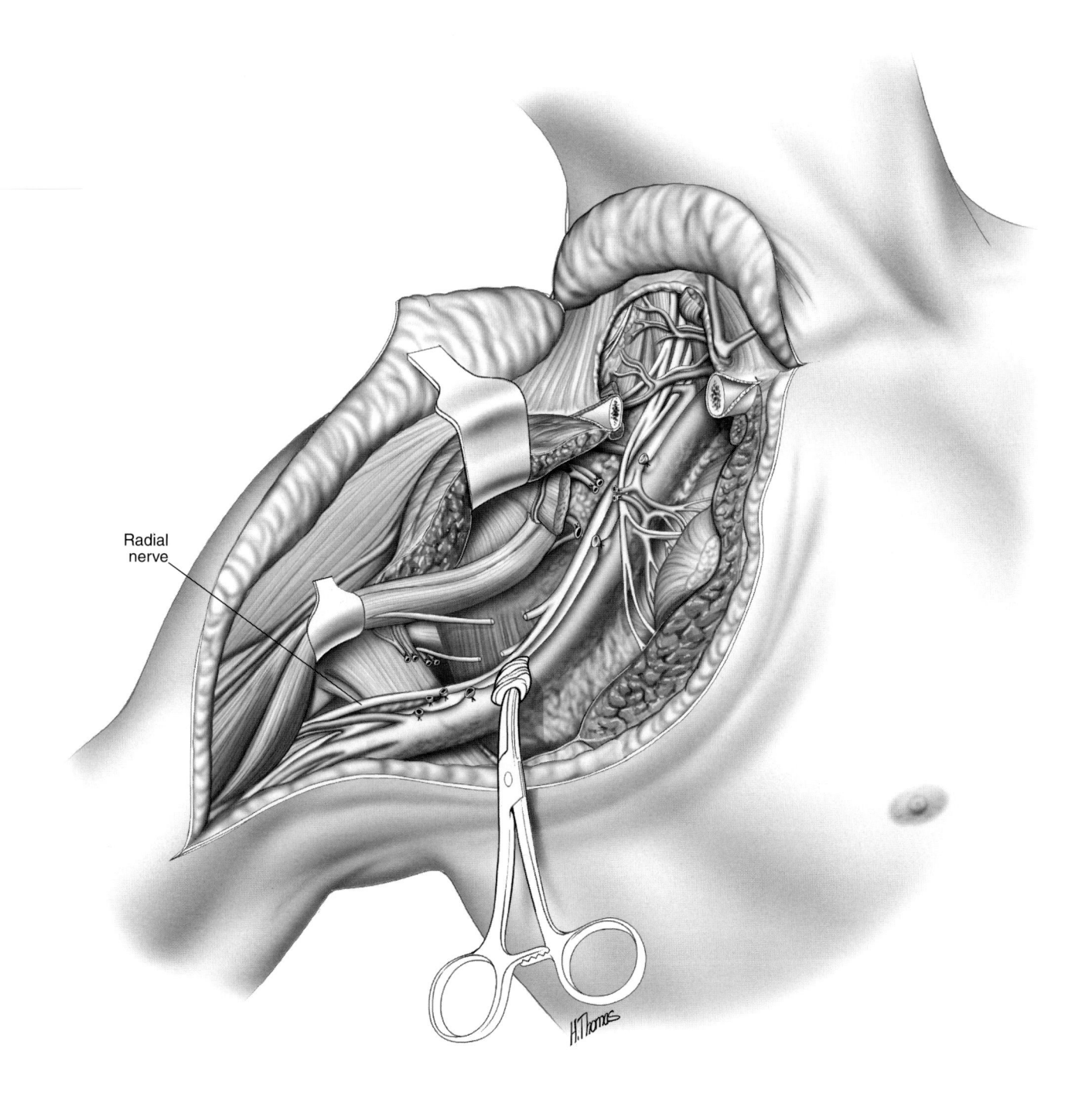

Figure 49–6 • The circumflex humeral vessels, axillary nerve, musculocutaneous nerve, and transverse scapular vessels are divided. The radial nerve is identified as it passes over the latissimus dorsi insertion and enters the spiral groove.

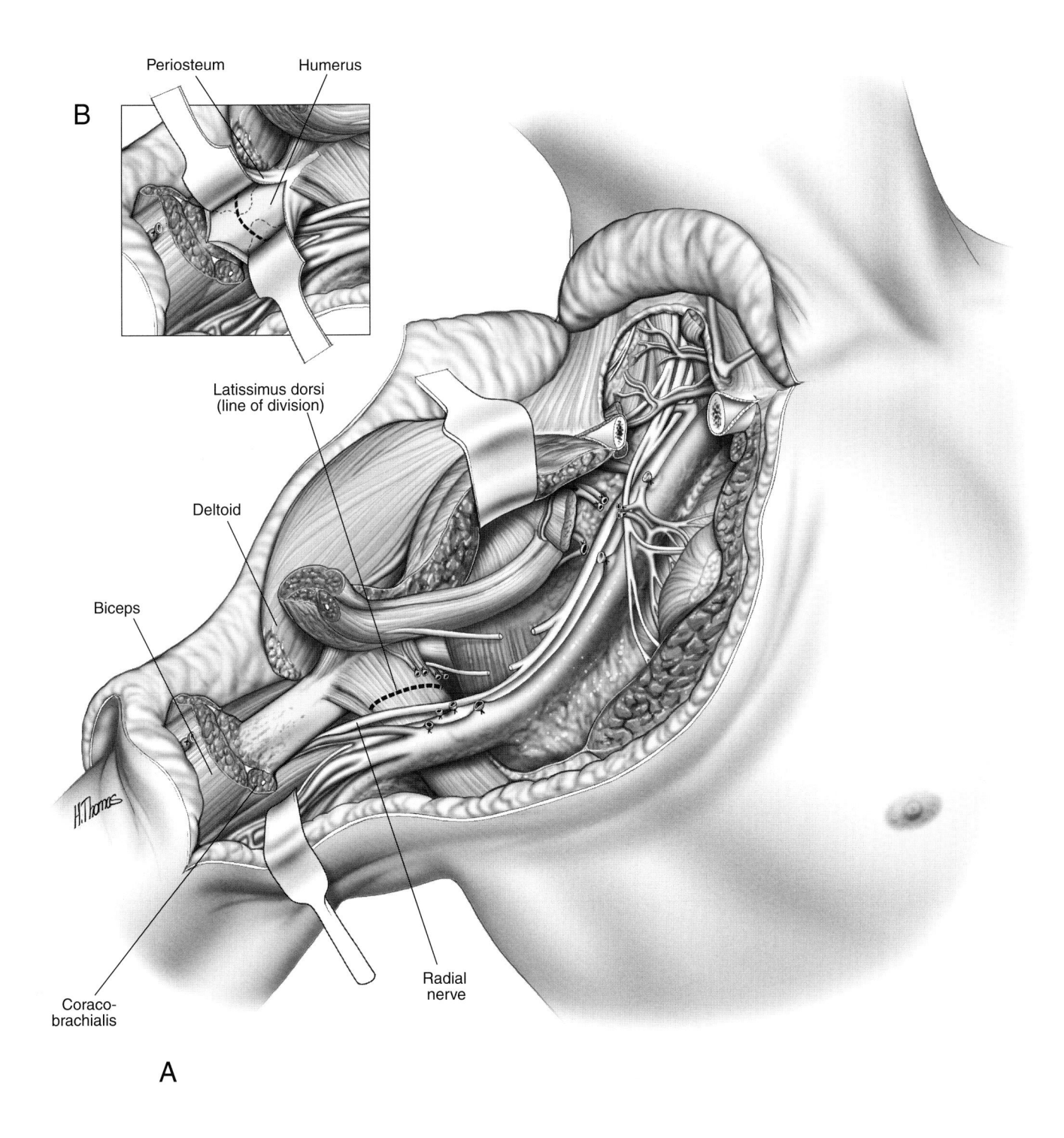

Figure 49-7 • **A,** The biceps, coracobrachialis, and deltoid are divided at the line of resection on the humerus.

B, The periosteum on the humerus is incised, and the humeral neck is divided.

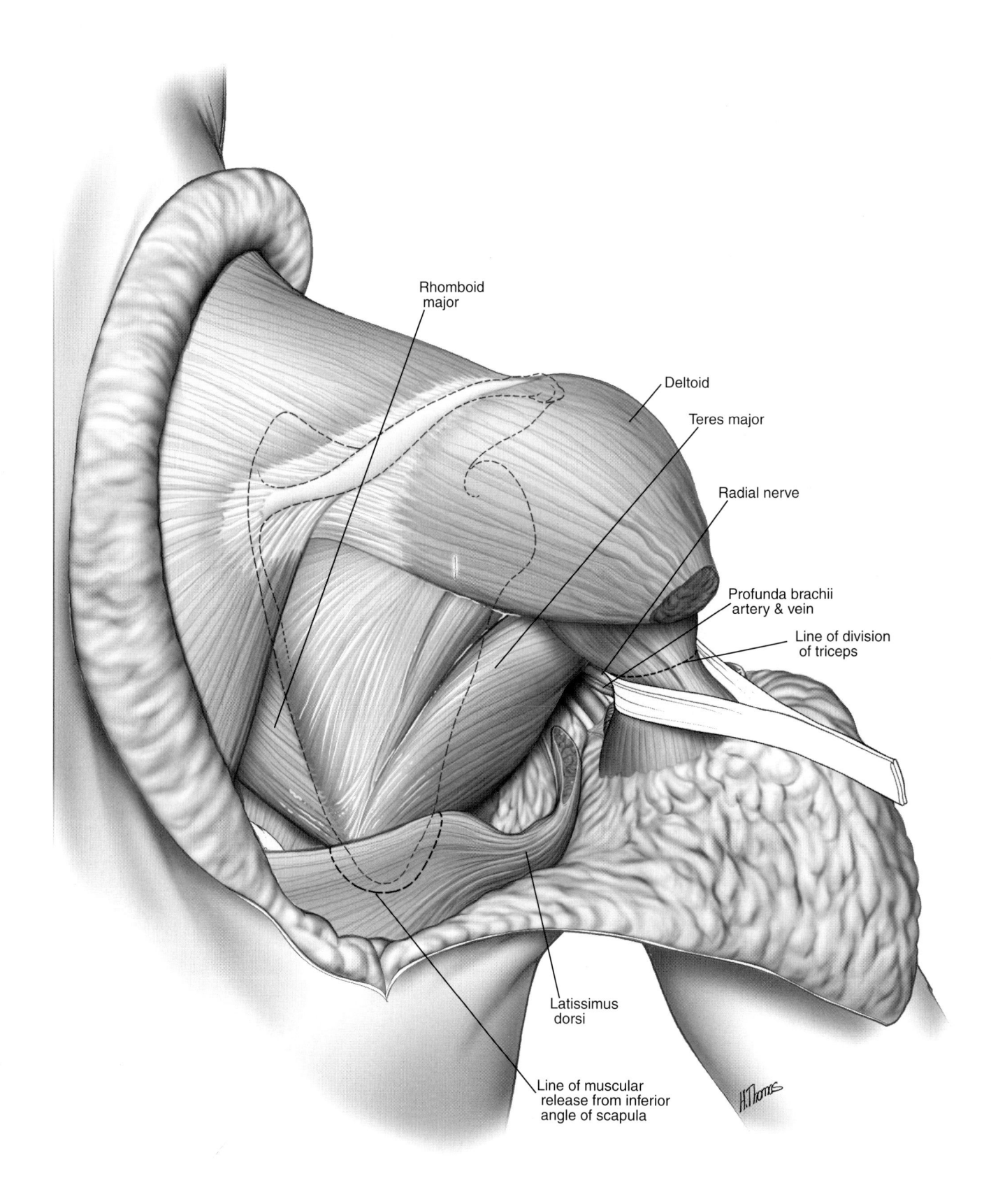

Figure 49-8 • The posterior skin flaps are completed. The deltoid and triceps muscles are divided.

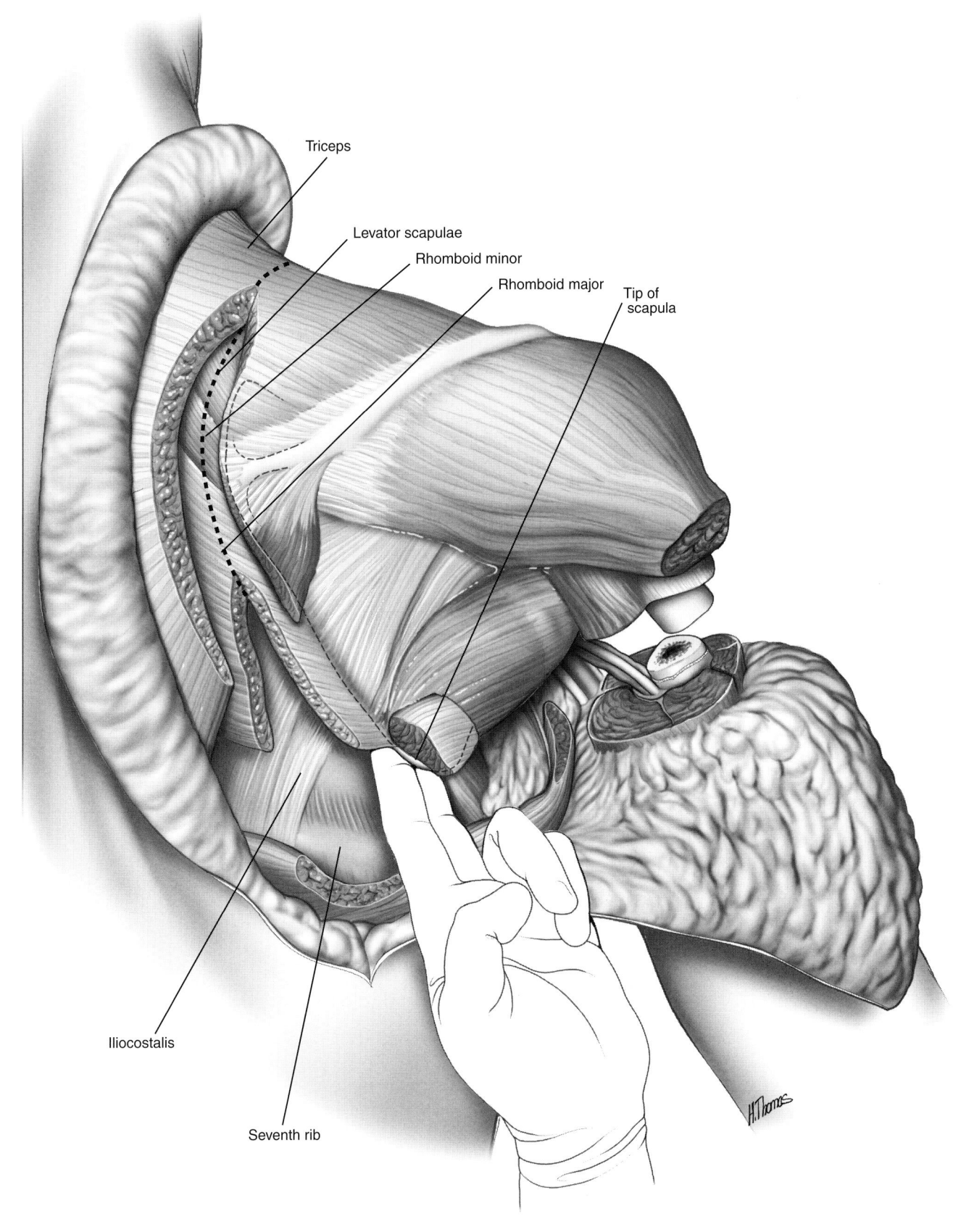

Figure 49-9 • The serratus is divided at the tip of the scapula, and, with a hand underneath the scapula, the rhomboids, levator scapulae, and trapezius are divided.

424 • Part V   RADICAL AMPUTATIONS

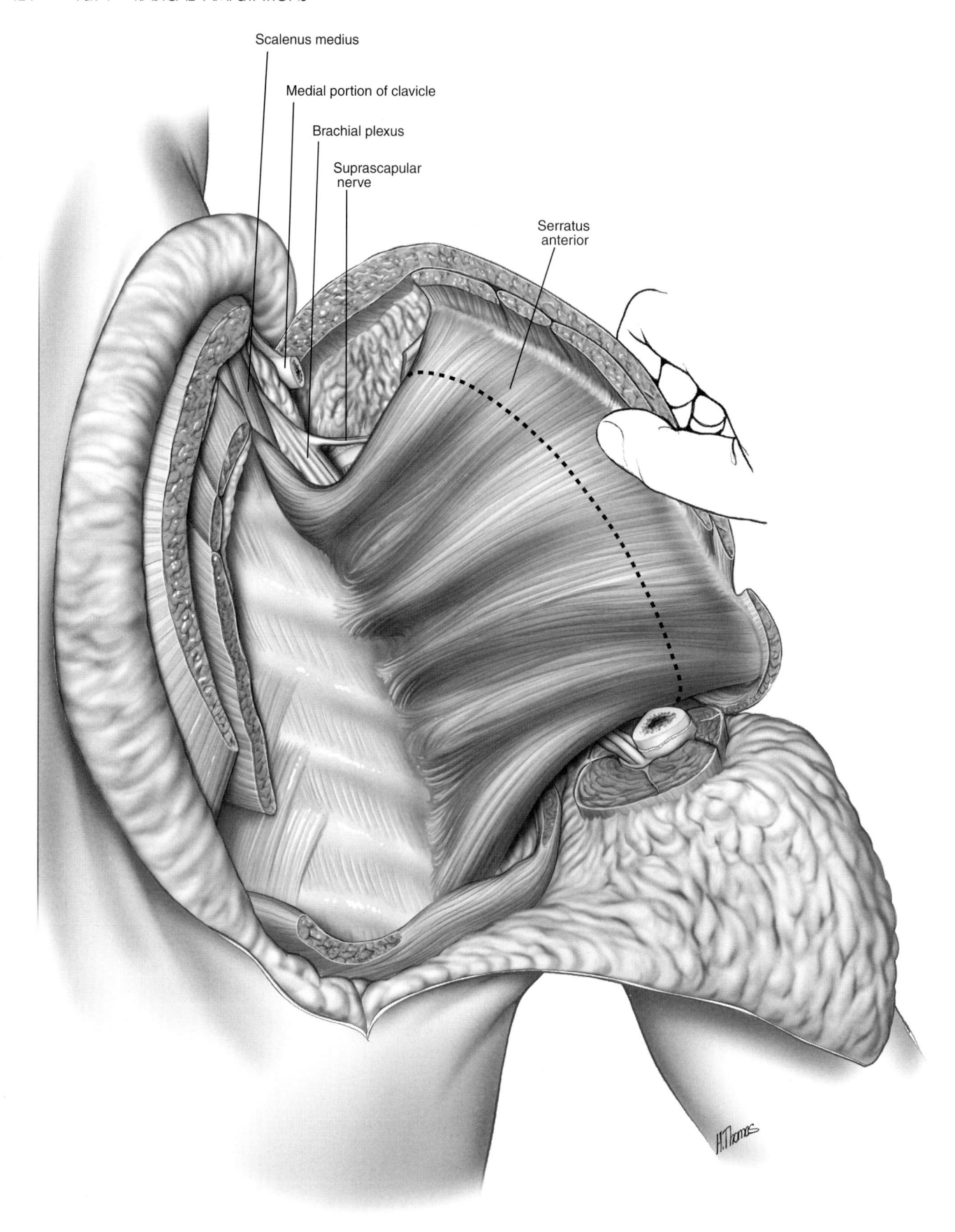

Figure 49–10 • The origins of the serratus posteriorly are removed from the chest wall. As this muscle seals the axilla if a chest wall resection is to be included, the inferior point of entry into the chest is defined by this muscle.

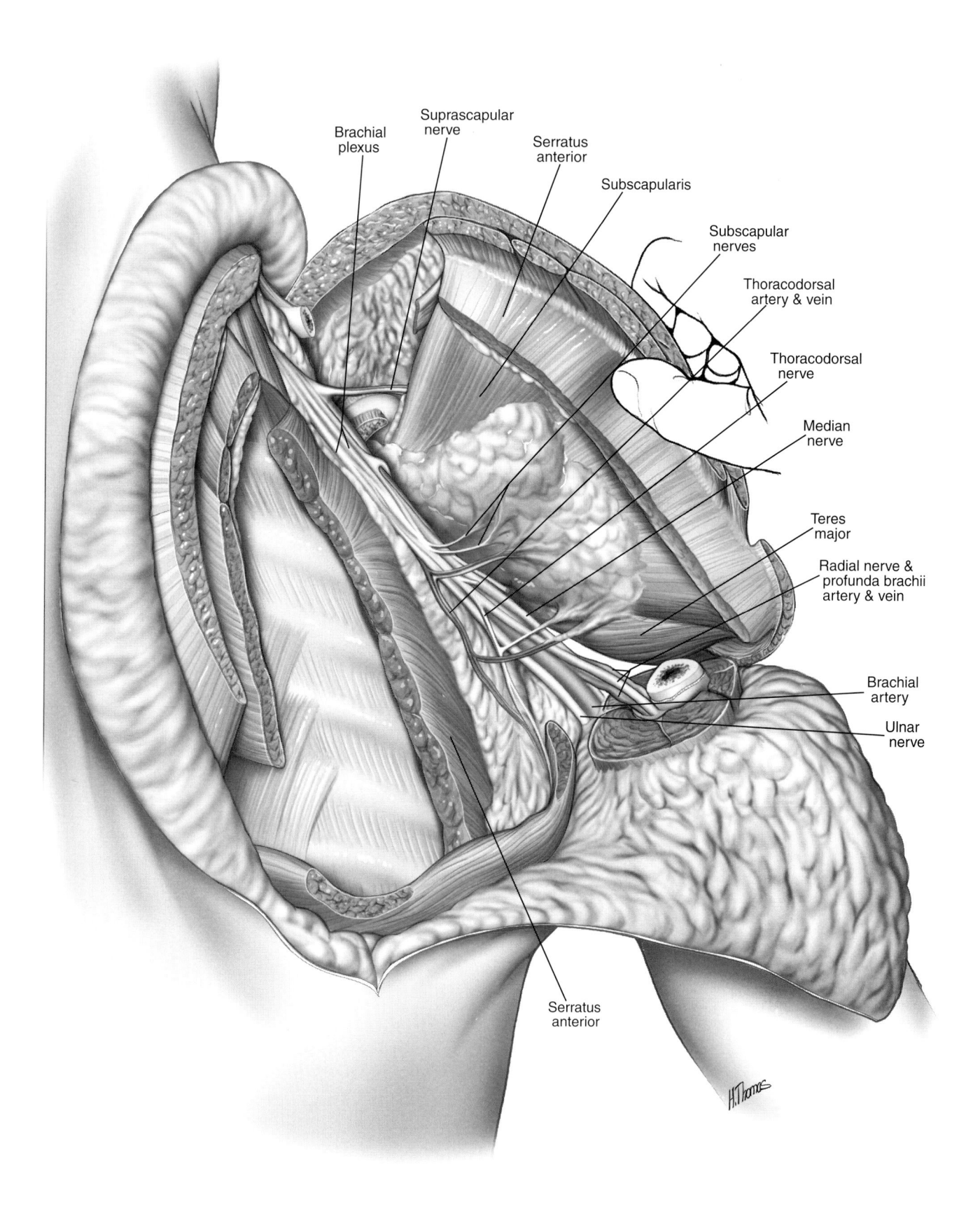

Figure 49–11 • The radial nerve is clearly demonstrated, as are the main trunks of the brachial plexus.

426 • Part V RADICAL AMPUTATIONS

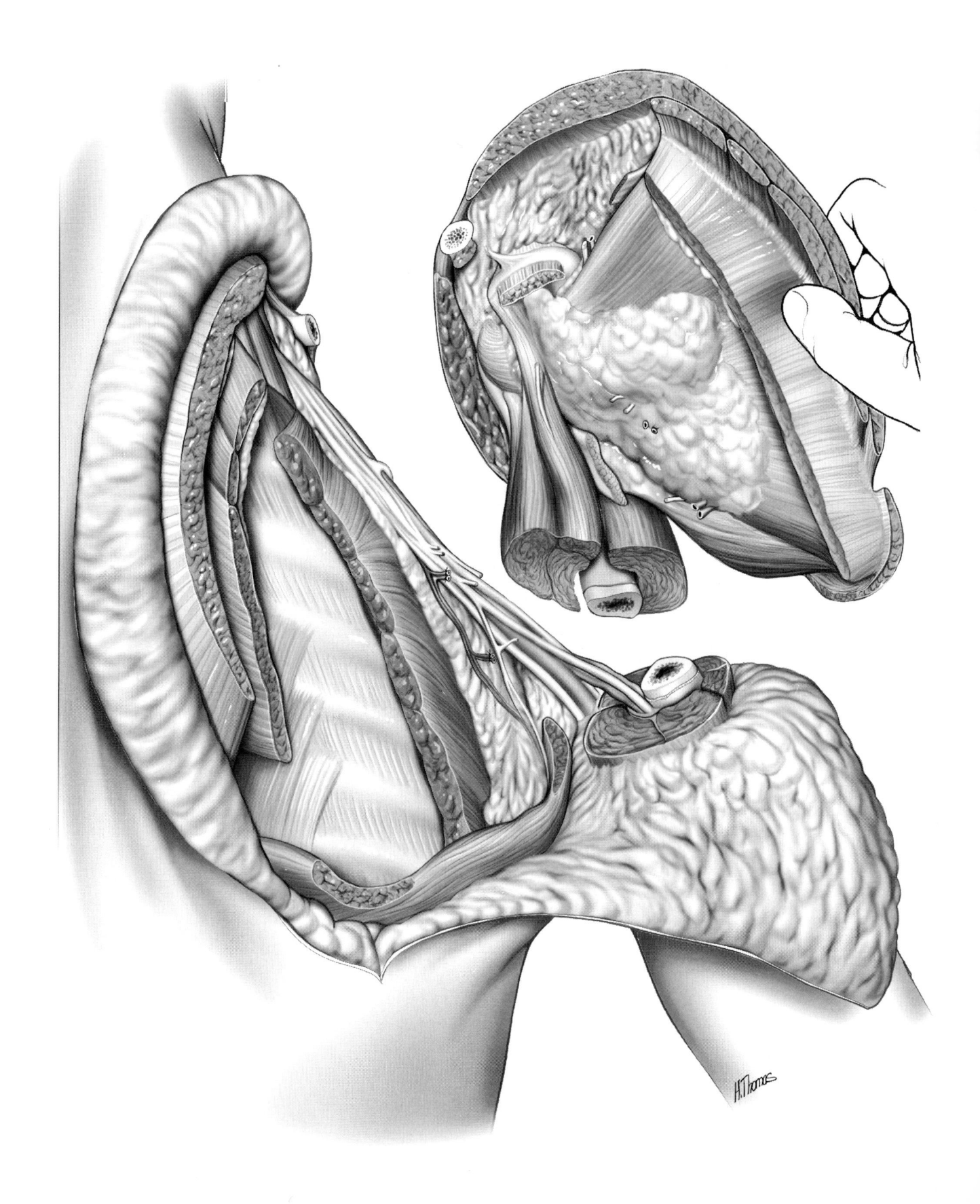

Figure 49–12 • The resection is completed.

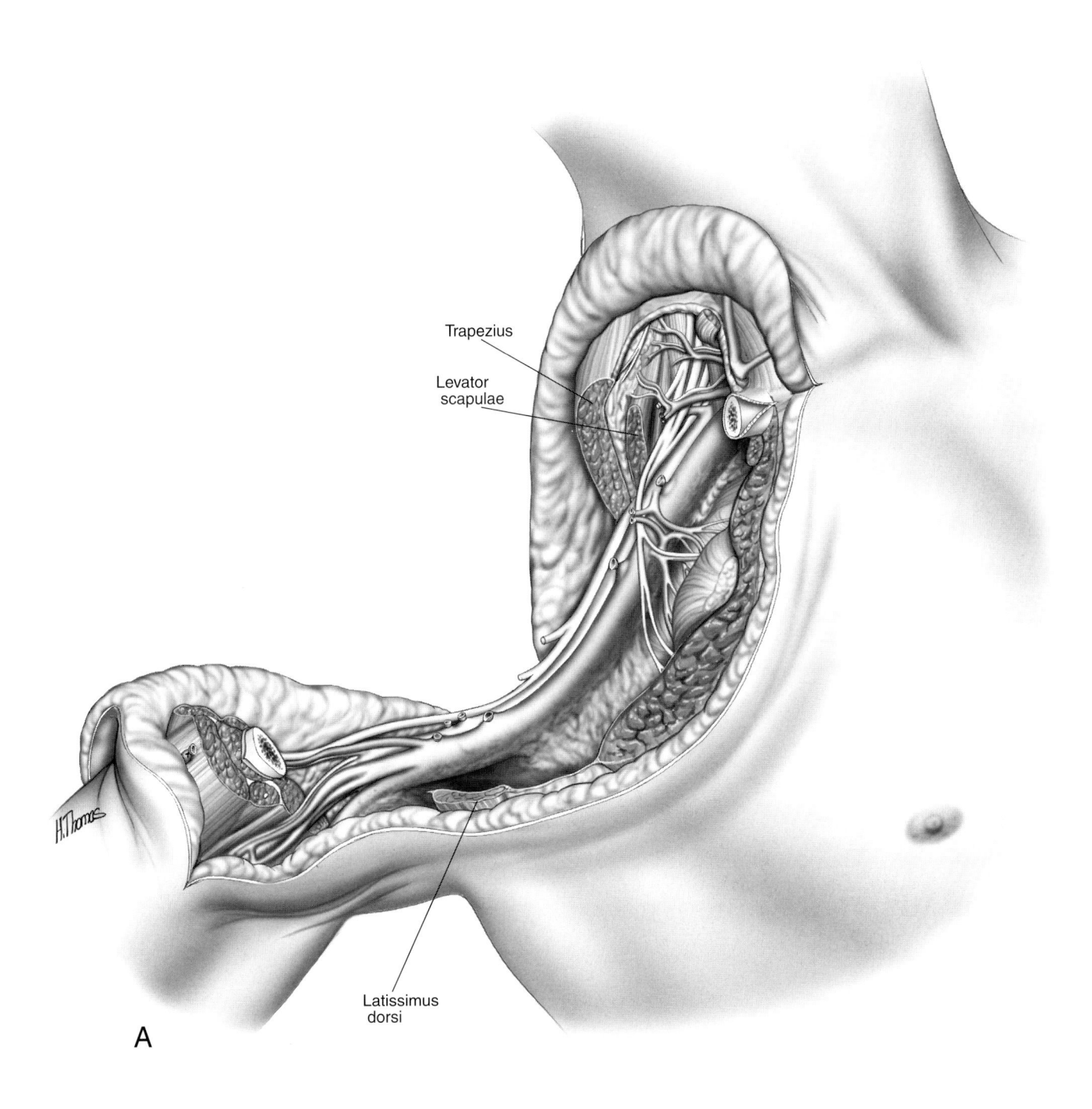

Figure 49–13 • **A,** Anterior view of resulting deficit.
   B, Prior to closure of the skin, Marlex mesh is secured between the cut ends of the triceps and biceps distally and the trapezius, levator scapulae, and clavicle superiorly to add support to the upper extremity.

Illustration continued on following page

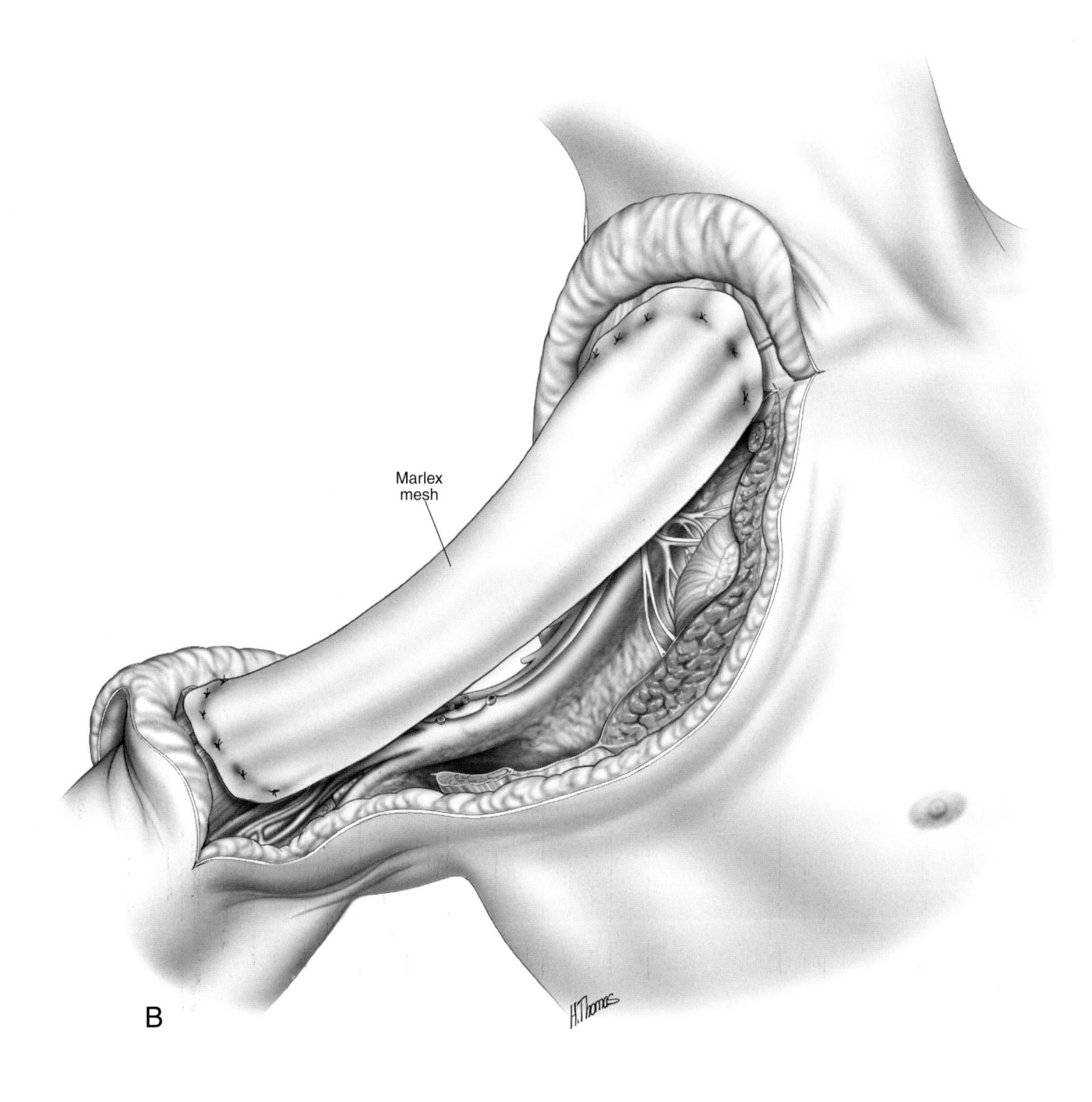

Figure 49–13B • *Continued*

Chapter 50
Surgical Anatomy of the Pelvis

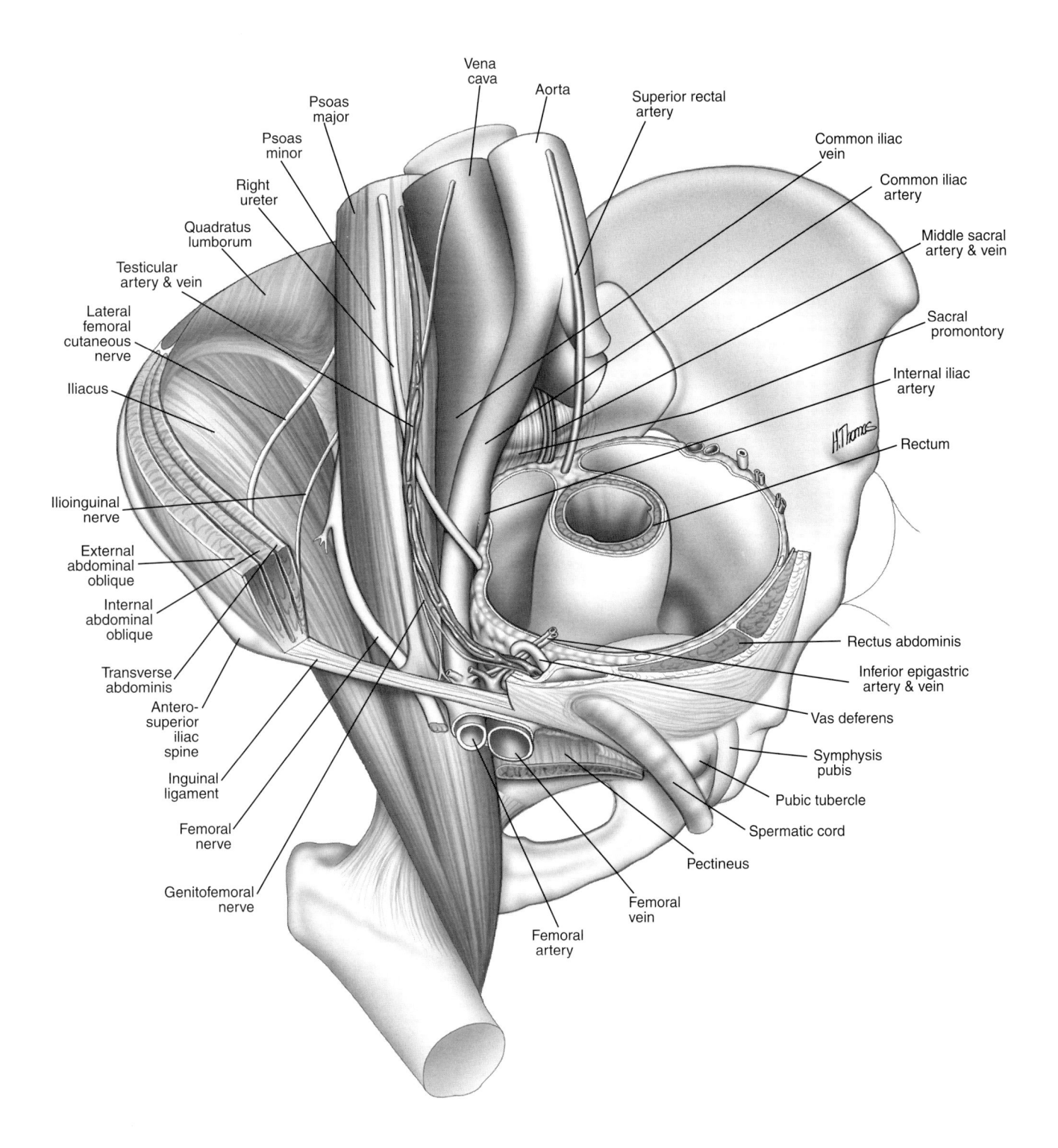

Figure 50–1 • In the orientation of the operating surgeon, the pelvic anatomy is depicted.

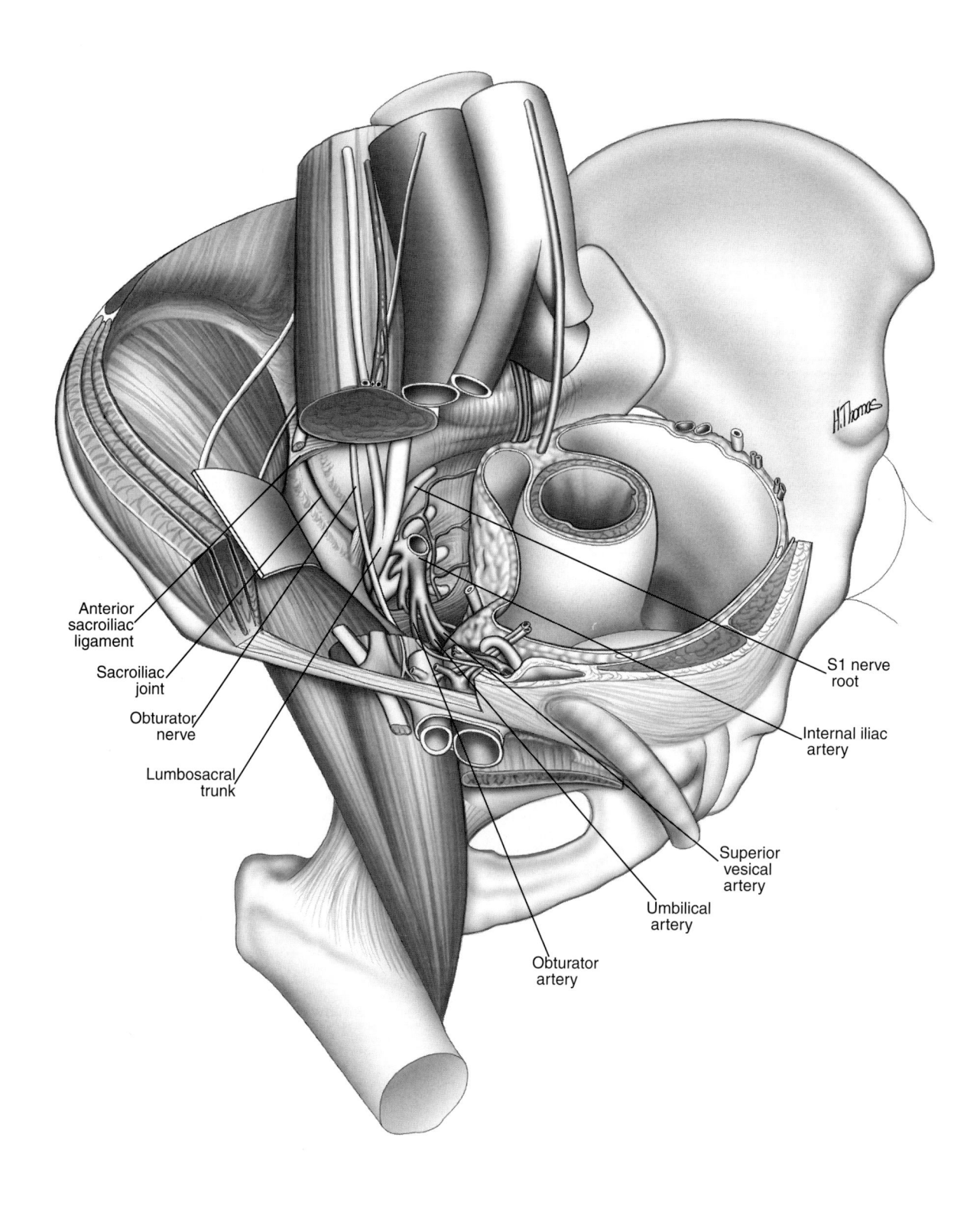

Figure 50-2 • With the psoas muscle removed as well as a section of the common iliac vessels, the sciatic nerve and vascularity around the sacroiliac joint are depicted.

Surgical Anatomy of the Pelvis • 431

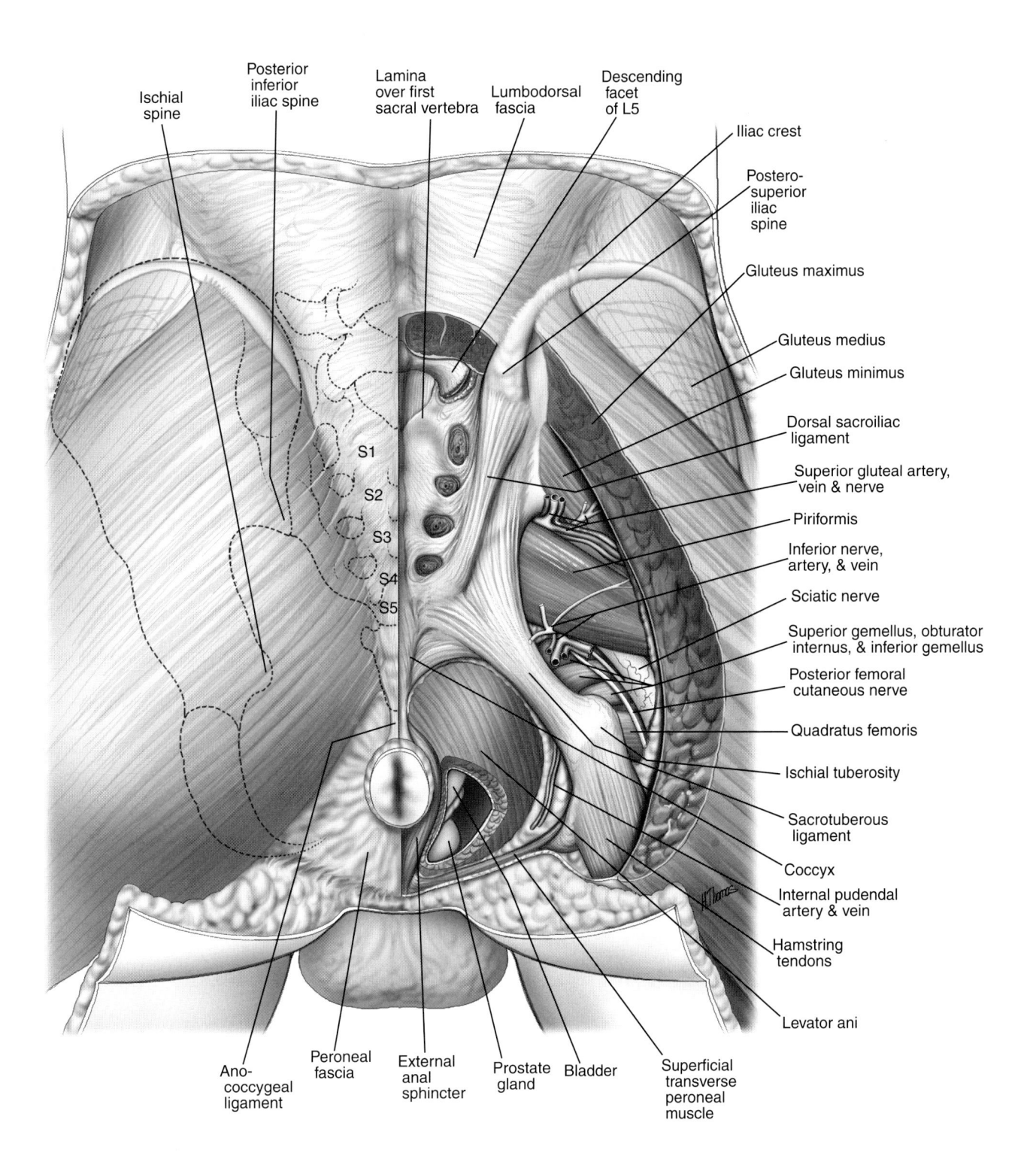

Figure 50–3 • The perineal anatomy around the sacroiliac joint is depicted.

Chapter 51
Hemipelvectomy

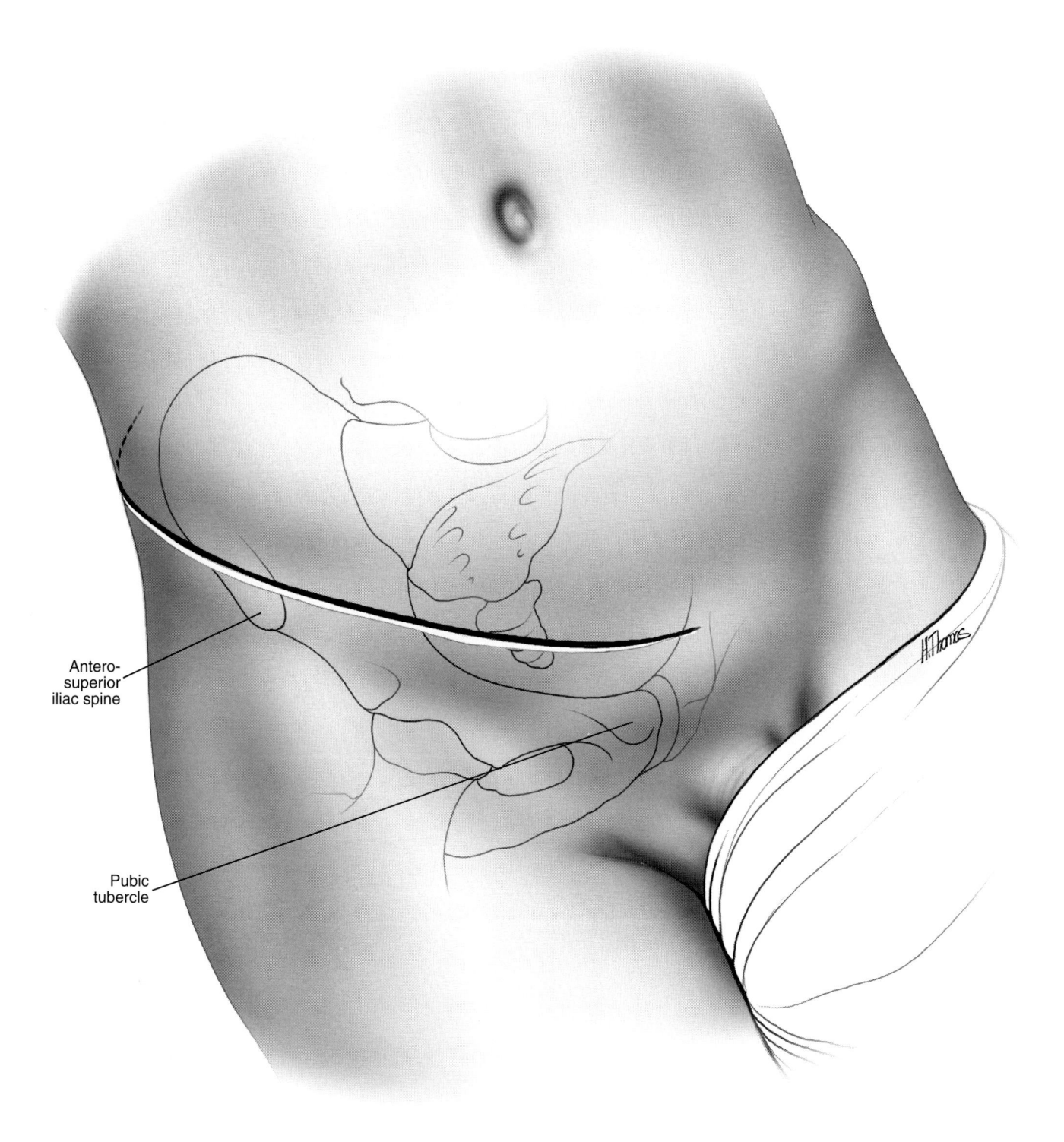

Figure 51–1 • An oblique incision is made 2 fingerbreadths above the inguinal ligament.

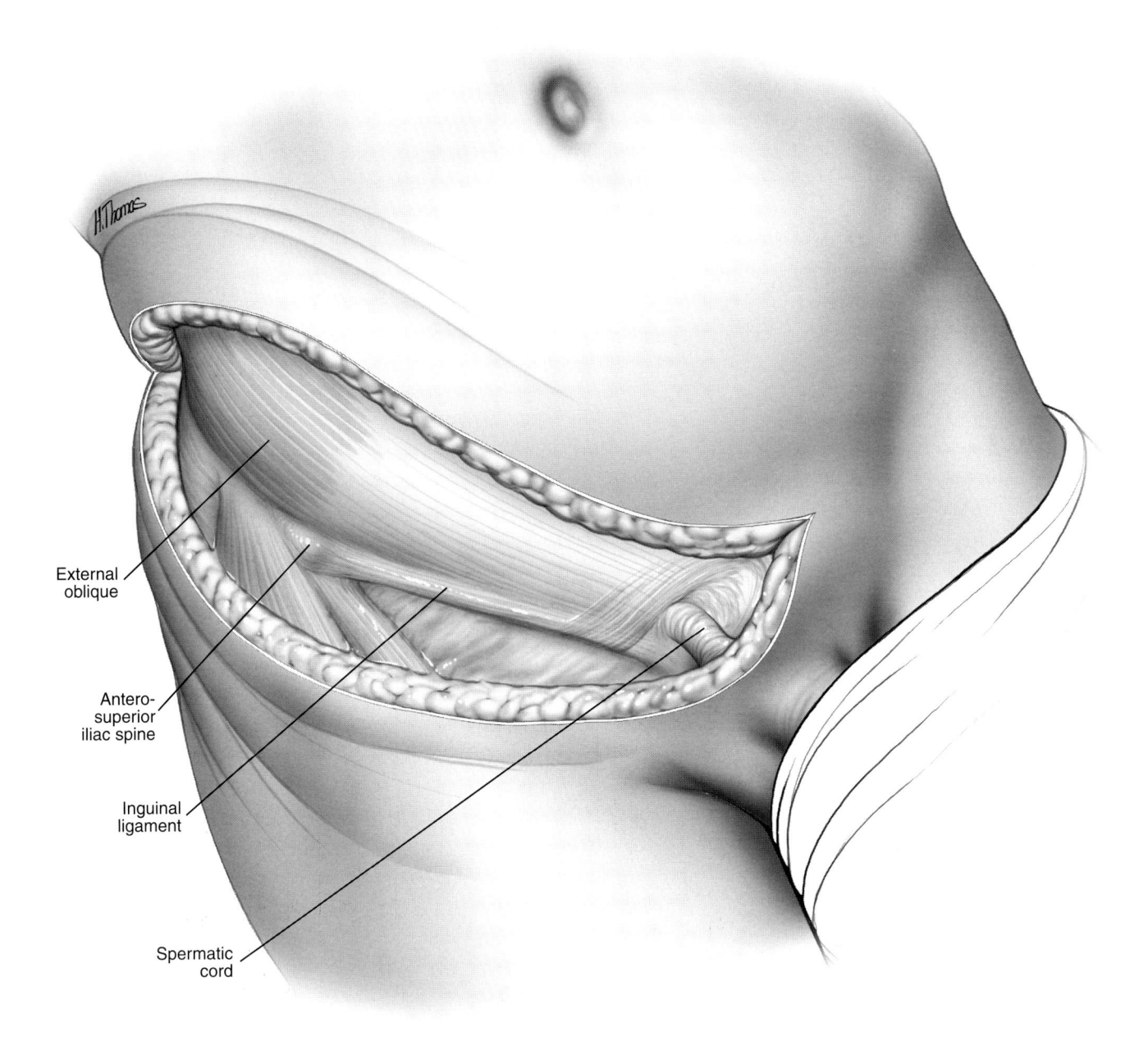

Figure 51–2 • The anatomy of the abdominal wall is depicted.

434 • Part V RADICAL AMPUTATIONS

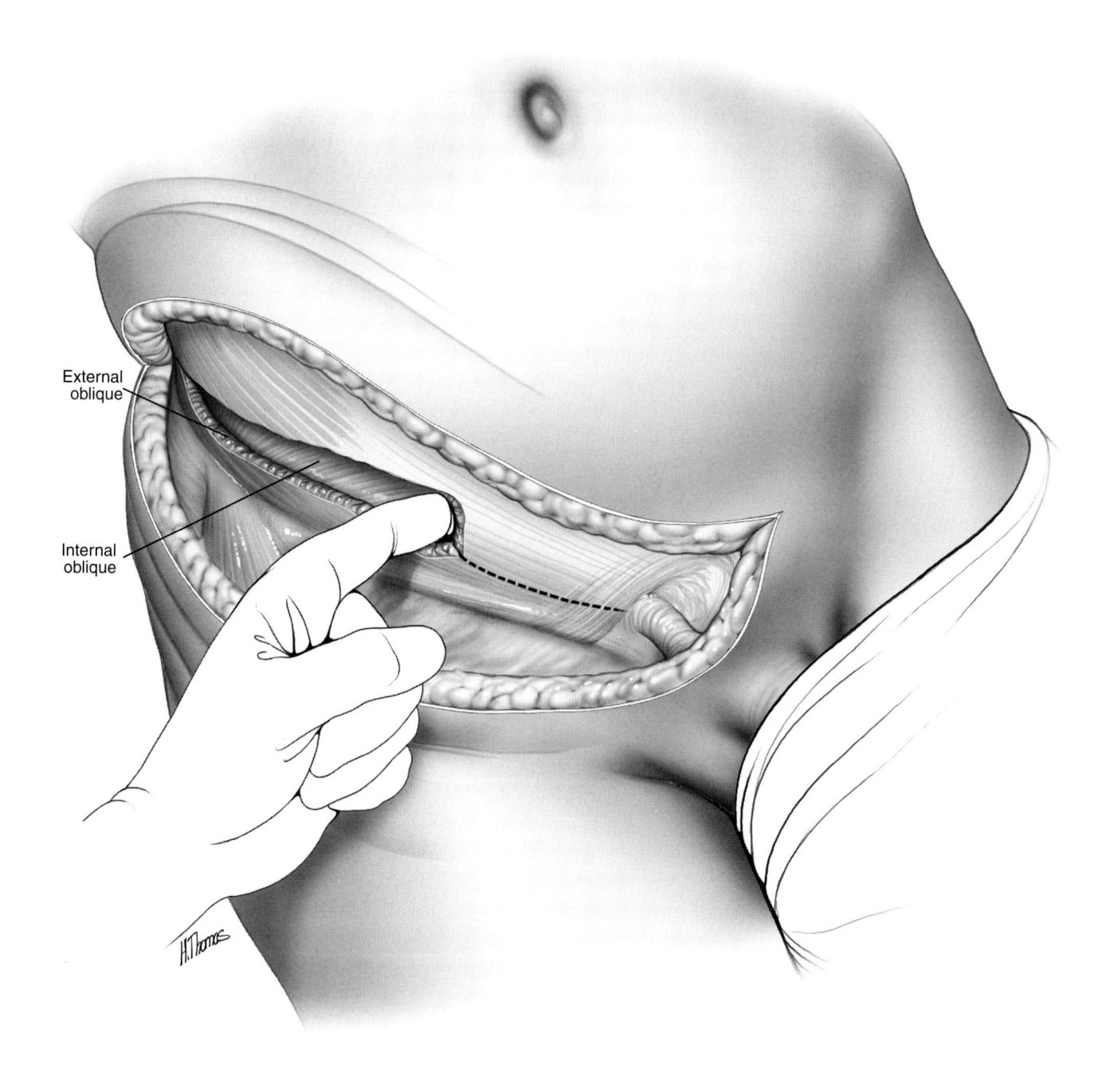

Figure 51–3 • The external oblique muscle is divided.

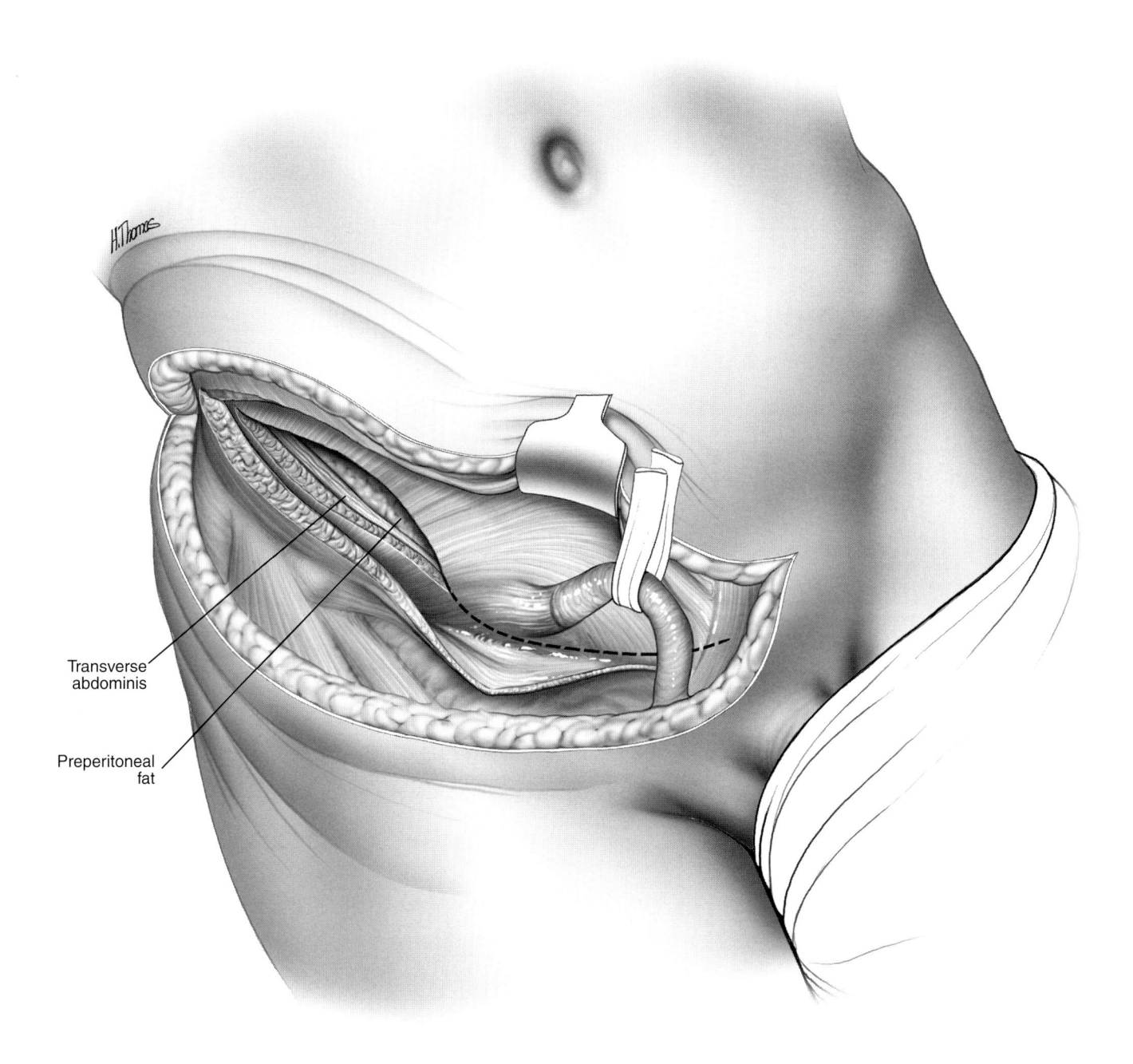

Figure 51–4 • The internal oblique and transverse abdominis muscles are divided to gain access into the retroperitoneal space. The line of resection is carried distal to the spermatic cord, which is preserved.

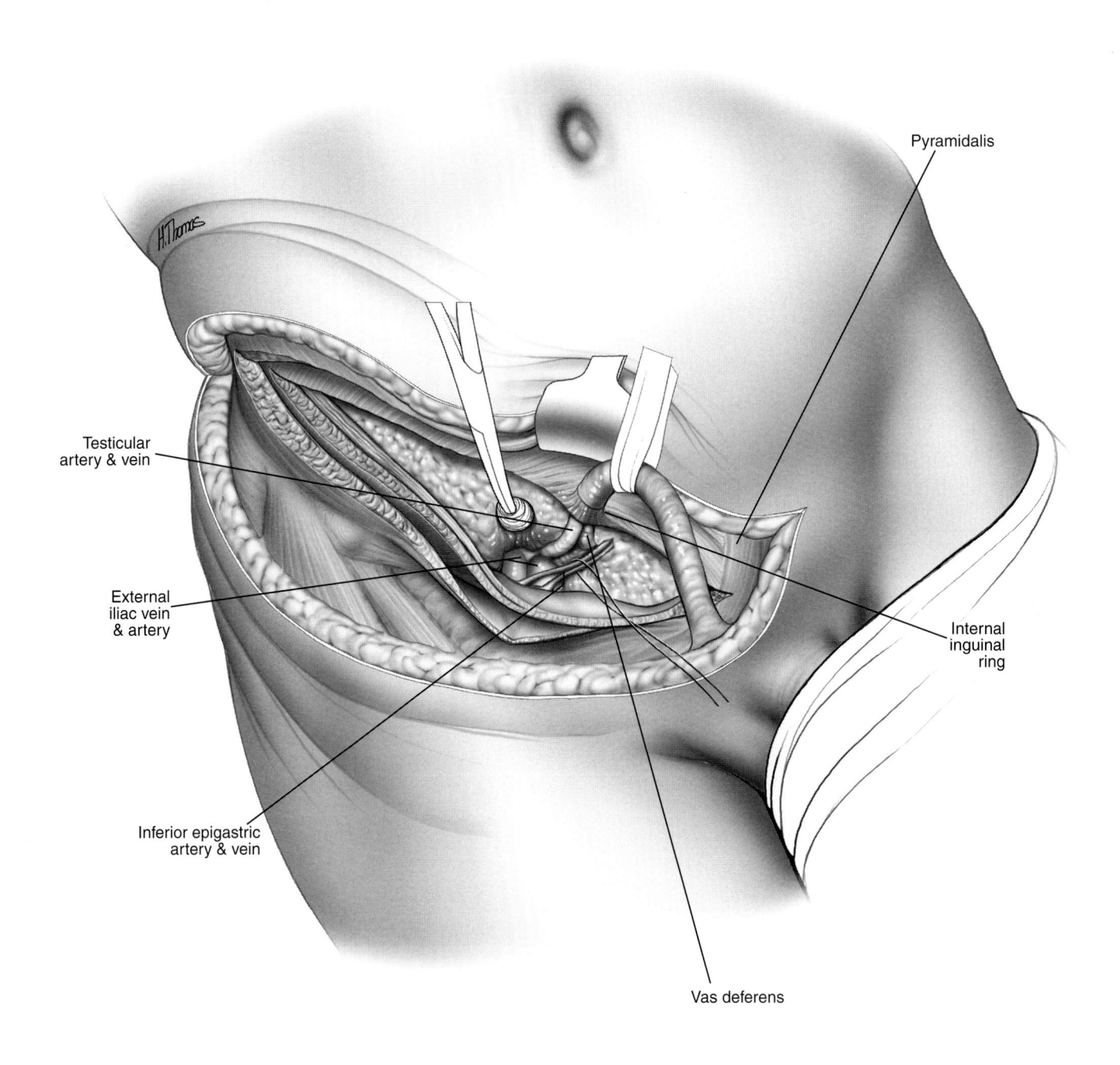

Figure 51-5 • The peritoneal envelope is bluntly dissected off the iliacus and psoas muscles, identifying the iliac vessels.

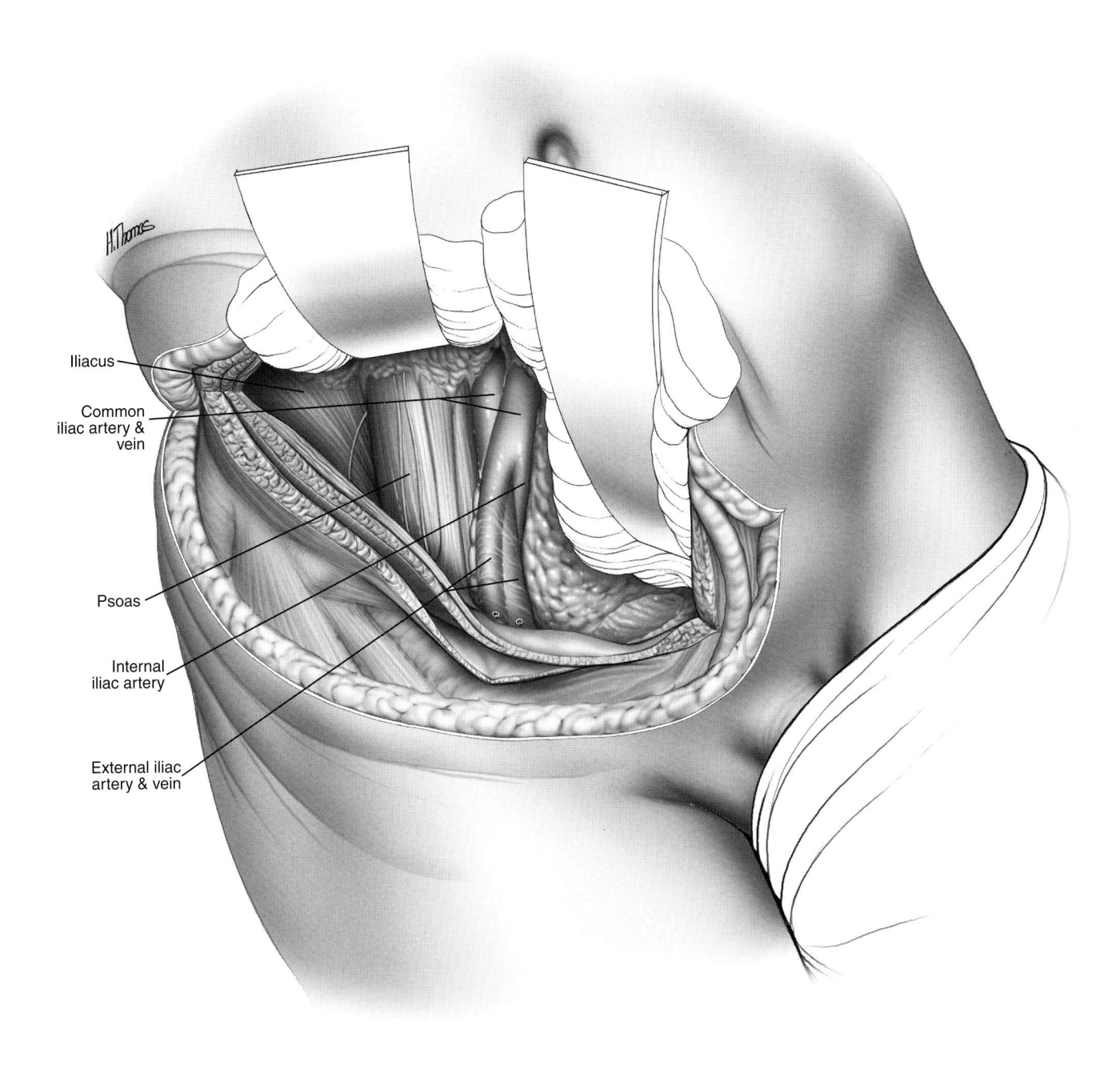

Figure 51–6 • The inferior epigastric vessels are divided, and the common iliac vessels are identified.

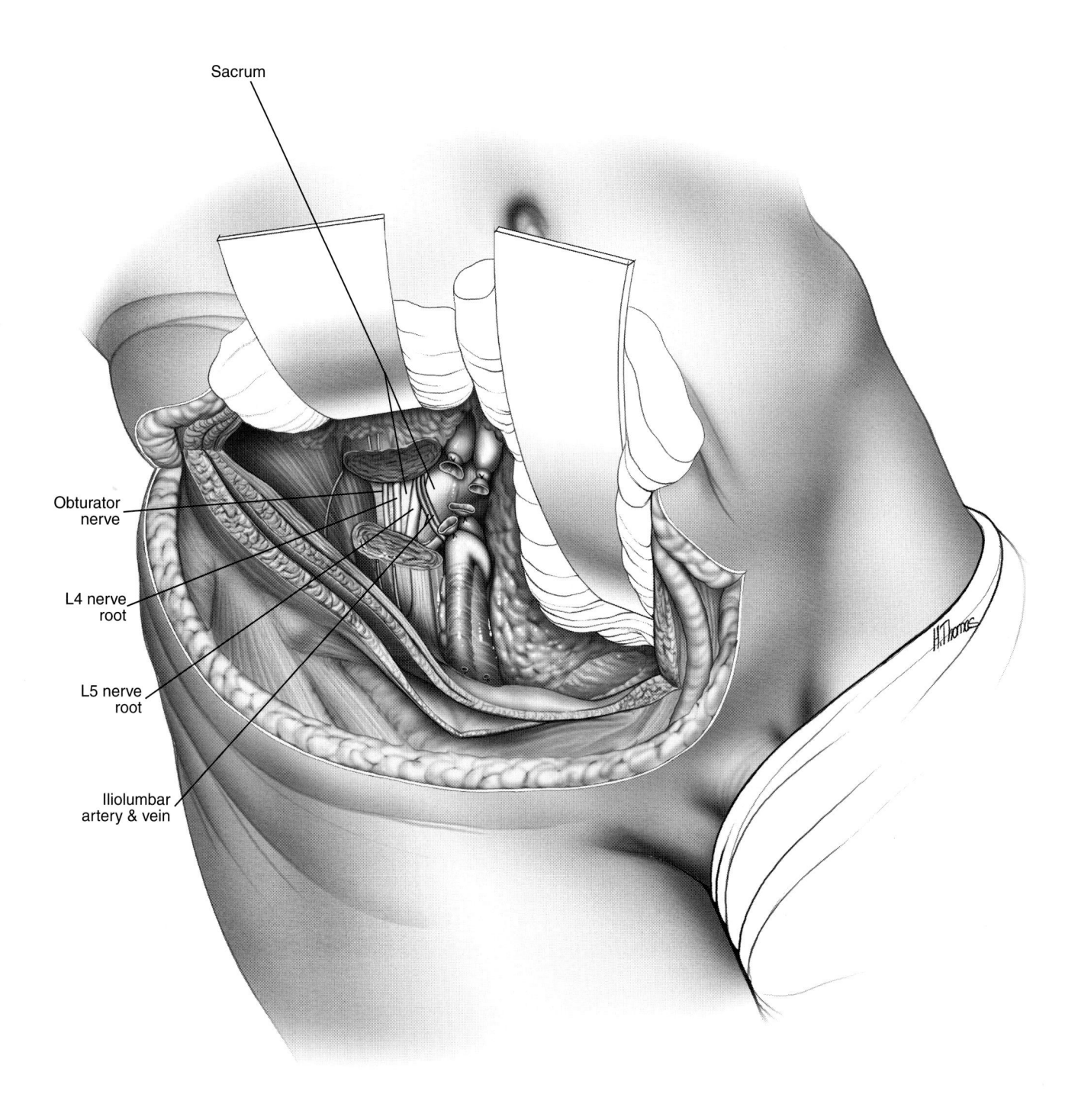

Figure 51-7 • The psoas muscle is divided, identifying the main roots of the sciatic nerve. The common iliac artery and vein are divided.

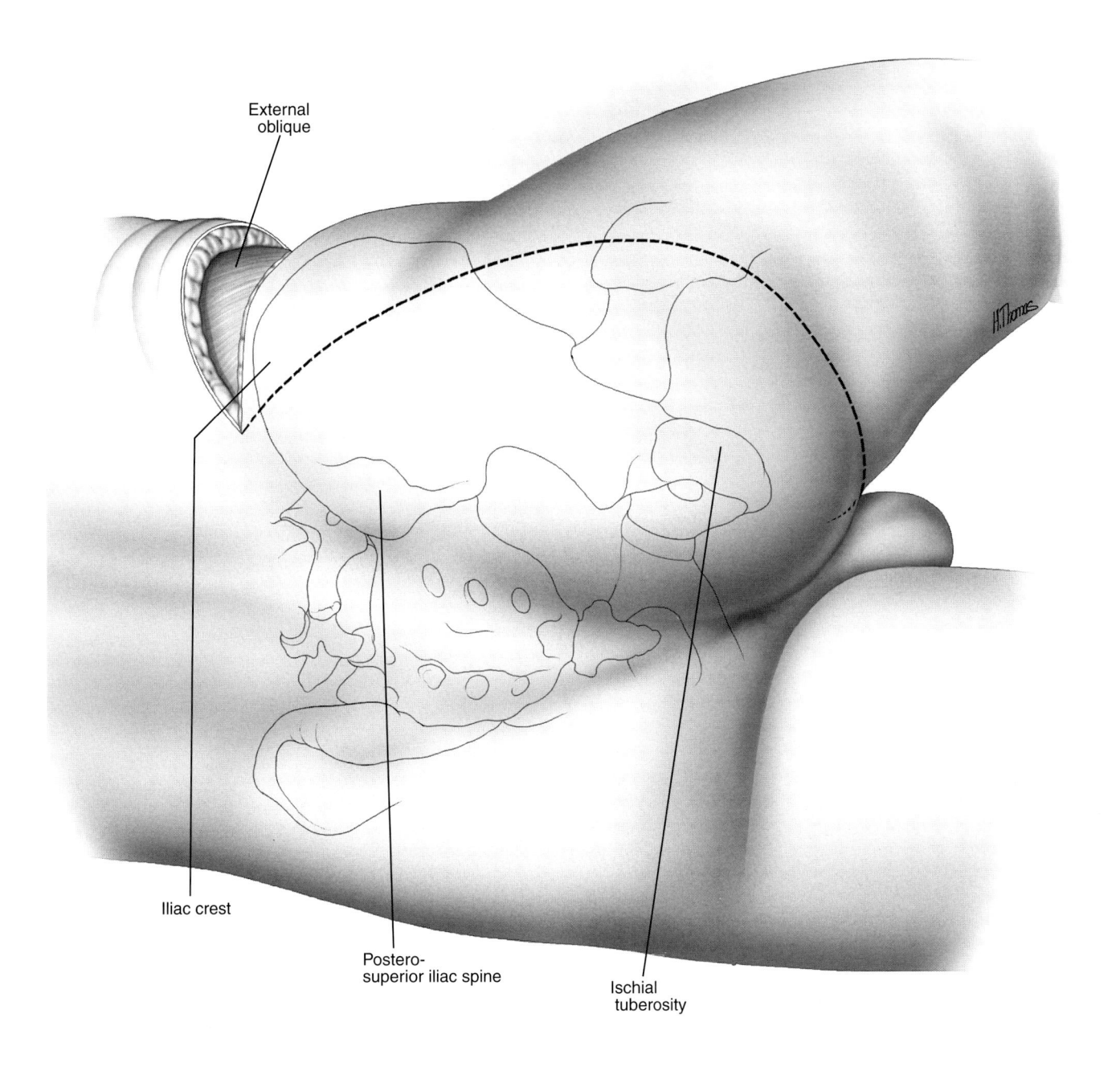

Figure 51–8 • The posterior skin flaps are defined.

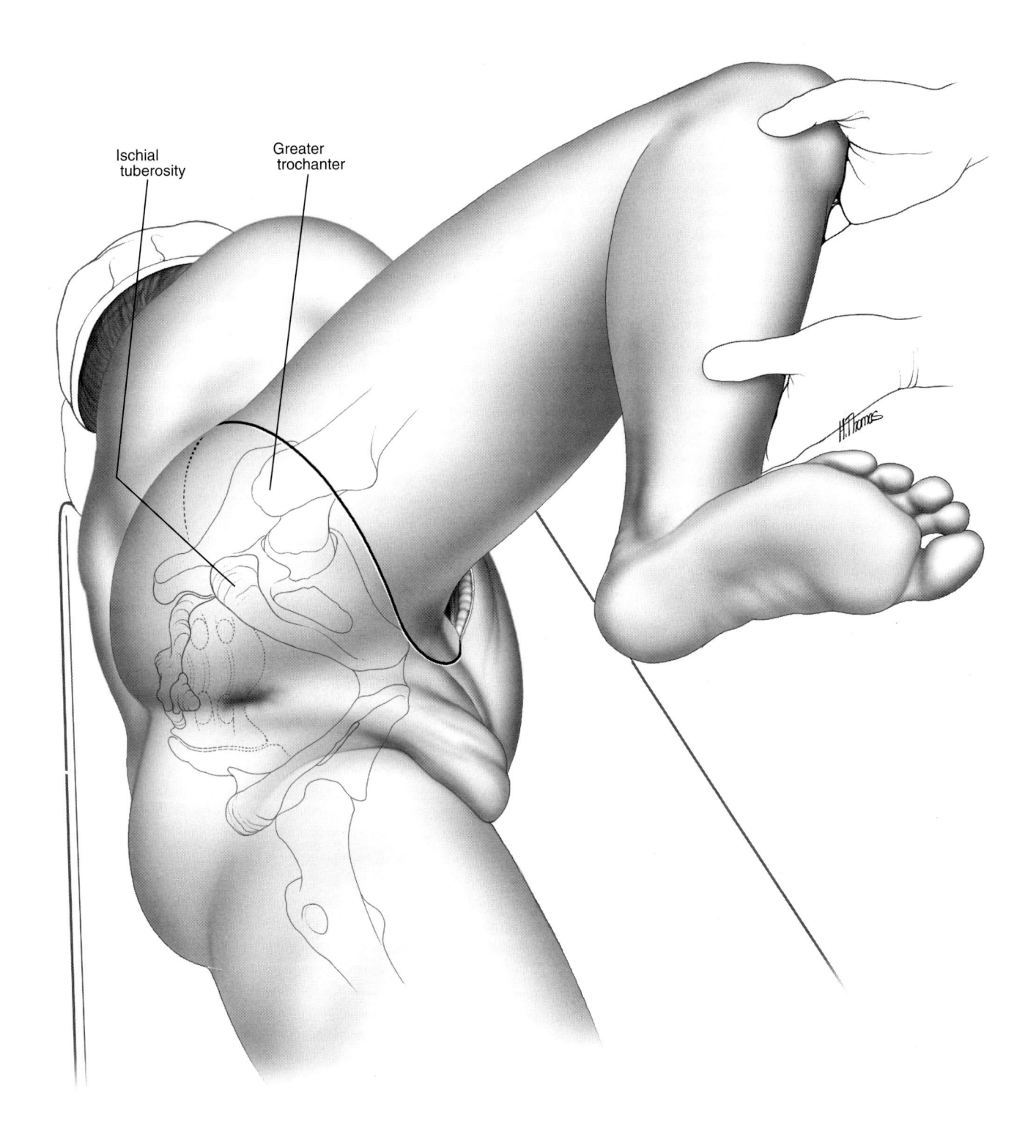

Figure 51-9 • The skin incision is carried distal to the greater trochanter and around the leg toward the symphysis pubis.

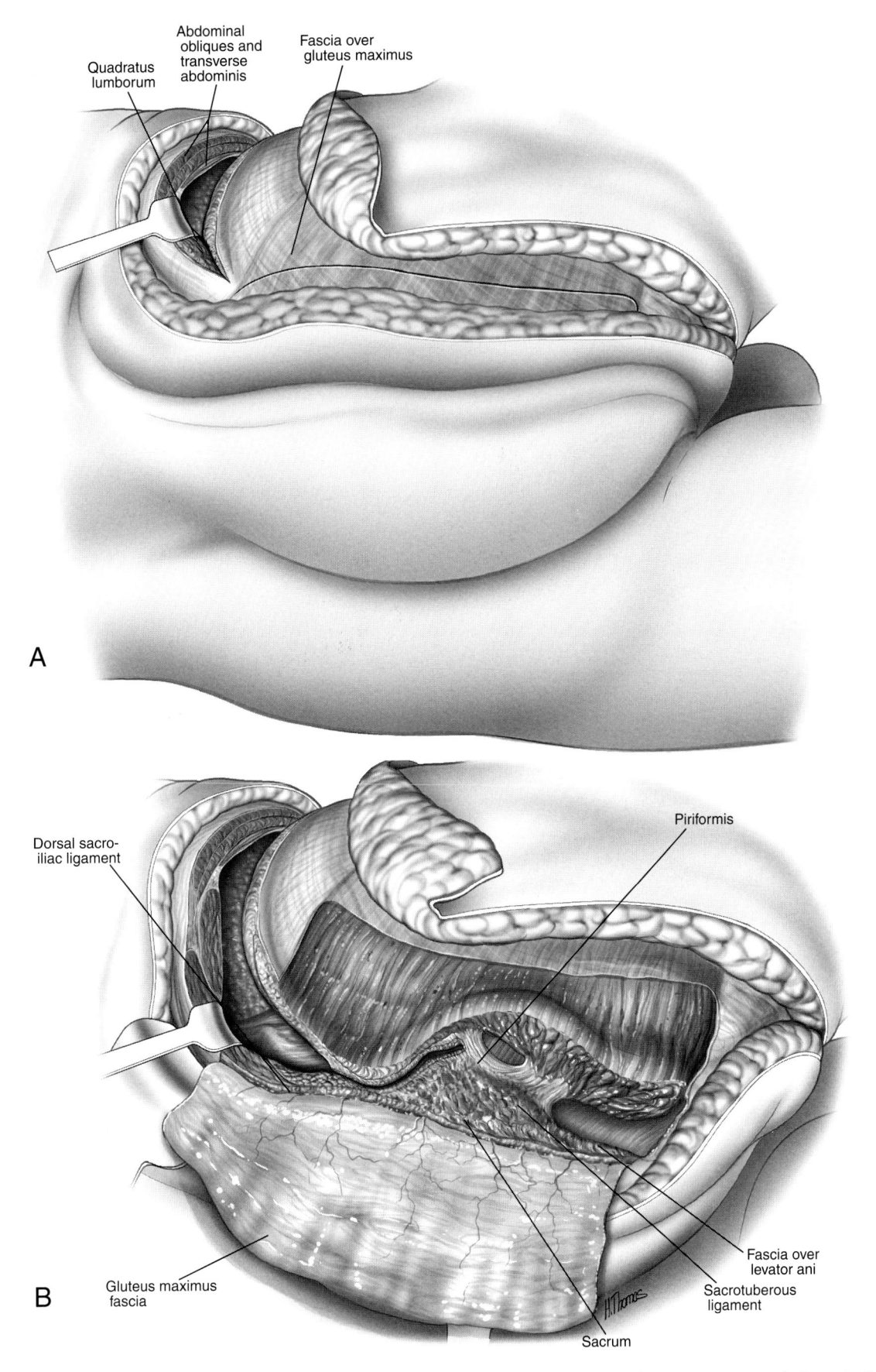

Figure 51–10 • **A,** The remaining portions of the obliques and transverse abdominis muscles are divided, as is the quadratus lumborum, exposing the L5 transverse process.

B, The gluteus muscles are divided, exposing the sacrum and the piriformis muscle.

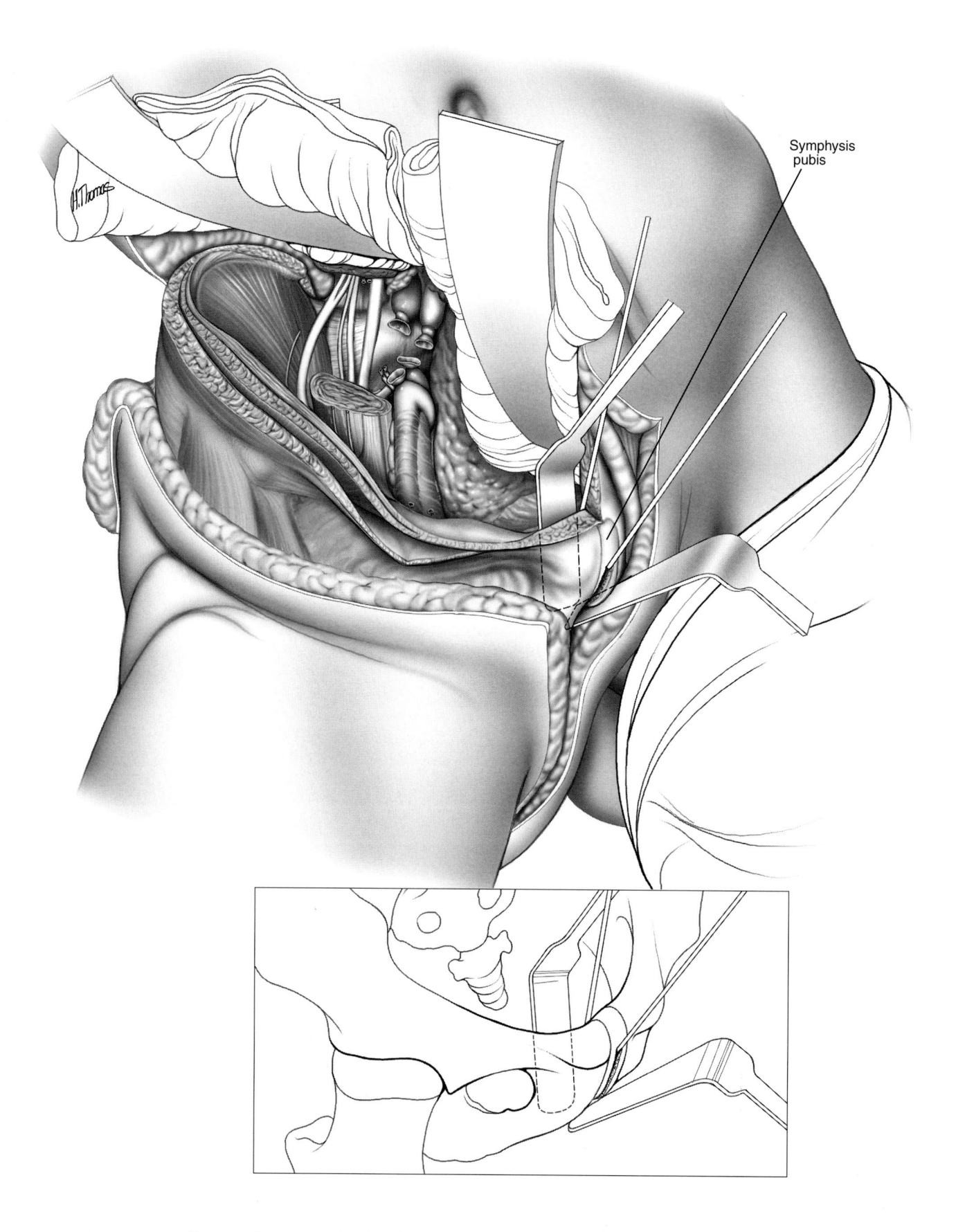

Figure 51–11 • Returning anteriorly, the symphysis pubis is divided with a Gigli saw.

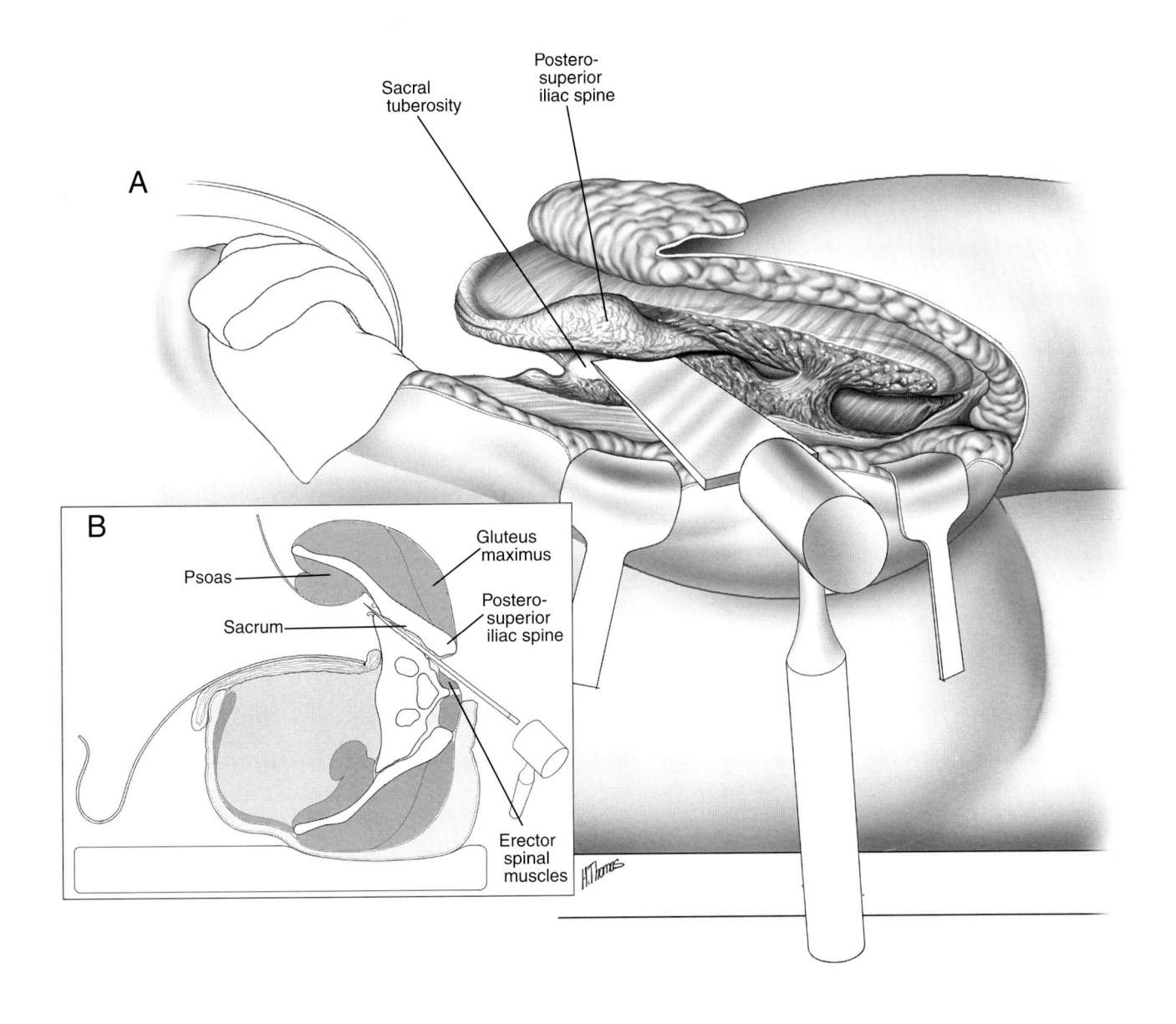

Figure 51–12 • **A,** The sacroiliac joint is osteotomized from posterior to anterior.
B, The proper angle of the joint is depicted. If desired, a portion of the sacral ala can be included.

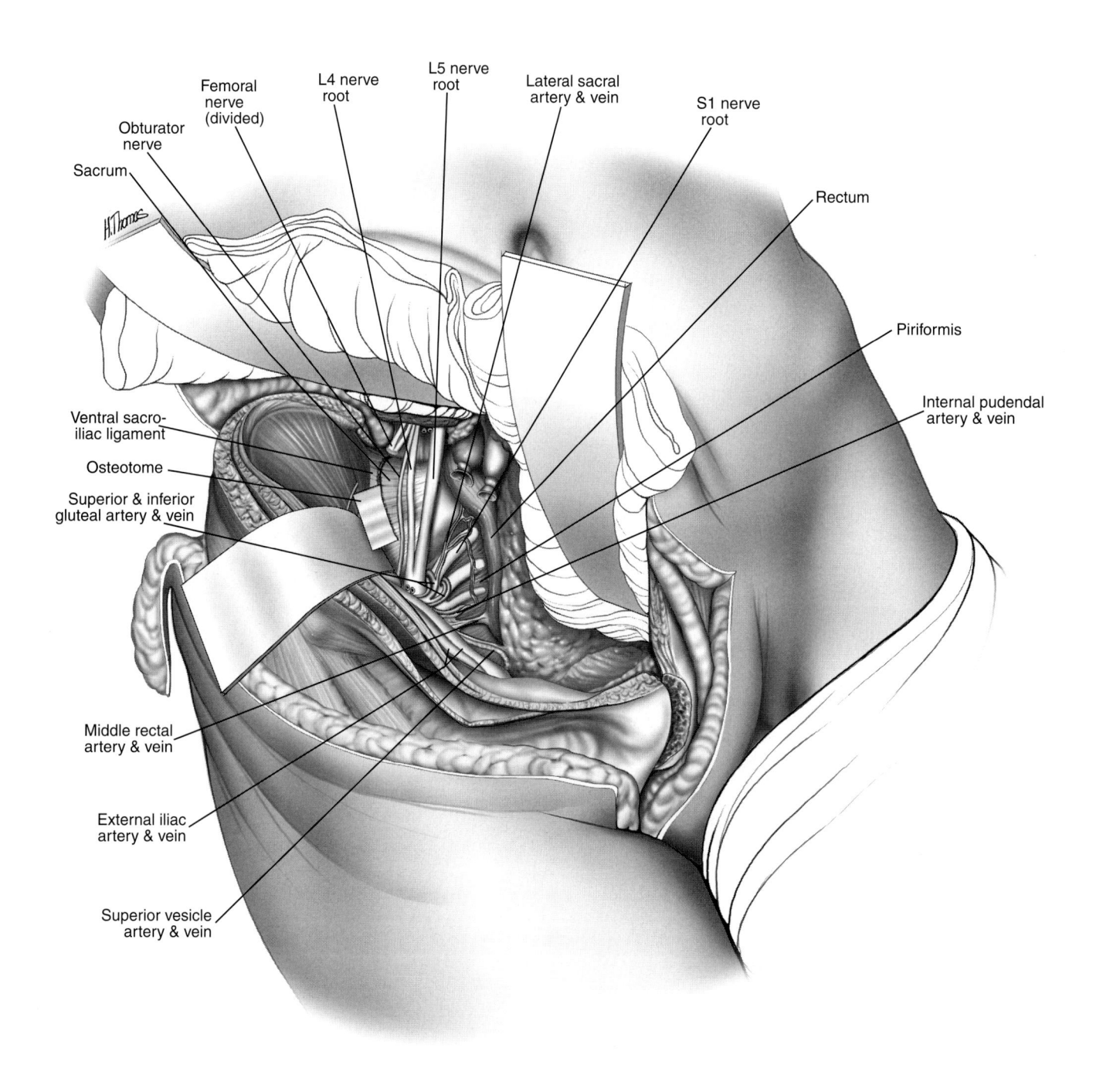

Figure 51–13 • An anterior view showing the osteotome coming through the sacroiliac joint.

Hemipelvectomy • 445

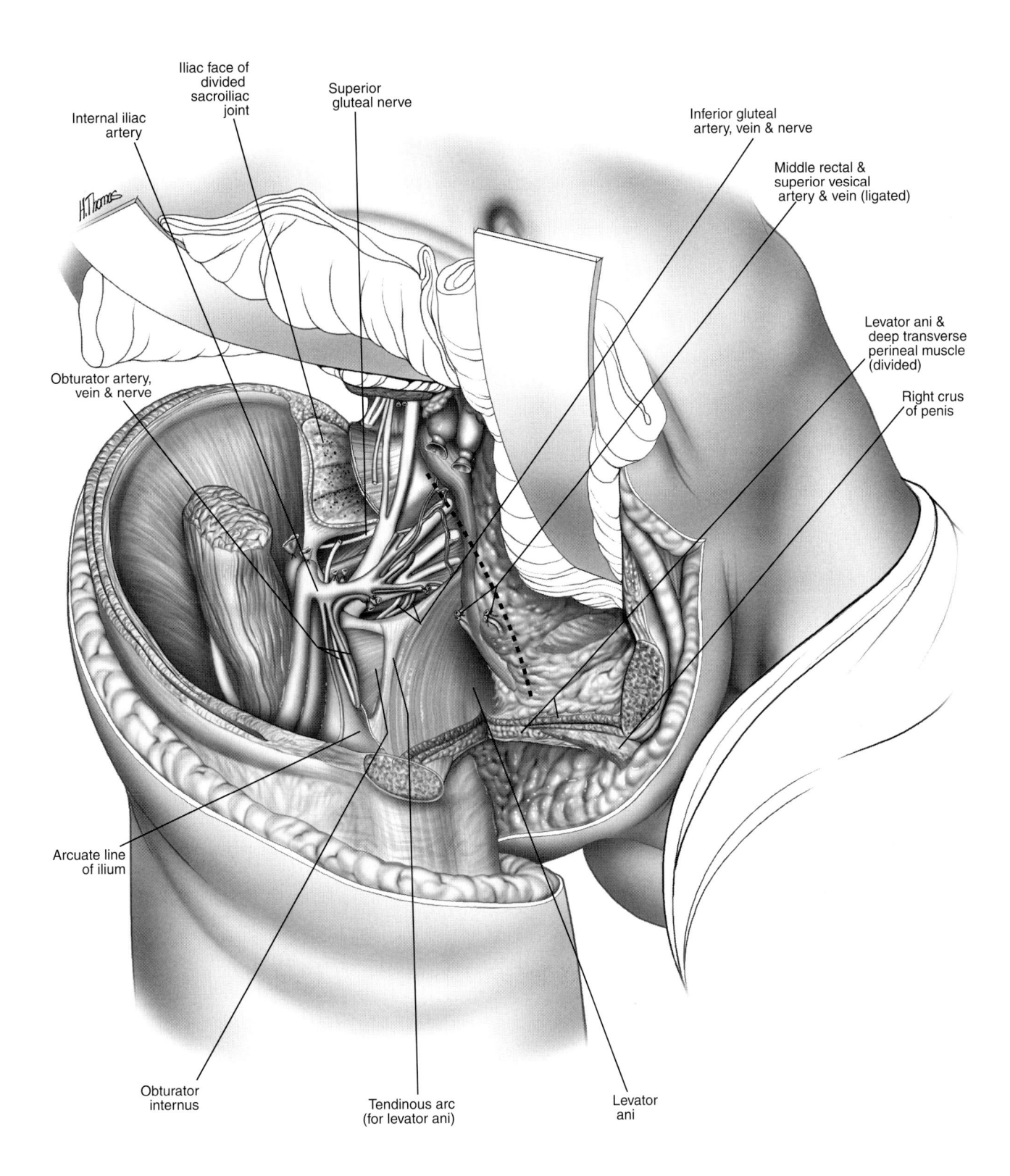

Figure 51–14 • Division of the nerve roots is commenced, as well as division of several branches off the hypogastrics.

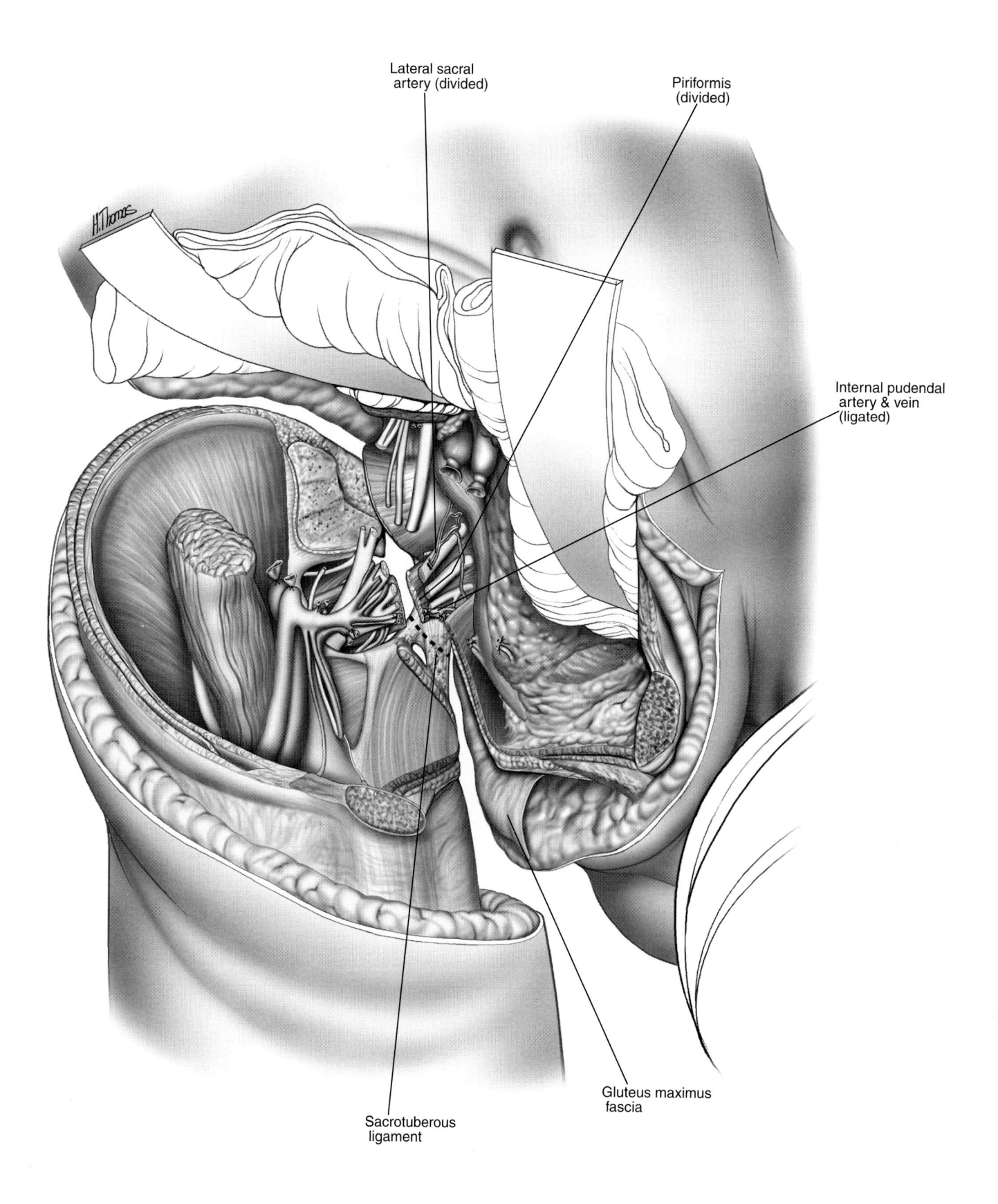

Figure 51–15 • After division of the levator ani and piriformis, the sacrotuberous ligament is the remaining attachment.

Hemipelvectomy • 447

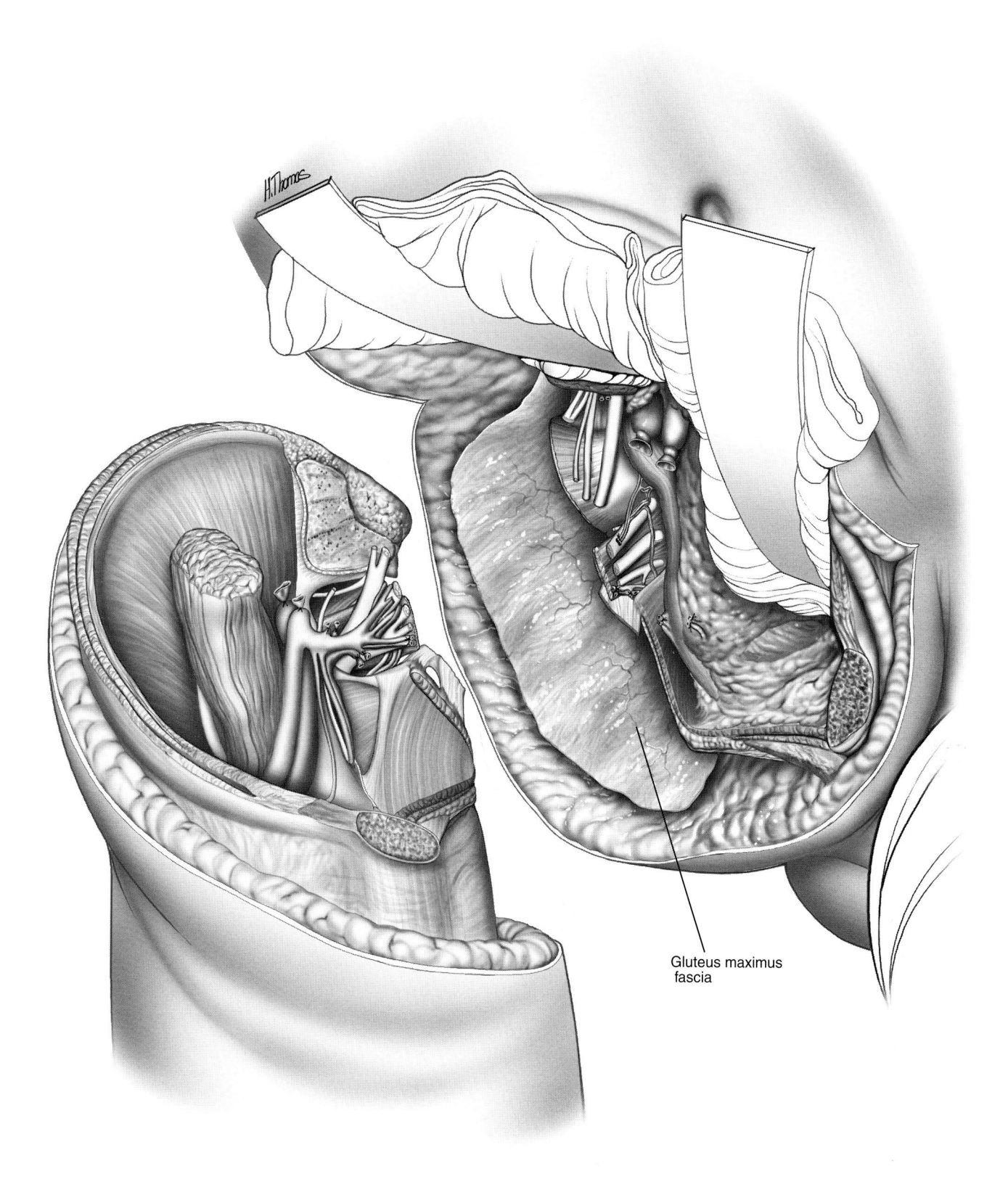

Gluteus maximus fascia

Figure 51–16 • The specimen is removed. There is usually some bleeding from the venous plexus around the bladder wall, which can be controlled with suture ligatures.

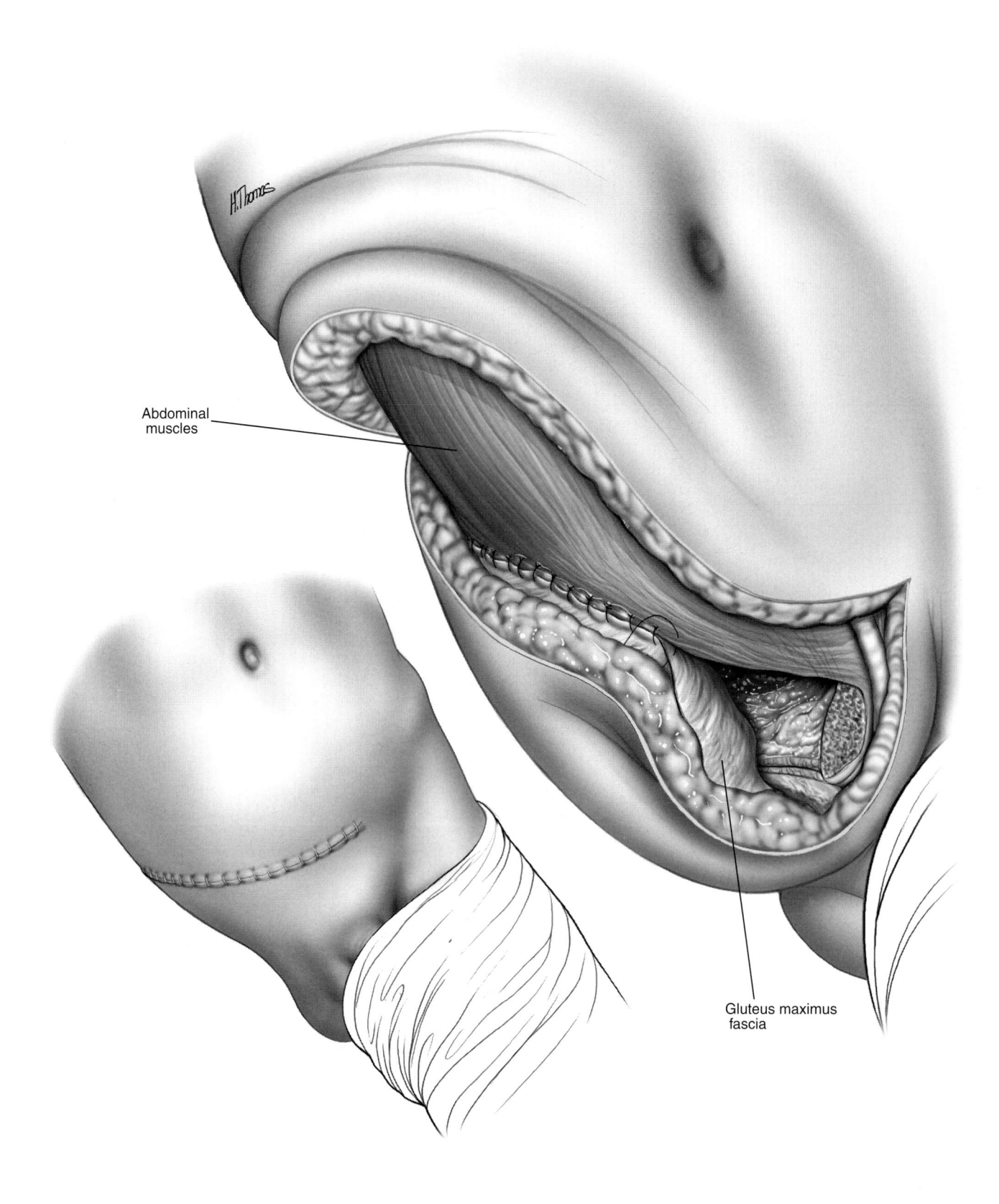

Figure 51–17 • The resulting defect is closed by attaching the cut ends of the gluteals to the abdominal wall musculature. The skin and subcutaneous tissue are then closed. No drains are used.

Chapter 52
Clinical Case: Chondrosarcoma of the Pubis

Norman Bloom

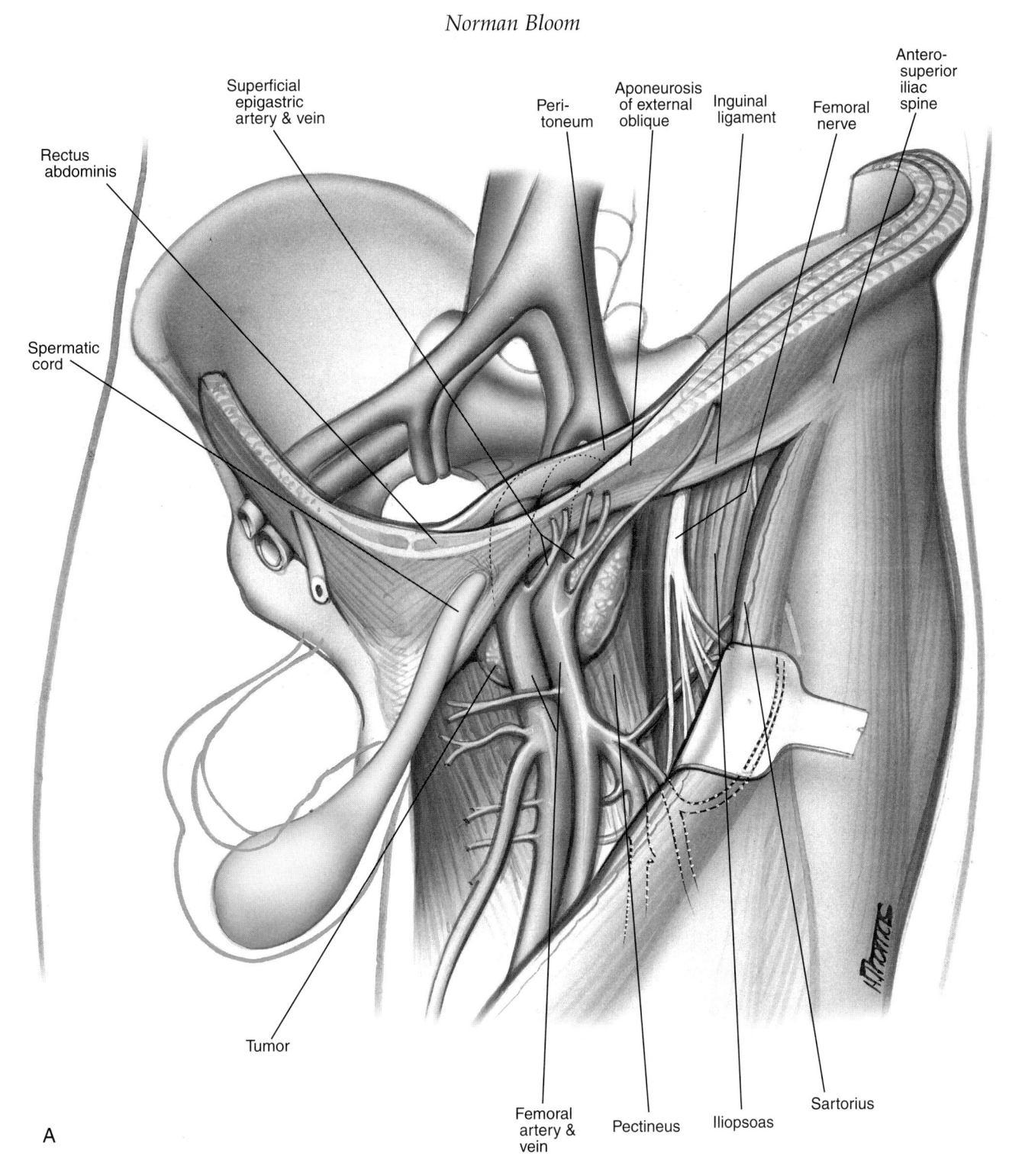

Figure 52–1 • **A,** A 32-year-old man presented with a chondrosarcoma arising from the superior ramus of the pubis. The patient underwent a Type III internal hemipelvectomy, removing the superior pubic ramus and the entire obturator space.

Illustration continued on next page

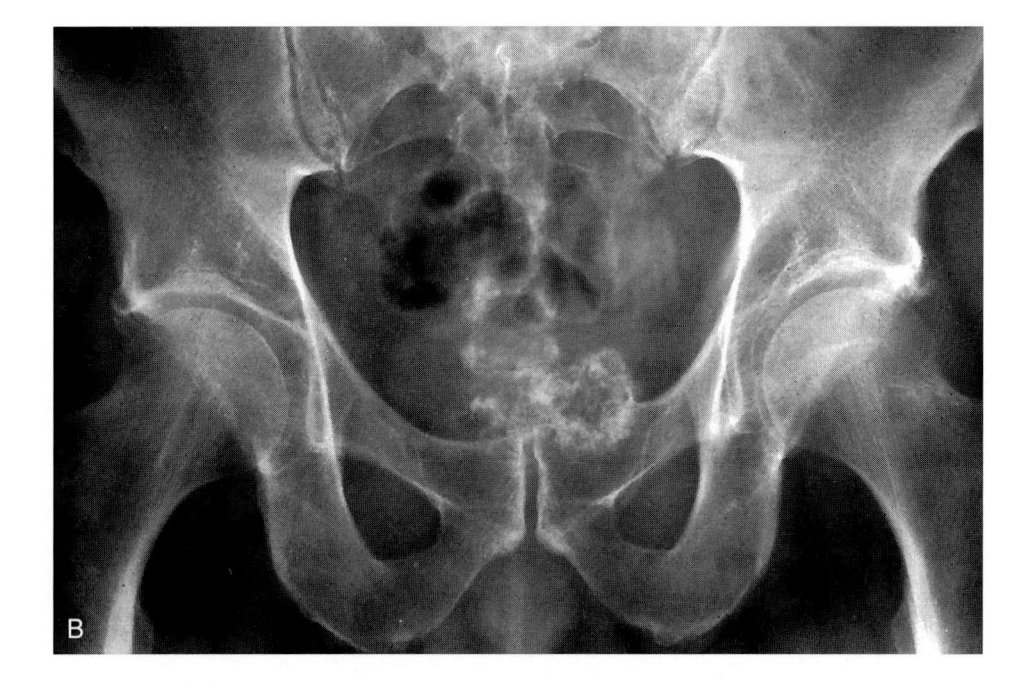

Figure 52–1 *Continued* • **B,** X-ray showing the chondrosarcoma arising from the superior ramus on the left.

Clinical Case: Chondrosarcoma of the Pubis • 451

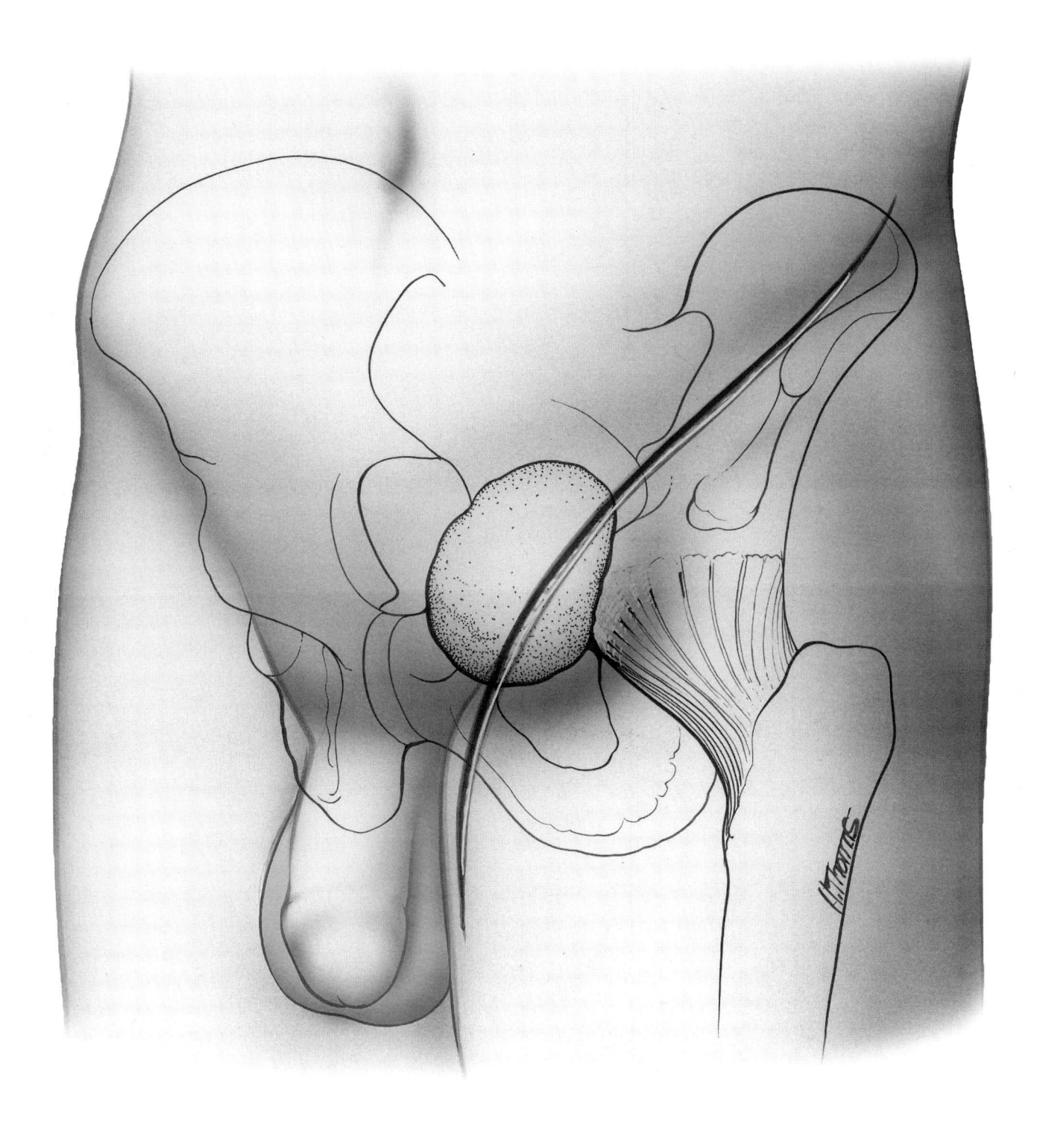

Figure 52–2 • An ilioinguinal incision is performed, and the retroperitoneal space is entered.

452 • Part V RADICAL AMPUTATIONS

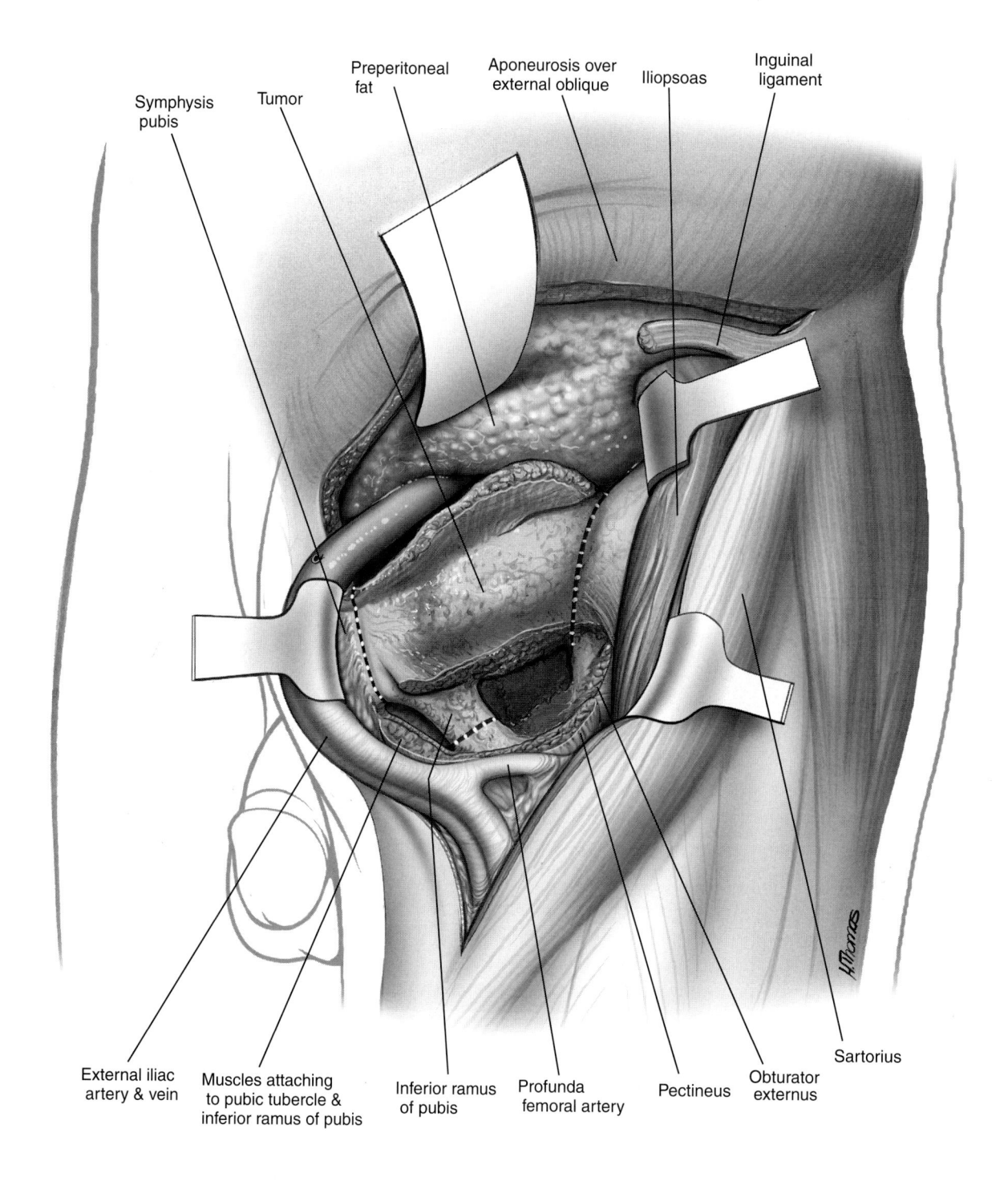

Figure 52–3 • The inguinal ligament is divided medially, and the iliac artery and vein are mobilized completely medially. The bony lines of resection are depicted.

Clinical Case: Chondrosarcoma of the Pubis • 453

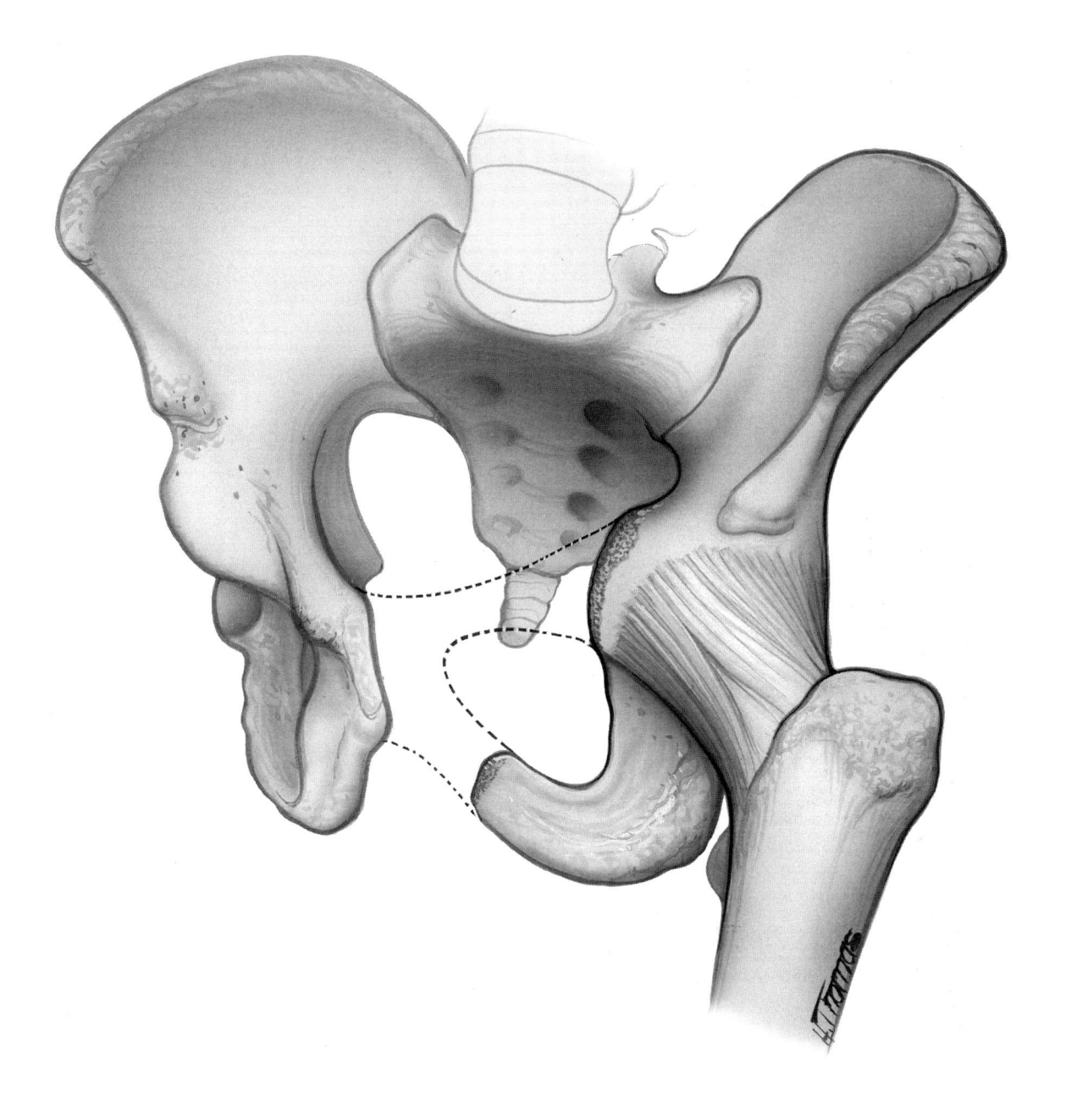

Figure 52–4 • After division of the obturator nerve, artery, and vein, the bony resection is completed.

454 • Part V RADICAL AMPUTATIONS

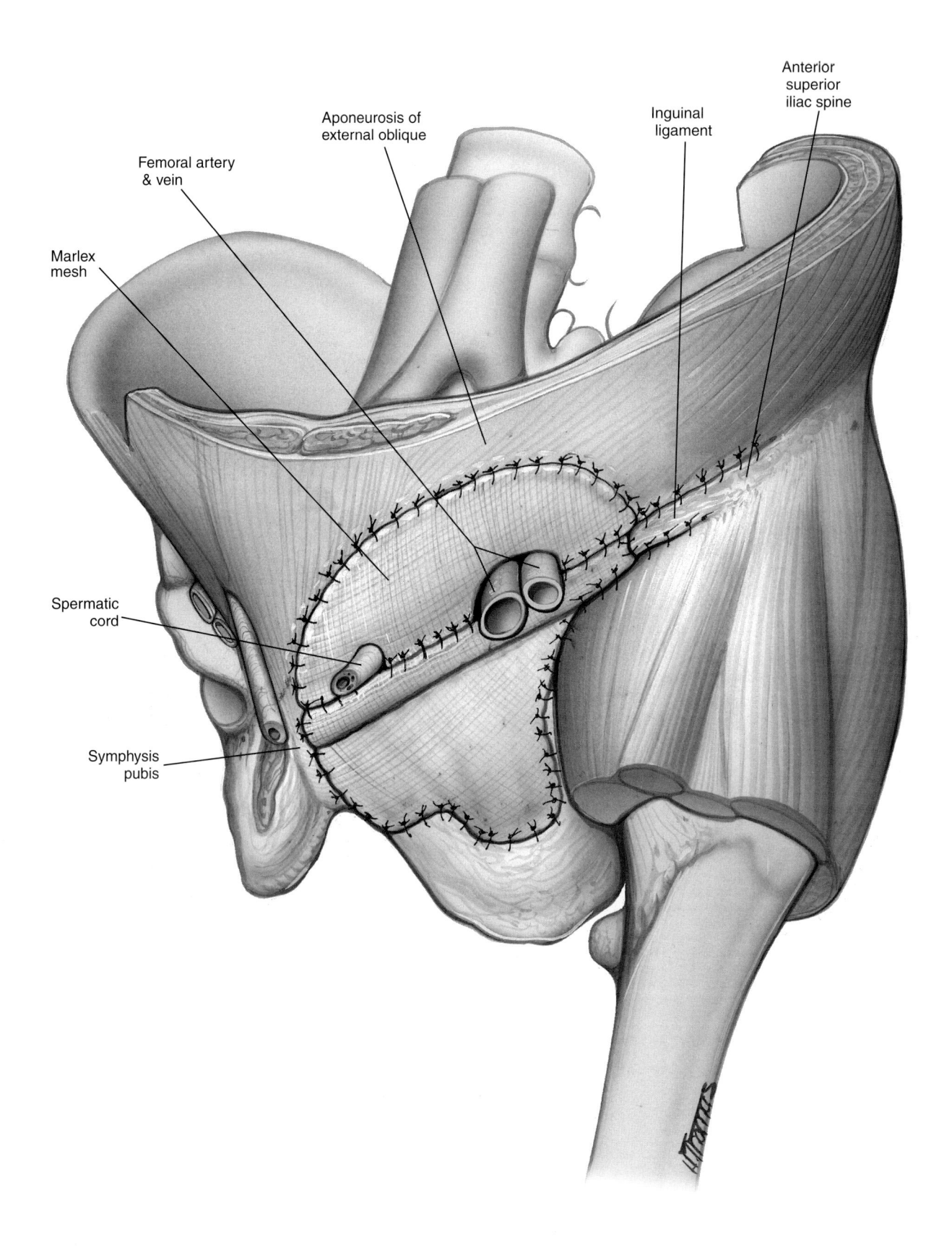

Figure 52–5 • Marlex mesh is used to reconstruct the pelvis.

Chapter 53
Clinical Case: Chondrosarcoma of the Iliac Wing

Norman Bloom

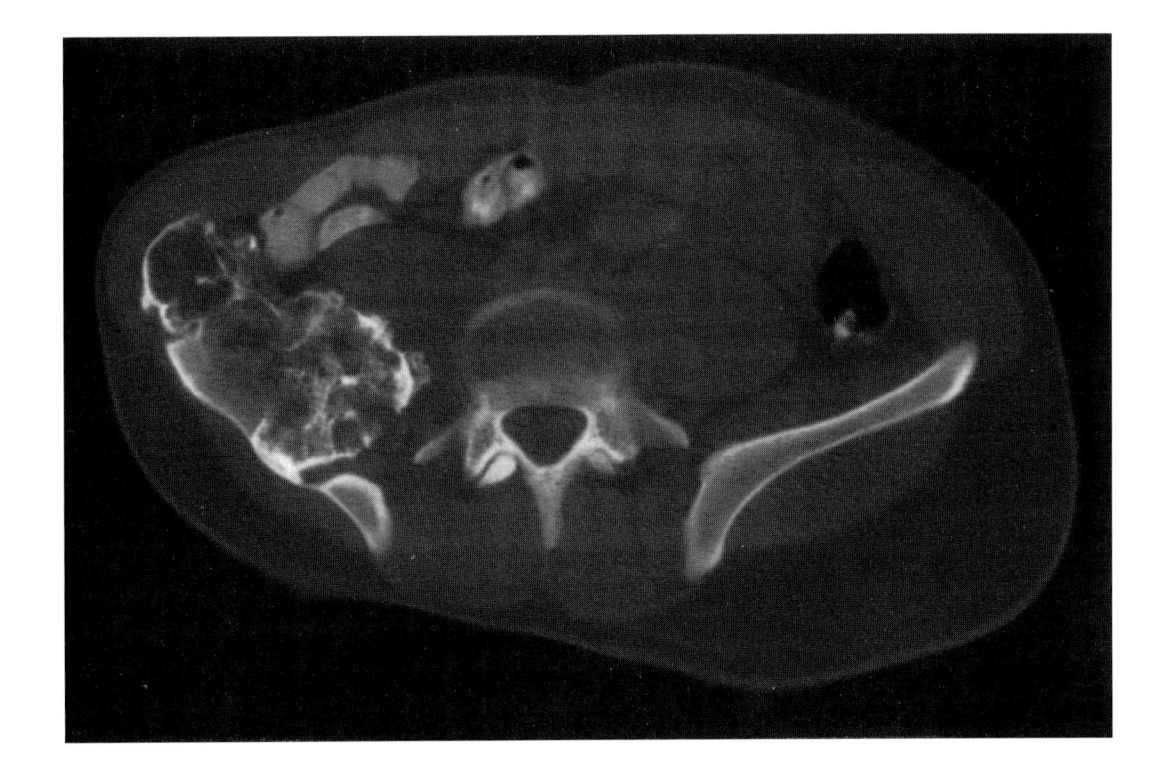

Figure 53–1 • A 36-year-old man presented with a chondrosarcoma of the iliac wing. This tumor arose in a giant benign osteochondroma that underwent malignant degeneration.

456 • Part V RADICAL AMPUTATIONS

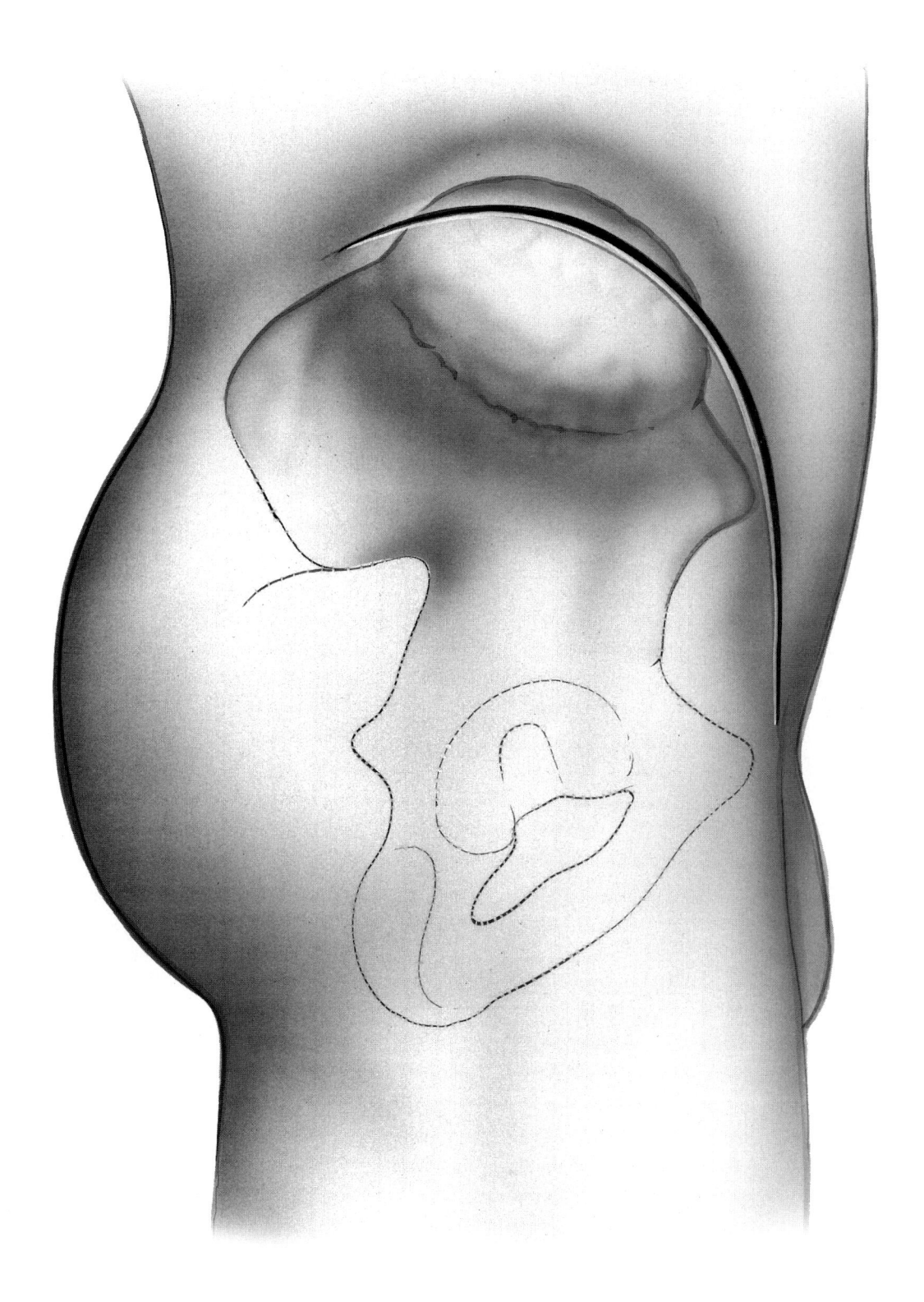

Figure 53–2 • An ilioinguinal incision was made in order to perform a Type I internal hemipelvectomy.

Clinical Case: Chondrosarcoma of the Iliac Wing • 457

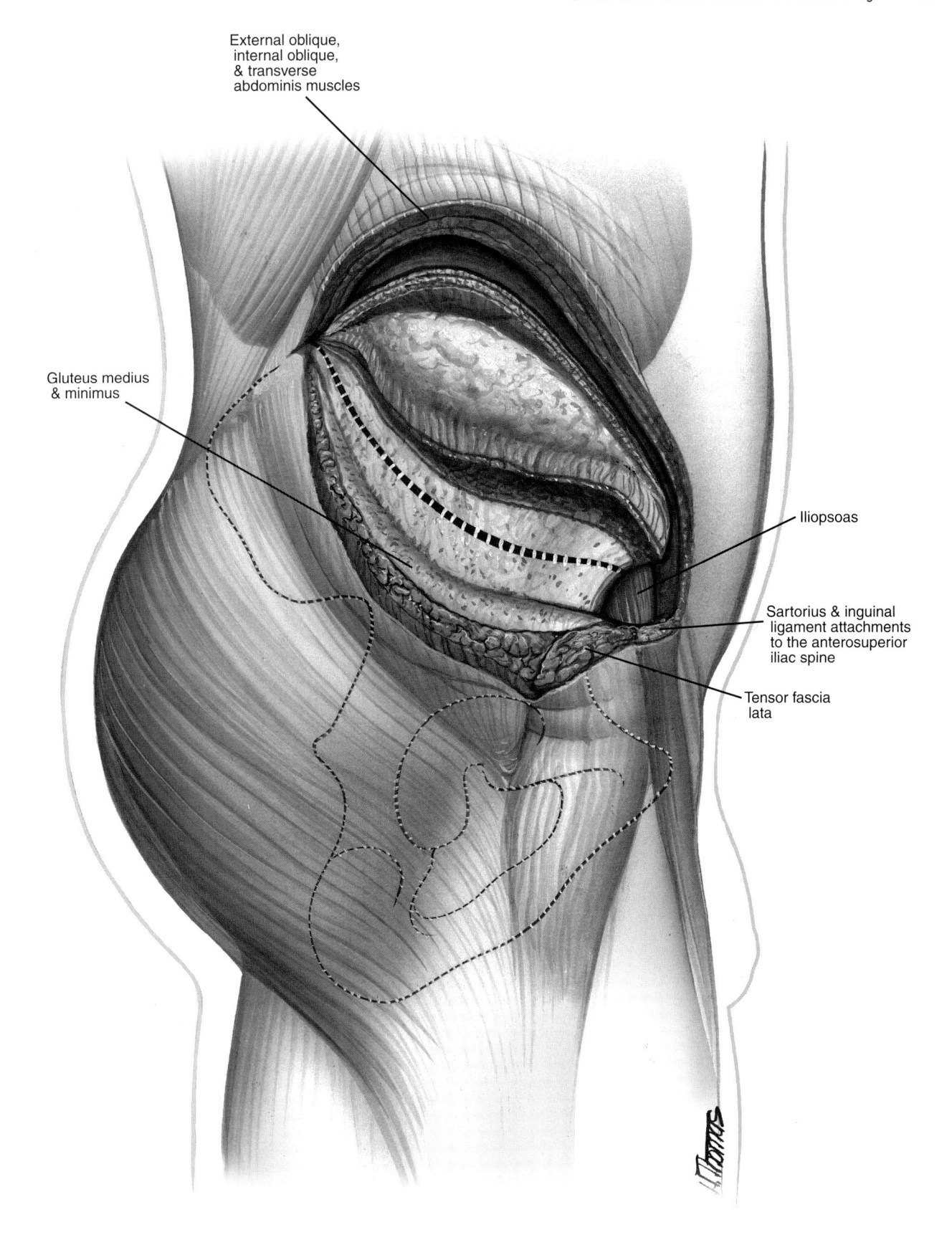

Figure 53–3 • Following entry into the retroperitoneal space, the peritoneal envelope is mobilized off the iliacus. Externally, the gluteal muscles are divided at the line of resection on the bony pelvis.

458 • Part V RADICAL AMPUTATIONS

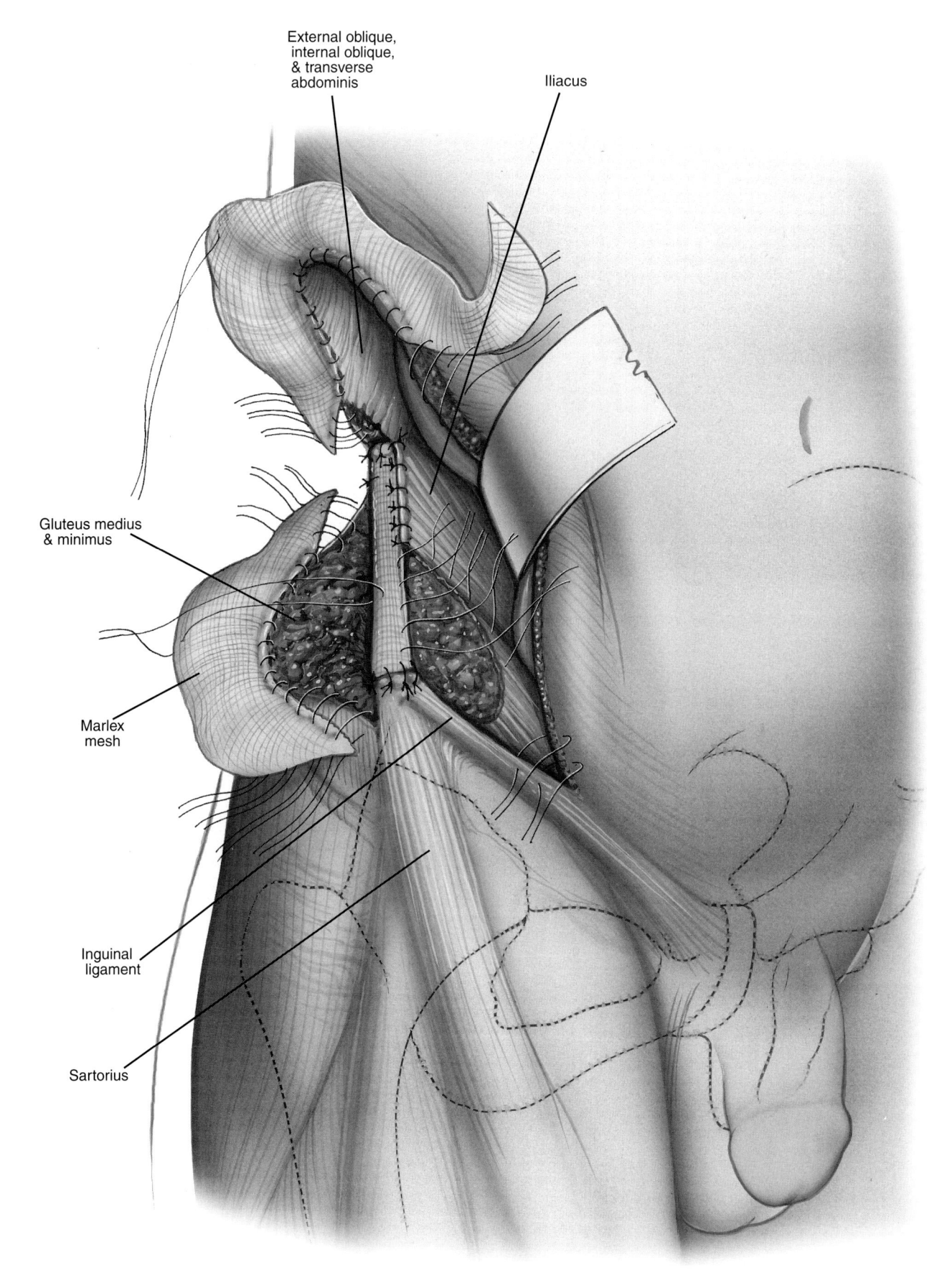

Figure 53-4 • Following the completed resection, Marlex mesh is used to reconstruct the defect.

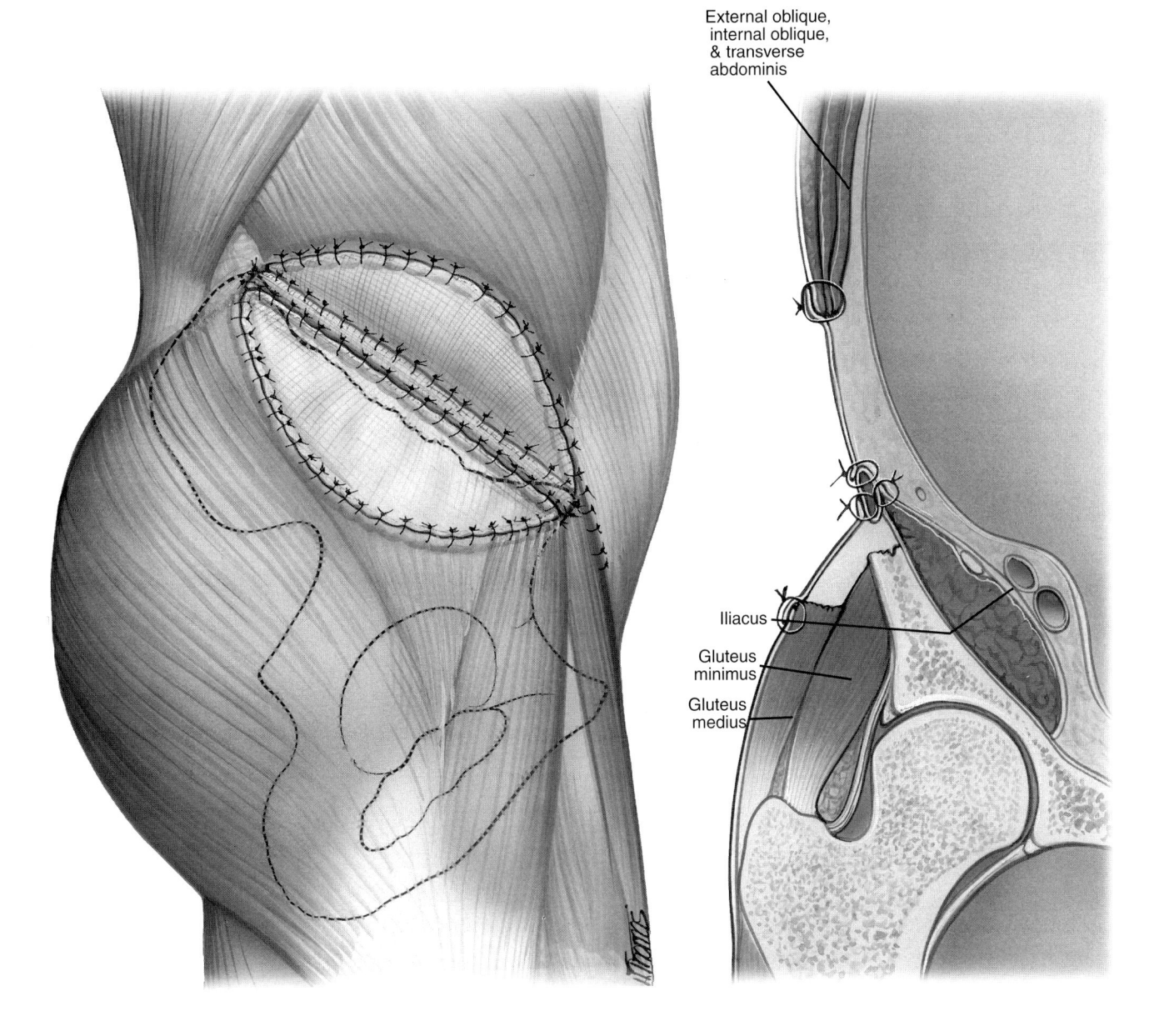

Figure 53–5 • The completed reconstruction shows the abdominal wall musculature and the gluteals reattached to an inguinal ligament fashioned of mesh and directly attached to the remaining bony pelvis.

Part VI

BREAST AND SOFT TISSUE TUMORS

Chapter 54
Surgical Anatomy of the Breast

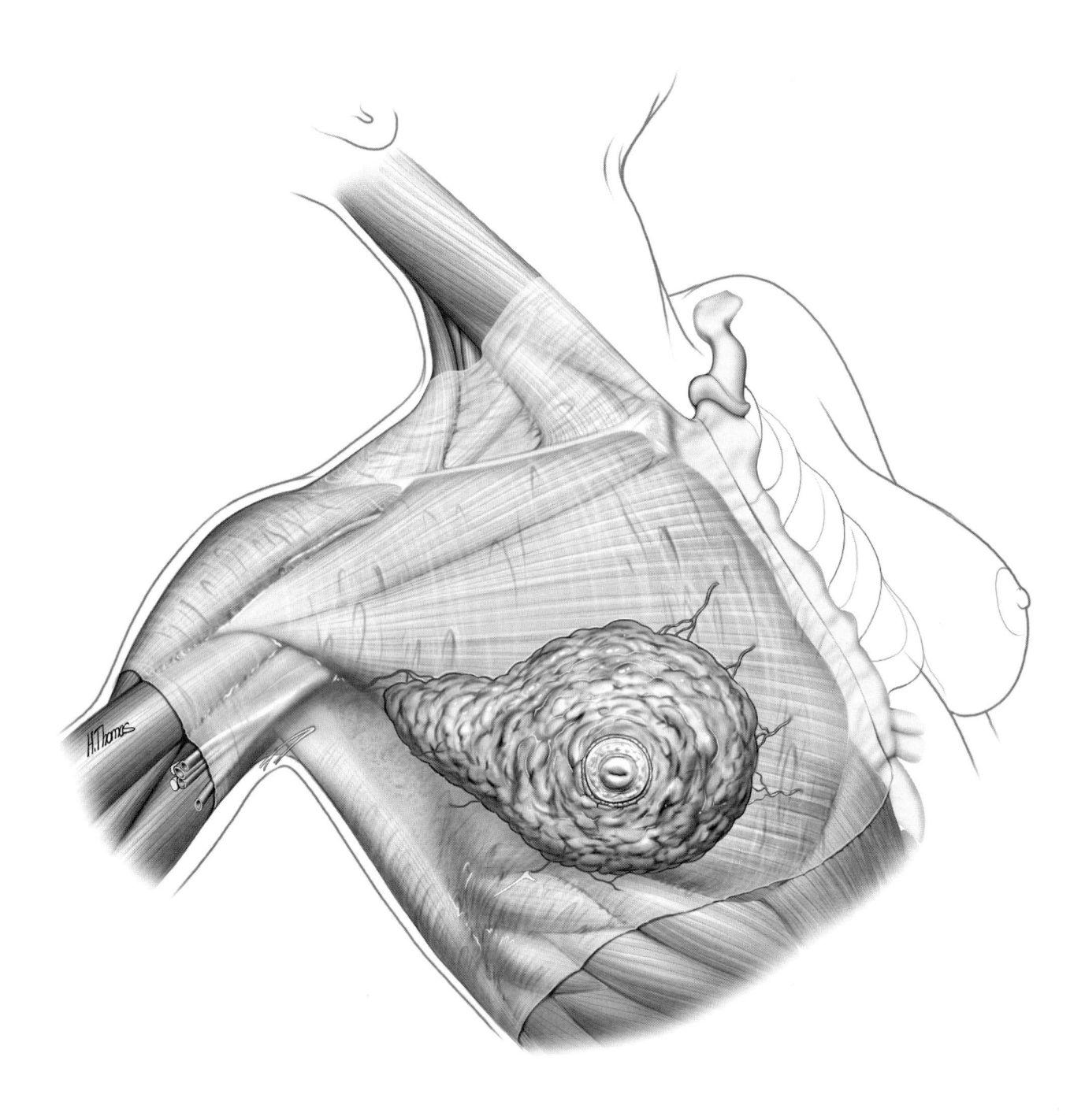

Figure 54–1 • The breast and associated underlying anatomy is depicted.

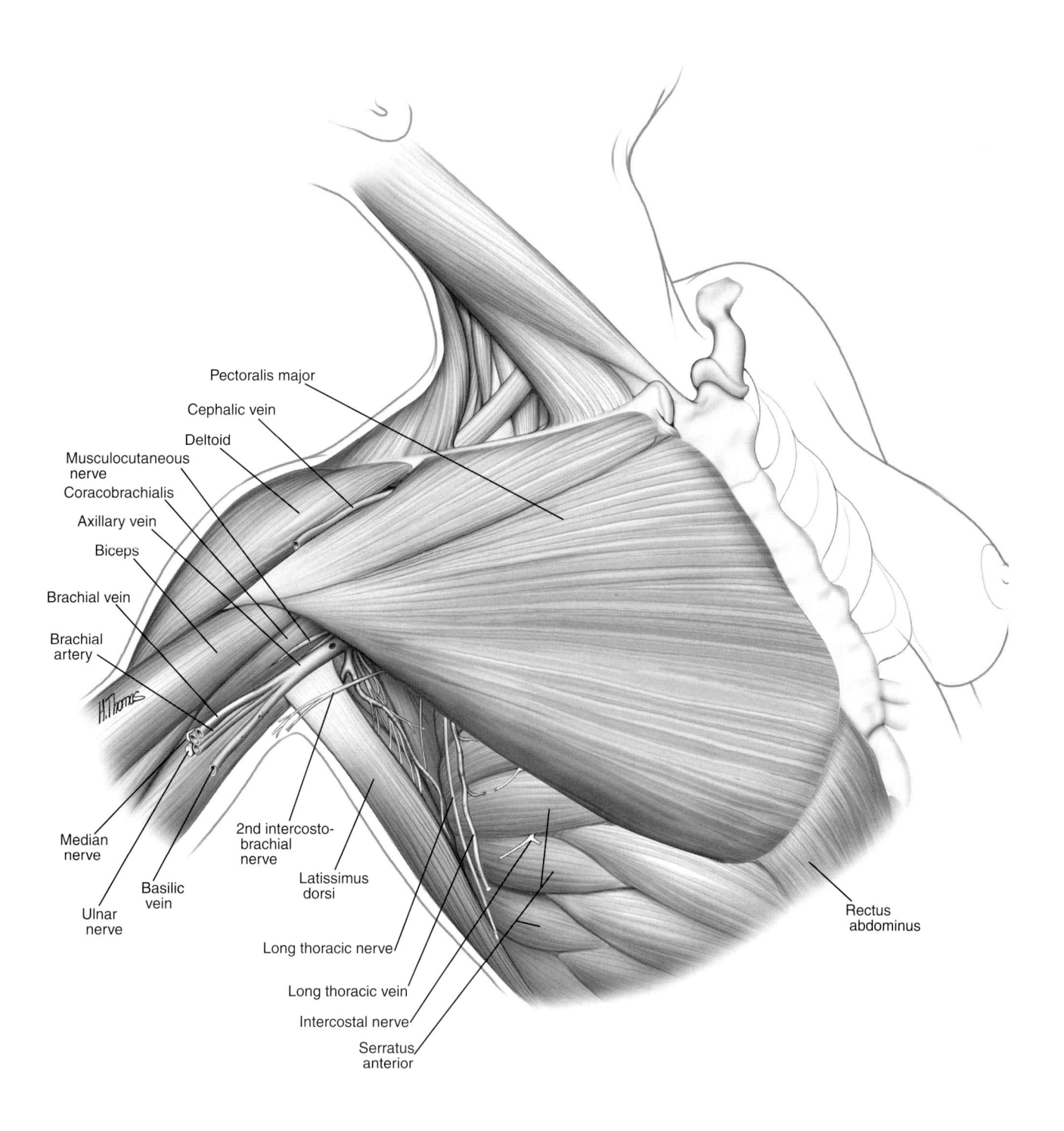

Figure 54–2 • With the skin and breast removed, the muscular anatomy is emphasized.

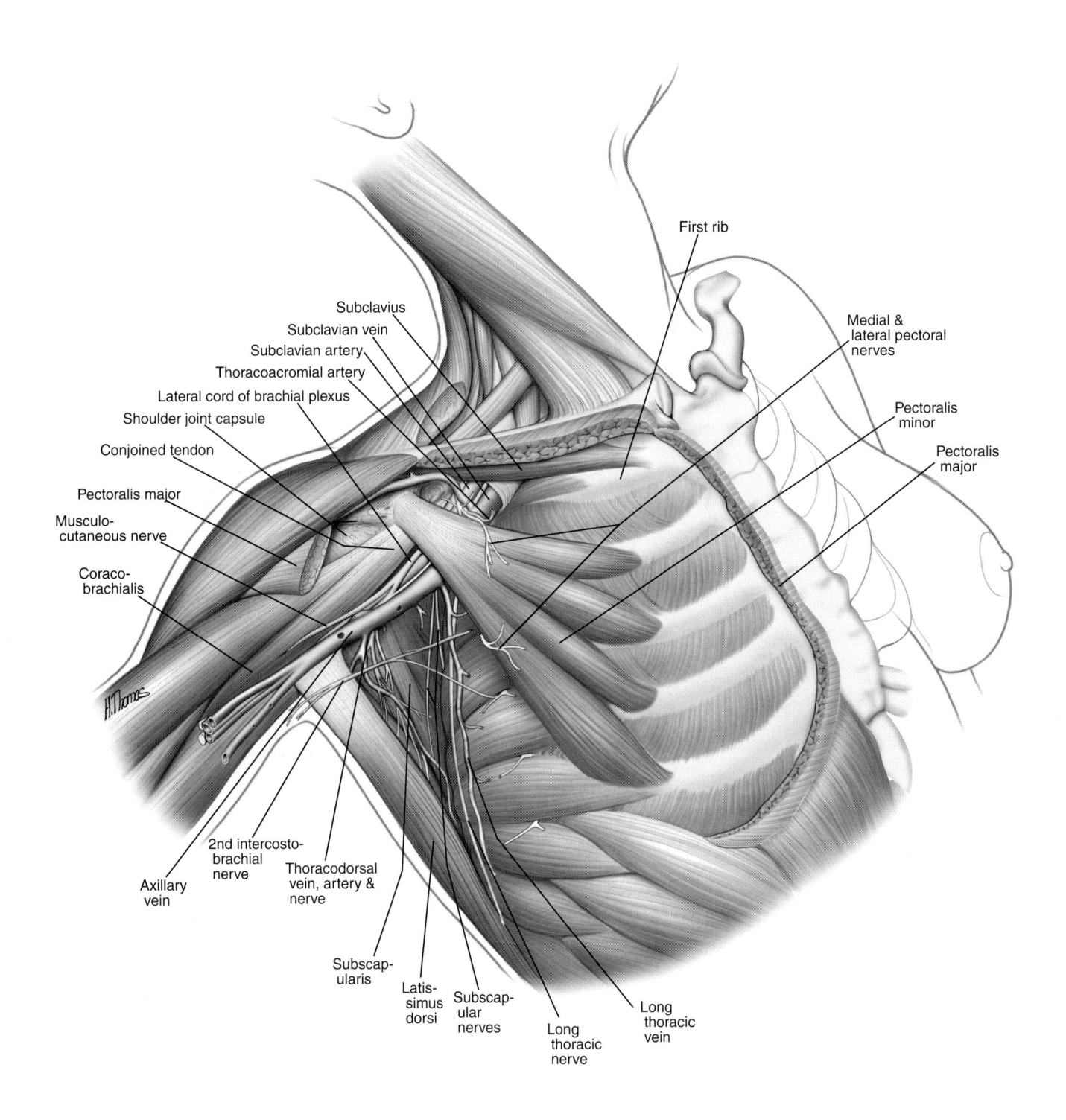

Figure 54–3 • The neurovascular anatomy of the axilla is depicted.

Chapter 55
Modified Radical Mastectomy

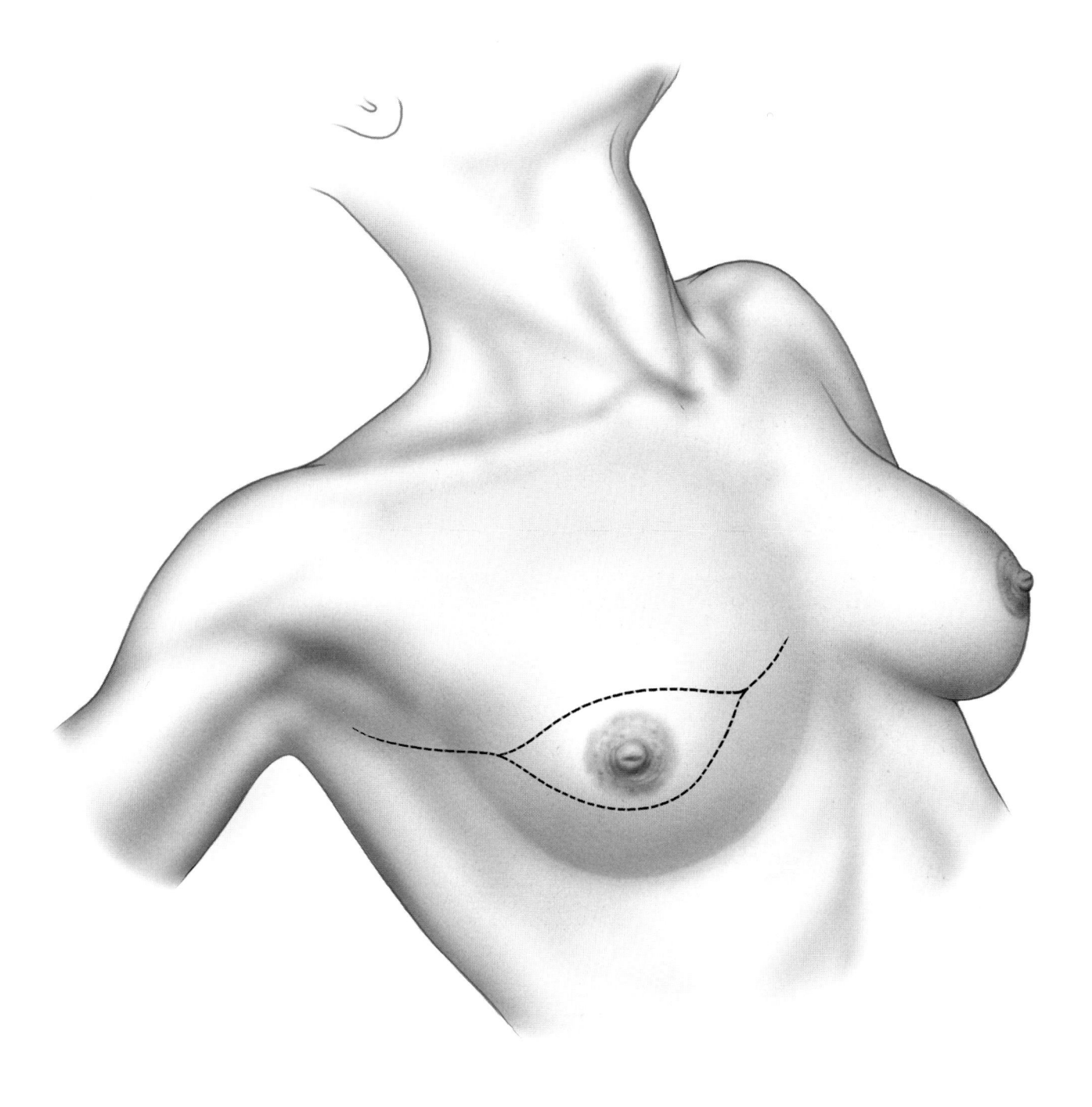

Figure 55–1 • A transverse incision allows for better reconstruction options. The size and exact location are dictated by tumor location and personal preference.

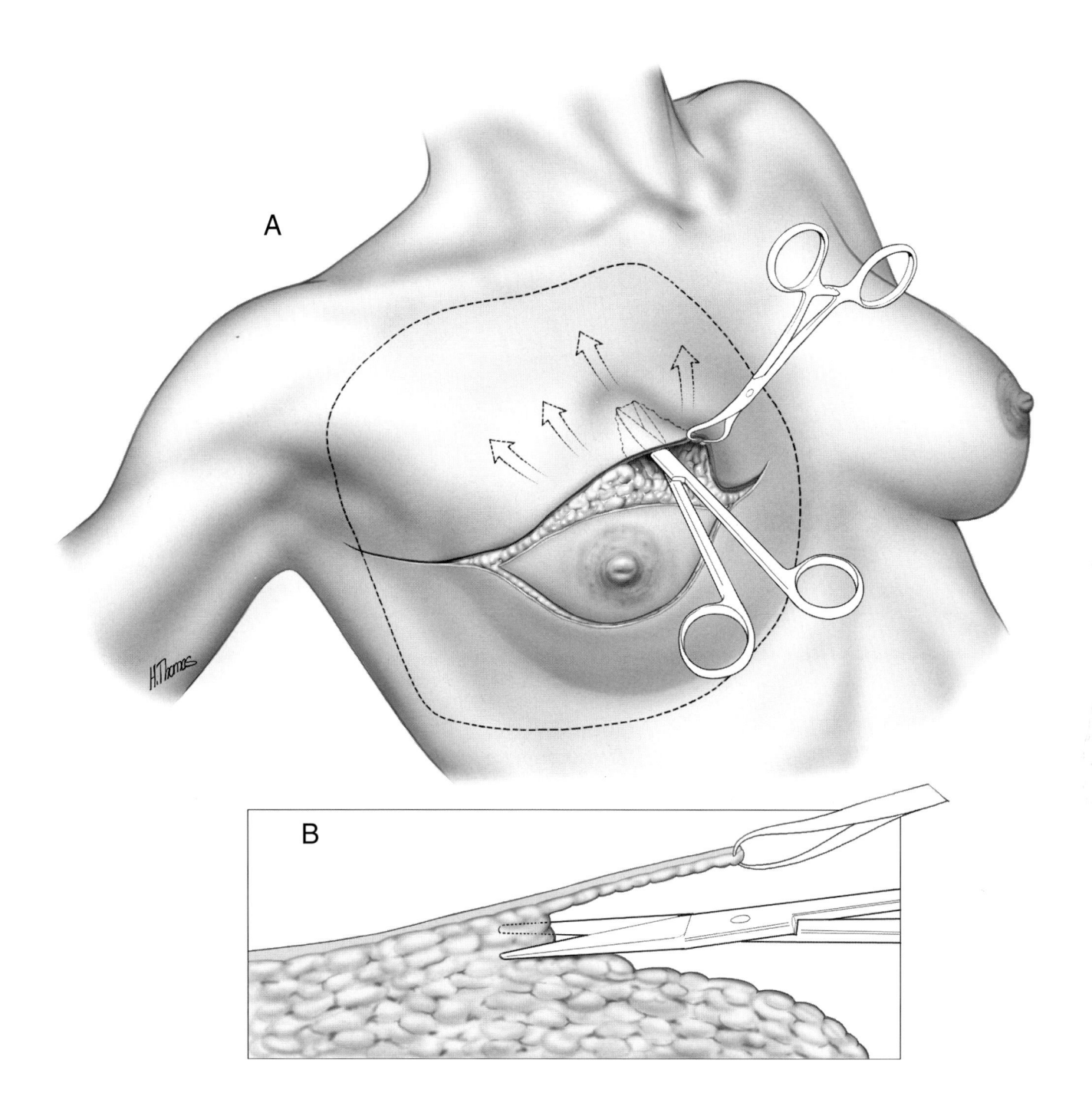

Figure 55–2 • **A,** Skin flaps are elevated to the indicated lines. Laterally there is no need to elevate the skin beyond the edge of the latissimus.

B, A technique for elevating the skin flaps utilizing a Metzenbaum scissors is illustrated.

Modified Radical Mastectomy • 467

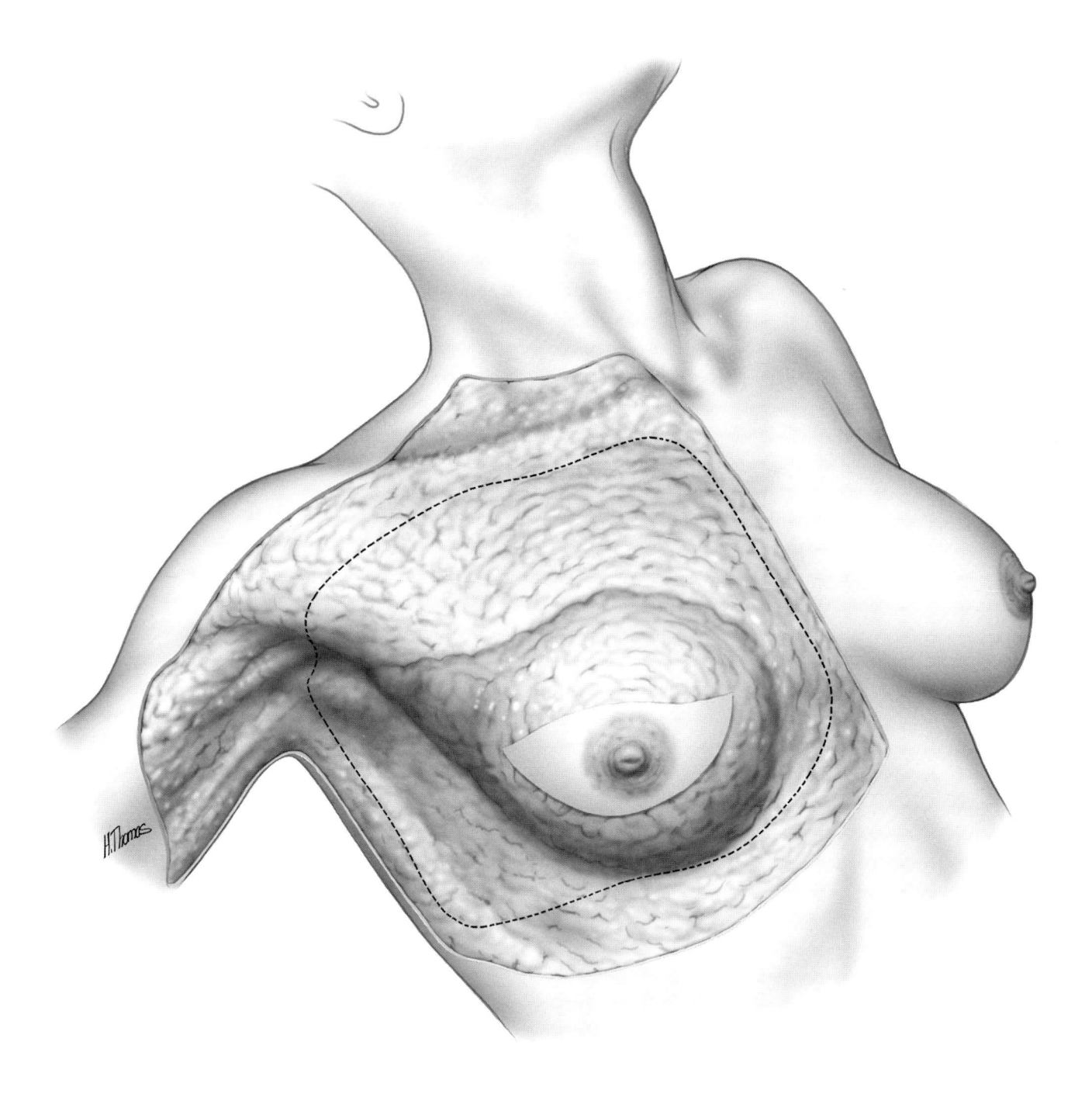

Figure 55–3 • The breast is depicted with the skin flaps removed rather than being retracted.

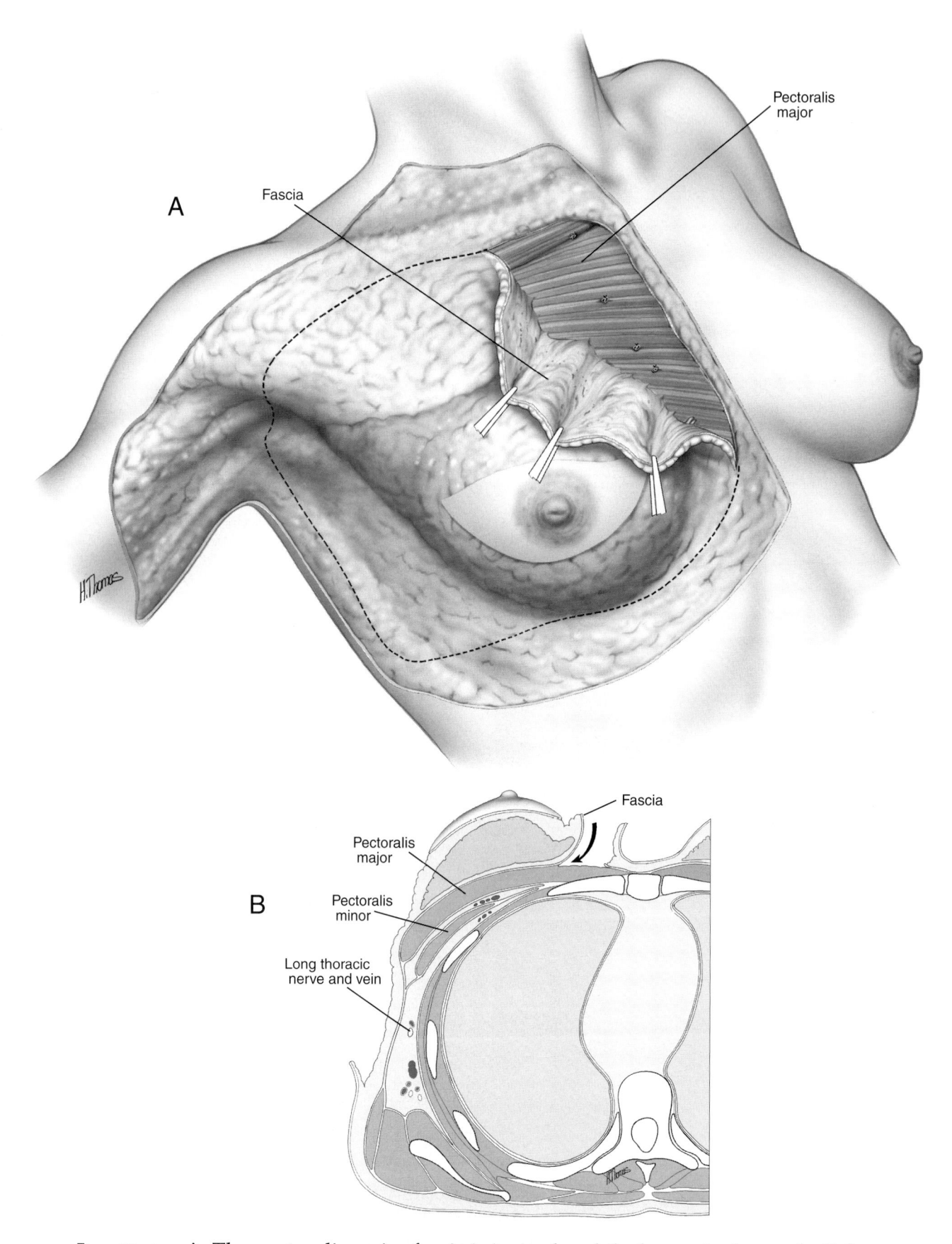

Figure 55–4 • **A,** The pectoralis major fascia is incised and the breast is elevated off the underlying muscle from anterior and medial to inferior and lateral. **B,** A cross-sectional view of the dissection.

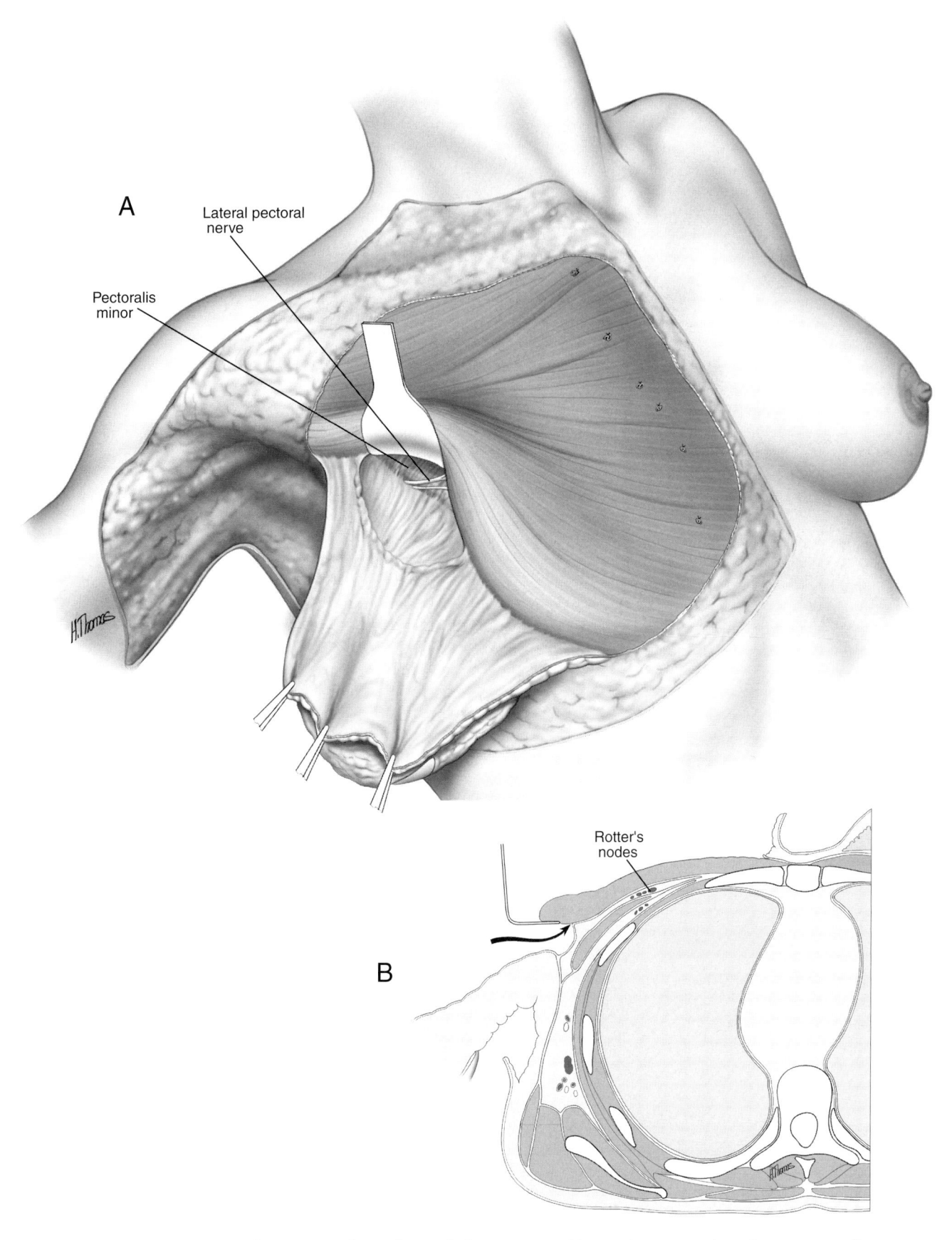

Figure 55–5 • **A,** By elevating the edge of the pectoralis major muscle, the pectoralis minor fascia can be removed in continuity along with Rotter's nodes (*B*). **B,** A cross-sectional view of the dissection.

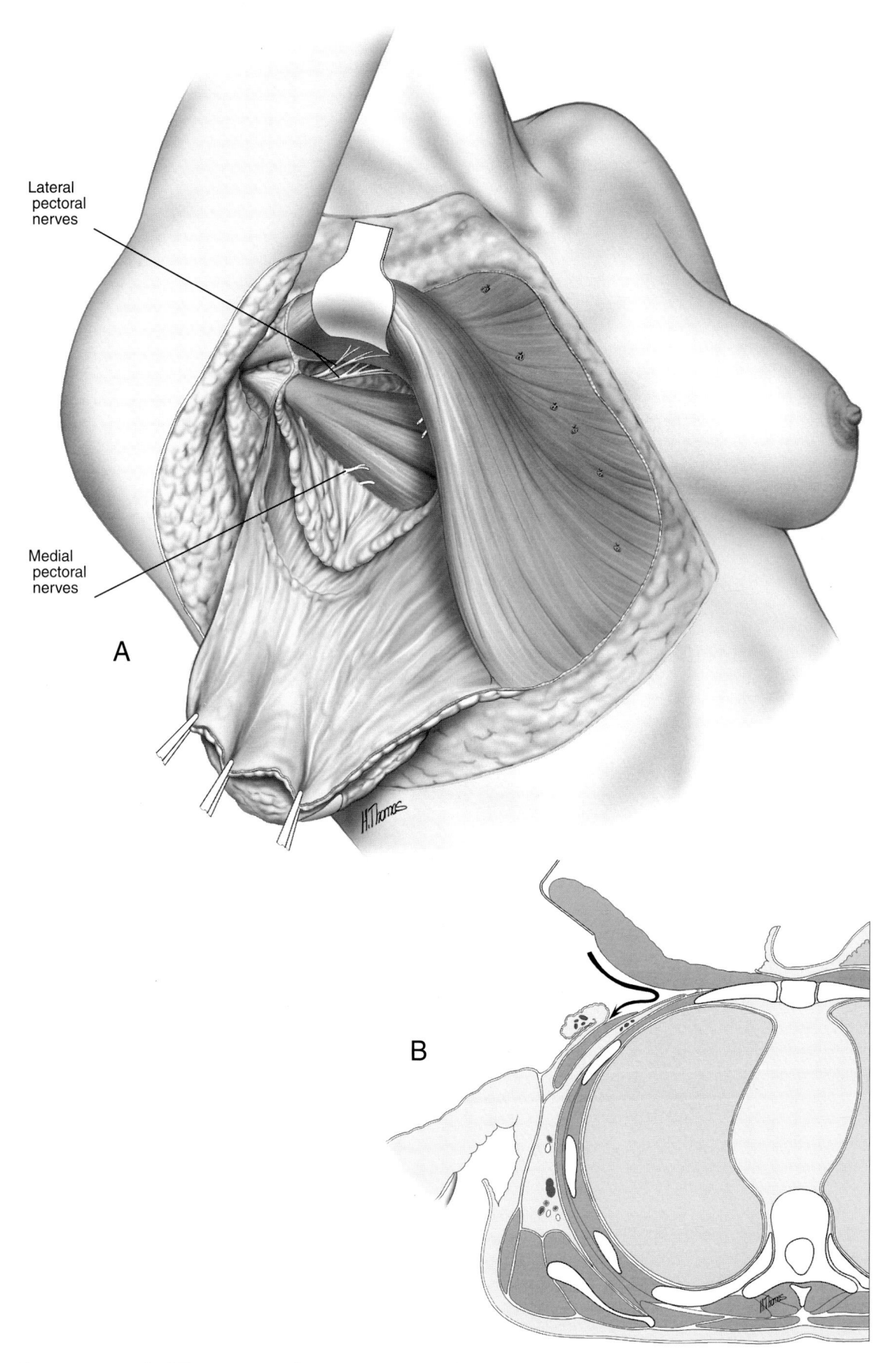

Figure 55–6 • **A,** The pectoralis minor muscle can be preserved. The medial pectoral nerve can be divided to facilitate elevation of the muscle.
B, A cross-sectional view defines the planes of dissection clearly.

470

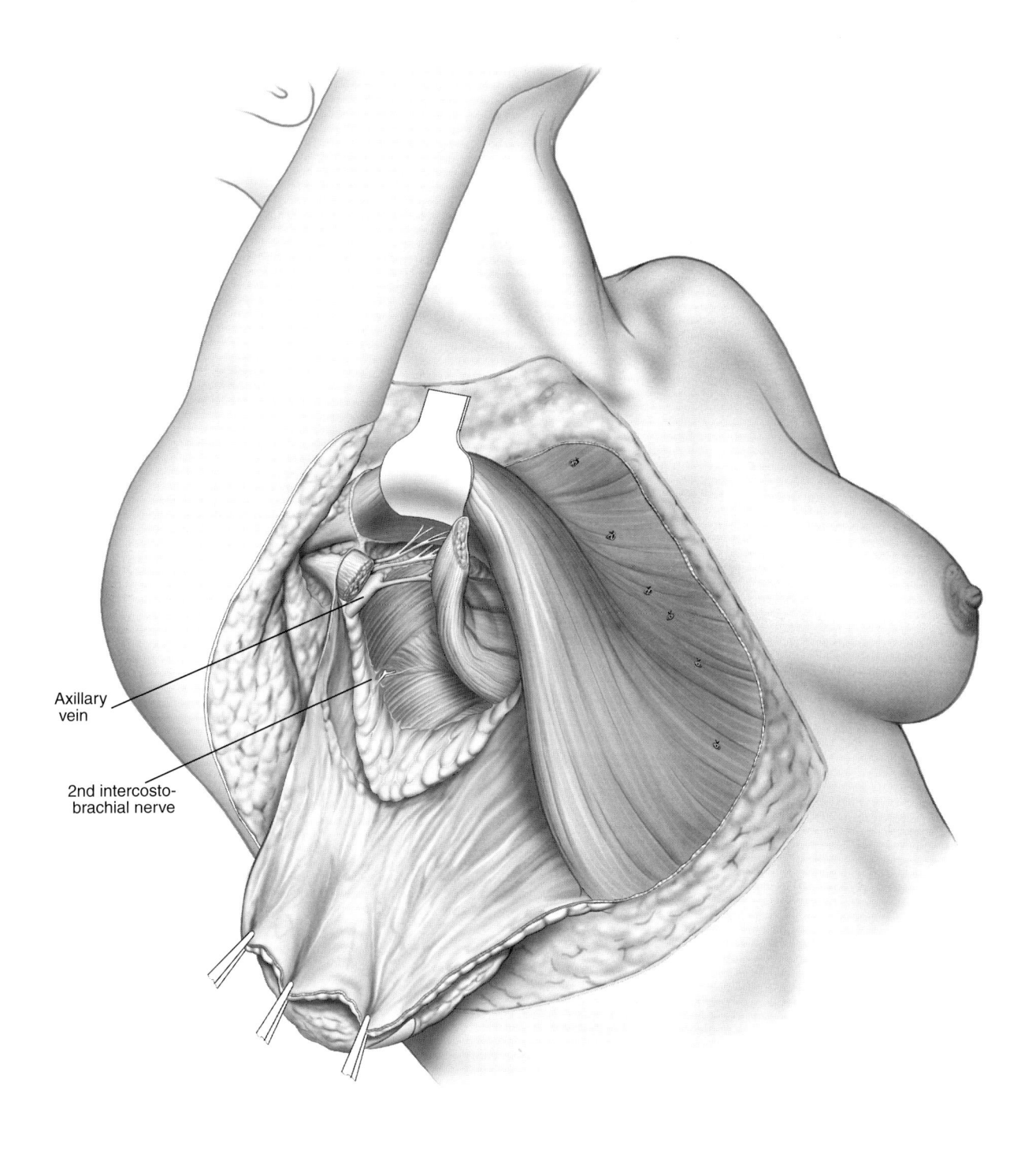

Figure 55–7 • Another option is to divide the pectoralis minor at its insertion and reattach it after completion of the axillary dissection. The 2nd intercostobrachial nerve is identified.

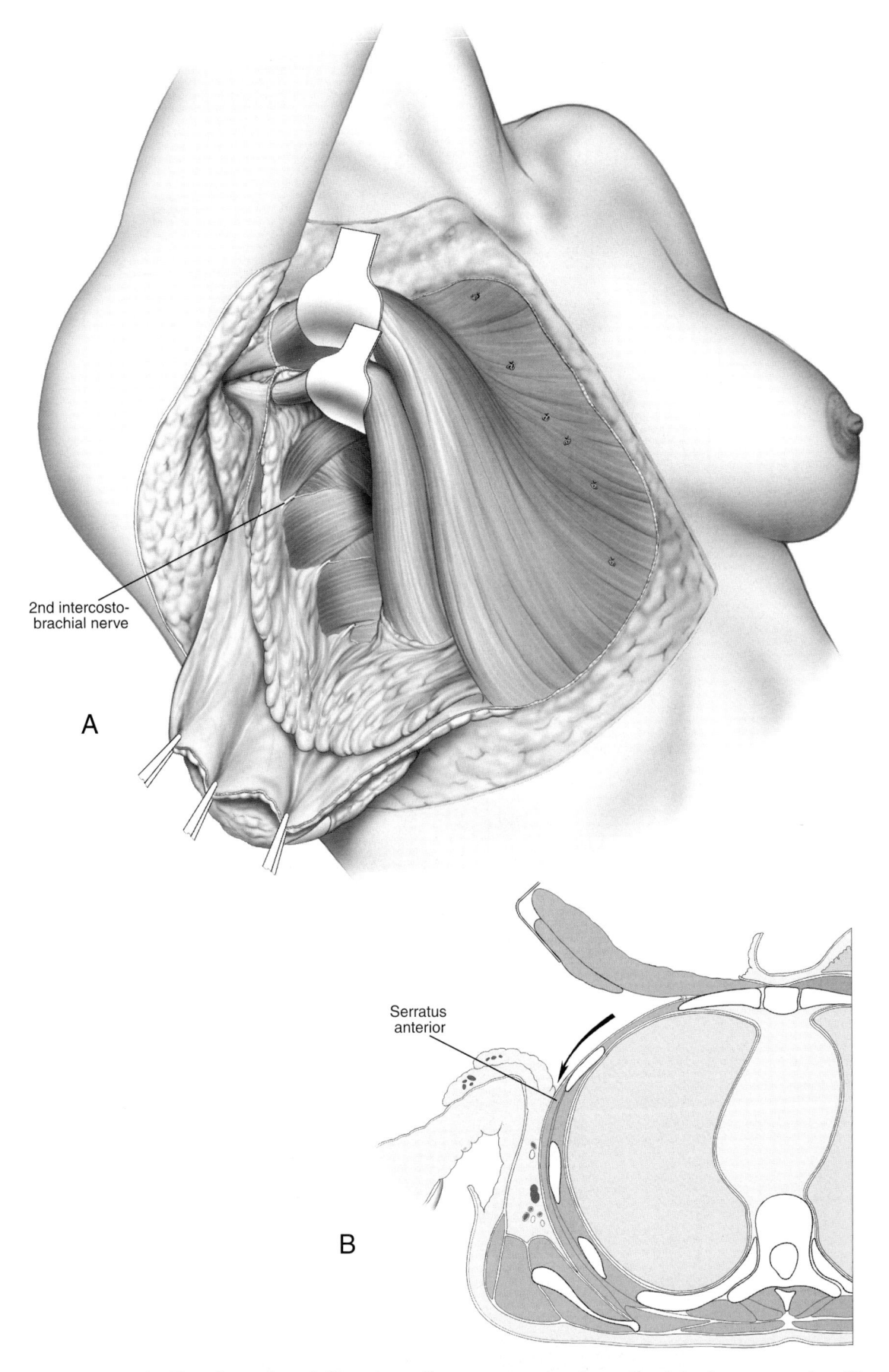

Figure 55–8 • **A,** Continued mobilization allows access to the tail of the breast and axilla. **B,** Once again, a cross-sectional view highlights the plane of dissection.

Modified Radical Mastectomy • 473

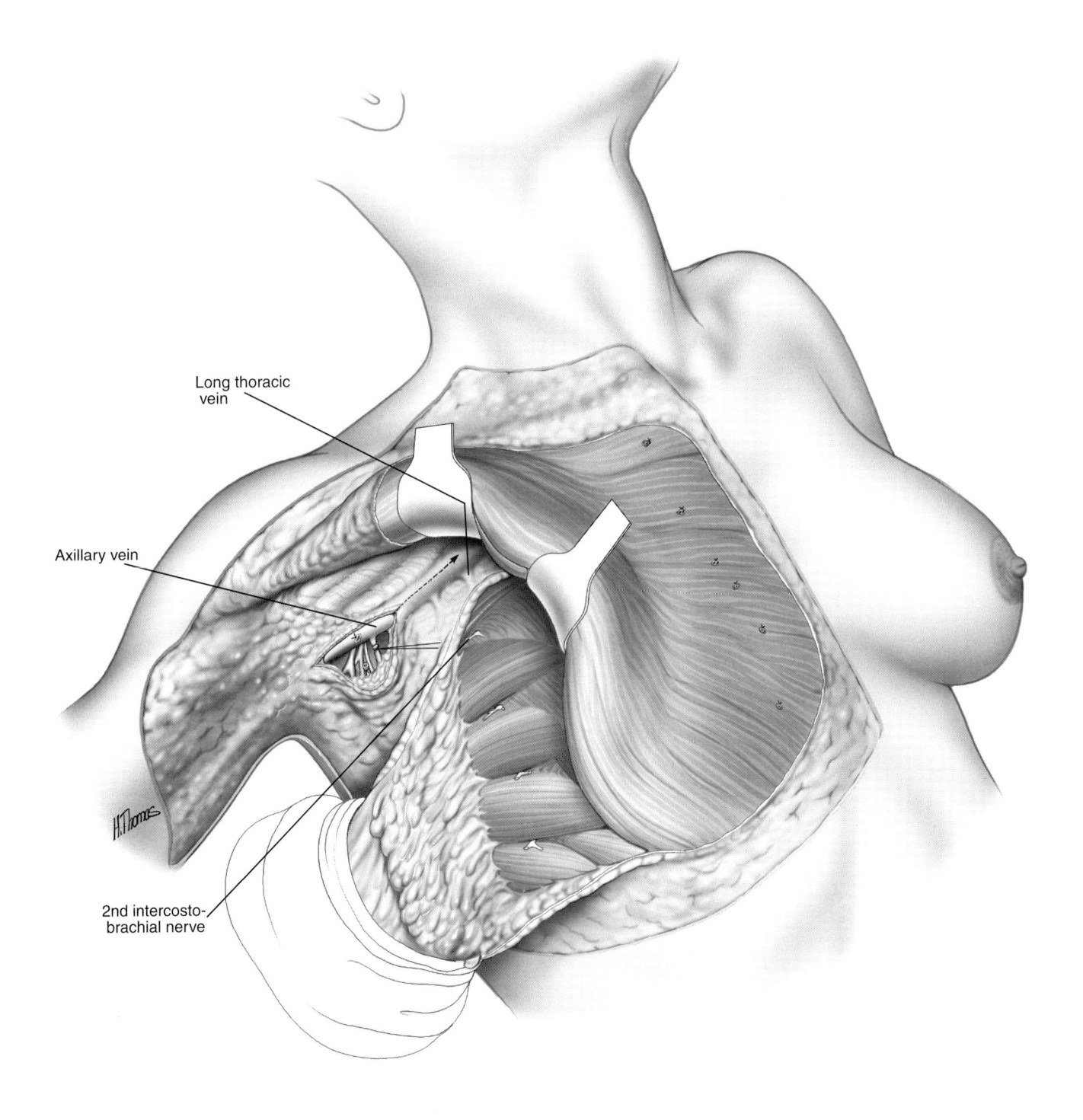

Figure 55-9 • Continued dissection along the chest wall involves dividing the 2nd intercostobrachial nerve. The superior extent of the axillary dissection is defined by dividing the clavipectoral fascia and exposing the vein.

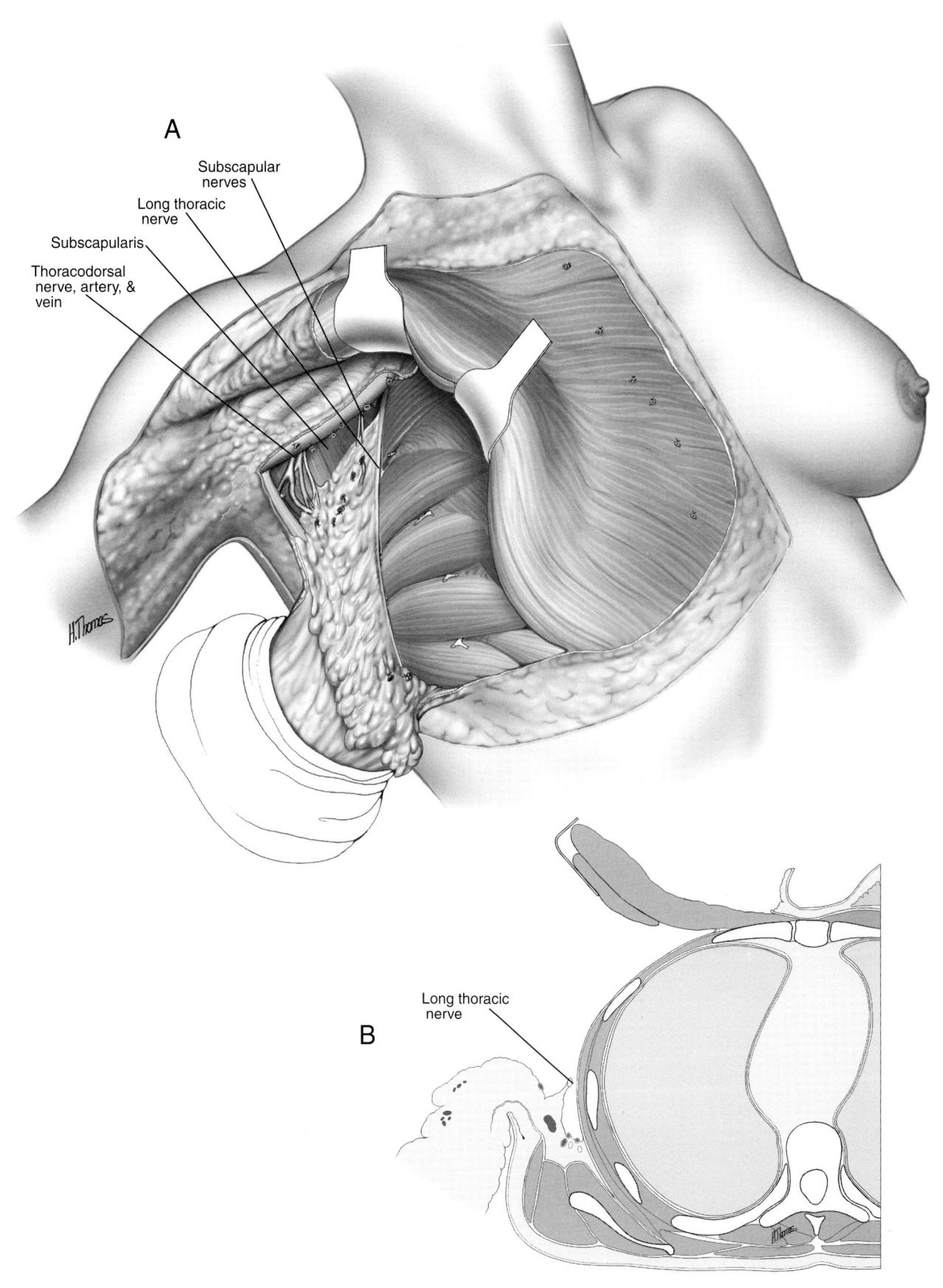

Figure 55–10 • **A,** The thoracodorsal nerve, artery, and vein define the lateral extent of the axillary dissection. The long thoracic nerve defines the medial extent. The latter is identified in the fat of the subscapular space as the entire package is dissected off the chest wall.

B, A cross-sectional view of the dissection.

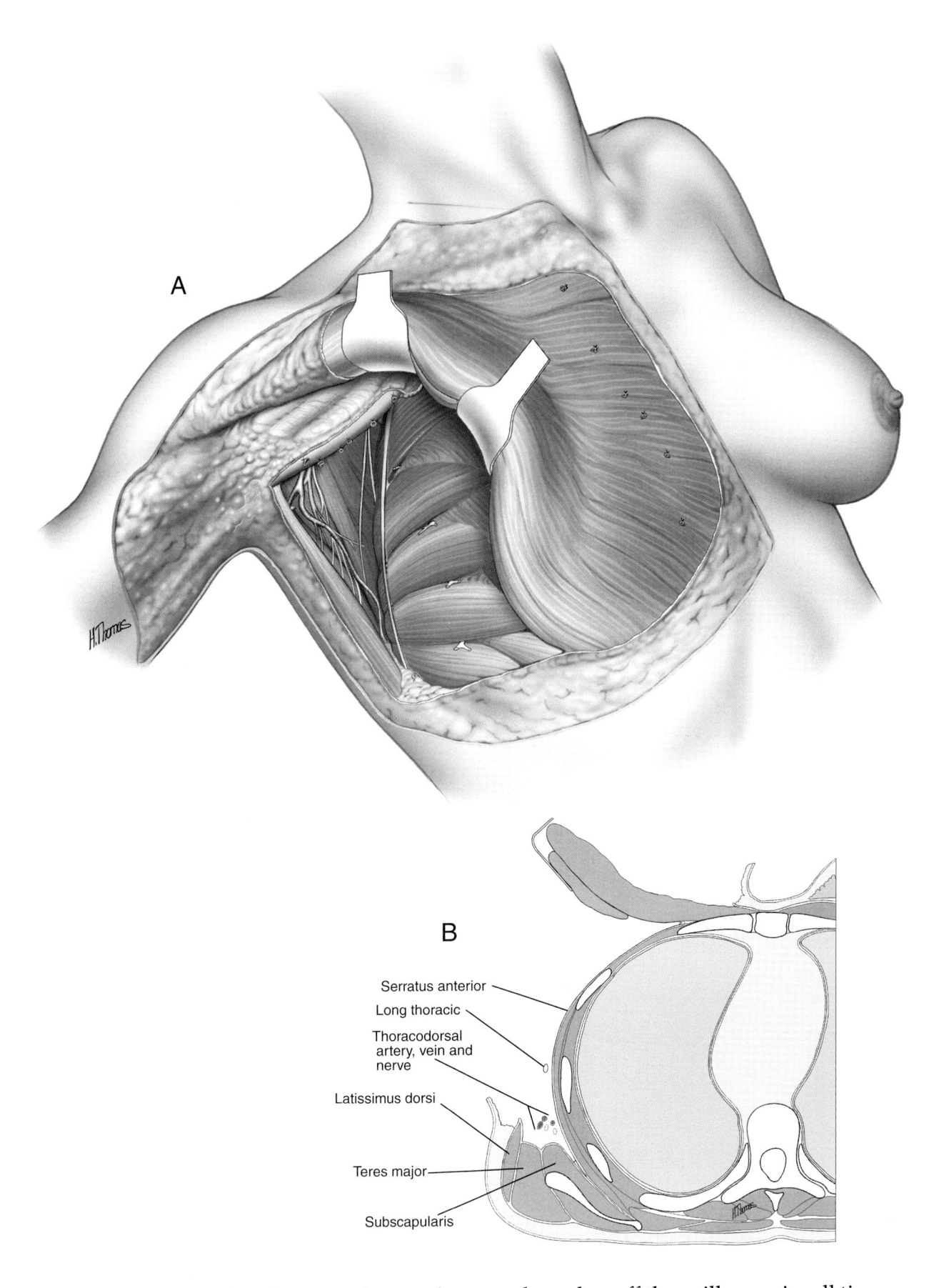

Figure 55–11 • **A,** After division of several venous branches off the axillary vein, all tissue occupying the subscapular space between the thoracodorsal nerve and long thoracic nerve is removed.

B, A cross-sectional view of the dissection.

Chapter 56
Radical Mastectomy

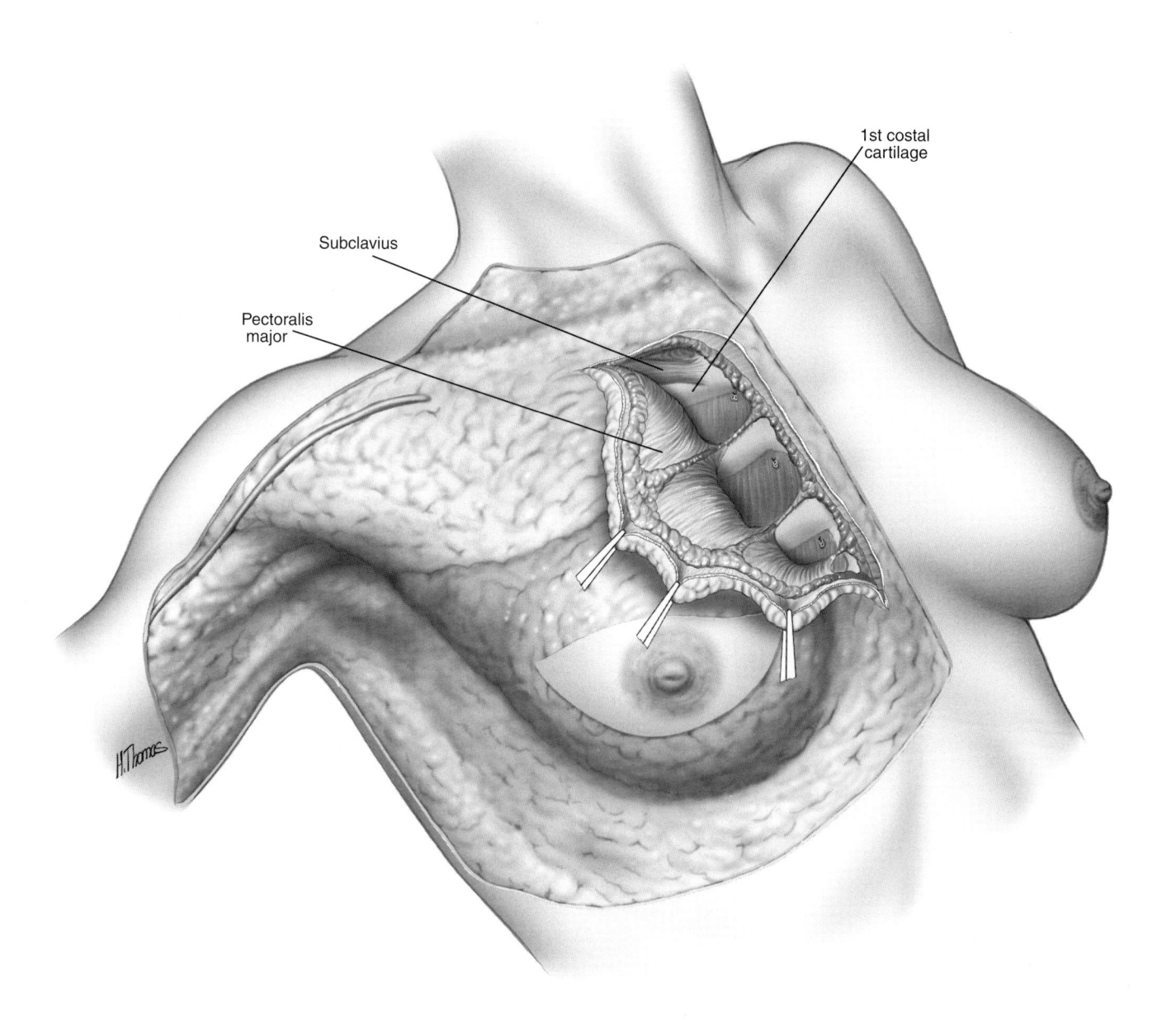

Figure 56–1 • Although the radical mastectomy is seldom performed, nonetheless it is indicated in selected cases. Removal of both the pectoralis major and minor muscles makes the axillary dissection easier to perform and more complete. After elevation of the skin flaps, the pectoralis major muscle origins are taken off the chest wall medially.

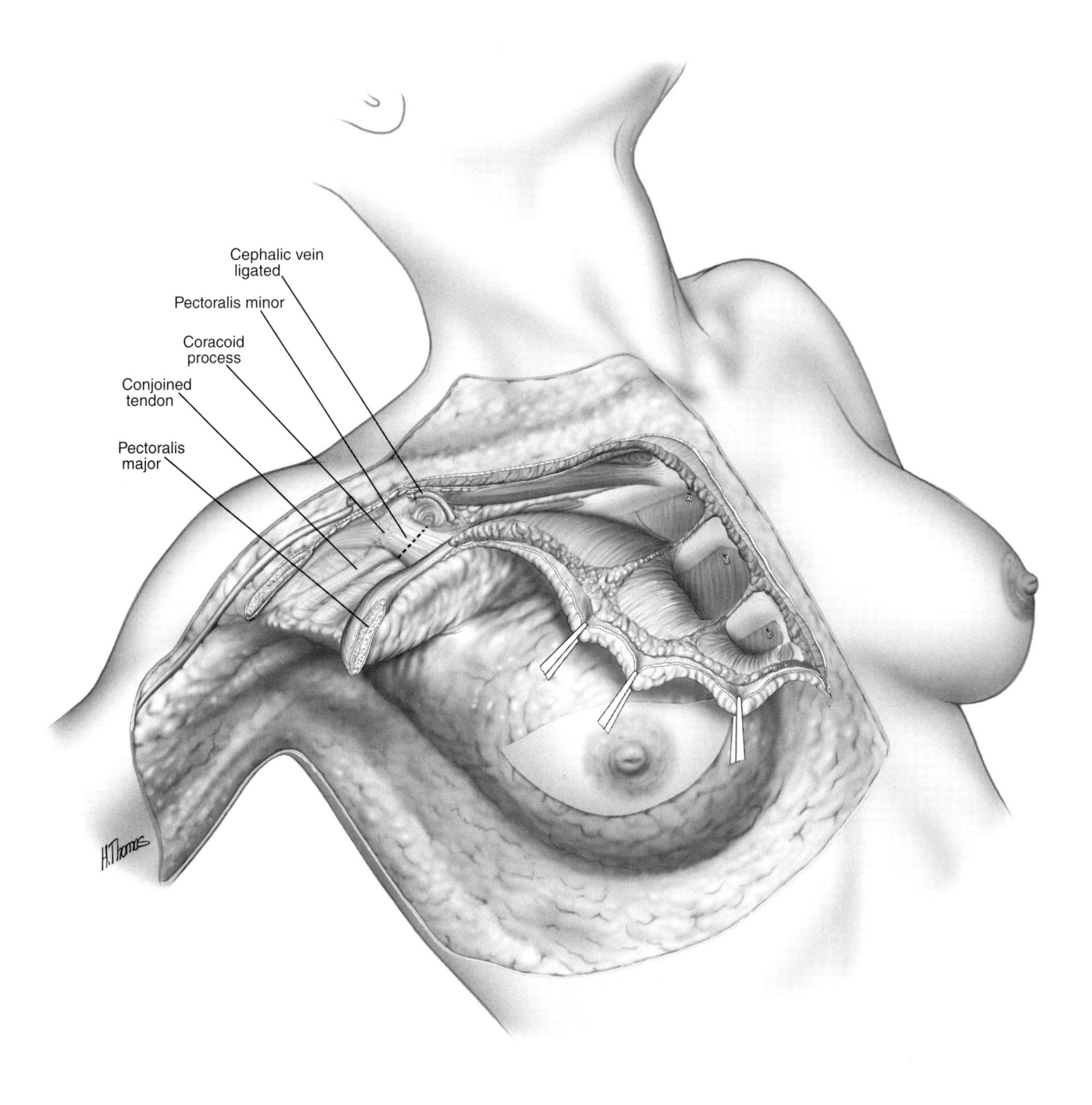

Figure 56–2 • The transverse fibers of the pectoralis major are divided from medial to lateral and the insertion of the muscle on the head of the humerus is divided. The head of the pectoralis minor is divided close to the coracoid process of the scapular.

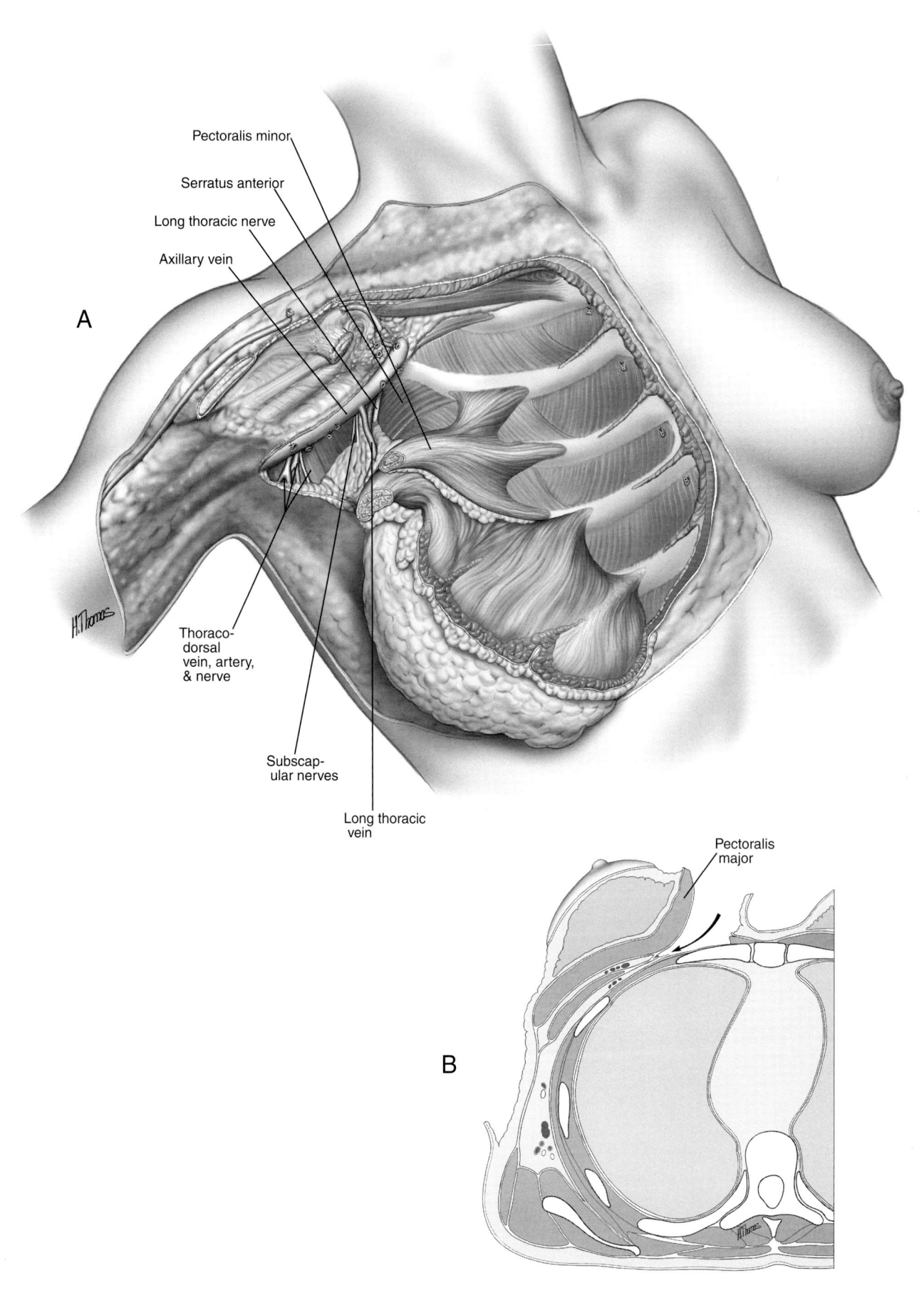

Figure 56–3 • **A,** The medial origins of the pectoralis minor are divided.
B, A cross-sectional view is depicted.

Radical Mastectomy • 479

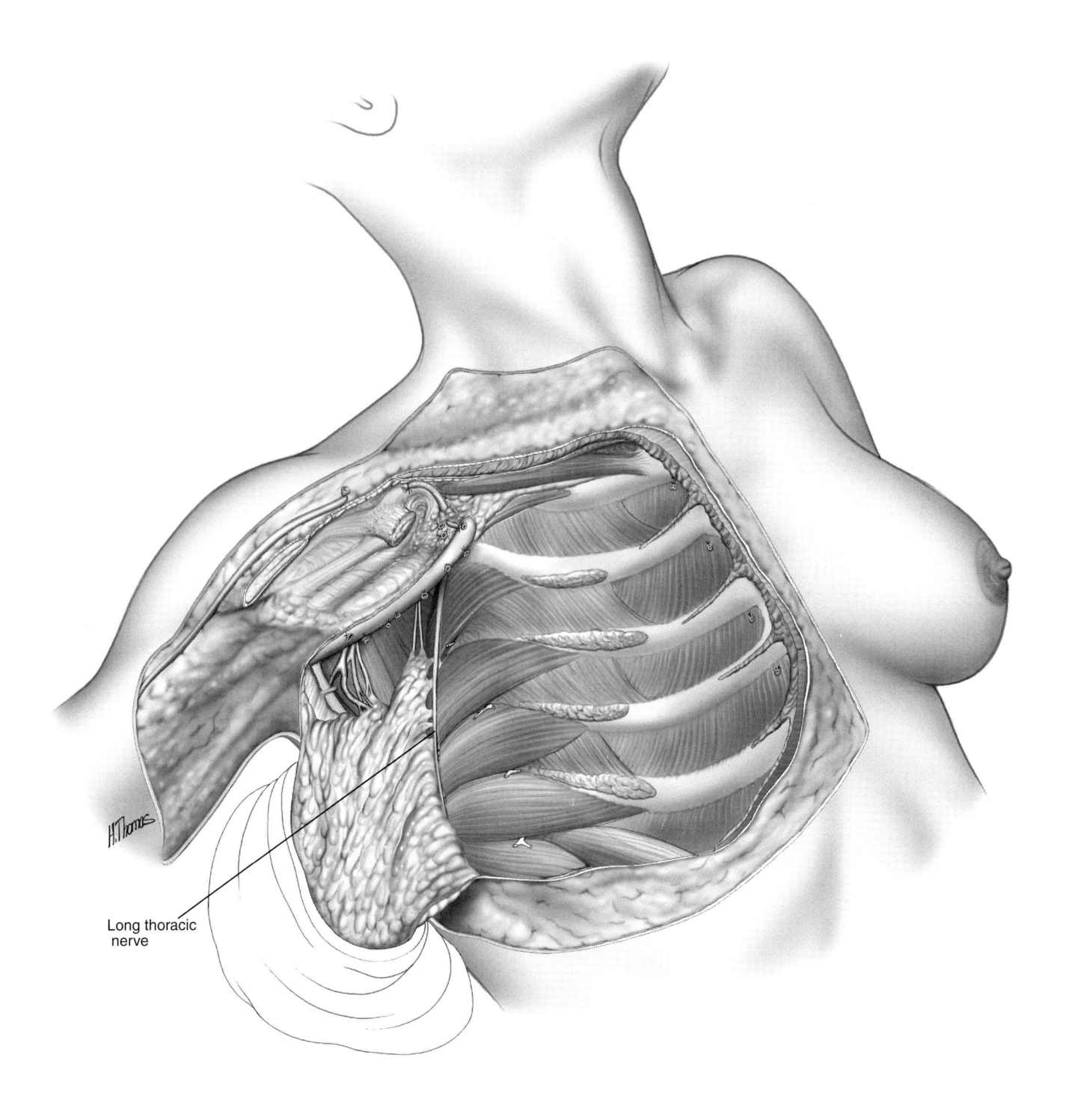

Figure 56–4 • The clavipectoral fascia is incised as described previously and the axillary dissection is completed.

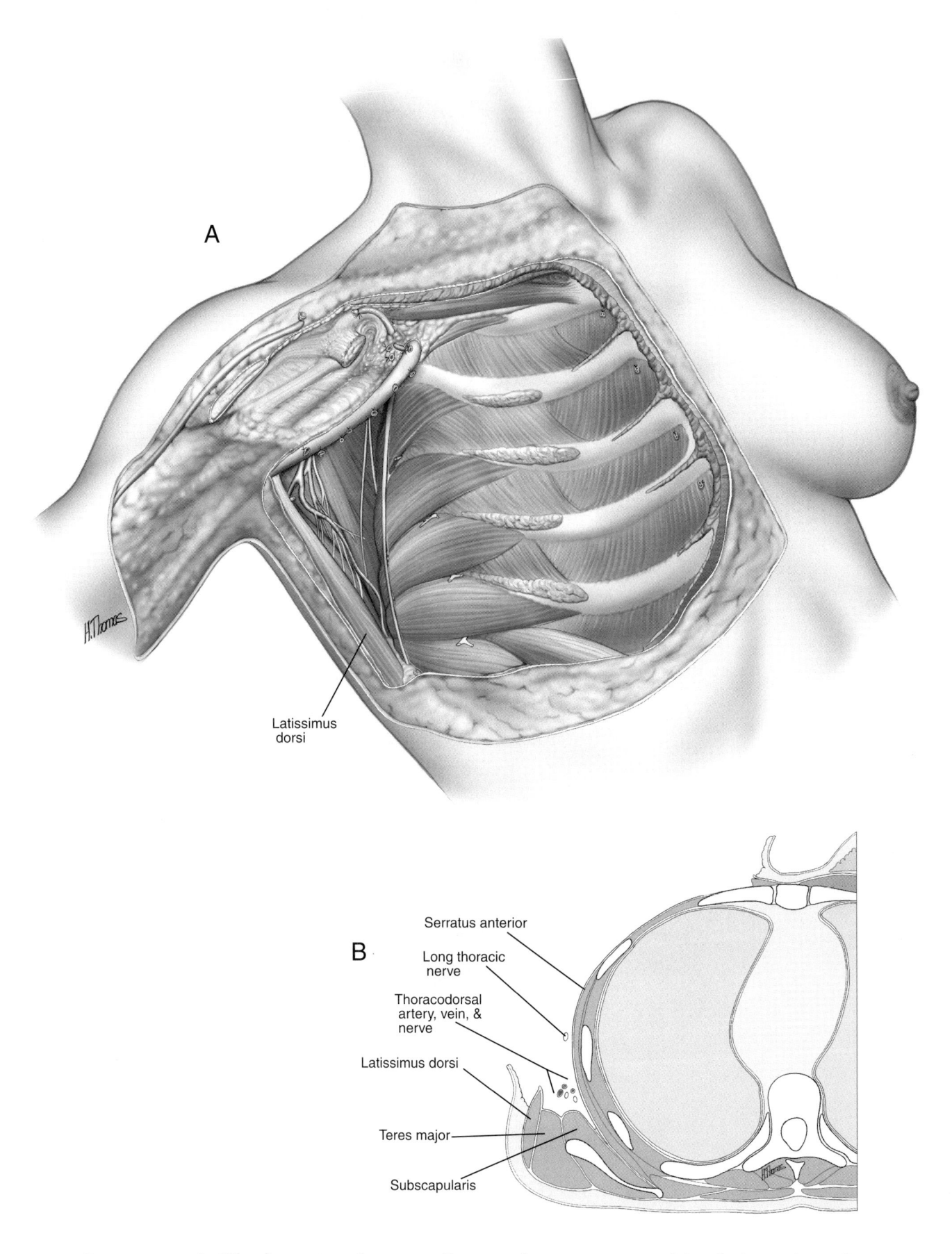

Figure 56–5 • **A,** The breast and pectoralis muscles are removed in their entirety by skeletonizing the edge of the latissimus dorsi from inferior to superior and exposing the serratus anterior.

B, A cross-sectional view is depicted.

480

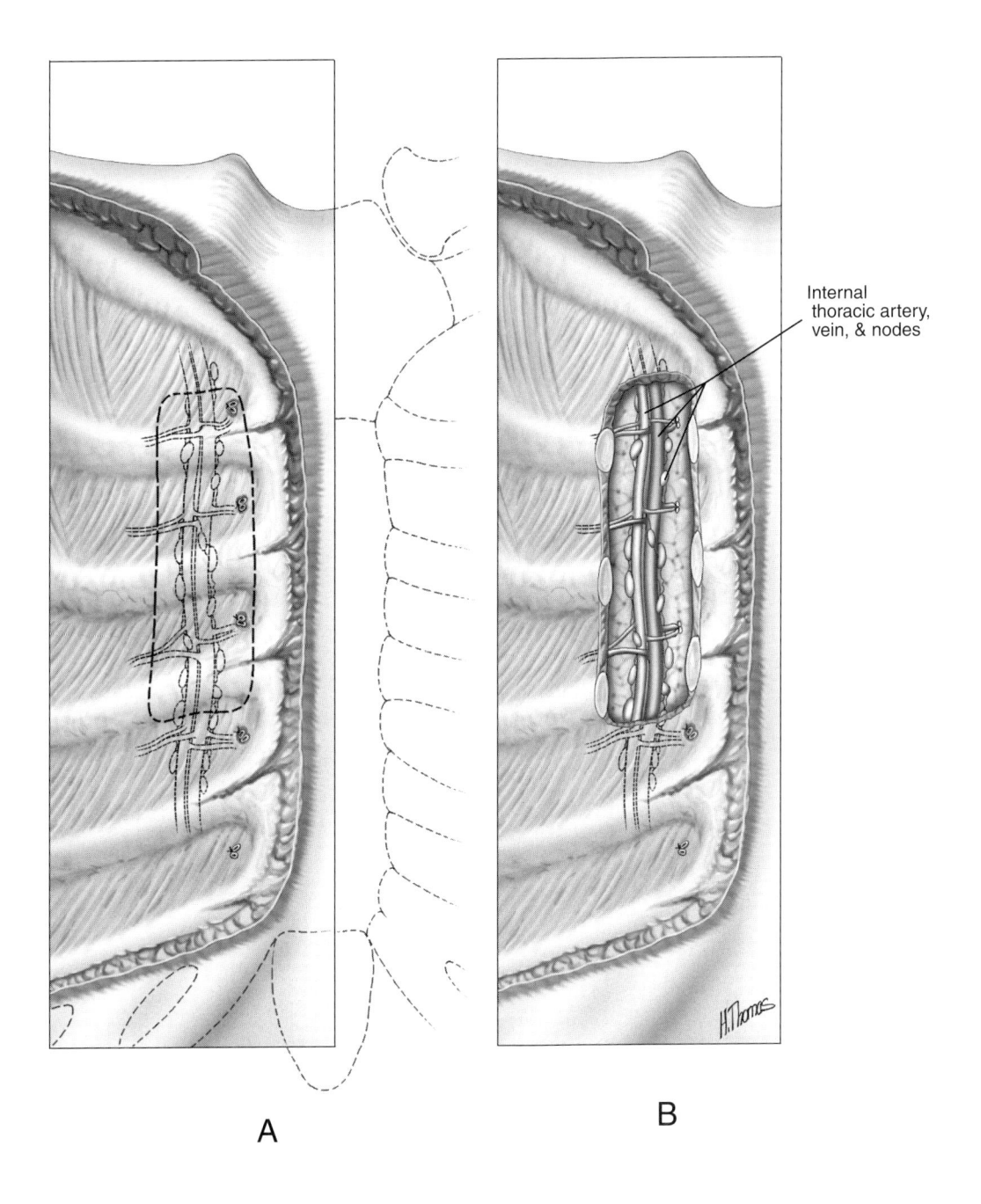

Figure 56–6 • **A,** An internal mammary node sampling is performed by removing the cartilaginous insertions of the second, third, and fourth ribs.
B, The nodes are associated with the internal mammary artery and vein and are removed en bloc.

Chapter 57
Surgical Anatomy of the Groin

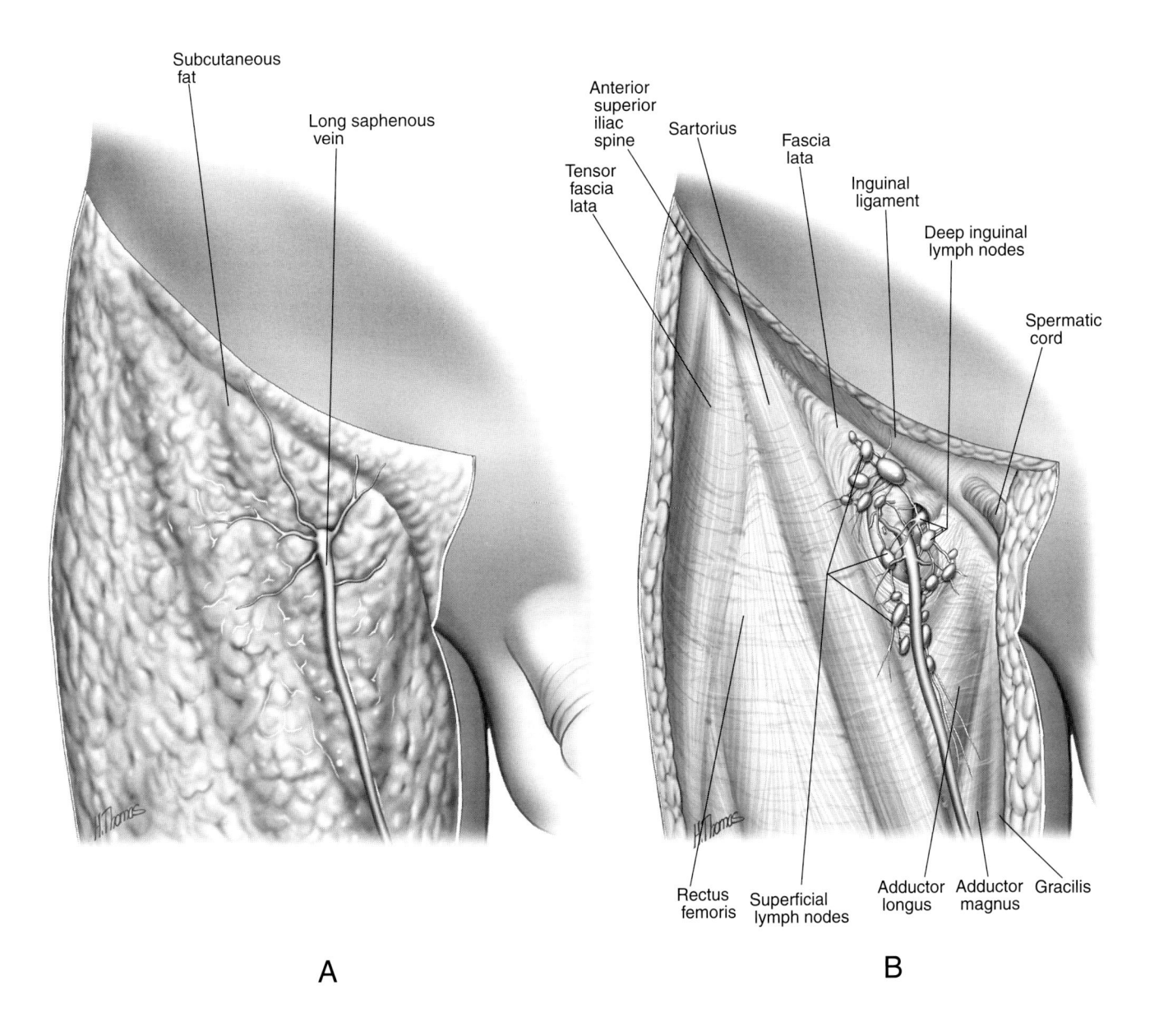

Figure 57–1 • **A,** With the skin elevated the saphenous vein is depicted coursing toward the foramen ovale.
B, The muscular anatomic boundaries of the groin are depicted.

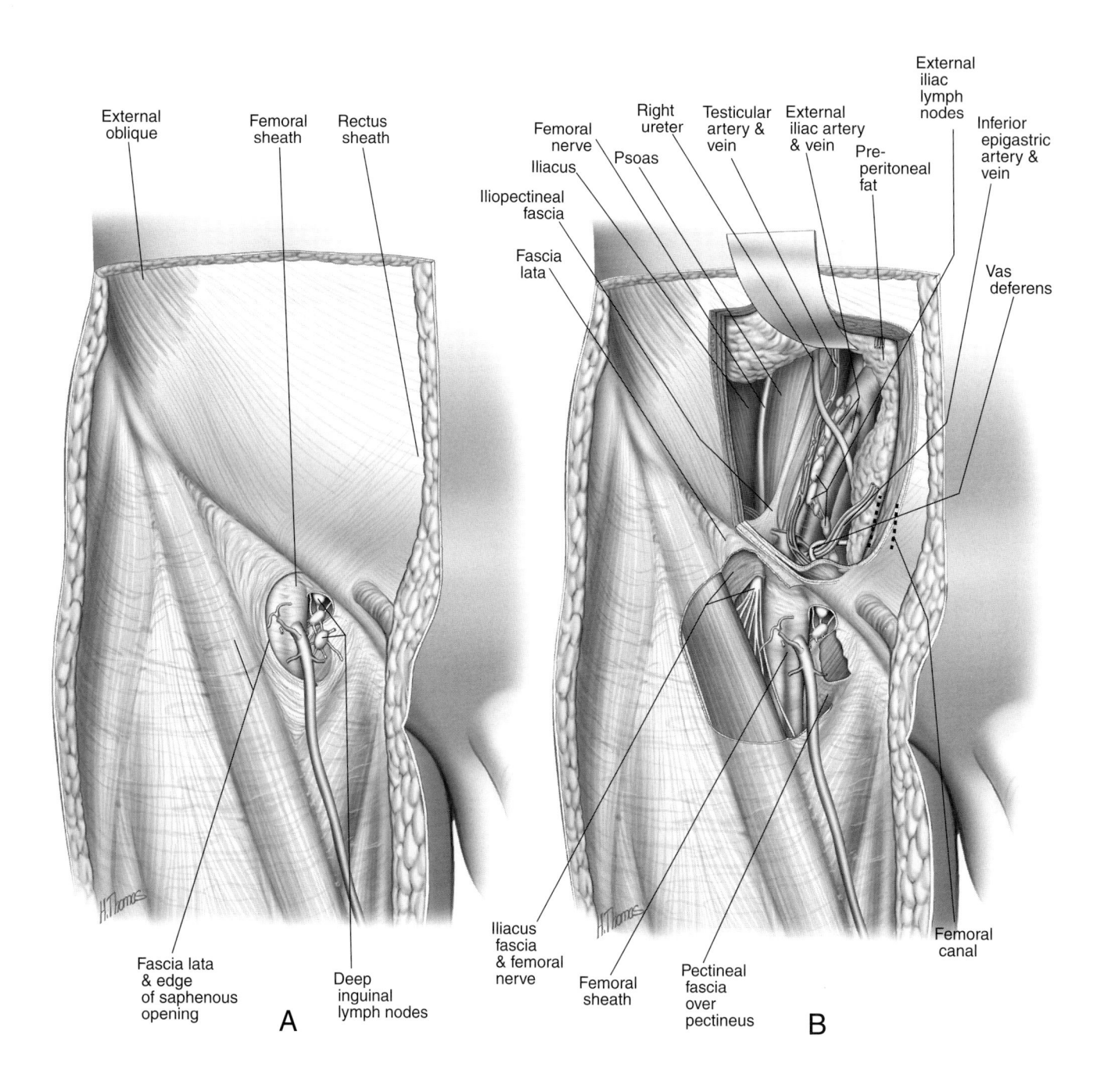

Figure 57–2 • **A,** The anatomy around the femoral ring is depicted.
B, The deep inguinal anatomy is defined.

Chapter 58
Groin Dissection

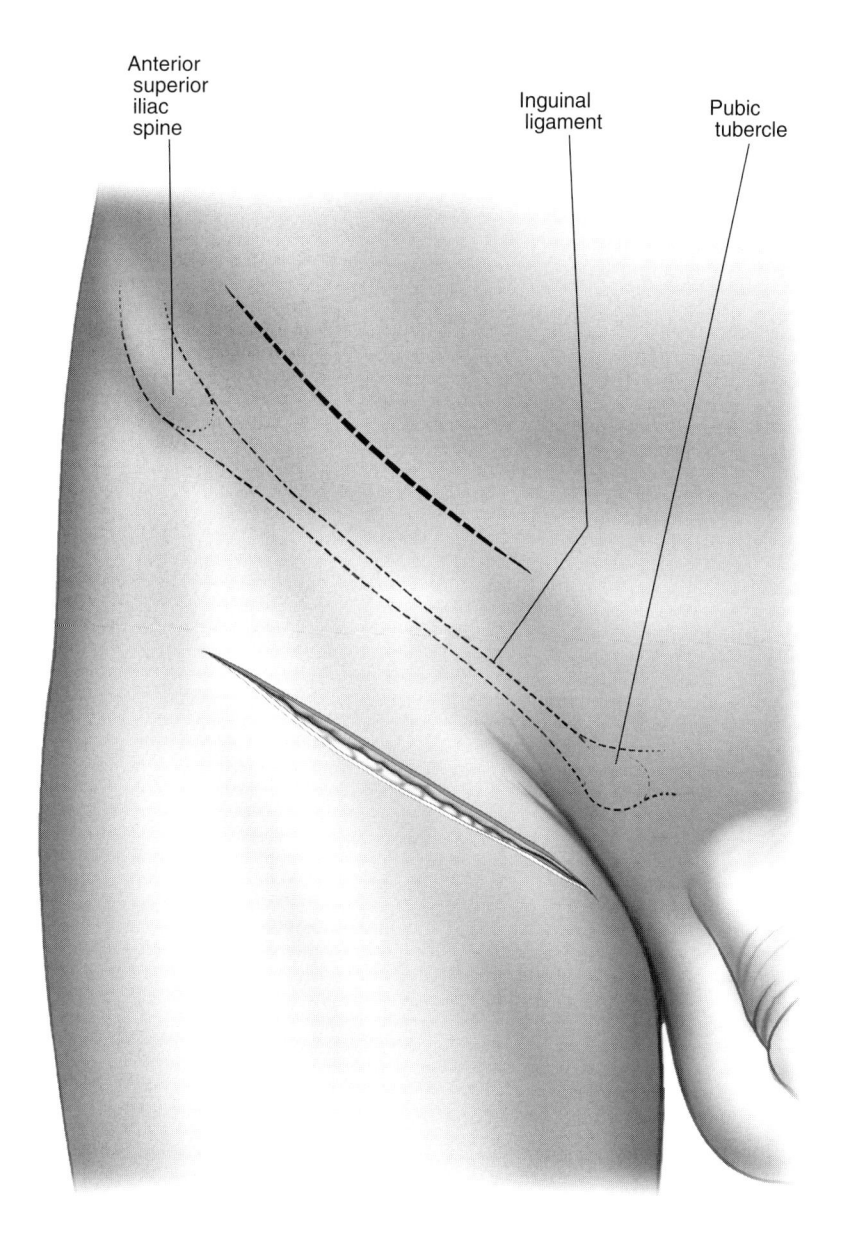

Figure 58–1 • A skin incision is made parallel to the inguinal ligament on the thigh. If a deep node dissection is to be performed as well, a separate parallel incision is made above the inguinal ligament.

486 • Part VI BREAST AND SOFT TISSUE TUMORS

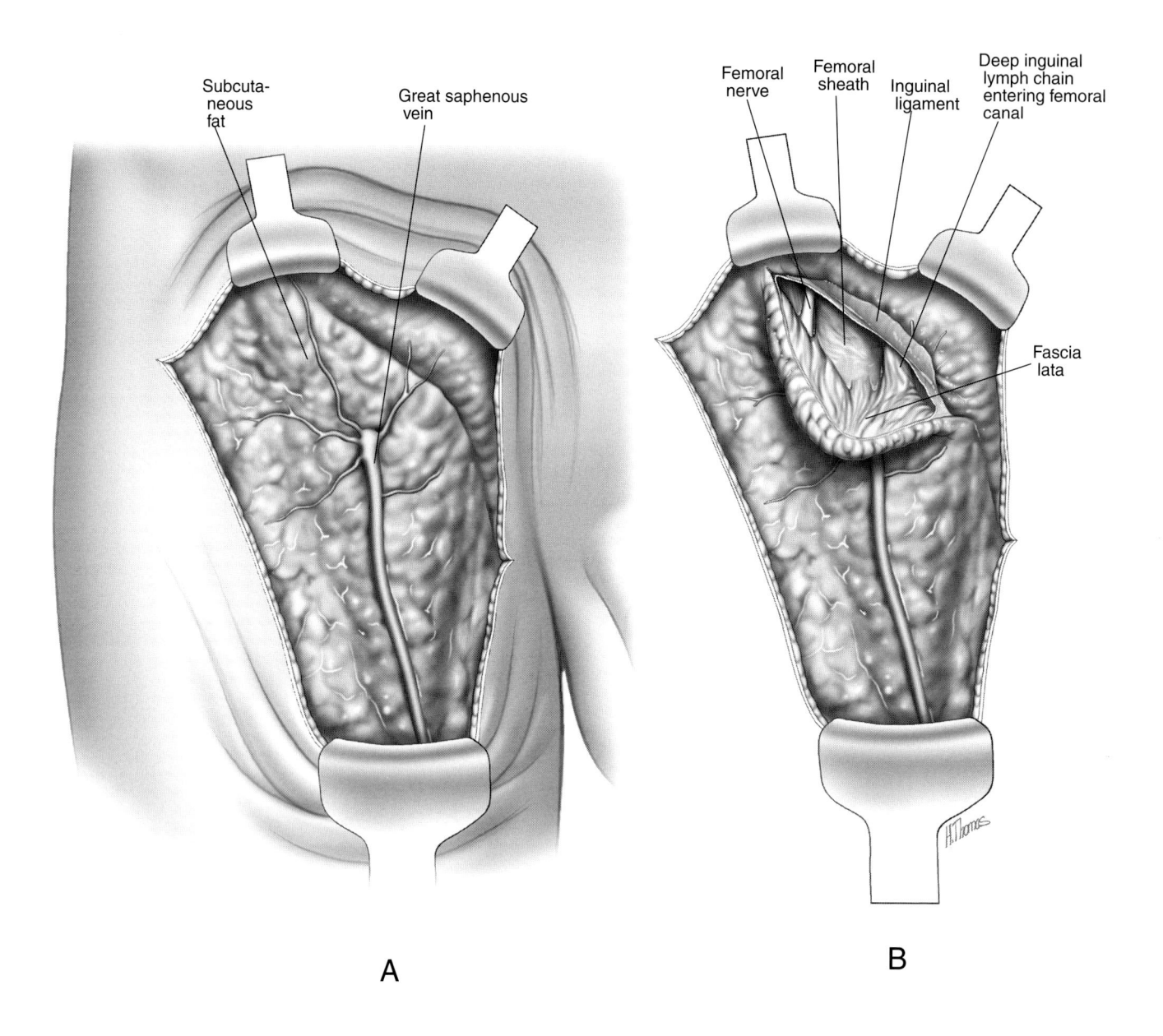

Figure 58–2 • **A,** The skin flaps are elevated above the inguinal ligament and inferiorly to the point where the saphenous vein will be divided.
B, The subcutaneous tissue is dissected off the inguinal ligament, exposing the femoral canal.

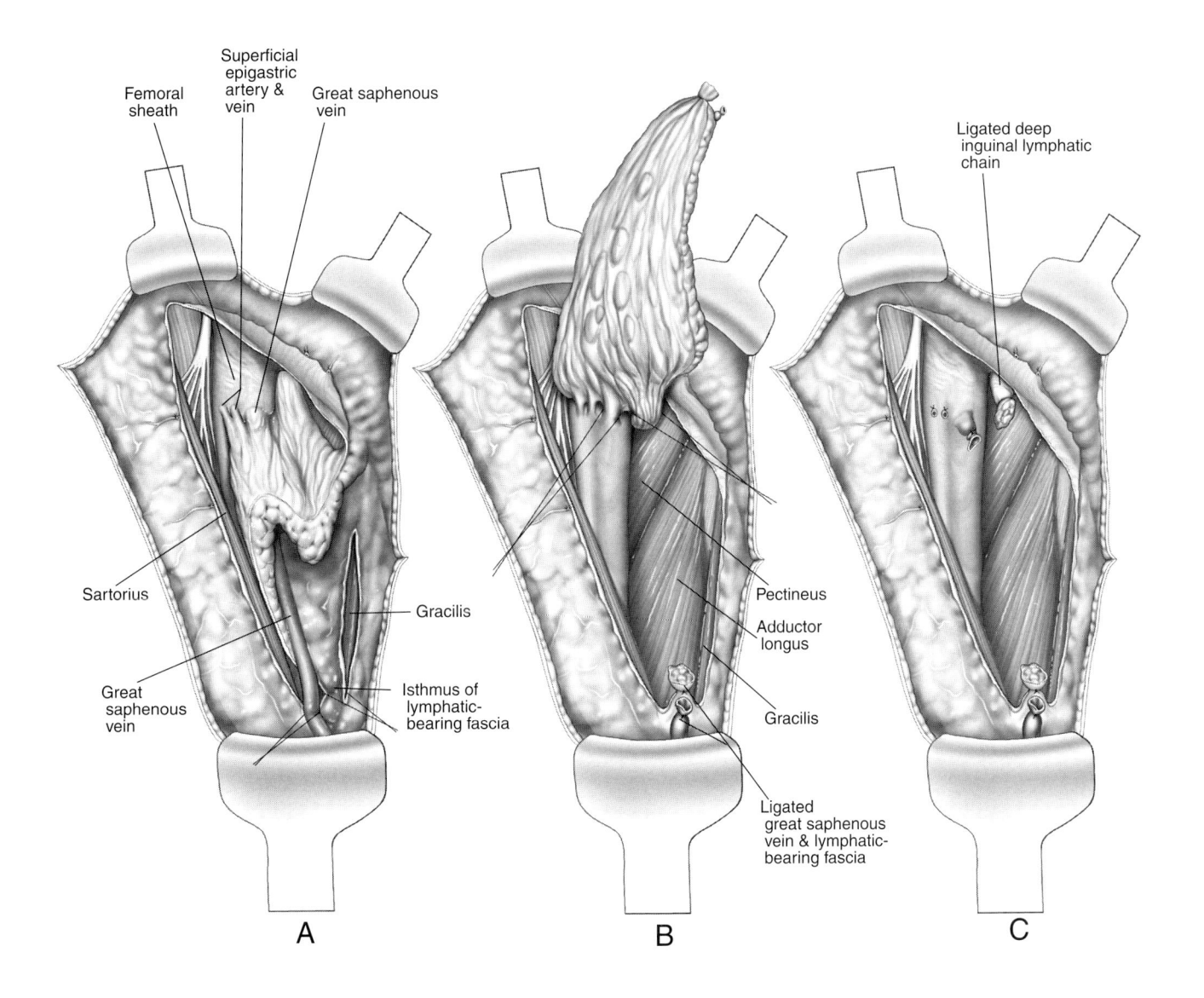

Figure 58–3 • **A,** The subcutaneous tissue is dissected medially off the gracilis and laterally off the sartorius.

B, The saphenous vein is divided, and all the lymphatic tissue is dissected off the femoral vessels, identifying the confluence of the saphenous vein with the femoral vein.

C, The saphenofemoral junction is divided. If a superficial node dissection is to be done only, the operation is completed by ligating and dividing the lymphatic chain.

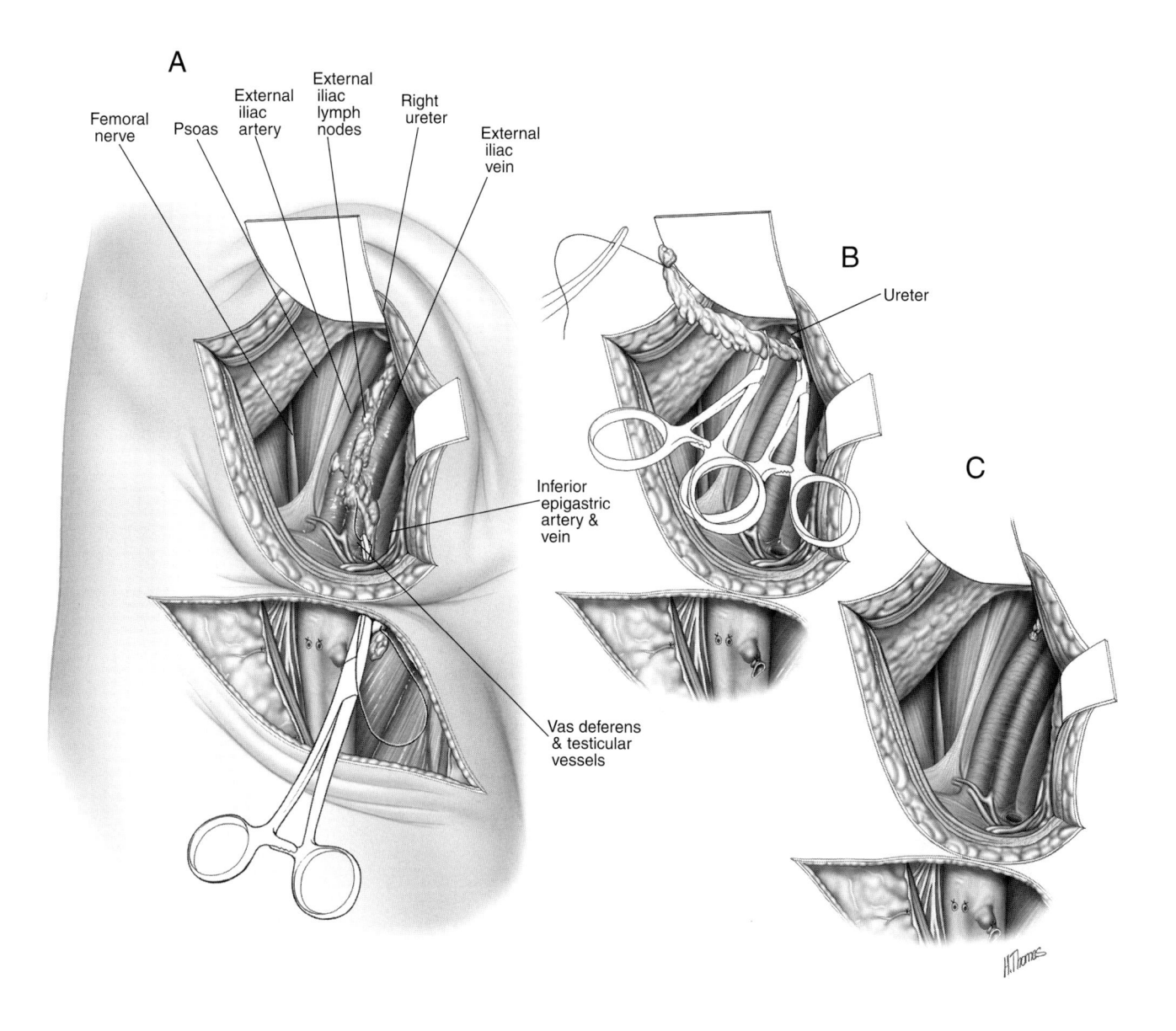

Figure 58–4 • **A,** If a deep node dissection is to be performed, the abdominal incision is completed by dividing the external and internal obliques and the transversus abdominis muscle to gain entry into the retroperitoneal space. The peritoneal envelope is bluntly dissected superiorly, exposing the external iliac vessels.

B, All nodal tissue is then dissected from inferiorly to superiorly along the external iliacs.

C, The completed deep node dissection. Beware of the ureter at the apex of the dissection.

Index

Abdomen, lower, anatomy of, 274–278
  upper, after division of falciform ligament and hepatic elevation, 147
    anatomy of, 146–152
    blood supply to stomach in, 148
    branches of vena cava in, 152
    exposure of, in gastric surgery, 155
    exposure of lesser sac in, 149
    structures in, 146
    vascular anatomy of, 151
Abdominal incision. See *Incision(s)*.
Abdominal wall, anatomy of, in hemipelvectomy, 433
  muscles of, reattachment of, in resection of chondrosarcoma of iliac wing, 459
Abdominosacral resection, 377–394
  advancement of gluteus muscles in, 394
  creation of ileal conduit and colostomy in, 383
  division of ureters and urethra in, 381
  entering peritoneal cavity in, 390
  full-thickness flaps in, 388
  incisions for, 378–379
  laminectomy in, 389
  lap pads used in, 384
  lateral view of, 385, 393
  mobilization of sigmoid and rectum in, 380
  posterior incision in, 386–387
  reconstruction of pelvic floor in, 392
  specimen removal in, 391
  staged procedure in, 382
  utilization of Vicryl mesh in, 383
Adductor longus muscle, 483
Adductor magnus muscle, 333, 483
Adrenal gland, 152
Adrenal vein, 152
  ligation of, in adrenalectomy, 266, 271
Adrenalectomy, left, 268–271
  division of splenophrenic ligament in, 269
  ligation of adrenal vein and removal of gland in, 271
  mobilization of colonic flexure in, 268
  right, 264–267
    identification of kidney and inferior vena cava in, 265
    ligation of adrenal vein and removal of gland in, 266
    mobilization of hepatic flexure in, 264
Amputations, of upper extremity, forequarter, 401–414. See also *Forequarter amputation*.
  surgical anatomy for, 396–399
Anal sphincter, 333, 370
Anastomosis, colorectal, in lower anterior resection, 331
  gastroesophageal, in thoracic esophagectomy, 133
  in left hemicolectomy, 300
  in sigmoid colectomy, 319
  in transhiatal resection of esophagus and gastric pull-up, 123

Anastomosis (*Continued*)
  in transverse colectomy, 310
  rectal, in female pelvic exenteration, 357
  Roux-en-Y, in extended gastrectomy with radical lymphadenectomy, 181
    in Whipple procedure, 253
  stapled, in esophagogastrectomy, 143
    in right hemicolectomy, 291
Anococcygeal ligament, 333, 370
  division of, in perineal resection, 336
Antecolic gastrojejunostomy, 166
Anterior triangle, of neck, 29
Aorta, 152
  ascending, 81
  descending, 81
Apicoposterior, artery, 50
Axilla, access to, in modified radical mastectomy, 472
  neurovascular anatomy of, 464
Axillary artery, 396, 398
Axillary vein, 398, 463
Azygos vein, 48, 49, 61
  ligation of, in thoracic esophagectomy, 131

Basilar arterial branches, in lower left lung lobectomy, exposure of, 96
  ligation of, 97
Basilic vein, 396, 463
Biceps muscle, 396, 397, 463
  division of, in Tikoff-Lindberg procedure, 421
Bile duct, common, 148
Bladder, 277
  female, 342, 344
  male, 369
Bladder neck, division of, in male pelvic exenteration, 374
Brachial artery, 463
Brachial vein, 396
Brachialis muscle, 396
Breast, muscular anatomy of, 464
  surgical anatomy of, 462–464
  tail of, access to, in modified radical mastectomy, 472
Bronchus(i), anterior oblique view of, 53
  left, 50
  right, 48, 50
    approach to, 50
    three-dimensional relationship of, to lung, 51, 52
Bronchus intermedius, 50
Buccinator muscle, 21

Cardinal ligament, division of, in female pelvic exenteration, 353
Carotid artery(ies), 2, 4
Carotid sheath, 4
Celiac trunk, 148, 152
Cephalic vein, 396, 463
Cervical. See also *Neck*.

Cervical fascia, deep, 3
Cervical incision, for transhiatal resection of esophagus and gastric pull-up, 118
Cervical roots, sensory, division of, in radical neck dissection, 38
Chest. See also *Thoracic* entries.
  entering of, in esophagogastrectomy, 139
  placement of stomach in, esophagectomy and, 132
  esophagogastrectomy and, 141
  right, surgical anatomy of, 48–55
Chest wall, dissection along, in modified radical mastectomy, 473
Cholecystectomy, in vascular isolation technique of hepatic lobectomy, 220
  radical, 232–240
    dissection of nodal tissue in, 236, 237
    dissection of porta hepatis in, 235
    division of cystic artery in, 236
    division of cystic duct in, 237
    division of falciform ligament in, 233
    incision for, 232
    marking of liver portion to be resected in, 238
    mobilization of hepatic lobe in, 234
    resection of hepatic parenchyma in, 239–240
Chondrosarcoma, of iliac wing, 455–459
  resection of, division of gluteal muscles in, 457
    incision for, 456
    Marlex mesh used in reconstruction of defect following, 458
    mobilization of peritoneal envelope in, 457
    reattachment of gluteal muscles and abdominal wall muscles following, 459
  of pubis, 449–454
    resection of, division of inguinal ligament in, 452
      division of inguinal obturator nerve, artery, and vein in, 453
      incision for, 451
      Marlex mesh used in reconstruction of pelvis following, 454
      x-ray of, 450
  of sternum, 106–112
    CT scan of, 106
    resection of, 108–109
      incision in, 107
      pectoralis major muscle advancement following, 112
Clamp removal, in vascular isolation technique of hepatic lobectomy, 231
Clavicle, 396, 397
  removal of, in forequarter amputation, 404
    in Tikoff-Lindberg procedure, 418
Clavipectoral fascia, incision of, in radical mastectomy, 479
  in Tikoff-Lindberg procedure, 418
Coccyx, 370

Colectomy, sigmoid, 278, 311–319
　abdominal incision for, 311
　anastomosis in, 319
　division and ligation of sigmoid
　　branches in, 316–317
　identification of ureter in, 315
　incision along colic gutter in, 312–313
　mobilization of splenic flexure in, 314, 319
　transverse, 301–310
　　abdominal incision for, 301
　　anastomosis in, 310
　　detachment of greater omentum in, 302
　　division of transverse mesocolon in, 308
　　mobilization of greater omentum in, 303
　　mobilization of hepatic flexure in, 305
　　mobilization of left colon in, 306
　　mobilization of right colon in, 304
　　mobilization of splenic flexure in, 307
　　preservation of vascular vessels in, 309
Colic artery, 149, 277
　division of, in right hemicolectomy, 288
Colic (colonic) gutter, 276
　incision along, in sigmoid colectomy, 312–313
　to splenic flexure, in left hemicolectomy, 295
Colic vein, 149
Colon, left, mobilization of, in transverse colectomy, 306
　mobilization of, along line of Toldt, in lower anterior resection, 322
　in left hemicolectomy, 296
　in right hemicolectomy, 283, 287
　resections of, type of, 278
　right, mobilization of, in transverse colectomy, 304
　sigmoid, division of, in female pelvic exenteration, 353
　　in male pelvic exenteration, 374
　　mobilization of, in abdominosacral resection, 380
　　in female pelvic exenteration, 350
　transverse, 274
Colonic alternative, to transhiatal resection of esophagus and gastric pull-up, 124–125
Colonic flexure, mobilization of, in distal pancreatectomy, 254
　in left adrenalectomy, 268
　right, 146
Colorectal anastomosis, in lower anterior resection, 331
Colostomy, creation of, in abdominosacral resection, 383
Computed tomography, of chondrosarcoma, of sternum, 106
Coracobrachialis muscle, 396, 397, 463
　division of, in Tikoff-Lindberg procedure, 421
Coracoid process, 397
Cricoid cartilage, 2, 4
Cricopharyngeus muscle, 5
Cricothyroid muscle, 4
Cystic artery, division of, in radical cholecystectomy, 236
Cystic duct, division of, in radical cholecystectomy, 237

Deflation, of left lung, for lobectomy, 93
Deltoid muscle, 396, 397, 399, 463
　division of, in Tikoff-Lindberg procedure, 421

Desmoid tumor, of thoracic inlet, 43–45
　resection of, 44
　vascular and nerve grafting for, 45
Devascularization, in left hepatic lobectomy, 203
Diaphragm, 152
Duodenum, 147, 276
　division of, in gastric surgery, 159
　identification of, in right hemicolectomy, 286
　kocherization of, in extended gastrectomy with radical lymphadenectomy, 172
　in Whipple procedure, 247

Epigastric vessels, inferior, division of, in hemipelvectomy, 437
Esophagectomy, thoracic, 126–133
　division of gastric artery and vein in, 129
　division of gastrohepatic ligament in, 128
　gastroesophageal anastomosis in, 133
　incision for, 127
　incision of parietal pleura in, 130
　ligation of azygos vein in, 131
　mobilization and placement of stomach in chest in, 132
　patient position for, 126
　pyloroplasty in, 129
Esophagogastrectomy, 134–143
　division of gastric artery and vein in, 137
　entering of chest in, 139
　incision for, 135
　mobilization of esophagus in, 140
　mobilization of liver and stomach in, 136
　mobilization of spleen and pancreas in, 138
　patient position for, 134
　placement of stomach into chest in, 141
　pyloroplasty in, 137
　stapled anastomosis in, 143
Esophagus, 6, 148
　mobilization of, in esophagogastrectomy, 140
　in transhiatal resection of esophagus and gastric pull-up, 119
　transhiatal resection of, and gastric pull-up, 113–125
　　abdominal incision for, 114
　　anastomosis in, 123
　　colonic alternative to, 124–125
　　gastrohepatic ligament incision in, 115
　　mobilization of esophagus in, 119
　　mobilization of stomach in, 116
　　neck incision in, 118
　　patient position for, 113
　　placement of stomach in neck in, 122
　　pyloroplasty in, 117
Extremity, upper, amputations of, surgical anatomy for, 396–399

Facial artery, 21
　ligation of, in radical neck dissection, 32
Facial nerve, 21
　dissection of, in parotidectomy, 24–25
　relationship of, to deep lobe following parotidectomy, 27
Facial vein, 4, 21
　ligation of, in radical neck dissection, 32
Falciform ligament, 146
　division of, in radical cholecystectomy, 233
　in right hepatic lobectomy, 183–184
　in trisegmentectomy, 206

Fallopian tube, 342
Fascia, cervical, deep, 3
　clavipectoral, incision of, in radical mastectomy, 479
　　in Tikoff-Lindberg procedure, 418
　Gerota's, identification of, in right hemicolectomy, 286
　perineal, 333
　reflection and incision of, in radical neck dissection, 35
Fascia lata, 483
Femoral artery, 342
Femoral ring, anatomy around, 484
Femoral vein, 342
Foramen of Winslow, assessment of, in Whipple procedure, 249
Forequarter amputation, 401–414
　anterior and posterior views of, 411–412
　division of latissimus and serratus in, 407, 409, 410
　division of pectoralis major and minor in, 403
　division of subclavius and omohyoid in, 405
　division of teres, levator scapulae, and trapezius in, 408
　exposure of pectoralis major in, 402
　exposure of second and third ribs in, 413
　incisions for, 401
　ligation of subclavian vessels in, 414
　mobilization of vessels in, 406
　removal of clavicle in, 404
　Tikoff-Lindberg procedure in, 415–428. See also *Tikoff-Lindberg procedure.*
Full-thickness flaps, in abdominosacral resection, 388

Gallbladder, 148
　removal of, in extended gastrectomy with radical lymphadenectomy, 176
　in left hepatic lobectomy, 198
　in right hepatic lobectomy, 186
Gastrectomy, extended, with radical lymphadenectomy, 168–181
　completed resection in, 180
　creation of Roux-en-Y anastomosis in, 181
　dissection of hepatoduodenal ligament in, 175
　dissection of nodal tissue in, 174
　dissection of paraaortic lymph nodes in, 177–178
　exposure of intraabdominal organs in, 169
　incision for, 168
　kocherization of duodenum in, 172
　mobilization of greater omentum in, 171
　mobilization of hepatic flexure in, 170
　mobilization of splenophrenic ligament in, 173
　removal of gallbladder in, 176
　total, esophageal resection for, 161
　esophagojejunostomy following, 167
　with splenectomy, 163
　without splenectomy, 162
　type of, 153
Gastric. See also *Stomach.*
Gastric artery(ies), 148
　division of, in esophagogastrectomy, 137
　in gastric surgery, 160
　in thoracic esophagectomy, 129
Gastric surgery, 153–167
　abdominal incision for, 154
　antecolic gastrojejunostomy in, 166
　detachment and mobilization of greater omentum in, 156–157

Gastric surgery (Continued)
  division of duodenum in, 159
  division of gastric arteries in, 160
  division of splenic artery and vein in, 165
  exposure of lesser sac in, 157
  exposure of upper abdomen in, 155
  mobilization of lesser curvature in, 158
  mobilization of spleen and pancreas in, 164
  total gastrectomy in, esophageal resection for, 161
    esophagojejunostomy following, 167
    with splenectomy, 163
    without splenectomy, 162
  types of, 153
Gastric vein(s), 148
  division of, in esophagogastrectomy, 137
    in thoracic esophagectomy, 129
Gastrocolic mesentery, incision of, in Whipple procedure, 243
Gastroduodenal artery, 149
Gastroepiploic artery, 148
Gastroesophageal anastomosis, in thoracic esophagectomy, 133
Gastrohepatic ligament, 148
  division of, in left hepatic lobectomy, 199
    in thoracic esophagectomy, 128
  incision of, in transhiatal resection of esophagus and gastric pull-up, 115
    in Whipple procedure, 242
Gastrojejunostomy, antecolic, 166
Gastrosplenic ligament, 150
Gerota's fascia, identification of, in right hemicolectomy, 286
Gluteal artery, superior, 343, 344
Gluteus maximus muscle, 333, 370
Gluteus medius muscle, 370
Gluteus minimus muscle, 370
Gluteus muscles, advancement of, in abdominosacral resection, 394
  division of, in hemipelvectomy, 441
    in resection of chondrosarcoma of iliac wing, 457
  reattachment of, in resection of chondrosarcoma of iliac wing, 459
Gracilis muscle, 483
Greater omentum, 146, 274
  detachment of, in gastric surgery, 156–157
    in transverse colectomy, 302
  elevation of, in left hemicolectomy, 294
  mobilization of, in extended gastrectomy with radical lymphadenectomy, 171
    in gastric surgery, 156–157
    in right hemicolectomy, 281–282
    in transverse colectomy, 303
Groin, dissection of, 485–488
  division of saphenofemoral junction in, 487
  division of saphenous vein in, 487
  elevation of skin flaps in, 486
  incision for, 485
  nodal, 488
  removal of subcutaneous tissue in, 486–487
  muscular anatomic boundaries of, 483
  surgical anatomy of, 483–484

Hamstring tendons, 370
Hemiazygos vein, 81
Hemicolectomy, 278
  left, 293–300
    abdominal incision for, 293
    anastomosis in, 300
    division of transverse mesocolon in, 298
    elevation of greater omentum in, 294

Hemicolectomy (Continued)
    incision along colic gutter to splenic flexure in, 295
    mobilization of colon in, 296
    mobilization of splenic flexure in, 297
  right, 279–291
    abdominal incision for, 279
    alignment of small bowel with transverse colon in, 290
    clamping of mesenteric attachments at hepatic flexure in, 285
    division of colic and ileocolic vessels in, 288
    identification of Gerota's fascia and duodenum in, 286
    inspection of liver in, 280
    mobilization of colon in, 283, 287
    mobilization of greater omentum in, 281–282
    mobilization of hepatic flexure in, 284
    stapled anastomosis in, 291
Hemipelvectomy, 432–448
  abdominal wall anatomy in, 433
  closure of defect in, 448
  dissection of peritoneal envelope in, 436
  division of nerve roots in, 445
  division of gluteus muscles in, 441
  division of inferior epigastric vessels in, 437
  division of levator ani and piriformis in, 446
  division of oblique muscle in, 434–435
  division of psoas muscle in, 438
  division of symphysis pubis in, 442
  incision for, 432
  incisions for, distal to greater trochanter, 440
  osteomization of sacroiliac joint in, 443–444
  removal of specimen in, 447
  Type I, for chondrosarcoma of iliac wing, 455–459
  Type III, for chondrosarcoma of pubis, 449–454
Hemorrhoidal artery(ies), 277, 344, 369
  clipping of, in lower anterior resection, 326
  division of, in female pelvic exenteration, 353
    in lower anterior resection, 329
Hemorrhoidal vein(s), 369
  clipping of, in lower anterior resection, 326
  division of, in female pelvic exenteration, 353
    in lower anterior resection, 329
Hepatic. See also Liver.
Hepatic artery(ies), common, 148
  division of, in left hepatic lobectomy, 201
  identification and division of, in right hepatic lobectomy, 191
Hepatic duct, division of, in left hepatic lobectomy, 201
  identification and division of, in right hepatic lobectomy, 191
Hepatic flexure, clamping of mesenteric attachments at, in right hemicolectomy, 285
  mobilization of, in extended gastrectomy with radical lymphadenectomy, 170
    in right adrenalectomy, 264
    in right hemicolectomy, 284
    in transverse colectomy, 305
Hepatic hilum, 147
Hepatic lobe, mobilization of, in radical cholecystectomy, 234

Hepatic lobectomy, left, 196–205
  abdominal incision for, 196
  devascularization of lobe in, 203
  division of gastrohepatic ligament in, 199
  division of hepatic artery, hepatic duct, and portal vein in, 201
  division of hepatic parenchyma in, 204
  division of hepatic vein in, 202
  exposure of hepatic veins in, 197
  removal of gallbladder in, 198
  removal of lobe in, 205
  right, 182–195
    abdominal incision for, 182
    completion of, 195
    division and incision of falciform ligament in, 183–184
    division of hepatic parenchyma in, 193–194
    division of vena cava branches in, 190
    exposure of porta hepatis in, 185
    exposure of vena cava in, 188
    identification and division of hepatic artery, hepatic duct, and portal vein in, 191
    ligation of hepatic vein in, 189
    removal of gallbladder in, 186
  vascular isolation technique of, 218–231
    cholecystectomy in, 220
    clamp removal in, 231
    clamping of inferior vena cava in, 225, 227
    clamping of porta hepatis in, 226
    division of right lobe in, 228
    exposure of tumor in, 219
    exposure of vena cava in, 221–224
    extension of tumor into vena cava in, 229
    ligation of hepatic veins in, 229
    MR image of tumor and, 218
    oversewing of hepatic vein in, 231
    removal of tumor in, 230
    repair of vena cava in, 230
Hepatic parenchyma, division of, in left hepatic lobectomy, 204
  in right hepatic lobectomy, 193–194
  in trisegmentectomy, 213–215
  resection of, in radical cholecystectomy, 239–240
Hepatic vein(s), division of, in left hepatic lobectomy, 202
  exposure of, in left hepatic lobectomy, 197
    in trisegmentectomy, 207
  ligation of, in right hepatic lobectomy, 189
    in trisegmentectomy, 216
    in vascular isolation technique of hepatic lobectomy, 229
  oversewing of, in vascular isolation technique of hepatic lobectomy, 231
Hilum, hepatic, 147
  of lung, 49
    anatomy of, cephalic, 82
      from rear, 84
      inferior, 86
    cephalad approach to, in upper left lung lobectomy, 87
    visualization of, following lower left lung lobectomy, 100
Hyoid bone, muscles of, 2

Ileal conduit, creation of, in abdominosacral resection, 383
  in urinary diversion, 365
  ileum segment for, 366
Ileocolic artery, 277
  division of, in right hemicolectomy, 288

Iliac artery, 342, 343, 344, 369
Iliac crest, 370
Iliac spine, 370, 483
Iliac vein, 342, 343, 344, 369
Iliac wing, chondrosarcoma of, 455–459. See also *Chondrosarcoma, of iliac wing.*
Iliocostalis muscle, 399
Incision(s), for abdominosacral resection, 378–379
  posterior, 386–387
 for esophagogastrectomy, 135
 for extended gastrectomy with radical lymphadenectomy, 168
 for female pelvic exenteration, 347
 for forequarter amputation, 401
 for gastric surgery, 154
 for hemipelvectomy, 432
  distal to greater trochanter, 440
 for left hemicolectomy, 293
 for left hepatic lobectomy, 196
 for lower anterior resection, 321
  in peritoneal reflection between bladder and rectum, 327
  mesenteric, from sacral promontory to iliac vessels, 324
 for male pelvic exenteration, 371–372
 for modified radical mastectomy, 465
  pectoralis major fascia and, 468
 for parotidectomy, 23
 for perineal resection, 335
 for radical cholecystectomy, 232
 for radical neck dissection, 31–32
 for resection of chondrosarcoma, of iliac wing, 456
  of pubis, 451
  of sternum, 107
 for right hemicolectomy, 279
 for right hepatic lobectomy, 182
 for sigmoid colectomy, 311
  along colic gutter, 312–313
 for thoracic esophagectomy, 127
 for thyroid lobectomy, 7
 for Tikoff-Lindberg procedure, 415
 for transhiatal resection of esophagus and gastric pull-up, abdominal, 114
  cervical, 118
 for transverse colectomy, 301
 for Whipple procedure, 241
 in groin dissection, 485
 mediastinal pleural, for right upper lung lobectomy, 62, 70
 of clavipectoral fascia, in radical mastectomy, 479
 thoracic, 57–58
Inferior vena cava. See also *Vena cava.*
 clamping of, in vascular isolation technique of hepatic lobectomy, 225, 227
 identification of, in adrenalectomy, 265
Infraspinatus muscle, 399
Inguinal anatomy, 484
Inguinal ligament, 483
 division of, resection of chondrosarcoma of pubis, 452
Inguinal lymph nodes, 483
Intercostal artery, 59
Intercostal muscles, 59
Intercostal nerve, 59, 463
Intercostal vein, 59
Intercostobrachial nerve, 463
Intraabdominal organs, exposure of, in extended gastrectomy with radical lymphadenectomy, 169
Ischial spine, 370
Ischial tuberosity, 333
Isthmus, division of, in thyroid lobectomy, 17

Jejunum, 152
Jugular vein(s), external, 21, 396
 internal, 2, 4
  division and ligation of, in radical neck dissection, 37

Kidney, 276
 identification of, in adrenalectomy, 265

Laminectomy, in abdominosacral resection, 389
Lap pads, in abdominosacral resection, 384
Large intestines, vascular anatomy of, 277
Laryngeal cartilage, 2
Laryngeal nerve(s), course of, 5
 recurrent, dissection of, 13
  identification of, 11
 superior, 3
Latissimus dorsi muscle, 57, 396, 398, 399, 463
 division of, in forequarter amputation, 407, 410
Lesser curvature, mobilization of, in gastric surgery, 158
Lesser omentum, 147
Lesser sac, exposure of, 149
 in gastric surgery, 157
Levator ani muscle, 333, 344, 370
 division of, in hemipelvectomy, 446
 in perineal resection, 336–337
Levator scapulae muscle, division of, in forequarter amputation, 408
 in Tikoff-Lindberg procedure, 423
Ligament of Treitz, 151, 277
Liver, 146. See also *Hepatic* entries.
 inspection of, in right hemicolectomy, 280
 marking of, for resection, in radical cholecystectomy, 238
 mobilization of, in esophagogastrectomy, 136
Lobectomy, hepatic, left, 196–205. See also *Hepatic lobectomy, left.*
 right, 182–195. See also *Hepatic lobectomy, right.*
 vascular isolation technique for, 218–231. See also *Hepatic lobectomy, vascular isolation technique of.*
 of lower left lung, 93–100
  anterior retraction of lobe in, 98
  deflation of left lung in, 93
  dissection of pleura in, 94
  exposure of basilar arterial branches in, 96
  ligation of basilar arterial branches in, 97
  opening of sheath over pulmonary artery in, 95
  visualization of hilum following, 100
 of lower right lung, 75–80
  identification of pulmonary artery branches in, 76
  lateral approach to, 75
  stapling of lower lobe bronchus in, 77
 of upper left lung, 87–92
  cephalad approach to hilum in, 87
  dissection around pulmonary artery branches in, 89
  identification and ligation of pulmonary vein in, 91
  ligation of pulmonary artery branches in, 90
  opening of pleura in, 88
  removal of lobe in, 92

Lobectomy (*Continued*)
 of upper right lung, 62–74
  exposure of pulmonary artery in, 67
  freeing of pulmonary artery in, 63
  freeing of upper bronchus in, 66
  incision of longitudinal fissure in, 69
  incision of mediastinal pleura in, anterior, 62
  posterior, 65
  ligation and division of upper lobe in, 70
  ligation of pulmonary artery in, 68
  stapling of upper lobe bronchus in, 72
  stretching at confluence of three lobes in, 64
  venous draining from upper and middle lobes in, 73–74
 thyroid, 7–19. See also *Thyroid lobectomy.*
Lung. See also *Pulmonary* entries.
 bronchi, arteries, and veins supplying, 51, 52
 fissures of, 53
  incomplete, 54
 hilum of. See *Hilum, of lung.*
 left lower, lobectomy of, 93–100. See also *Lobectomy, of lower left lung.*
 left upper, lobectomy of, 87–92. See also *Lobectomy, of upper left lung.*
 retraction of, visualization of azygos vein after, 61
 right lower, lobectomy of, 75–80. See also *Lobectomy, of lower right lung.*
 right upper, lobectomy of, 62–74. See also *Lobectomy, of upper right lung.*
 surgical anatomy of, 81–86
Lymph nodes, dissection of, from groin, 488
 in extended gastrectomy with radical lymphadenectomy, 174, 177–178
 in radical cholecystectomy, 236, 237
 inguinal, 483
Lymphadenectomy, radical, extended gastrectomy with, 168–181. See also *Gastrectomy, extended, with radical lymphadenectomy.*

Magnetic resonance imaging, of vascular tumor, 218
Mammary node sampling, in radical mastectomy, 481
Mandible, 21
Marlex mesh, in reconstruction of chest deformity, 45
 in reconstruction of defect, following resection of chondrosarcoma of iliac wing, 458
 in reconstruction of pericardium and sternum, 110–111
 in reconstruction of pubis, 454
Masseter muscle, 21
Mastectomy, radical. See *Radical mastectomy.*
Mastoid process, 21
Median nerve, 396, 463
Mediastinum, anterior, cross-sectional anatomy of, 102
 mass in, 101. See also *Thymoma.*
Mesenteric vessels, incision of, in Whipple procedure, 245–246
Mesocolon, incision of, in Whipple procedure, 244
 sigmoid, 276
 transverse, 149, 275, 276
  division of, in left hemicolectomy, 298
  in transverse colectomy, 308
Musculocutaneous nerve, 398, 463
Musculocutaneous vein, 397

Neck. See also *Cervical* entries.
  anteroposterior view of, 2
  course of laryngeal nerves in, 5
  location of parathyroid glands in, 6
  oblique view of, 3
  placement of stomach in, transhiatal resection of esophagus and gastric pull-up and, 122
  radical dissection of, 31–42
    closure of skin flaps in, 42
    division and ligation of internal jugular vein in, 37
    division of medial attachments in, 41
    division of omohyoid in, 35
    division of spinal accessory nerve in, 40
    division of sternocleidomastoid in, 36
      at origin, 39
    division of venous branches and sensory cervical roots in, 38
    division of Wharton's duct in, 33
    incisions for, 31–32
    posterior triangle dissection in, 36
    reflection and incision of fascia in, 35
    submaxillary gland dissection in, 34
    submaxillary triangle dissection in, 33
    surgical anatomy and, 28–30
    removal of strap muscles from, 4
    submaxillary, anterior, and posterior triangles of, 29
Nerve grafts, in resection of desmoid tumor, 45
Nerve roots, division of, in hemipelvectomy, 445
Nodal tissue, dissection of, in extended gastrectomy with radical lymphadenectomy, 174, 177–178
  in radical cholecystectomy, 236, 237

Oblique muscle, division of, in hemipelvectomy, 434–435
Obturator artery, 343, 344, 369
  division of, in resection of chondrosarcoma of pubis, 453
Obturator nerve, 343, 344, 369
  division of, in resection of chondrosarcoma of pubis, 453
Obturator vein, 343, 344, 369
  division of, in resection of chondrosarcoma of pubis, 453
Omentum, greater. See *Greater omentum.*
Omohyoid muscle, 2, 3
  division of, in forequarter amputation, 405
  in radical neck dissection, 35
  identification of, in forequarter amputation, 402
Ovarian artery, 342
  division of, in pelvic exenteration, 352
Ovarian vein, 342
  division of, in pelvic exenteration, 352
Ovary, 342

Pancreas, 148, 149
  division of, in Whipple procedure, 251
  mobilization of, in esophagogastrectomy, 138
  in gastric surgery, 164
Pancreatectomy, distal, 254–257
  division of phrenosplenic ligament in, 255
  division of splenic and gastric attachments in, 256
  transection of pancreas in, 257
  regional, for retroperitoneal sarcoma, 258–263

Pancreatectomy (*Continued*)
  Whipple procedure in, 241–253. See also *Whipple procedure.*
Pancreaticoduodenal artery, division of, in Whipple procedure, 251
Paraaortic lymph nodes, dissection of, in extended gastrectomy with radical lymphadenectomy, 177–178
Parathyroid gland(s), inferior, 6
  dissection of, 12
  location of, 6
  superior, 5
Parotid gland, surgical anatomy of, 21–22
Parotidectomy, 23–27
  dissection of facial nerve in, 24–25
  incisions for, 23
  ligation of Stensen's duct in, 26
  relationship of facial nerve to deep lobe following, 27
Pectoral nerve(s), 397
  median, division of, in modified radical mastectomy, 470
Pectoralis major muscle, 396, 463
  division of, in forequarter amputation, 403
  in radical mastectomy, 477–478
  in Tikoff-Lindberg procedure, 417
  exposure of, in forequarter amputation, 402
  in Tikoff-Lindberg procedure, 416
Pectoralis minor fascia, removal of, in modified radical mastectomy, 469
Pectoralis minor muscle, 397
  division of, in forequarter amputation, 403
  in radical mastectomy, 477–478
  in Tikoff-Lindberg procedure, 417
Pelvic exenteration, female, 347–363
  division of cardinal ligament, hemorrhoidal vessels, and sigmoid colon in, 353
  division of ovarian vessels in, 352
  incision for, 347
  mobilization of rectum in, 354
  mobilization of sigmoid colon in, 350
  mobilization of small bowel in, 348
  perineal closure following, 363
  perineal defects following, 362
  posterior, 358
    lines of resection in, 361
    rectal anastomosis in, 357
    specimen removal in, 356
  total, 359
    lines of resection in, 361
    specimen removal in, 360
  male, 371–376
    division of sigmoid colon and bladder neck in, 374
    division of sigmoid colon in, 374
    division of ureters in, 373
    incisions for, 371–372
    pelvic defect in, 376
    rectal transection and specimen removal in, 375
Pelvic floor, reconstruction of, in abdominosacral resection, 392
Pelvis, anatomy of, female, 341–345
  male, 369–370
  surgical, 429–431
Perineum, anatomy of, 333
  female, 345
  male, 370
  closure of, following female pelvic exenteration, 363
  defects of, following female pelvic exenteration, 362

Perineum (*Continued*)
  resection of, 335–339
    circumferential incision in, 335
    closure in, 339
    delivery of specimen in, 337–338
    division of anococcygeal ligament in, 336
    division of levator ani in, 336–337
Periosteum, humeral, incision of, in Tikoff-Lindberg procedure, 421
Peritoneal cavity, entering, in abdominosacral resection, 390
Peritoneum, dissection of, in hemipelvectomy, 436
Phrenic nerve, 48, 49
Phrenosplenic ligament, division of, in distal pancreatectomy, 255
Piriformis muscle, 369
  division of, in hemipelvectomy, 446
Pleura, dissection of, in lower left lung lobectomy, 94
  incision of, in thoracic esophagectomy, 130
  opening of, in upper left lung lobectomy, 88
Porta hepatis, clamping of, in vascular isolation technique of hepatic lobectomy, 226
  dissection of, in radical cholecystectomy, 235
  exposure of, in right hepatic lobectomy, 185
  identification of, in trisegmentectomy, 208
Portal vein, and pancreas, assessment of plane between, in Whipple procedure, 250
  assessment of, in Whipple procedure, 248
  identification and division of, in left hepatic lobectomy, 201
  in right hepatic lobectomy, 191
  left, 148
Posterior triangle, of neck, 29
  dissection of, 36
Profunda brachii artery, 398
Profunda brachii vein, 398
Prostate gland, 369, 370
Psoas muscle, 342
  division of, in hemipelvectomy, 438
  exposure of, in lower anterior resection, 323
Pubis, chondrosarcoma of, 449–454. See also *Chondrosarcoma, of pubis.*
Pulmonary. See also *Lung.*
Pulmonary artery, 48, 49
  in lower left lung lobectomy, opening of sheath over, 95
  in right upper lung lobectomy, exposure of, 67
    freeing of, 63
    ligation of, 68
  in upper left lung lobectomy, dissection around, 89
    ligation of, 90
Pulmonary ligament, inferior, 48, 49
Pulmonary vein, identification and ligation of, in upper left lung lobectomy, 91
  inferior, 48, 49, 50
  superior, 48
Pyloroplasty, in esophagogastrectomy, 137
  in thoracic esophagectomy, 129
  in transhiatal resection of esophagus and gastric pull-up, 117
Pylorus, 147
Pylorus-preserving procedure, in Whipple procedure, 252

Quadratus femoris muscle, 370

Radial artery, 398
Radical cholecystectomy, 232–240. See also *Cholecystectomy, radical.*
Radical mastectomy, 476–481
　division of pectoralis major and minor muscles in, 477–478
　incison of clavipectoral fascia in, 479
　mammary node sampling in, 481
　modified, 465–475
　　access to tail of breast and axilla in, 472
　　cross-sectional veiws of, 468–470, 472, 474–475
　　dissection along chest wall in, 473
　　division of median pectoral nerve in, 470
　　elevation of skin flaps in, 466
　　incision for, 465
　　incision of pectoralis major fascia in, 468
　　removal of pectoralis minor fascia in, 469
　　removal of tissue occupying subscapular space in, 475
　removal of pectoralis major and minor muscles in, 480
Radical neck dissection. See *Neck, radical dissection of.*
Rectal anastomosis, in female pelvic exenteration, 357
Rectal artery, 333
Rectal nerve, 333
Rectal vein, 333
Rectum, mobilization of, in abdominosacral resection, 380
　in female pelvic exenteration, 354
　in lower anterior resection, 325
　transection of, in male pelvic exenteration, 375
Rectus abdominis muscle, 463
Rectus femoris muscle, 483
Resection, lower anterior, 321–331
　clipping of hemorrhoidal vessels in, 326
　colorectal anastomosis in, 331
　division of hemorrhoidal artery and vein in, 329
　exposure of psoas and ureter in, 323
　incision for, 321
　incision of mesentery from sacral promontory to iliac vessels in, 324
　incision of peritoneal reflection between bladder and rectum in, 327
　mobilization of colon along line of Toldt in, 322
　mobilization of rectum in, 325
Retroperitoneal fat, 152
Retroperitoneal sarcoma, regional pancreatectomy for, 258–263
Rhomboid muscle, 399
　division of, in Tikoff-Lindberg procedure, 423
Rib(s), exposure of, in forequarter amputation, 413
　relationship of intercostal artery, vein, and nerve to, 59
Rib spreader, 60
Roux-en-Y anastomosis, creation of, in extended gastrectomy with radical lymphadenectomy, 181
　in Whipple procedure, 253

Sacroiliac joint, osteomization of, in hemipelvectomy, 443–444
　perineal anatomy of, 431
　vascular anatomy of, 430
Sacroiliac ligament, 370
Saphenofemoral junction, division of, in groin dissection, 487
Saphenous vein, 483
　division of, in groin dissection, 487
Sarcoma, retroperitoneal, regional pancreatectomy for, 258–263
Sartorius muscle, 483
Scapula, division of, in Tikoff-Lindberg procedure, 423
　retraction of, 58
Sensory cervical roots, division of, in radical neck dissection, 38
Serratus muscle, 57, 396, 397, 463
　division of, in forequarter amputation, 407, 409
　removal of, from chest wall, in Tikoff-Lindberg procedure, 424
Shoulder, axillary anatomy of, 398
　muscular anatomy of, 399
　neural and vascular anatomy of, 397
　surgical anatomy of, 396
Sigmoid colectomy. See *Colectomy, sigmoid.*
Sigmoid colon, division of, in female pelvic exenteration, 353
　in male pelvic exenteration, 374
　mobilization of, in abdominosacral resection, 380
　in female pelvic exenteration, 350
Skin flaps, closure of, in radical neck dissection, 42
　elevation of, in groin dissection, 486
　in modified radical mastectomy, 466
Small bowel, alignment of, with transverse colon, in right hemicolectomy, 290
　mesentery of, 276
　mobilization of, in female pelvic exenteration, 348
　vascular anatomy of, 277
Spermatic cord, 483
Spinal accessory nerve, division of, in radical neck dissection, 40
Spleen, 147, 276
　mobilization of, in esophagogastrectomy, 138
　in gastric surgery, 164
Splenic artery, 148, 151
　division of, in gastric surgery, 165
Splenic flexure, mobilization of, in left hemicolectomy, 297
　in sigmoid colectomy, 314, 319
　in transverse colectomy, 307
Splenic vein, 151
　division of, in gastric surgery, 165
Splenophrenic ligament, division of, in left adrenalectomy, 269
　mobilization of, in extended gastrectomy with radical lymphadenectomy, 173
Stapled anastomosis, in esophagogastrectomy, 143
　in right hemicolectomy, 291
Stensen's duct, 21
　ligation of, in parotidectomy, 26
Sternocleidomastoid muscle, 396
　division of, in radical neck dissection, 36
　at origin, 39
Sternohyoid muscle, 2, 3, 4
Sternothyroid muscle, 2, 3, 4
Sternotomy, partial, 103
　resection of thymic tumors after, 104
Sternum, chondrosarcoma of, 106–112. See also *Chondrosarcoma, of sternum.*

Stomach, 146, 274. See also *Gastric* entries.
　cervical placement of, for transhiatal resection of esophagus and gastric pull-up, 122
　mobilization of, in esophagogastrectomy, 136
　in thoracic esophagectomy, 132
　in transhiatal resection of esophagus and gastric pull-up, 116
　thoracic placement of, in esophagectomy, 132
　in esophagogastrectomy, 141
Subclavian artery, ligation of, in forequarter amputation, 414
Subclavian vein, ligation of, in forequarter amputation, 414
Subclavius muscle, 397
　division of, in forequarter amputation, 405
Subcutaneous tissue, removal of, in groin dissection, 486–487
Submaxillary gland, dissection of, in radical neck dissection, 34
Submaxillary triangle, of neck, 29
　deep structures in, 30
　dissection of, 33
Subscapular nerves, 397
Subscapular space, removal of tissue occupying, in modified radical mastectomy, 475
Subscapularis tendon, 397
Superior vena cava, 48, 49. See also *Vena cava.*
Symphysis pubis, 345
　division of, in hemipelvectomy, 442

Temporal artery, superficial, 21
Tensor fascia lata, 483
Teres muscle(s), division of, in forequarter amputation, 408
　major, 398, 399
　minor, 399
Testicular artery, 277
Testicular vessels, 369
Thoracic. See also *Chest.*
Thoracic esophagectomy, 126–133. See also *Esophagectomy, thoracic.*
Thoracic incisions, 57–58
Thoracic inlet, desmoid tumor of, 43–45
　resection of, 44
　vascular and nerve grafting for, 45
Thoracic nerve, 463
Thoracoacromial artery, 397
Thoracoacromial vein, 397
Thymoma, 101–105
　partial sternotomy for, 103
　resection of, 104
　specimen of, 105
Thyrohyoid ligament, 2
Thyrohyoid muscle, 4
Thyroid artery, superior, 2, 3
　division of, in thyroid lobectomy, 15
Thyroid gland, blood supply to, 4
　surgical anatomy of, 2–6
Thyroid lobectomy, 7–19
　cervical incision for, 7
　dissection of recurrent laryngeal nerve in, 13
　division of isthmus in, 17
　division of thyroid vessels in, 15
　exposure of trachea in, 14
　identification and division of thyroid vein in, 10
　identification of recurrent laryngeal nerve in, 11

Thyroid lobectomy (*Continued*)
  inferior parathyroid dissection in, 12
  midline exposure of thyroid in, 8
  mobilization of strap muscles in, 9
  wound closure in, 19
Thyroid vein, inferior, 2, 4
  middle, 4, 10
  superior, 2, 3
    division of, in thyroid lobectomy, 15
Tikoff-Lindberg procedure, 415–428.
  anterior view of defect in, 427–428
  completion of, 426
  division of biceps, coracobrachialis, and deltoid in, 421
  division of blood vessels and nerves in, 419–420
  division of pectoralis major and minor in, 417
  division of scapula, rhomboid, levator scapulae, and trapezius in, 423
  exposure of pectoralis major in, 416
  incision for, 415
  incision of clavipectoral fascia in, 418
  incision of humeral periosteum in, 421
  removal of clavicle in, 418
  removal of serratus from chest wall in, 424
Trachea, 2
  exposure of, in thyroid lobectomy, 14
Transhiatal resection, of esophagus, and gastric pull-up, 113–125. See also *Esophagus, transhiatal resection of, and gastric pull-up*.
Transverse colectomy, 278
Trapezius muscle, 57, 396, 397, 399
  division of, in forequarter amputation, 408
  in Tikoff-Lindberg procedure, 423
Triangular ligament, incision of, in trisegmentectomy, 209
Triceps muscle, 396, 399
Trisegmentectomy, 206–217
  completion of, 217
  division of falciform ligament in, 206
  exposure of hepatic veins in, 207
  exposure of vena cava in, 210
  hepatic parenchyma in, 213–215

Trisegmentectomy (*Continued*)
  identification of porta hepatis in, 208
  incision of triangular ligament in, 209
  ligation of hepatic vein in, 216
  ligation of vena cava in, 212
Tumor(s). See also specific tumor, e.g., *Chondrosarcoma*.
  desmoid, of thoracic inlet, 43–45
  vascular, isolation technique for removal of, 218–231. See also *Hepatic lobectomy, vascular isolation technique of*.

Ulnar nerve, 396, 463
Umbilical artery, 369
Upper extremity, amputations of, forequarter, 401–414. See also *Forequarter amputation*.
  surgical anatomy for, 396–399
Ureter(s), 277
  division of, in abdominosacral resection, 381
  in male pelvic exenteration, 373
  exposure of, in lower anterior resection, 323
  identification of, in sigmoid colectomy, 315
Urethra, division of, in abdominosacral resection, 381
Urethral opening, 345
Urinary diversion, 365–368
  creation of ileal conduit in, 365
  ileum segment for, 366
Uterine artery, 343, 344
Uterus, 342

Vagina, 344, 345
Vagus nerve, 4, 48
Vas deferens, 369
Vascular grafts, in resection of desmoid tumor, 45
Vascular isolation technique, hepatic lobectomy using, 218–231. See also *Hepatic lobectomy, vascular isolation technique of*.
Vascular tumor, removal of, isolation technique for, 218–231. See also *Hepatic lobectomy, vascular isolation technique of*.
Vascular vessels, preservation of, in transverse colectomy, 309
Vena cava, branches of, 152
  division of, in right hepatic lobectomy, 190
  exposure of, in right hepatic lobectomy, 188
  in trisegmentectomy, 210
  in vascular isolation technique of hepatic lobectomy, 221–224
  inferior, clamping of, in vascular isolation technique of hepatic lobectomy, 225, 227
  identification of, in adrenalectomy, 265
  ligation of, in trisegmentectomy, 212
  repair of, in vascular isolation technique of hepatic lobectomy, 230
  superior, 48, 49
Venous branches, division of, in radical neck dissection, 38
Vicryl mesh, use of, in abdominosacral resection, 383

Wharton's duct, division of, in radical neck dissection, 33
Whipple procedure, 241–253
  abdominal incision for, 241
  assessment of foramen of Winslow in, 249
  assessment of plane between portal vein and pancreas in, 250
  assessment of portal vein in, 248
  division of pancreas in, 251
  division of pancreaticoduodenal artery in, 251
  incision in mesenteric vessels in, 245–246
  incision in mesocolon in, 244
  incision of gastrocolic mesentery in, 243
  incision of gastrohepatic ligament in, 242
  kocherization of duodenum in, 247
  pylorus-preserving procedure in, 252
  Roux-en-Y anastomosis in, 253

X-ray, of chondrosarcoma of pubis, 450